MRI Normal Variants and Pitfalls

MRI
Normal Variants
and Pitfalls

Laura W. Bancroft, MD

Associate Professor
Mayo Clinic Florida
Jacksonville, Florida

Mellena D. Bridges, MD

Assistant Professor
Mayo Clinic Florida
Jacksonville, Florida

Wolters Kluwer | Lippincott Williams & Wilkins
Health

Philadelphia • Baltimore • New York • London
Buenos Aires • Hong Kong • Sydney • Tokyo

Acquisitions Editor: Lisa McAllister
Managing Editor: Kerry Barrett
Project Manager: Nicole Walz
Manufacturing Coordinator: Kathleen Brown
Marketing Manager: Angela Panetta
Creative Director: Doug Smock
Cover Designer: Itzhack Shelomi
Production Services: Laserwords Private Limited, Chennai, India

**WN
185
M9395
2009**

Library of Congress Cataloging-in-Publication Data
MRI normal variants and pitfalls / edited by Laura W. Bancroft and Mellena D. Bridges.
    p. ; cm.
  Includes bibliographical references and index.
  ISBN-13: 978-0-7817-8314-9
  ISBN-10: 0-7817-8314-3
  1. Magnetic resonance imaging. I. Bancroft, Laura W. II. Bridges, Mellena D., M.D.
III. Title: Magnetic resonance imaging normal variants and pitfalls.
  [DNLM: 1. Magnetic Resonance Imaging—methods. 2. Artifacts. 3. Diagnostic Errors—prevention & control. 4. Image Interpretation, Computer-Assisted. WN 185 M9395 2009]
  RC78.7.N83M759 2009
  616.07′548—dc22

                                                                            2008009240

Care has been taken to confirm the accuracy of the information presented and to describe generally accepted practices. However, the authors, editors, and publisher are not responsible for errors or omissions or for any consequences from application of the information in this book and make no warranty, expressed or implied, with respect to the currency, completeness, or accuracy of the contents of the publication. Application of this information in a particular situation remains the professional responsibility of the practitioner.

The authors, editors, and publisher have exerted every effort to ensure that drug selection and dosage set forth in this text are in accordance with current recommendations and practice at the time of publication. However, in view of ongoing research, changes in government regulations, and the constant flow of information relating to drug therapy and drug reactions, the reader is urged to check the package insert for each drug for any change in indications and dosage and for added warnings and precautions. This is particularly important when the recommended agent is a new or infrequently employed drug.

Some drugs and medical devices presented in this publication have Food and Drug Administration (FDA) clearance for limited use in restricted research settings. It is the responsibility of health care providers to ascertain the FDA status of each drug or device planned for use in their clinical practice.

To purchase additional copies of this book, call our customer service department at (800) 638-3030 or fax orders to (301) 223-2320. International customers should call (301) 223-2300.

Visit Lippincott Williams & Wilkins on the Internet: at www.LWW.com. Lippincott Williams & Wilkins customer service representatives are available from 8:30 AM to 6 PM, EST.

10 9 8 7 6 5 4 3 2

◼ Contents

Contents

List of Contributors

LAURA W. BANCROFT, MD
Associate Professor of Radiology
Department of Radiology
Mayo Clinic Florida
Jacksonville, Florida

THOMAS H. BERQUIST, MD, FACR
Professor of Radiology
Department of Radiology
Mayo Clinic Florida
Jacksonville, Florida

MELLENA D. BRIDGES, MD
Assistant Professor of Radiology
Department of Radiology
Mayo Clinic Florida
Jacksonville, Florida

JOSEPH G. CERNIGLIARO, MD
Assistant Professor of Radiology
Department of Radiology
Mayo Clinic Florida
Jacksonville, Florida

ELIZABETH R. DePERI, MD
Assistant Professor of Radiology
Department of Radiology
Mayo Clinic Florida
Jacksonville, Florida

JOHN E. KIRSCH, PhD
Senior Scientist
Magnetic Resonance Division
Siemens Medical Solutions, Inc.
Cary, North Carolina

MARK J. KRANSDORF, MD, FACR
Professor of Radiology
Department of Radiology
Mayo Clinic Florida
Jacksonville, Florida

RONALD S. KUZO, MD
Associate Professor of Radiology
Department of Radiology
Mayo Clinic
Rochester, Minnesota

PATRICK T. LIU, MD
Associate Professor of Radiology
Department of Radiology
Mayo Clinic Arizona
Scottsdale, Arizona

J. MARK McKINNEY, MD
Assistant Professor of Radiology
Department of Radiology
Mayo Clinic Florida
Jacksonville, Florida

DEBBIE J. MERINBAUM, MD
Chairman and Medical Director of Imaging
Department of Radiology
Wolfson Children's Hospital
Jacksonville, Florida

DAVID A. MILLER, MD
Assistant Professor of Radiology
Department of Radiology
Mayo Clinic Florida
Jacksonville, Florida

WILLIAM B. MORRISON, MD
Associate Professor of Radiology
Department of Radiology
Thomas Jefferson University
Philadelphia, Pennsylvania

JEFFREY J. PETERSON, MD
Associate Professor of Radiology
Department of Radiology
Mayo Clinic Florida
Jacksonville, Florida

ROBERT A. POOLEY, PhD
Assistant Professor of Radiology
Department of Radiology
Mayo Clinic Florida
Jacksonville, Florida

ERIC M. WALSER, MD
Professor of Radiology
Department of Radiology
Mayo Clinic Florida
Jacksonville, Florida

◼ Preface

MRI Normal Variants and Pitfalls was conceived as a reference for magnetic resonance imaging features of normal variations that may simulate disease, as well as a showcase for MRI pitfalls. The inspirations for this project have been Dr. Keats' monumental and indispensable radiographic reference, the *Atlas of Normal Roentgen Variants That May Simulate Disease*, and Dr. Bergman and colleagues' anatomic reference, *Compendium of Human Anatomic Variation*.

MRI Normal Variants and Pitfalls is a reference book that facilitates recognition of normal structures, artifacts, and mimickers of pathology on MRI. The scope of *MRI Normal Variants and Pitfalls* includes the gamut of neuroradiology, breast imaging, vascular, cross-sectional and musculoskeletal radiology.

We have organized the information into chapters based on anatomic location. Within each chapter are examples of normal anatomy, variations, common incidental or benign conditions, and imaging features that may be confused with other disease processes. Figure legends have been kept concise in order to facilitate rapid identification of imaging characteristics. Examples of common MRI artifacts have been distributed by anatomic location, with brief explanations from physicists in language that is understandable to the practicing radiologist. The target audience of this book includes practicing radiologists, radiologists in training, and other physicians for whom MRI has become clinically important.

■ Acknowledgments

We would like to thank our radiology colleagues, fellows, residents, technologists, and nurses for their dedication to radiology and their commitment to continuous learning. In particular, our MR technologists' tolerance of both challenge and change is the secret behind the excellent quality of many of these images. We also would like to thank John Hagen and Alice McKinney for their medical illustrations.

We would like to thank Lisa McAllister, Kerry Barrett, Ryan Shaw, and all of the staff at Lippincott Williams & Wilkins for their assistance in the production and editing of this book.

And, most importantly, we would like to thank our families for their patience and cheerfulness as we disappeared into a record-setting blizzard of arrows, images, and legends.

HEAD
AND NECK

Chapter 1

The Head

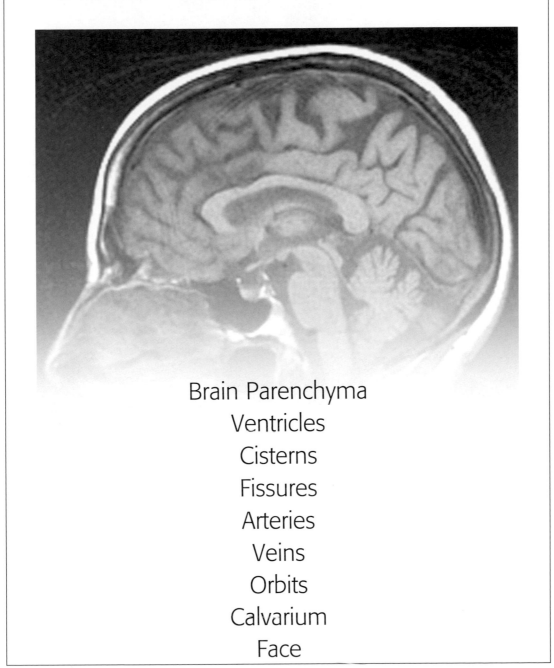

Brain Parenchyma
Ventricles
Cisterns
Fissures
Arteries
Veins
Orbits
Calvarium
Face

David A. Miller, Debbie J. Merinbaum, and John E. Kirsch

▪ Brain Parenchyma

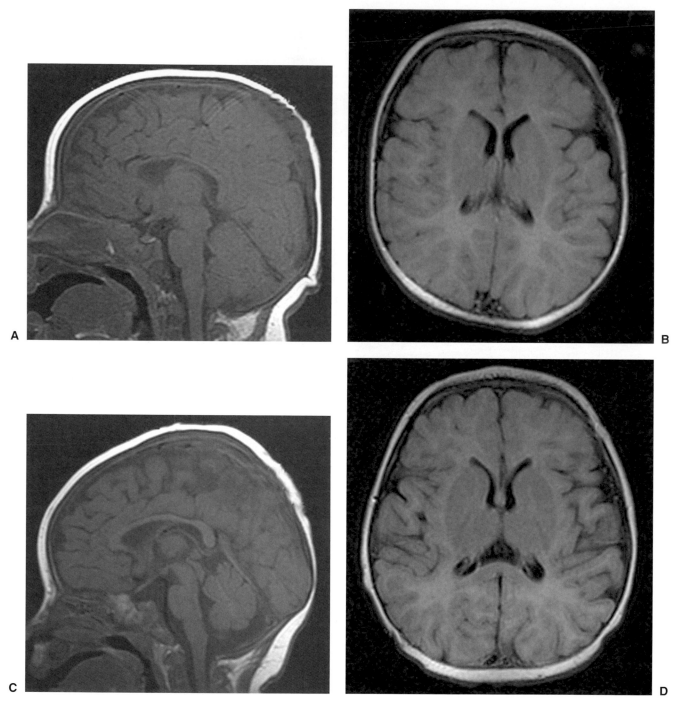

FIGURE 1-1   Normal pediatric myelination on T1-weighted images. A: Sagittal and **(B)** axial T1-weighted images in a healthy 4-month-old infant. **C:** Sagittal and **(D)** axial T1-weighted images in a healthy 7-month-old infant. Myelination patterns in the corpus callosum and brainstem in infants are best evaluated on T1-weighted images. The corpus callosum is isointense relative to white matter at birth and becomes progressively increased in signal until it reaches the intensity of the adult structure at approximately 7 to 8 months.

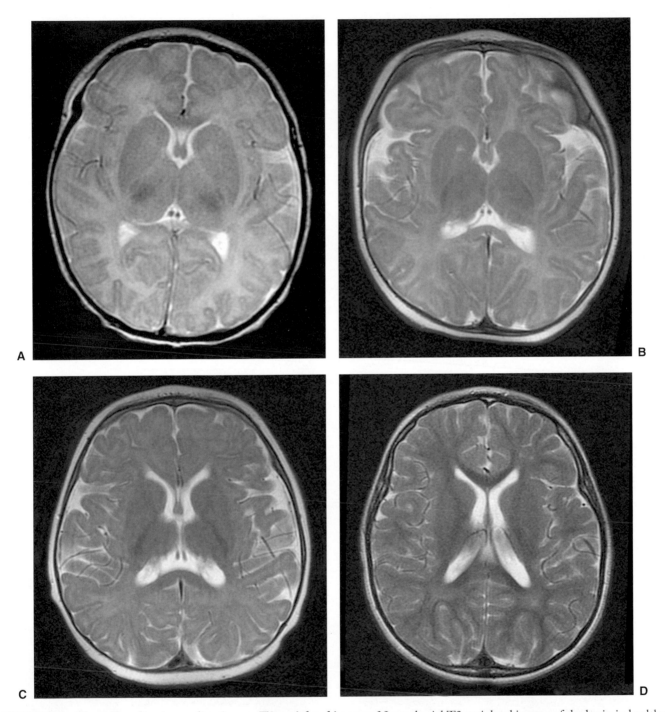

FIGURE 1-2 Normal pediatric myelination on T2-weighted images. Normal axial T2-weighted images of the brain in healthy **(A)** 3-day-old, **(B)** 4-month-old, **(C)** 7-month-old, and **(D)** 4-year-old children. At birth the signal intensities of gray and white matter are the reverse of that in the adult brain. White matter is of lower signal intensity than gray matter on T1-weighted images, and of higher signal intensity than gray matter on T2-weighted images. This persists until the age of approximately 6 months. After this the white matter becomes progressively brighter than gray matter on T1 and darker than gray matter on T2 until the adult pattern is reached.

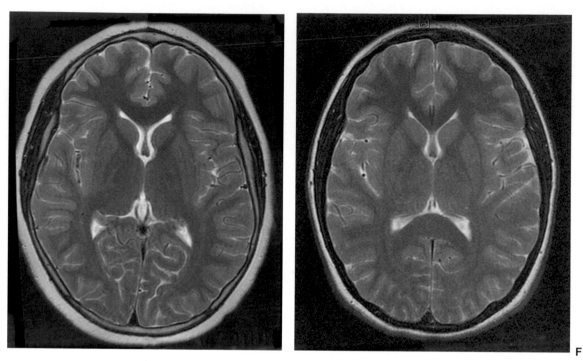

E

F

FIGURE 1-2 **Normal pediatric myelination on T2-weighted images.** (*continued*) Normal axial T2-weighted images of the brain in healthy (**E**) 8-year-old and (**F**) 16-year-old children.

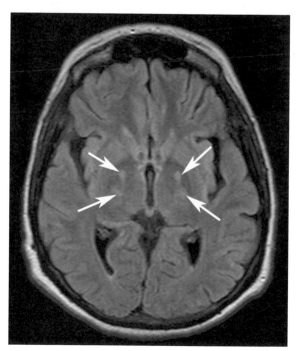

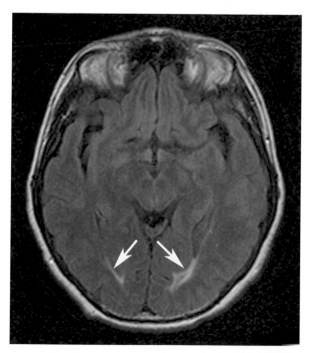

FIGURE 1-3 **Hyperintense posterior limb of the internal capsule, related to lack of myelination.** Axial fluid attenuation inversion recovery (FLAIR) image demonstrates increased signal in the posterior limbs of the internal capsule (*arrows*). Lack of myelination in this region is a normal variant.

FIGURE 1-4 **Hyperintense signal around the occipital horns.** Axial fluid attenuation inversion recovery (FLAIR) image demonstrates mildly asymmetric, hyperintense signal (*arrows*) around the occipital horns, which can be present in asymptomatic older adults.

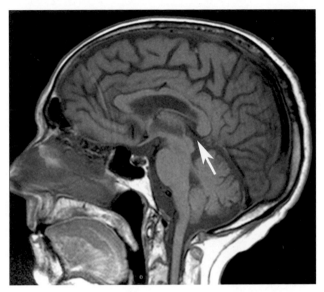

FIGURE 1-5   Aplastic rostrum of the corpus callosum. Sagittal T1-weighted image through the midline demonstrates absence of the most posterior portion of the corpus callosum (*arrow*), which can be seen as an asymptomatic developmental variant.

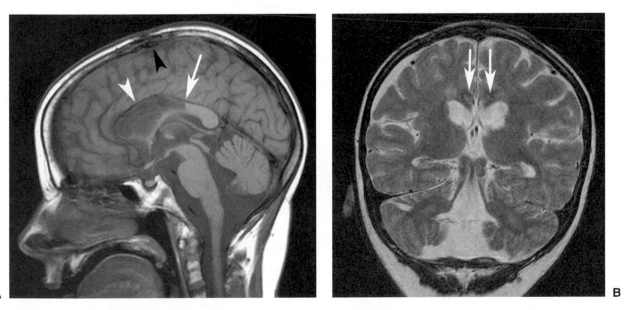

FIGURE 1-6   Corpus callosotomy. A: Sagittal T1-weighted image through the midline demonstrates the transition (*arrow*) between the transected corpus callosum (*white arrowhead*) and remaining normal posterior structure. Note the postoperative artifact from bur hole (*black arrowhead*). **B:** Coronal FSE T2-weighted fat-suppressed image shows the transected halves of the corpus callosum (*arrows*). These postsurgical changes should not be confused with agenesis of the corpus callosum.

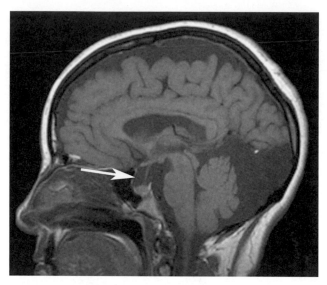

FIGURE 1-7 **Elongated sella.** Sagittal T1-weighted image through the midline demonstrates increased craniocaudal dimension of the sella turcica (*arrow*), a normal variant.

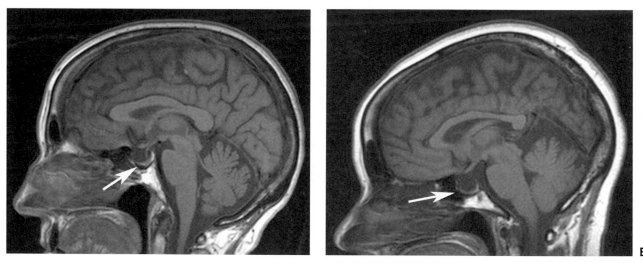

A   B

FIGURE 1-8 **Partially empty sella.** (**A** and **B**) Sagittal T1-weighted images in two different patients delineate diminutive, peripherally positioned pituitary glands (*arrows*) within the sella turcica.

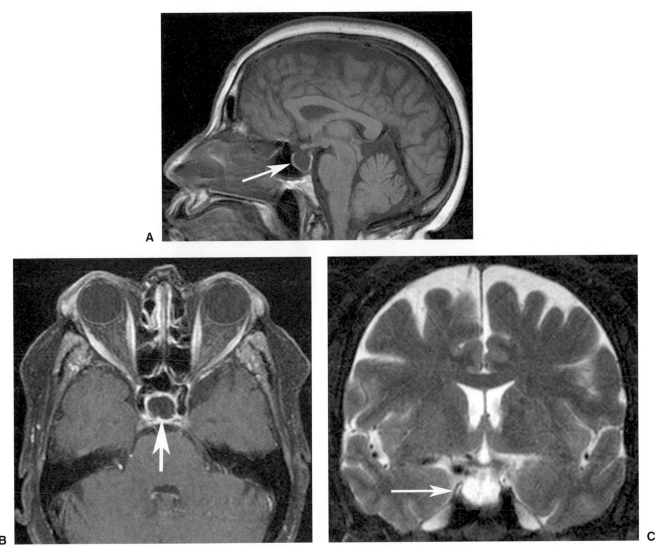

FIGURE 1-9   Empty sella. A: Sagittal T1-weighted, **(B)** axial enhanced and **(C)** coronal FSE T2-weighted images through the midline demonstrate complete absence of pituitary tissue within the sella turcica (*arrows*).

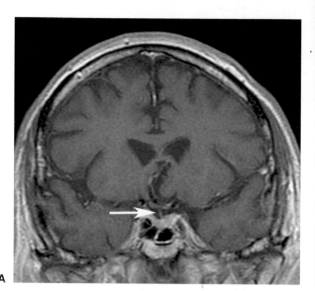

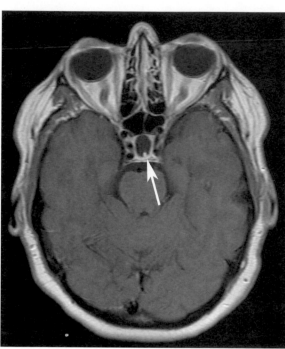

A
B

FIGURE 1-10 **Deviated pituitary stalk. A:** Coronal enhanced T1-weighted image through the pituitary stalk show deviation of stalk (*arrow*) to the right. **B:** Axial enhanced T1-weighted image demonstrates the enhancing stalk (*arrow*) deviated to the left of midline.

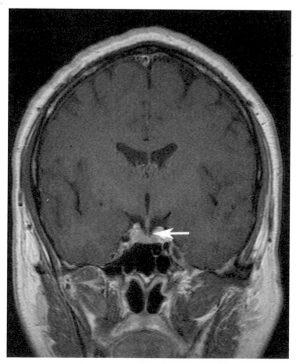

FIGURE 1-11 **Tapered infundibulum.** Coronal enhanced T1-weighted image through the infundibulum depicts slight tapering (*arrow*) of the inferior portion of the infundibulum.

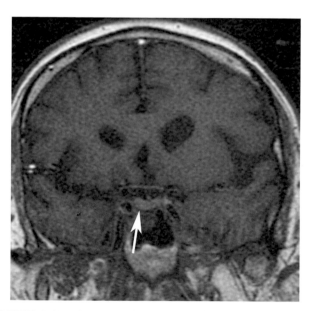

FIGURE 1-12 **Asymmetric pituitary gland.** Right lobe of the pituitary (*arrow*) is larger than the left in this patient. Dynamic pituitary imaging showed no evidence of adenoma.

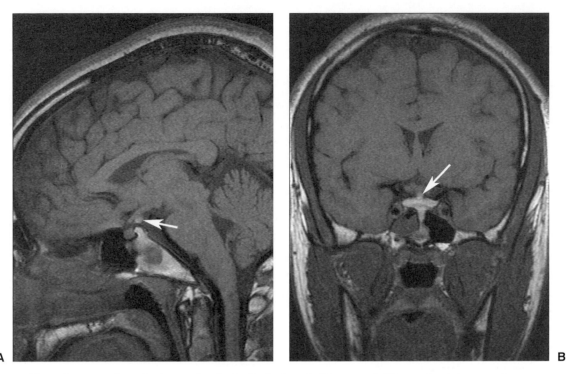

FIGURE 1-13 Ectopic posterior pituitary gland. A: Sagittal and **(B)** coronal T1-weighted images demonstrate posterior positioning of the posterior lobe (neurohypophysis or "bright spot") of the pituitary gland (*arrows*) within the floor of the third ventricle. Ectopic location of the pituitary gland may be accompanied by multiple endocrine deficiencies. Fat-suppressed images will allow differentiating of this entity from dermoid or lipoma.

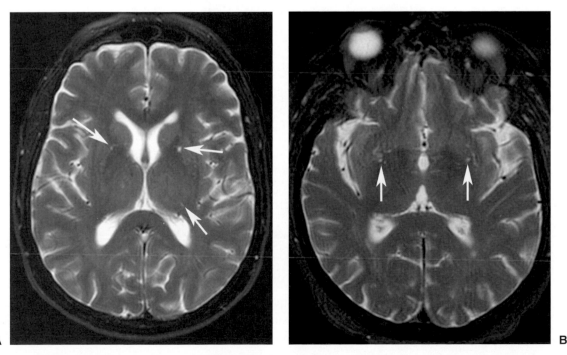

FIGURE 1-14 Virchow-Robbins spaces in the basal ganglia. A and **B:** Axial FSE T2-weighted fat-suppressed images in four different patients demonstrate various degrees of dilatation (*arrows*) about the axonal pathways of the basal ganglia.

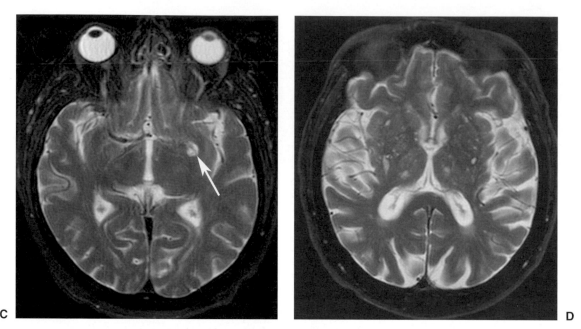

C   D

FIGURE 1-14 **Virchow-Robbins spaces in the basal ganglia.** (*continued*) **C** and **D:** Axial FSE T2-weighted fat-suppressed images in four different patients demonstrate various degrees of dilatation (*arrows*) about the axonal pathways of the basal ganglia.

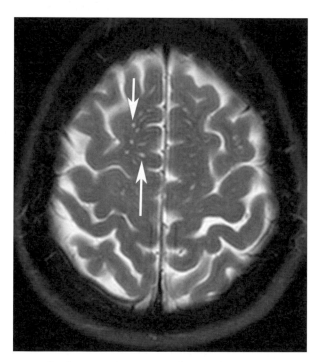

FIGURE 1-15 **Virchow-Robbins spaces in the centrum semiovale.** Axial FSE T2-weighted fat-suppressed image through the level of the centrum semiovale show prominent cerebrospinal fluid (CSF) or Virchow-Robbins spaces (*arrows*).

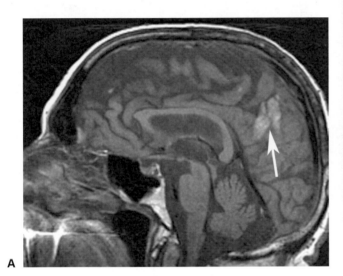

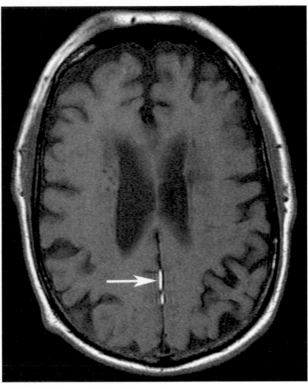

FIGURE 1-16 **Falcine lipoma. A:** Sagittal T1-weighted and **(B)** axial fluid attenuation inversion recovery (FLAIR) images demonstrate a bilobed lipoma (*arrows*) along the falx cerebrum.

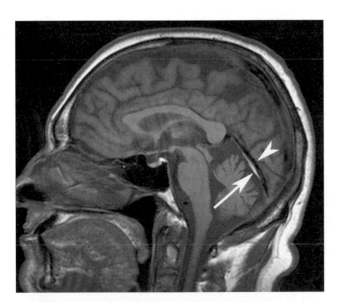

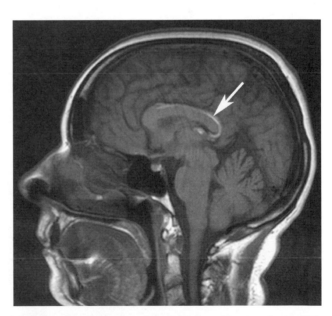

FIGURE 1-17 **Lipoma inferior to the straight sinus.** Sagittal T1-weighted image displays a linear lipoma (*arrow*) inferior to the straight sinus (*arrowhead*).

FIGURE 1-18 **Lipoma of the corpus callosum.** Sagittal T1-weighted image displays a curvilinear lipoma (*arrow*) wrapping around the corpus callosum.

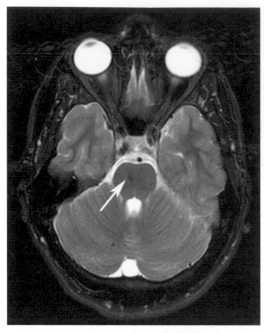

FIGURE 1-19 **Artifact through pons.** Axial FSE T2-weighted fat-suppressed image demonstrates a small hypointense focus in the right pons (*arrow*), which did not persist on additional sequences, and is artifactual.

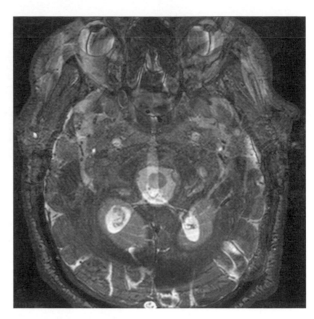

FIGURE 1-20 **Aliasing/wrap artifact.** Axial gradient-echo image through the level of the basal ganglia demonstrates superimposition of the more superior structures due to undersampling and aliasing in a superior-to-inferior direction.

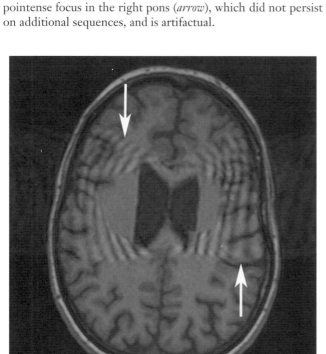

FIGURE 1-21 **Motion artifact.** Axial fluid attenuation inversion recovery (FLAIR) image has repeating artifact (*arrows*) along the phase-encoding direction due to motion artifact.

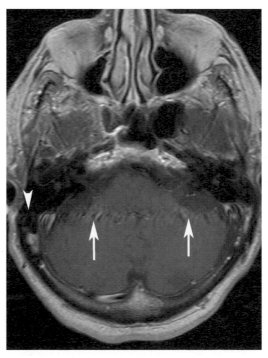

FIGURE 1-22 **Pulsatility artifact.** Axial enhanced T1-weighted image demonstrates pulsatility artifact (*arrows*) through the cerebellum from the jugular vein (*arrowhead*).

■ Ventricles

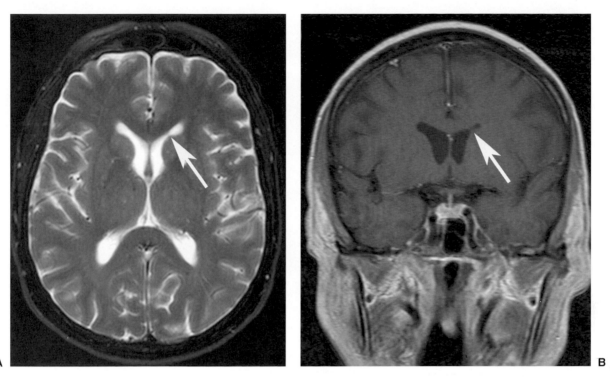

FIGURE 1-23 **Front horn coaptation. A:** Axial FSE T2-weighted fat-suppressed and **(B)** coronal T1-weighted enhanced images in the same patient demonstrate apposition of the left frontal horn (*arrow*).

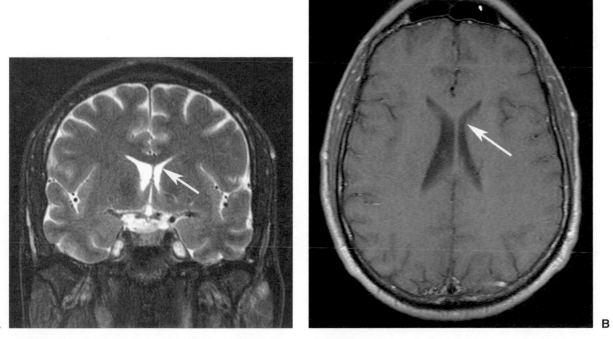

FIGURE 1-24 **Frontal horn asymmetry. A:** Coronal FSE T2-weighted fat-suppressed and **(B)** axial enhanced T1-weighted images in three different patients show the normal variant of relative narrowing of the left frontal horn (*arrows*).

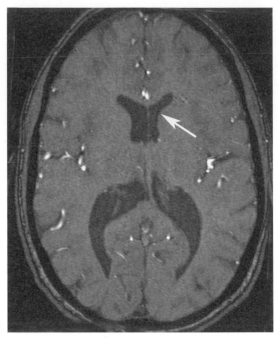

C

FIGURE 1-24   Frontal horn asymmetry. (*continued*) **C:** Axial enhanced T1-weighted images in three different patients show the normal variant of relative narrowing of the left frontal horn (*arrow*).

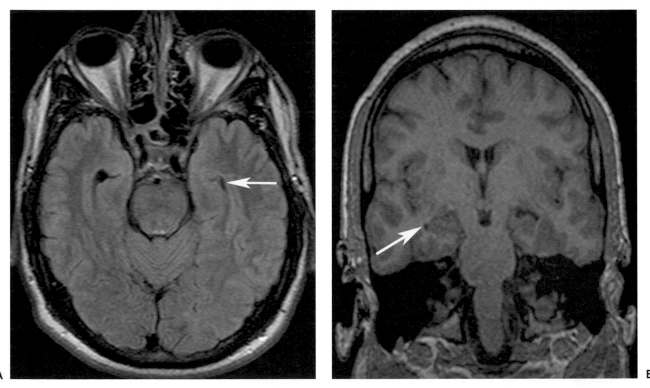

A   B

FIGURE 1-25   Temporal horn asymmetry. A: Axial fluid attenuation inversion recovery (FLAIR), **(B)** coronal T1-weighted enhanced images through the temporal horns depict the normal variation of temporal horn size (*arrows*) in different patients.

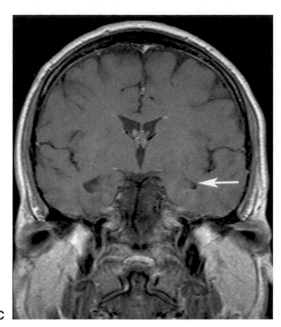

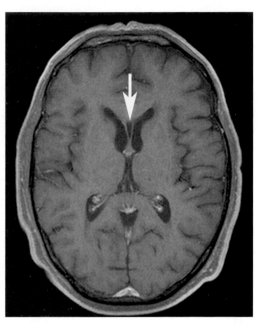

FIGURE 1-25 Temporal horn asymmetry. (*continued*) **C:** T1-weighted enhanced image through the temporal horns depict the normal variation of temporal horn size (*arrow*) in different patients.

FIGURE 1-26 Cavum septum pellucidum. Axial enhanced T1-weighted image demonstrates a normal variant, developmental cerebrospinal fluid (CSF)-filled space (*arrow*) between the frontal horns—termed the *cavum septum pellucidum.*

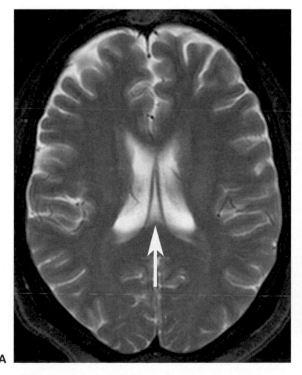

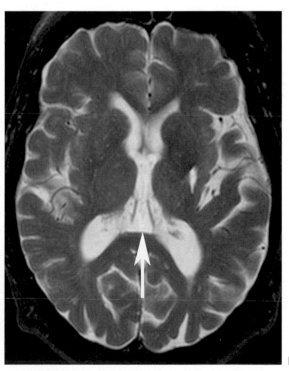

FIGURE 1-27 Cavum vellum interpositum. A and **B:** Axial FSE T2-weighted fat-suppressed images demonstrate a normal variant cerebrospinal fluid (CSF)-filled space (*arrows*) between the bodies and occipital horns of the ventricles—termed the *cavum vellum interpositum.*

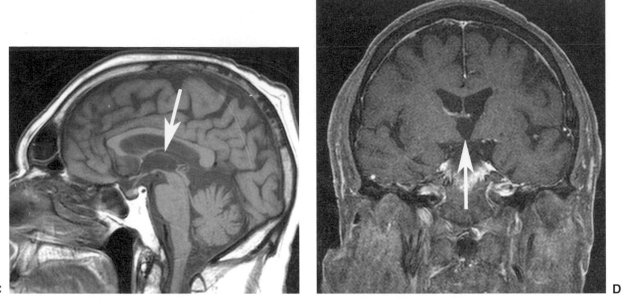

FIGURE 1-27   Cavum vellum interpositum. (*continued*) **C:** Sagittal T1-weighted and (**D**) coronal T1-weighted enhanced images demonstrate the corresponding location of the low-signal intensity fluid (*arrow*).

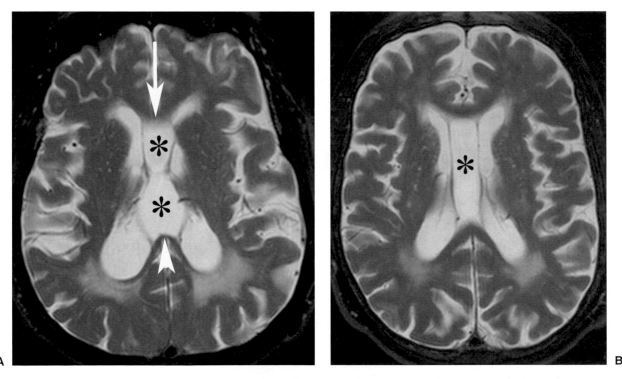

FIGURE 1-28   Cavum septum pellucidum et vergae. A and **B:** Axial FSE T2-weighted fat-suppressed images show a prominent cavum septum pellucidum et vergae (*asterisk*) extending anteriorly (*arrow*) and posteriorly (*arrowhead*) between the ventricles.

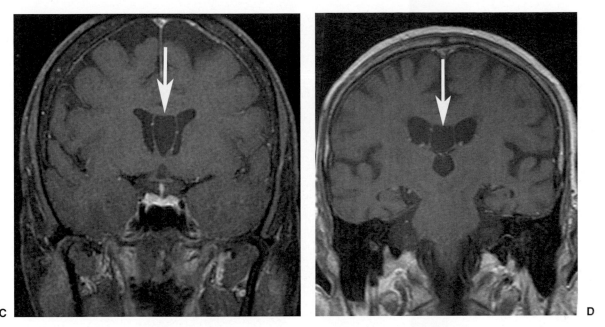

C   D

FIGURE 1-28 Cavum septum pellucidum et vergae. (*continued*) Coronal images show the variations **(C)** anteriorly through the pellucidum and **(D)** posteriorly through the vergae.

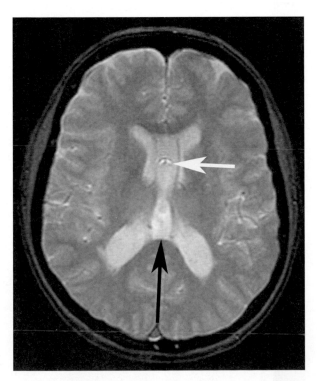

FIGURE 1-29 Artifact in cavum septum pellucidum et vergae. Axial FSE T2-weighted fat-suppressed image demonstrates flow artifact (*white arrow*) through the cavum septum pellucidum et vergae (*black arrow*).

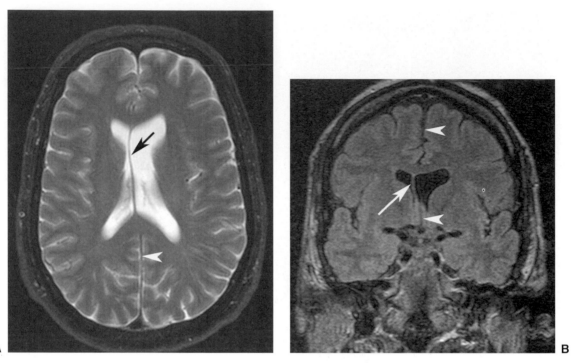

FIGURE 1-30 **Shifted septum. A:** Axial FSE T2-weighted fat-suppressed and **(B)** coronal fluid attenuation inversion recovery (FLAIR) images demonstrate incidental shift of the septum (*arrows*) to the right of midline (*arrowheads*).

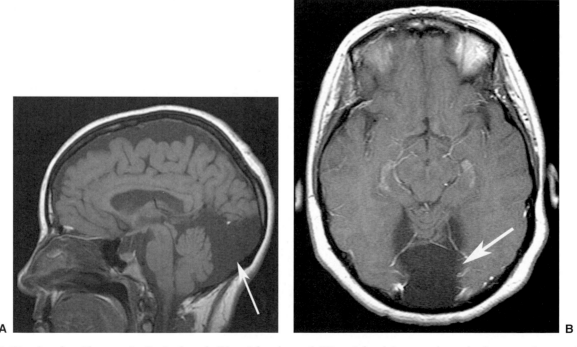

FIGURE 1-31 **Arachnoid cyst. A:** Sagittal and **(B)** axial enhanced T1-weighted images through the posterior cranial fossa demonstrate a large arachnoid cyst (*arrow*) between the cerebrum and cerebellum.

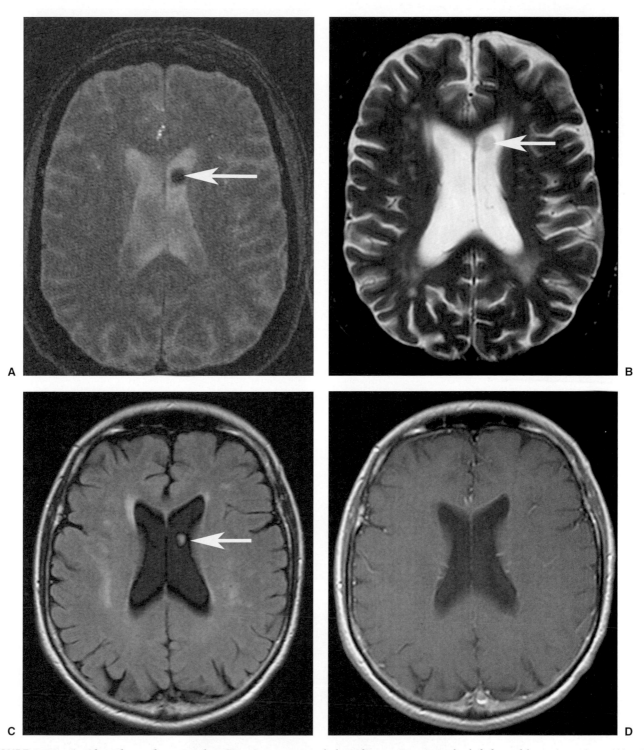

FIGURE 1-32 Artifact through ventricles. Hypointense, rounded artifact projects into the left frontal horn (*arrow*) on **(A)** axial proton density, **(B)** FSE T2-weighted fat-suppressed, and **(C)** fluid attenuation inversion recovery (FLAIR) sequences, but does not persist on **(D)** T1-weighted enhanced images.

▣ Cisterns

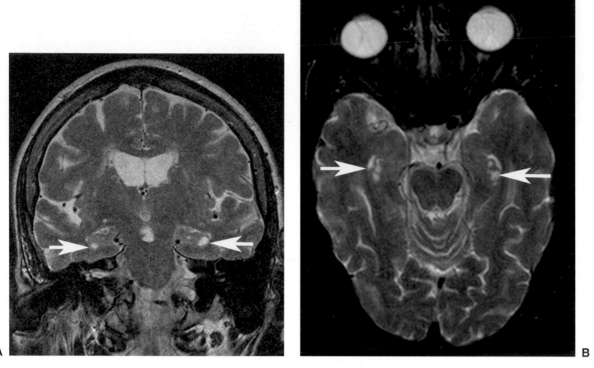

FIGURE 1-33 **Cystic foci in the hippocampal sulcal remnants. A:** Coronal and **(B)** axial FSE T2-weighted fat-suppressed images through the temporal lobes delineate small cystic foci (*arrows*) in the hippocampal sulcal remnants, normal developmental variants.

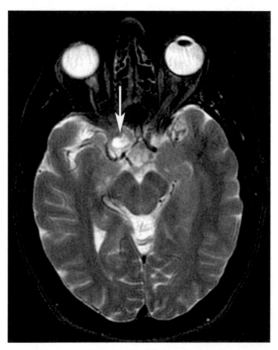

FIGURE 1-34 **Prominent cerebrospinal fluid posterolateral to the anterior clinoid process.** Axial FSE T2-weighted fat-suppressed image demonstrates a prominent focus of cerebrospinal fluid (CSF) posterior to the clinoid, representing asymmetry that is within normal limits.

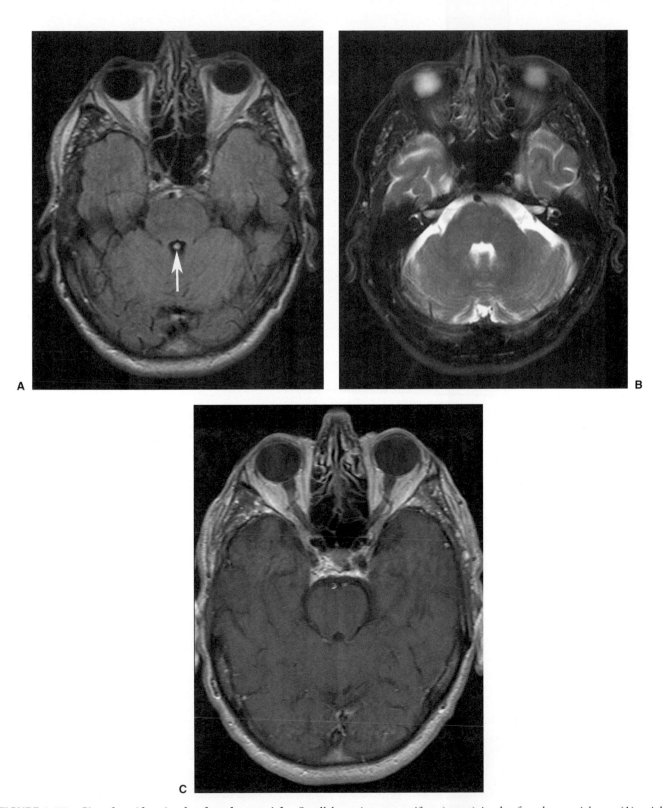

FIGURE 1-35 Signal artifact in the fourth ventricle. Small hyperintense artifact (*arrow*) in the fourth ventricle on **(A)** axial fluid attenuation inversion recovery (FLAIR) image does not persist on **(B)** FSE T2-weighted fat-suppressed or **(C)** enhanced T1-weighted sequences.

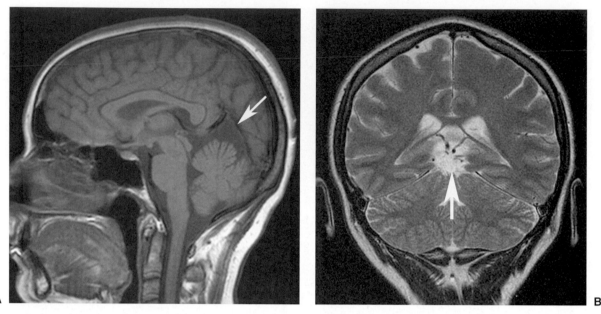

FIGURE 1-36 Fluid superior to the cerebellum. A: Sagittal T1-weighted and **(B)** coronal FSE T2-weighted fat-suppressed images demonstrate prominent cerebrospinal fluid (CSF) (*arrow*) superior to the cerebellum. The lack of focal loculation of the fluid contrasts with an arachnoid cyst, shown in Figure 1-37.

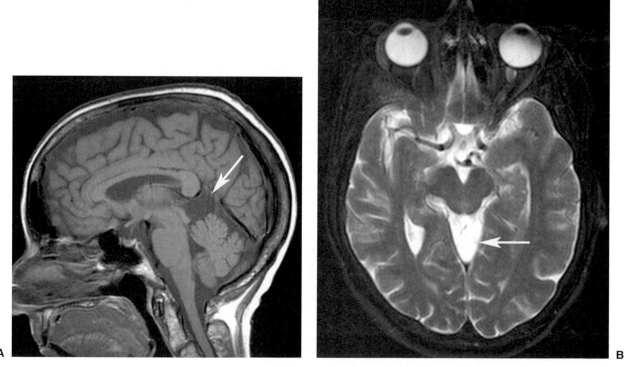

FIGURE 1-37 Arachnoid cyst in the suprasellar cistern. Sagittal T1-weighted **(A)** and axial FSE T2-weighted fat-suppressed **(B)** images show a focal collection of fluid (*arrows*) superior to the cerebellum, in contrast to Figure 1-36.

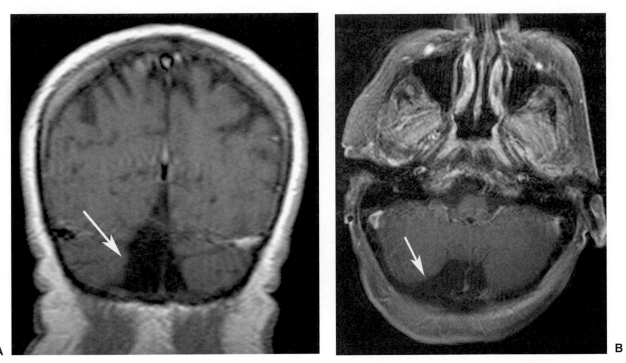

FIGURE 1-38 **Enlarged cisterna magna.** Enhanced T1-weighted coronal **(A)** and axial **(B)** images demonstrate an enlarged cisterna magna (*arrows*) posterior to the central and right portions of the cerebellum.

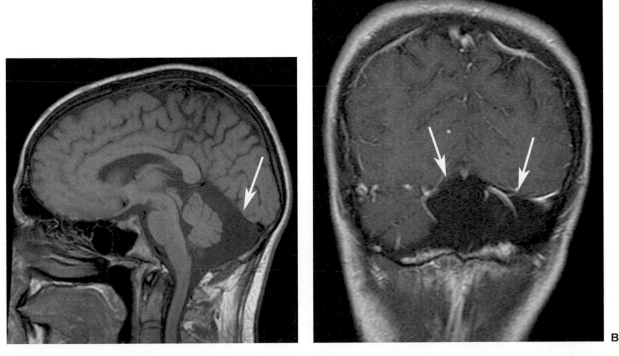

FIGURE 1-39 **Enlarged, asymmetric cisterna magna.** Enhanced T1-weighted coronal **(A)** and axial **(B)** images demonstrate a larger cisterna magna (*arrows*) than it was in Figure 1-35, with extension posterior to the left hemisphere of the cerebellum.

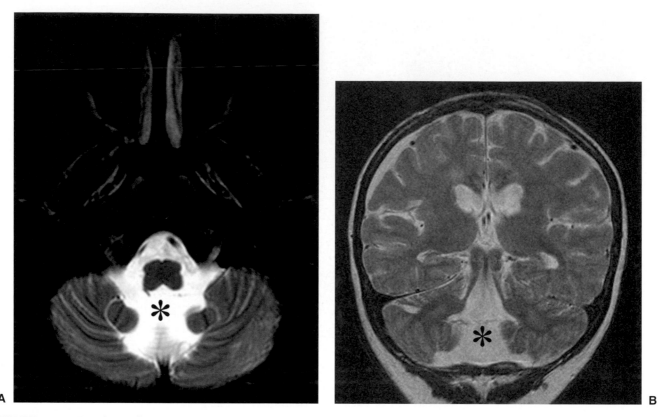

FIGURE 1-40 Dandy-Walker variant. Contrast normal variant in Figure 1-39 with the Dandy-Walker variant in this case. **A:** Axial and **(B)** coronal FSE T2-weighted fat-suppressed images delineate mild vermian hypoplasia with a cystic space (*asterisk*) caused by open communication of the posteroinferior fourth ventricle and cisterna magna through an enlarged vallecula.

■ Fissures

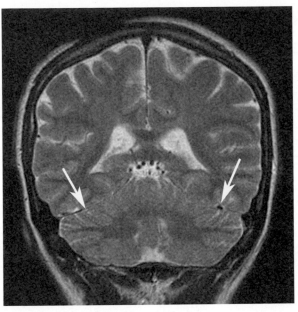

FIGURE 1-41 Choroidal fissure asymmetry. Coronal FSE T2-weighted fat-suppressed image through the temporal lobes demonstrates subtle asymmetry of the choroidal fissures (*arrows*), with the left being slightly more prominent than the right.

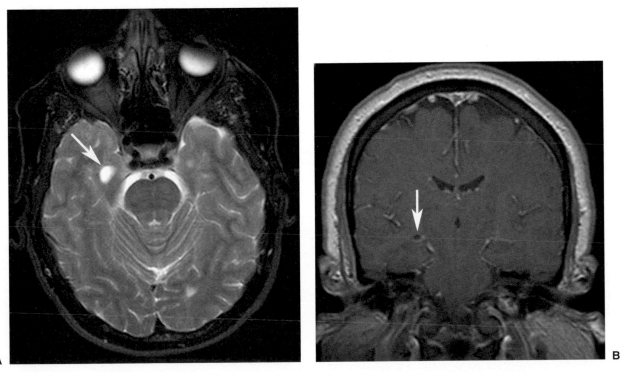

FIGURE 1-42 Choroidal fissure cyst. A: Axial FSE T2-weighted fat-suppressed image shows an oval cerebrospinal fluid (CSF)-like cystic focus (*arrow*) in the right choroidal fissure, representing a neuroepithelial cyst in the choroidal fissure. **B:** Coronal T1-weighted enhanced image in a different patient demonstrates a smaller choroidal fissure cyst (*arrow*).

Arteries

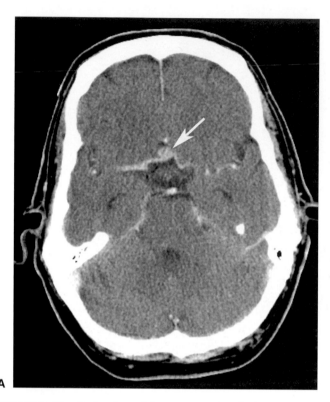

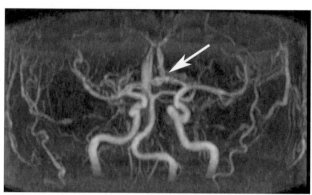

A

B

FIGURE 1-43 **Redundant A1 segment, simulating an aneurysm on CT. A:** A small, rounded focus of contrast enhancement on CT in the expected location of the anterior communicating artery was worrisome for aneurysm, and prompted evaluation of this region with MRA. **B:** The maximum intensity projection (MIP) of the circle of Willis shows no aneurysm, but rather a redundant A1 segment of the anterior cerebral artery (ACA) (*arrow*) in this location.

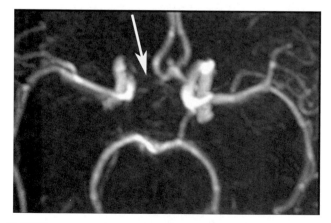

FIGURE 1-44 **Aplastic right A1 segment.** Maximum intensity projection (MIP) of the circle of Willis in the axial plane demonstrates an aplastic right A1 segment (*arrow*). More than 83 variations of the circle of Willis have been described in the literature.

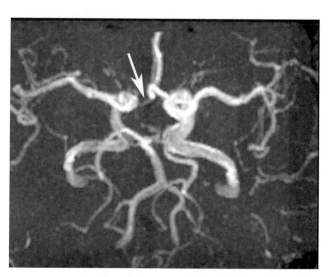

FIGURE 1-45 **Hypoplastic A1 segment.** Maximum intensity projection (MIP) of the circle of Willis shows a markedly hypoplastic right A1 segment (*arrow*) between the carotid artery and A2 segment.

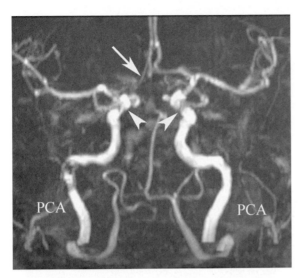

FIGURE 1-46 Hypoplastic A1 segment and fetal-type posterior cerebral arteries. Maximum intensity projection (MIP) of the circle of Willis shows a markedly hypoplastic right A1 segment (*arrow*). In addition, the posterior cerebral arteries (*PCA*) originate from the internal carotid arteries (*arrowheads*) rather than the basilar artery (called *fetal origin*). This common normal variant occurs in up to 20% of the population.

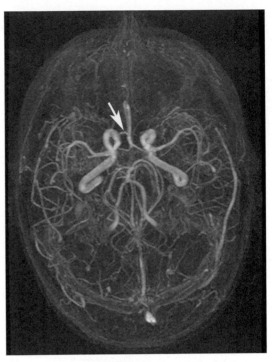

FIGURE 1-47 A2 segment originating from the mid portion of A1. Maximum intensity projection (MIP) of the circle of Willis demonstrates variant anatomy, with the right A2 segment (*arrow*) originating from the mid portion of the A1 segment.

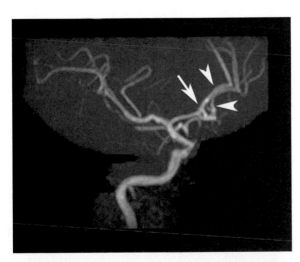

FIGURE 1-48 Fenestrated anterior communicating artery (ACOM). Maximum intensity projection (MIP) of the circle of Willis shows a fenestration (or apparent focal duplication) of the anterior communicating artery (*arrow*). Right and left A2 segments are designated with *arrowheads*.

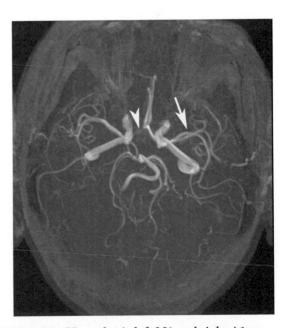

FIGURE 1-49 Hypoplastic left M1 and right A1 segments. Maximum intensity projection (MIP) of the circle of Willis shows two normal variants, a hypoplastic left M1 segment (*arrow*) and markedly hypoplastic right A1 segment (*arrowhead*).

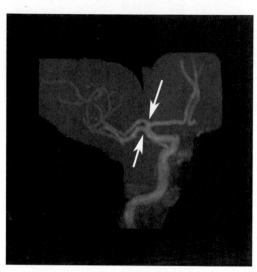

FIGURE 1-50   Duplicated right M1 segment. Maximum intensity projection (MIP) of the circle of Willis displays parallel, duplicated right M1 segments (*arrows*) of the middle cerebral artery (MCA).

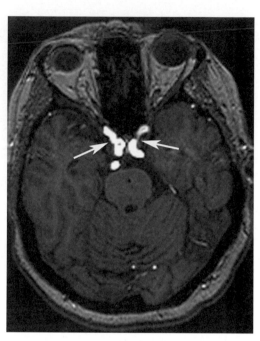

FIGURE 1-51   Medial cavernous and supraclinoid internal carotid artery (ICA). Axial source image for an MRA displays medial positioning of the cavernous and supraclinoid portions (*arrows*) of the internal carotid artery.

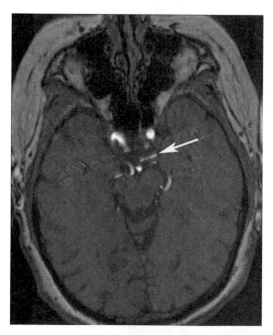

FIGURE 1-52   Medial course of left posterior communicating artery (PCOM). Axial source image for an MRA shows a medial course of the left posterior communicating artery (*arrow*).

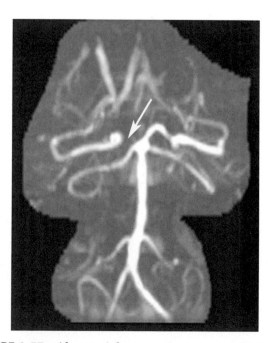

FIGURE 1-53   Absent right posterior communicating artery (PCOM). Maximum intensity projection (MIP) of the circle of Willis fails to show a right PCOM (*arrow*) between the middle and posterior cerebral arteries.

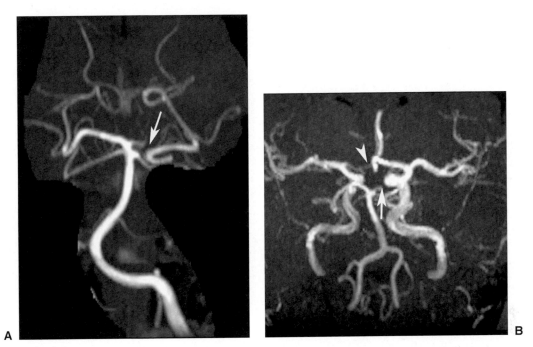

FIGURE 1-54 Hypoplastic left P1 and aplastic right A1 segments. A: Maximum intensity projection (MIP) of the posterior circulation shows a hypoplastic left P1 segment (*arrow*) of the posterior cerebral artery. **B:** MIP of the circle of Willis also demonstrates an aplastic right A1 segment (*arrowhead*) of the anterior cerebral artery (ACA).

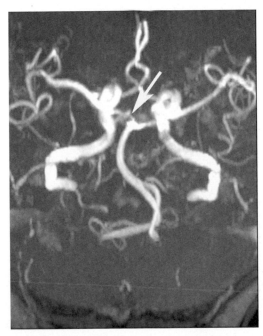

FIGURE 1-55 Hypoplastic right P1 segment with fetal-type right posterior cerebral artery (PCA). Maximum intensity projection (MIP) of the circle of Willis demonstrates a markedly hypoplastic right P1 segment (*arrow*) of the PCA, with near-complete supply of the right PCA by the right internal carotid artery.

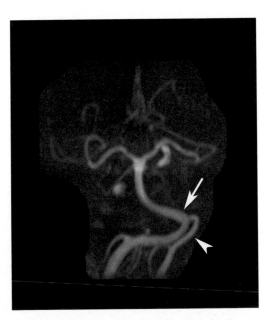

FIGURE 1-56 Tortuous distal right vertebral artery and proximal basilar artery. Maximum intensity projection (MIP) of the posterior circulation shows marked tortuosity of the distal right vertebral artery and vertebrobasilar junction (*arrow*). *Arrowhead* denotes smaller left vertebral artery.

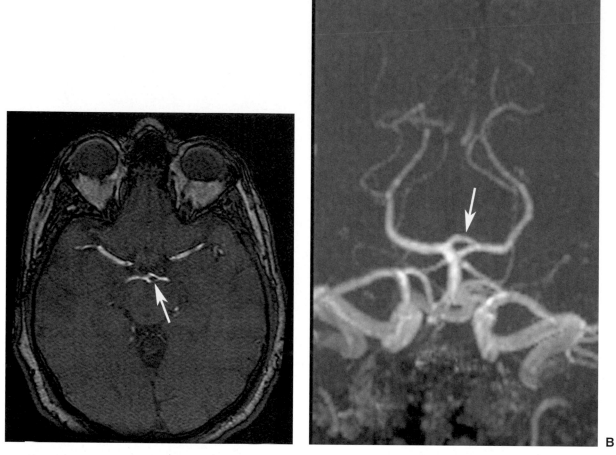

A **B**

FIGURE 1-57   Duplicated left P1 segment. A: Axial source image and **(B)** maximum intensity projection (MIP) of the circle of Willis demonstrate focal fenestration of the left posterior cerebral artery (PCA) (*arrow*).

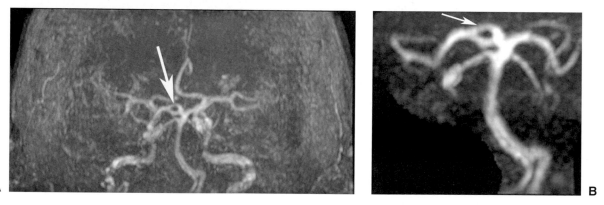

A **B**

FIGURE 1-58   Fenestrated right posterior cerebral artery (PCA). A and **B:** Maximum intensity projections (MIPs) of the circle of Willis demonstrate focal fenestration of the right PCA (*arrow*).

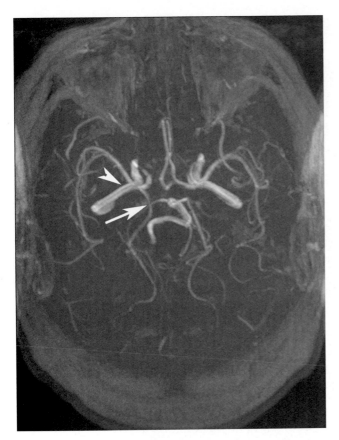

FIGURE 1-59 **Fetal circulation of the right posterior cerebral artery (PCA).** Maximum intensity projection (MIP) of the circle of Willis demonstrates normal variant blood supply of the right PCA (*arrow*) from the internal carotid artery (*arrowhead*).

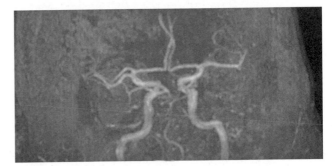

FIGURE 1-60 **Bilateral fetal-type circulation.** Maximum intensity projection (MIP) of the circle of Willis demonstrates normal variant blood supply of the bilateral posterior cerebral arteries (*arrows*) originating from the internal carotid arteries (*arrowheads*).

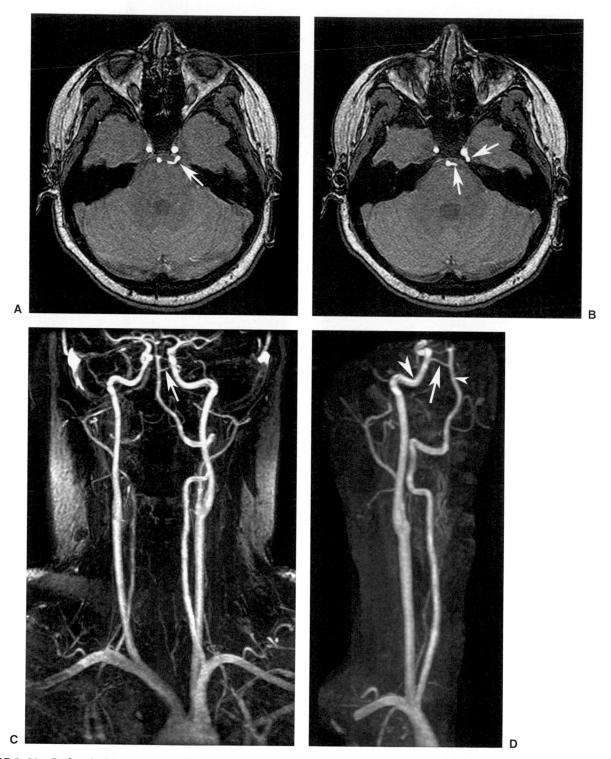

FIGURE 1-61 **Left primitive trigeminal artery. A** and **B:** Axial source, **(C)** coronal, and **(D)** oblique coronal projects from a MRA demonstrate a primitive left trigeminal artery (*arrows*). The embryonic trigeminal artery supplies the basilar artery before the posterior communicating artery and vertebral arteries develop. As these vessels develop, the primitive trigeminal artery normally disappears.

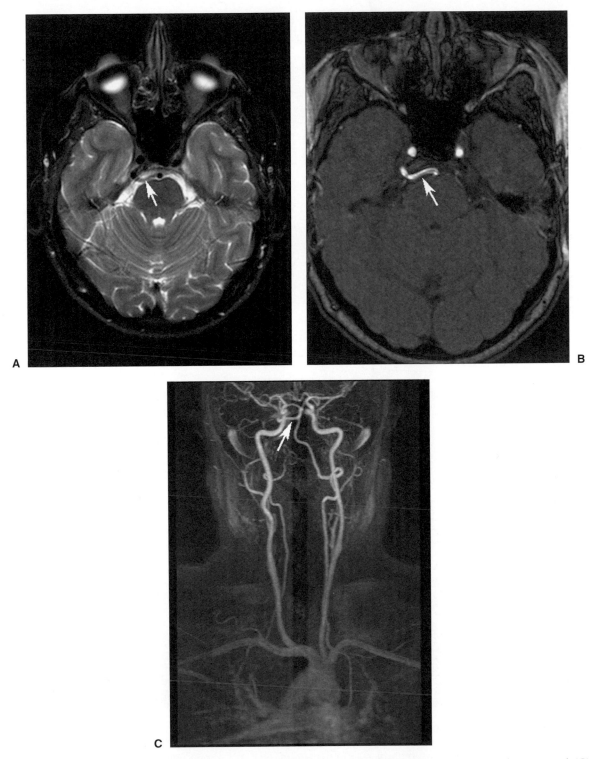

FIGURE 1-62 **Right primitive trigeminal artery. A:** Axial FSE T2-weighted fat-suppressed, **(B)** axial source and **(C)** coronal projection of the MRA demonstrate the most common carotid-basilar anastomosis, the primitive trigeminal artery (*arrows*), which occurs in up to 0.6% of angiograms.

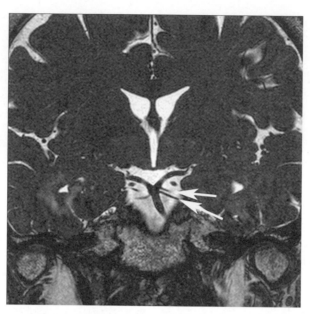

FIGURE 1-63 **Duplicated superior cerebellar arteries.** Coronal high-resolution constructive interference in steady state (CISS) image shows duplicated left superior cerebellar arteries (*arrows*), which originate near the basilar artery tip and curve posteriorly around the pons. The superior cerebellar arteries supply the superior surface of the vermis and cerebellar hemispheres.

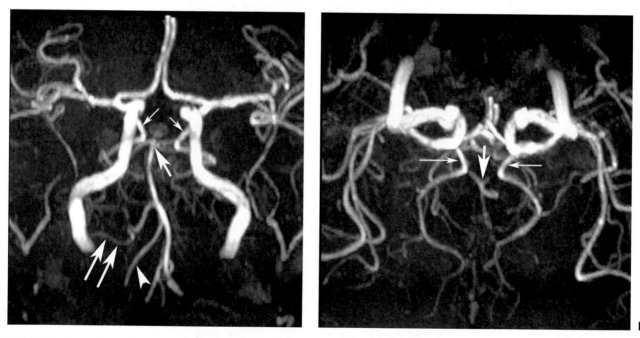

FIGURE 1-64 **Anterior inferior cerebellar artery-posterior inferior cerebellar artery (AICA-PICA) complex and fetal-type circulation. A** and **B:** Enlarged vessel representing the AICA and PICA combination (*double arrows*) coming off the basilar artery. Note no PICA off the right vertebral artery (*arrowhead*). In addition, there is bilateral fetal-type circulation, with hypoplastic P1 segments (*arrow*) and fetal-type origin of both posterior cerebral arteries (PCAs) (*small arrows*).

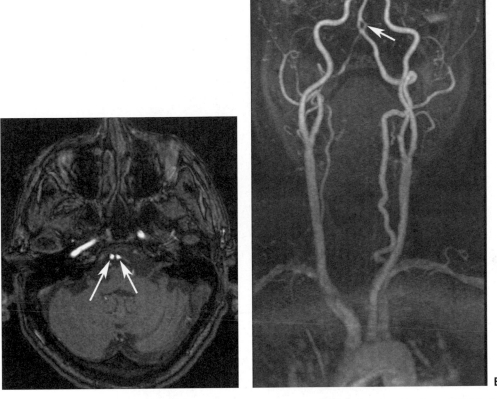

FIGURE 1-65 **Fenestration of the basilar artery.** A: Axial source image and **(B)** coronal projection of MRA demonstrate focal fenestration of the basilar artery (*arrows*).

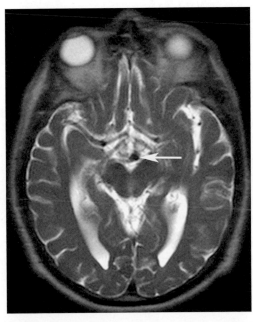

FIGURE 1-66 **Bulbous basilar tip.** Axial FSE T2-weighted fat-suppressed image above the skull base shows a prominent signal void (*arrow*) corresponding to a normal variant bulbous basilar tip.

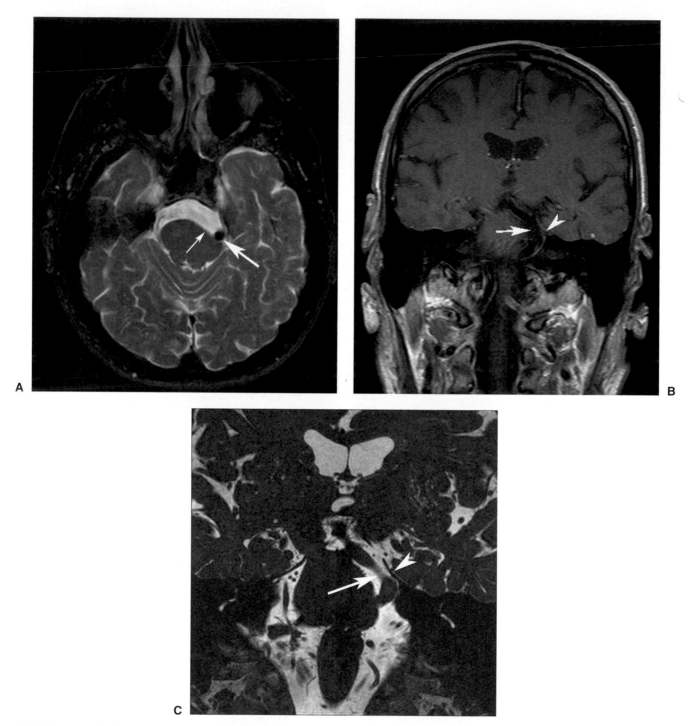

FIGURE 1-67 **Basilar artery dolicoectasia, resulting in left fifth nerve compression. A:** Axial FSE T2-weighted fat-suppressed, **(B)** coronal T1-weighted, and **(C)** high-resolution constructive interference in steady state (CISS) images demonstrate compression of the cisternal portion of the left fifth cranial nerve (*arrowhead*) by the dolicoectatic basilar artery (*arrows*). Also note the deformity of the left pons (*small arrow*) due to the mass effect in **(A)**.

■ Veins

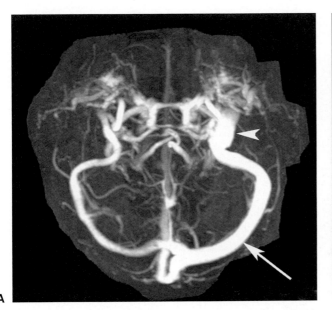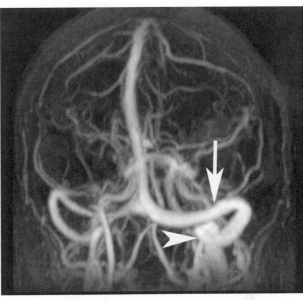

FIGURE 1-68 **Dominant left transverse sinus and jugular bulb. A** and **B:** Maximum intensity projection (MIP) of images obtained during the venous phase of an enhanced MRA demonstrates enlarged left transverse sinus (*arrow*) and jugular bulb (*arrowhead*).

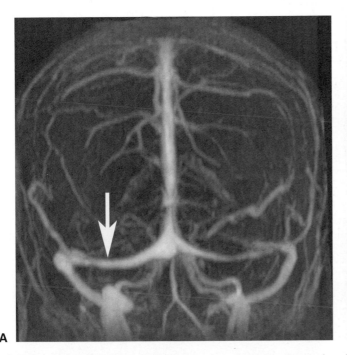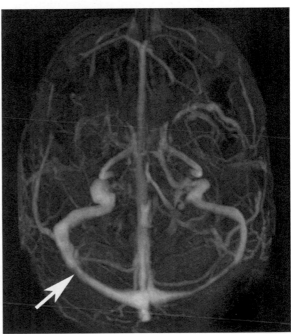

FIGURE 1-69 **Dominant right transverse sinus. A:** Coronal and **(B)** axial projections of images obtained during the venous phase of an enhanced MRA demonstrate a relatively enlarged right transverse sinus (*arrows*), indicating its dominance.

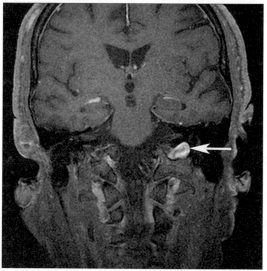

FIGURE 1-70 Dominant right transverse sinus and jugular bulb. Coronal projection of images obtained during the venous phase of an enhanced MRA demonstrates an enlarged right transverse sinus (*arrow*) and jugular bulb (*arrowhead*).

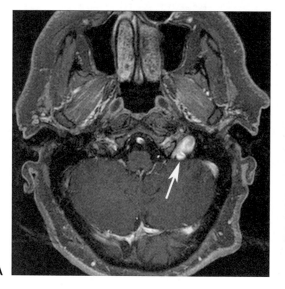

FIGURE 1-71 High position of the jugular bulb. A: Axial and **(B)** coronal enhanced T1-weighted images show a superiorly positioned left jugular bulb (*arrow*). A "high riding" jugular bulb is one that extends above the floor of the internal auditory canal (IAC) into the middle ear cavity. **C:** Coronal enhanced image in a different patient demonstrates a different orientation of a high riding left jugular bulb (*arrow*).

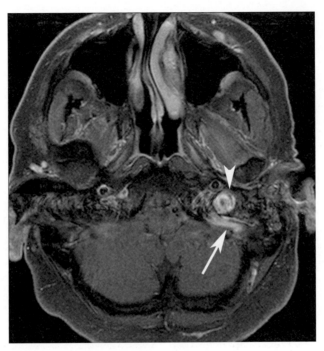

FIGURE 1-72 Prominent left sigmoid sinus and internal jugular vein (IJV). Axial enhanced T1-weighted image shows a superiorly positioned left jugular bulb (*arrowhead*) and a prominent left sigmoid sinus (*arrow*).

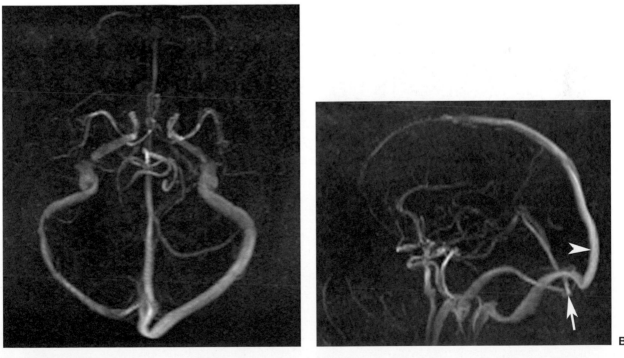

FIGURE 1-73 Superior sagittal sinus (SSS) drains into dominant left transverse sinus and straight sinus (SS) drains into smaller right transverse sinus. An obliqued posterior projection obtained during the venous phase of an enhanced MRA shows that the SSS drains into the dominant left transverse sinus (*arrowhead*), and the SS drains into the smaller right transverse sinus (*arrow*), which reflects a normal developmental variant.

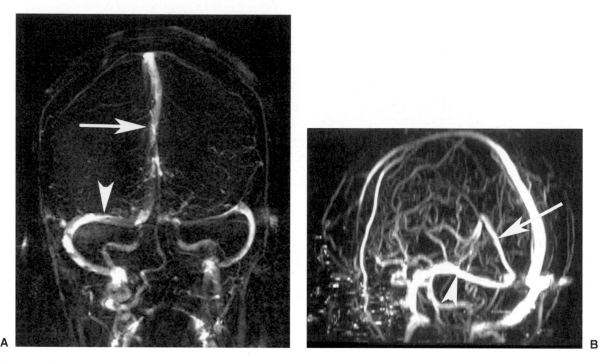

FIGURE 1-74 **Superior sagittal sinus (SSS) drains into dominant right transverse and straight sinus drains into left transverse sinus. A:** Coronal oblique image obtained during the venous phase of an enhanced MRA shows that the SSS (*arrow*) drains into the dominant right transverse sinus (*arrowhead*). **B:** Oblique image shows the straight sinus (*arrow*) draining into the left transverse sinus (*arrowhead*).

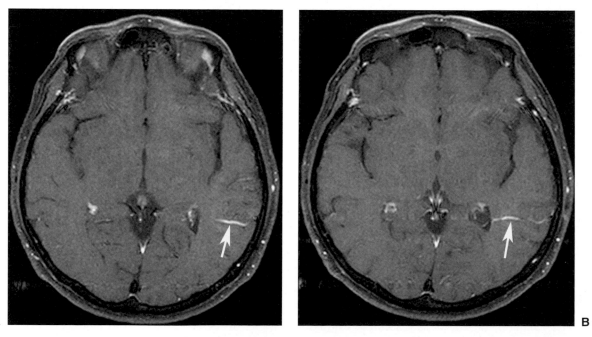

FIGURE 1-75 **Venous angioma. A** and **B:** Axial enhanced images demonstrate a linear enhancing vessel (*arrows*) extending through the left temporal lobe, consistent with a developmental anomaly, the venous angioma.

■ Orbits

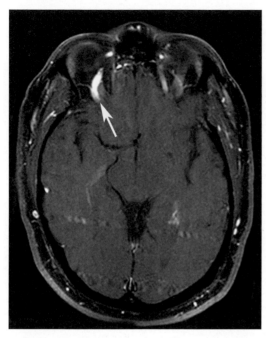

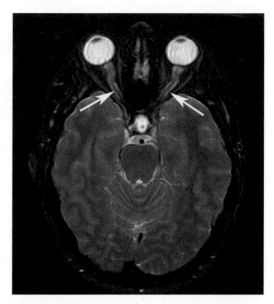

FIGURE 1-76 Enlarged superior ophthalmic vein. Axial enhanced T1-weighted image demonstrates asymmetric enlargement of the right superior ophthalmic vein (*arrow*), of no clinical consequence.

FIGURE 1-77 Optic nerve sheath fluid. Axial FSE T2-weighted fat-suppressed image through the orbits displays a tiny amount of fluid in the bilateral optic nerve sheaths (*arrows*), a normal variant.

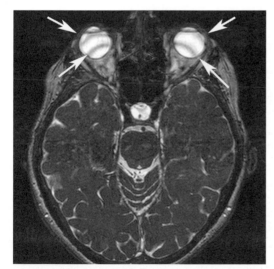

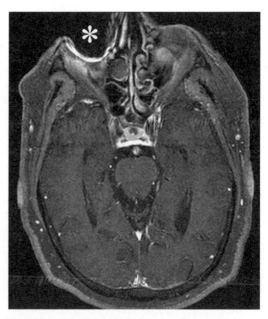

FIGURE 1-78 Banding artifact through the orbits. Axial FSE T2-weighted fat-suppressed image demonstrates several curvilinear artifacts through the orbits (*arrows*). In this steady state free precession sequence, in which multiple radio frequency (RF) pulses are used to create a steady state of the magnetization, the banding artifact is a representation of constructive/destructive interference between the signals from these RF pulses, caused by off-resonance effects of the main magnetic field due to metallic particles in eye makeup.

FIGURE 1-79 Artifact through the orbits and frontal scalp. Axial T1-weighted enhanced image demonstrates focal, marked field inhomogeneity which obscures the right orbit (*asterisk*) and adjacent scalp, due to small metallic foreign body.

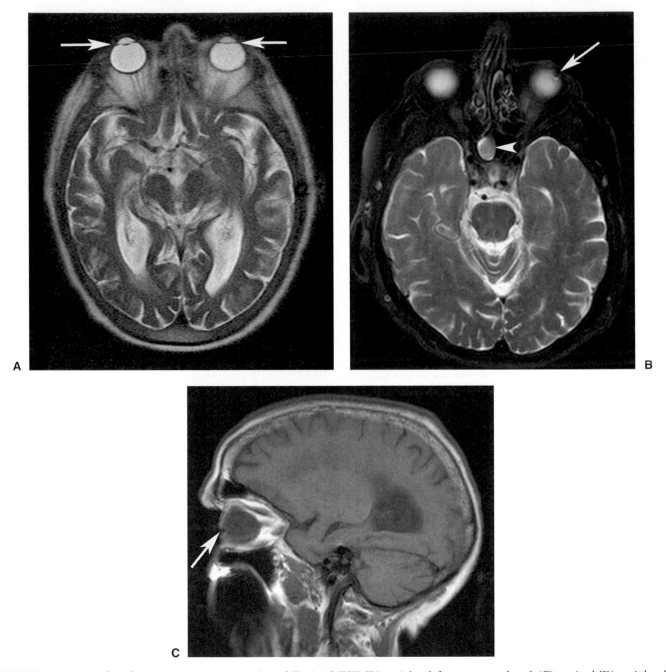

FIGURE 1-80 Artifact from cataract surgery. A and **B:** Axial FSE T2-weighted fat-suppressed and **(C)** sagittal T1-weighted images in different patients demonstrate focal susceptibility artifact (*arrows*) from prior cataract surgery (*Sphenoid sinus opacification = arrowhead*).

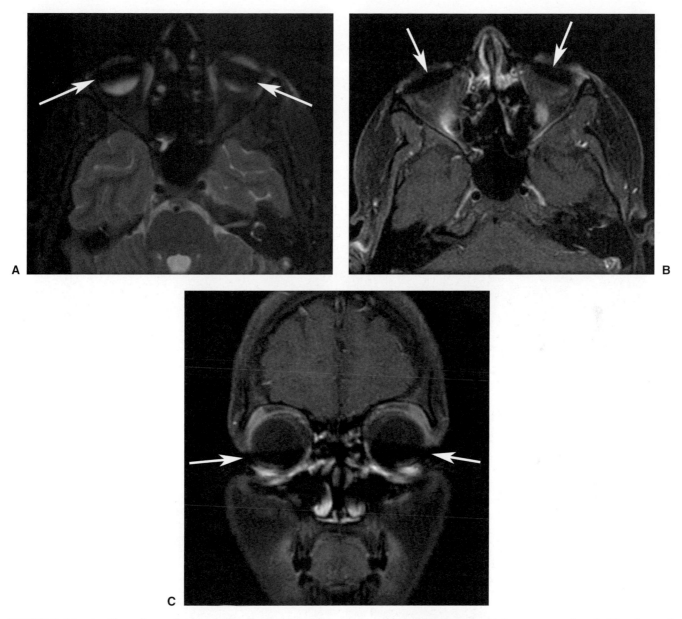

FIGURE 1-81 Artifact through the orbits from eye makeup. A: Axial FSE T2-weighted-fat suppressed and **(B)** enhanced T1-weighted images demonstrate focal shading artifact (*arrows*) through the orbits, which prove to be in the line of the eyelids on **(C)** coronal enhanced T1-weighted image. Artifact was due to metallic property of the patient's eye makeup.

■ Calvarium

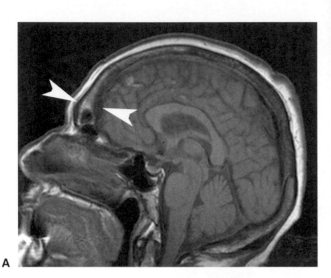
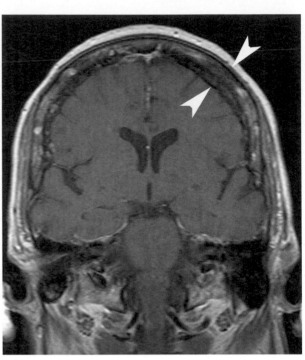

FIGURE 1-82   Thickened calvarium. A: Sagittal T1-weighted and **(B)** coronal enhanced T1-weighted images through the midline demonstrate a diffusely thickened calvarium, most marked involving the frontal bones (*arrowheads*).

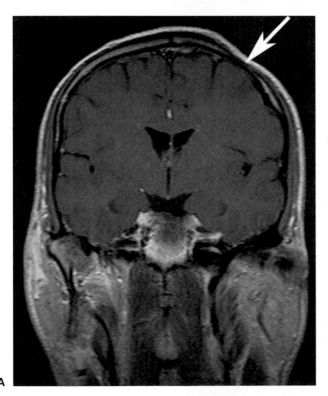
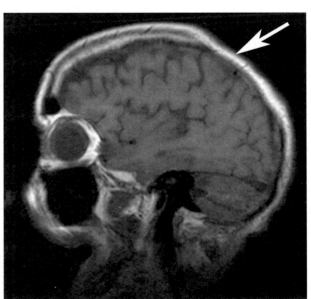

FIGURE 1-83   Thinned calvarium. A: Coronal and **(B)** sagittal images of different patients demonstrate asymmetric foci of calvarial thinning (*arrows*), which are normal variants and of no clinical significance.

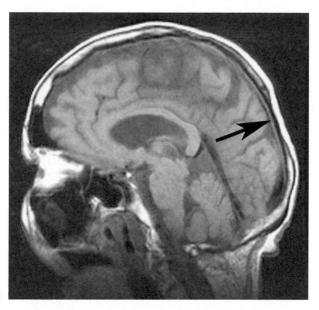

C

FIGURE 1-83 **Thinned calvarium.** (*continued*) **C:** Sagittal images of different patients demonstrate asymmetric foci of calvarial thinning (*arrows*), which are normal variants and of no clinical significance.

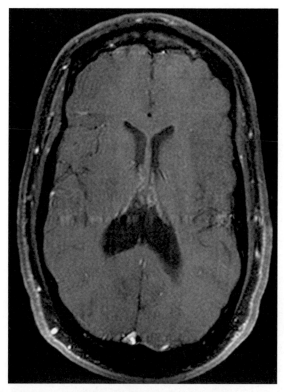

FIGURE 1-84 **Scaphocephaly.** Axial T1-weighted enhanced image through the mid-calvarium demonstrates increased anterior to posterior diameter of the skull, due to premature fusion of the sagittal suture. Compare with Figure 1-85.

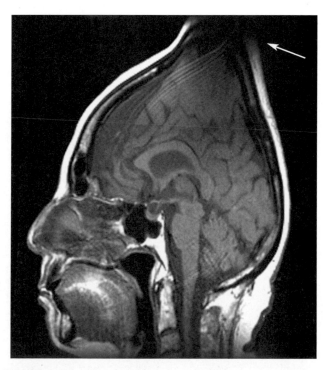

FIGURE 1-85 **Metal artifact from bobby pin.** Spin dephasing and distortion (*arrow*) is observed due to differences in magnetic susceptibility of a metal hairpin compared to that of tissue and air.

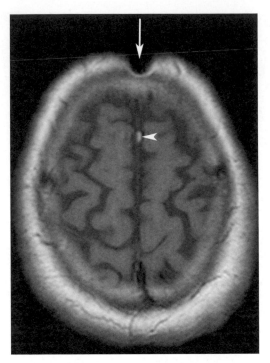

FIGURE 1-86 **Distortion.** The arrow points to an area of signal dephasing and distortion from an unknown source. This should not be confused with a true variation in calvarial contour (*Falcine lipoma = arrowhead*).

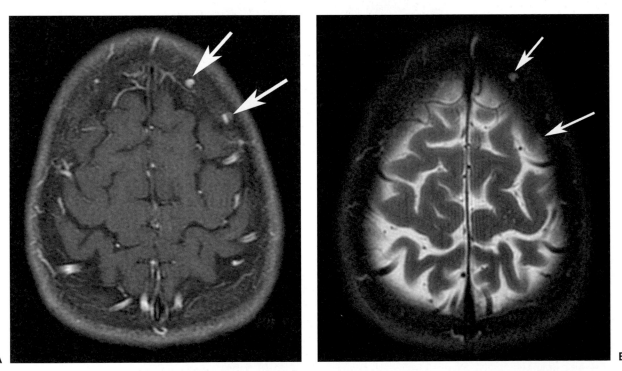

FIGURE 1-87 **Venous lake versus granulation tissue less frontal calvarium. A:** Axial enhanced T1-weighted and **(B)** FSE T2-weighted fat- suppressed images through the superior aspect of the head display two small enhancing foci in the left frontal calvarium (*arrows*), consistent with either venous lakes or granulation tissue.

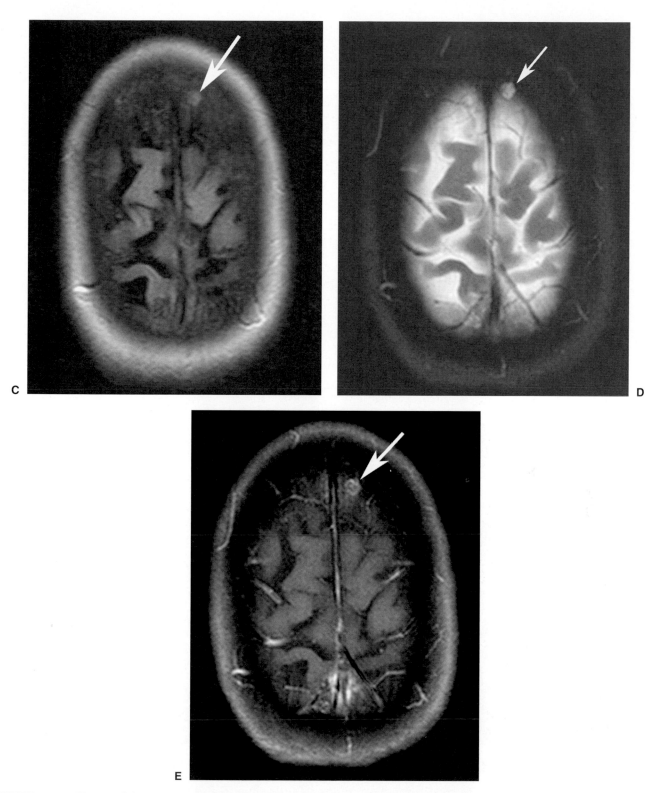

FIGURE 1-87 **Venous lake versus granulation tissue left frontal calvarium.** (*continued*) **C:** Axial fluid attenuation inversion recovery (FLAIR), (**D**) FSE T2-weighted fat-suppressed, and (**E**) enhanced T1-weighted images in a different patient demonstrate a similar enhancing focus in the left frontal calvarium.

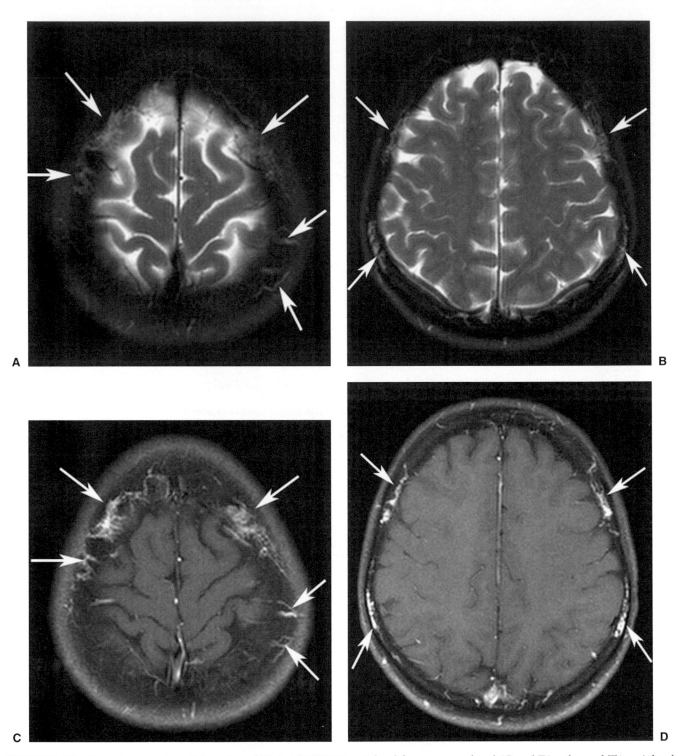

FIGURE 1-88 **Prominent venous lakes. A** and **B**: Axial FSE T2-weighted fat-suppressed and (**C** and **D**) enhanced T1-weighted images demonstrate symmetrically prominent venous lakes throughout the calvarium (*arrows*).

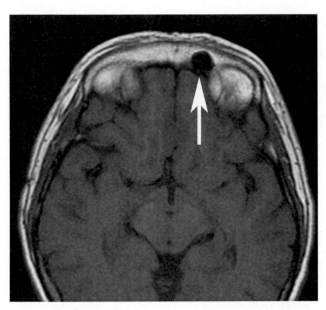

FIGURE 1-89 Asymmetric frontal sinuses. Axial fluid attenuation inversion recovery (FLAIR) image through the frontal sinuses demonstrates a left frontal sinus (*arrow*) that is larger and extends more superiorly than the right sinus.

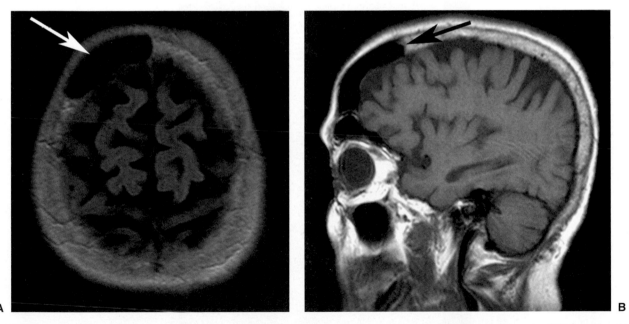

FIGURE 1-90 Enlarged frontal sinus. A: Axial fluid attenuation inversion recovery (FLAIR) and **(B)** sagittal T1-weighted images demonstrate marked enlargement of the right frontal sinus (*arrows*), which is a normal variant.

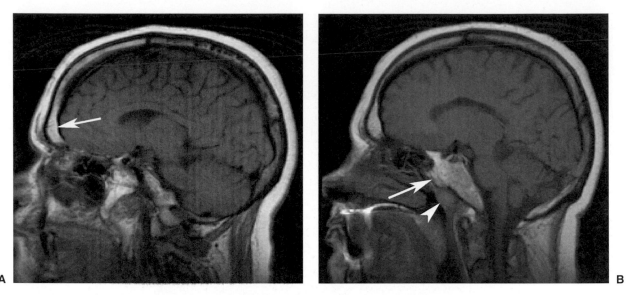

FIGURE 1-91   Nonpneumatized frontal and sphenoid sinuses. A: Sagittal T1-weighted image shows absence of the frontal sinus (*arrow*). **B:** Sagittal image in the same patient also shows lack of pneumatization of the sphenoid sinuses (*arrow*), with continuous marrow signal intensity. Note the incidental Tornwalt duct cyst (*arrowhead*).

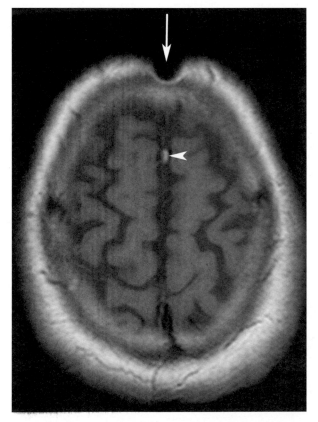

FIGURE 1-92   Artifact in the frontal scalp. Distortion (*arrow*) from a small metallic body in the frontal scalp obscures the adjacent scalp and outer diploe of the frontal calvarium. Note the incidental small falcine lipoma (*arrowhead*).

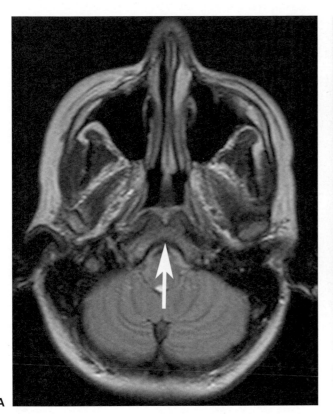

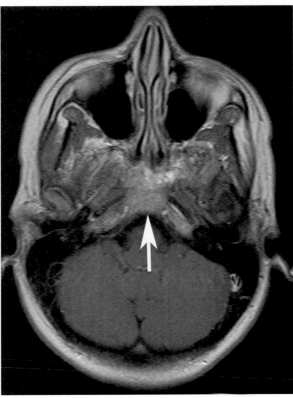

A **B**

FIGURE 1-93 **Heterogeneous clivus. A:** Axial fluid attenuation inversion recovery (FLAIR) image shows normal heterogeneity of the clivus (*arrow*), with diffuse enhancement on **(B)** enhanced T1-weighted image.

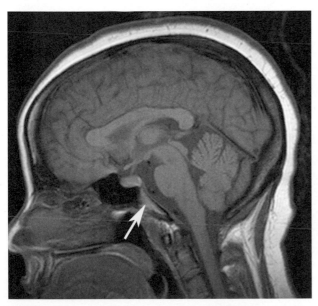

FIGURE 1-94 **Hypointense clivus on T1-weighted images.** Sagittal T1-weighted image through the midline shows a normal variant hypointense clivus (*arrow*).

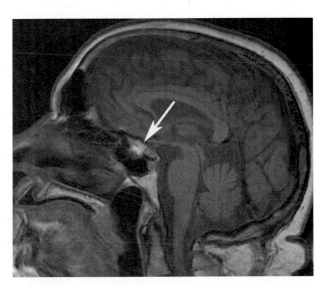

FIGURE 1-95 **Anterior sella turcica is less discernible on T1-weighted images.** Sagittal T1-weighted image demonstrates decreased conspicuity of the anterior sella turcica (*arrow*), relative to the posterior portion, which is a normal variant.

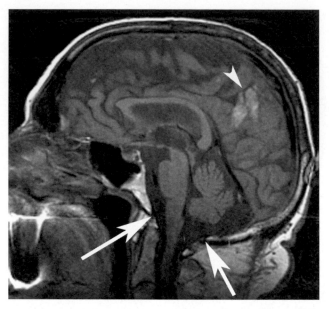

FIGURE 1-96 Large foramen magnum. Sagittal T1-weighted image (of the same patient in Fig. 1-13) shows a large foramen magnum (*arrows*), a normal variant. Incidental note is made of the lipoma along the falx (*arrowhead*).

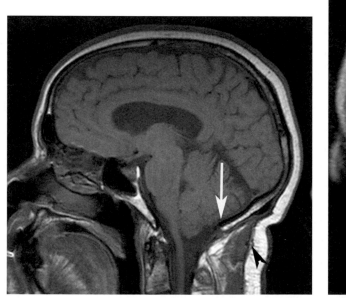

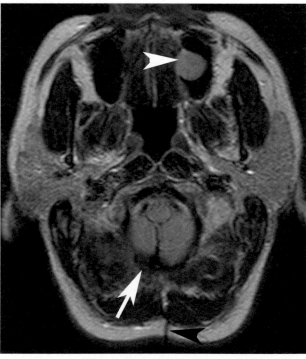

FIGURE 1-97 Occipital decompression. A: Sagittal T1-weighted and **(B)** axial fluid attenuation inversion recovery (FLAIR) images demonstrate the postsurgical appearance of occipital decompression, with abrupt transition of the resected posterior border of the foramen magnum (*arrows*). Note the susceptibility artifact (*black arrowheads*) in the posterior nuchal soft tissues from prior surgery and the low-lying cerebellar tonsils. Incidentally, there is a left maxillary sinus mucus retention cyst (*white arrowhead*).

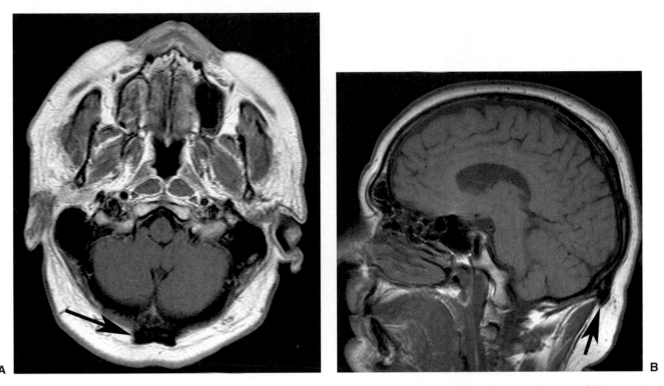

FIGURE 1-98 **Occipital protuberance.** **A:** Axial fluid attenuation inversion recovery (FLAIR) and **(B)** sagittal T1-weighted images through the midline show a focal signal voids (*arrow*) contiguous with the occipital calvarium, consistent with normal variant occipital protuberance. This finding is also commonly present in canines.

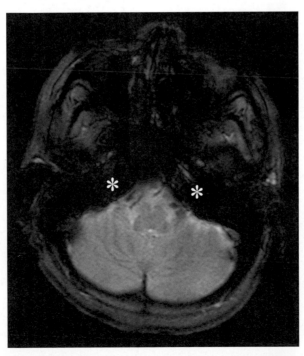

FIGURE 1-99 **Pneumatization of petrous apices.** Axial gradient echo image demonstrates extensive blooming artifact throughout the aerated petrous apices (*asterisk*) and paranasal sinuses.

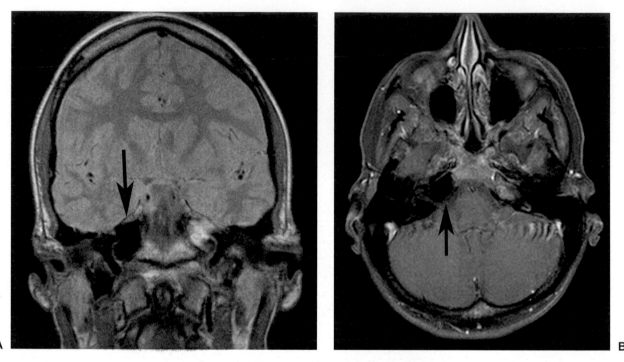

FIGURE 1-100 Asymmetric petrous apex pneumatization. A: Coronal T1-weighted and **(B)** axial FSE T2-weighted fat-suppressed images demonstrate asymmetric pneumatization of the right petrous apex (*arrows*).

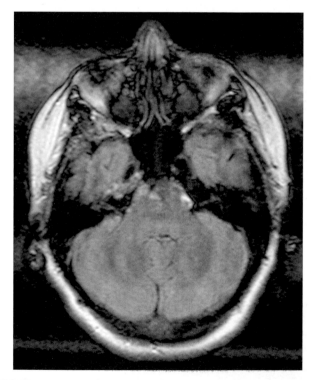

FIGURE 1-101 Ghosting. Ghosting/smearing most likely due to system related instabilities.

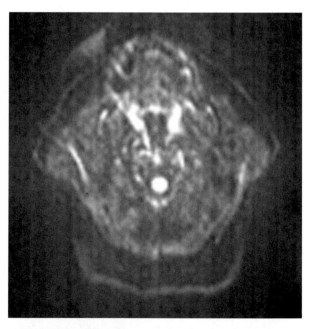

FIGURE 1-102 Receive path error. The vertical streaking in this image is consistent with an error in the receive path of the signal, for example, poor coil connection or receiver error. The global inhomogeneity is a consequence of the normalization process.

■ Face

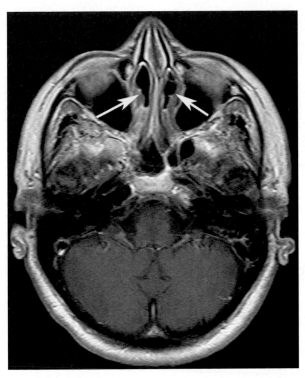

FIGURE 1-103   Concha bullosa. Axial enhanced T1-weighted image delineates bilateral concha bullosa (*arrows*), which are air cells that enlarge the middle turbinates. Although these are normal anatomic variants, they can lead to sinus obstruction if they become large enough, and require surgical decompression.

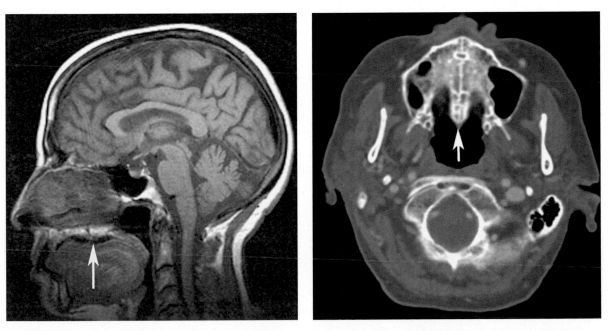

A   B

FIGURE 1-104   Torus palatine. A: Sagittal T1-weighted image through the midline demonstrates a prominent hypointense ridge (*arrow*) along the hard palate, consistent with a torus palatine. **B:** CT scan shows the axial appearance of a torus palatine (*arrow*).

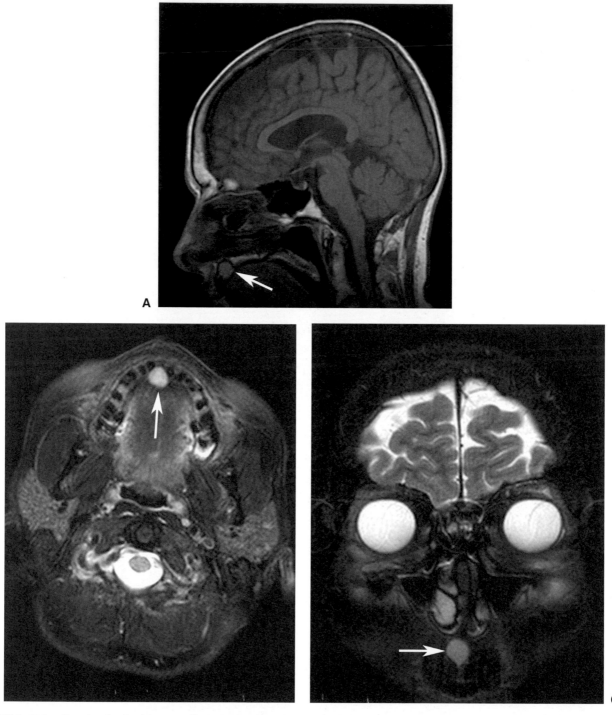

FIGURE 1-105 **Cyst in the incisive canal. A:** Sagittal T1-weighted, **(B)** axial T2-weighted, and **(C)** coronal FSE T2-weighted fat-suppressed image through the level of the temporal lobes demonstrates a small cyst (*arrow*) in the left incisive canal.

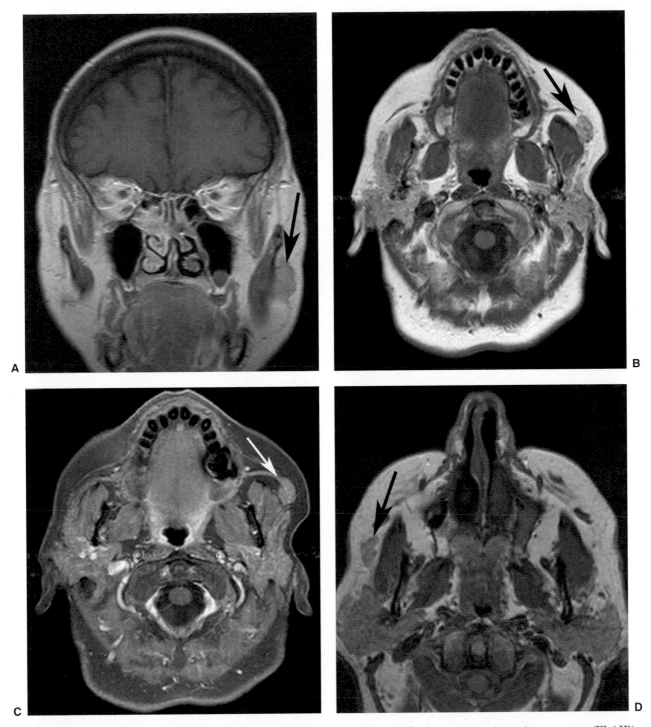

FIGURE 1-106 Accessory parotid tissue. A: Coronal T1-weighted, **(B)** axial fluid attenuation inversion recovery (FLAIR), and **(C)** enhanced T1-weighted images through the face demonstrate a soft tissue nodule (*arrows*) superficial to the left masseter muscle that is isointense to parotid tissue. Finding is consistent with accessory parotid tissue. **D:** Axial FLAIR T1-weighted images in different patients demonstrate the variable appearance and number of accessory parotid tissue foci (*arrows*).

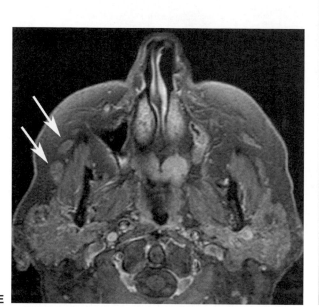

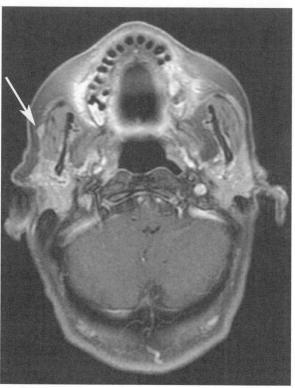

FIGURE 1-106 **Accessory parotid tissue.** (*continued*) **E** and **F:** Axial enhanced T1-weighted images in different patients demonstrate the variable appearance and number of accessory parotid tissue foci (*arrows*).

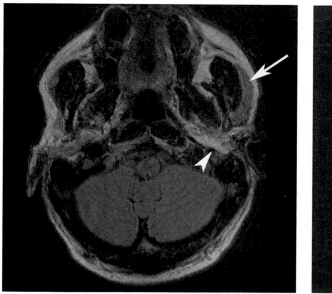

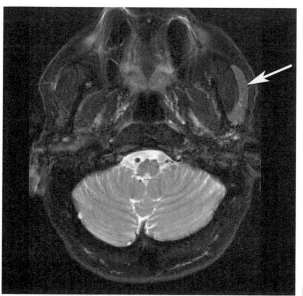

FIGURE 1-107 **Hypertrophied parotid tissue after left parotidectomy. A:** Axial fluid attenuation inversion recovery (FLAIR), **(B)** FSE T2-weighted fat-suppressed images delineate the postsurgical change, status after left parotidectomy (*arrowhead*). Notice the elliptical soft tissue (*arrows*) extending superficial to the left masseter muscle that is isointense to the contralateral parotid gland on all sequences, consistent with hypertrophied parotid tissue.

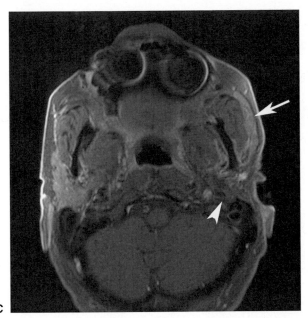

FIGURE 1-107 Hypertrophied parotid tissue after left parotidectomy. (*continued*) **C:** Enhanced images delineate the postsurgical change, status after left parotidectomy (*arrowhead*). Notice the elliptical soft tissue (*arrow*) extending superficial to the left masseter muscle that is isointense to the contralateral parotid gland on all sequences, consistent with hypertrophied parotid tissue.

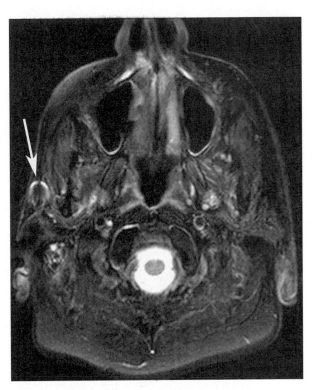

FIGURE 1-108 Artifact from parotid surgery. Axial FSE T2-weighted fat-suppressed image demonstrates a focus of susceptibility artifact (*arrow*) through the right parotid gland from prior surgery.

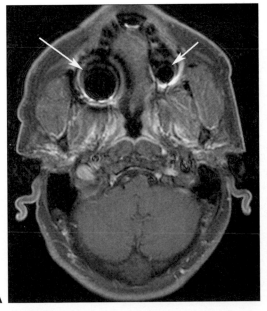

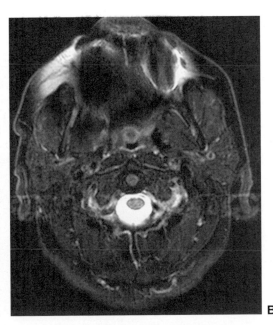

FIGURE 1-109 Artifact from dental hardware. Ferromagnetic artifact from dental hardware (*arrows*) on **(A)** axial T1-weighted enhanced and **(B)** FSE T2-weighted fat-suppressed images.

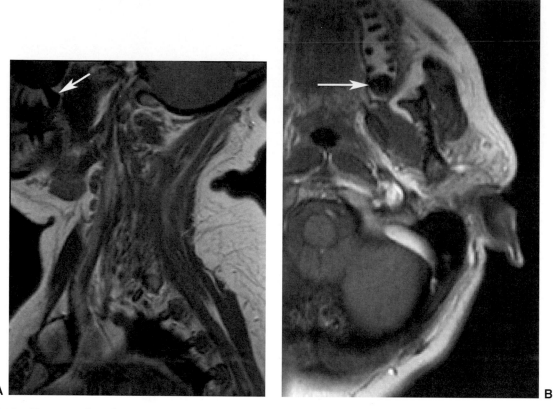

FIGURE 1-110 **Unerupted molar. A:** Coronal and **(B)** axial T1-weighted images demonstrate an angulated, unerupted molar (*arrow*).

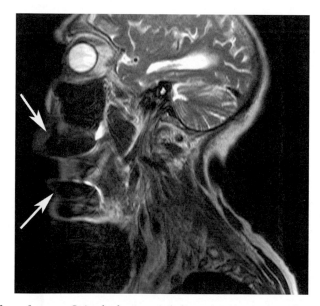

FIGURE 1-111 **Metal artifact from braces.** Spin dephasing and distortion (*arrows*) is observed due to differences in magnetic susceptibility of metal dental braces compared to that of tissue and air.

Suggested Readings

Adem C, Lafitte F, Jarquin S, et al. The persistence of a spheno-occipital synchondrosis in an adult. *J Radiol*. 1999;80:863–865.

Ahmadi H, Larsson EM, Jinkins JR. Normal pituitary gland: Coronal MRI of infundibular tilt. *Radiology*. 1990;177:389–192.

Ahmetoglu A, Kul S, Kuzeyli K, et al. Intracranial and subcutaneous lipoma associated with sagittal sinus fenestration and falcine sinus. *AJNR Am J Neuroradiol*. 2007;28:1034–1035.

Akita K, Shimokawa T, Sato T. Aberrant muscle between the temporalis and the lateral pterygoid muscles: M. pterygoideus proprius (Henle). *Clin Anat*. 2001;14:288–291.

Amonoo-Kuofi H, Darwish HH. Accessory levator muscle of the upper eyelid: Case report and review of the literature. *Clin Anat*. 1998;11:410–416.

Anik H, Anil Y, Koc K, et al. Agenesis of sphenoid sinuses. *Clin Anat*. 2006;18:217–219.

Ballasteros MC, Hansen PE, Soila K, et al. MRI of the developing human brain, part 2. *Neonatal Dev Radiographics*. 1993;13:611–622.

Barkovich AJ. MRI of the neonatal brain. *Neuroimaging Clin N Am*. 2006;16(1):17–35.

Bartha AI, Yap KRL, Miller SP, et al. The normal neonatal brain: MRI, diffusion tensor imaging, and 3D MR spectroscopy in healthy term neonates. *AJNR Am J Neuroradiol*. 2007;28:1015–1021.

Bayramoglu A, Aydingoz U, Hayran M, et al. Comparison of qualitative and quantitative analyses of age-related changes in clivus bone marrow on MRI. *Clin Anat*. 2003;16:304–308.

Becker DB, Cheverud JM, Govier DP, et al. Os parietale divisum. *Clin Anat*. 2005;18:452–456.

Benshoff ER, Katz BH. Ectopia of the posterior pituitary gland as a normal variant: Assessment with MRI. *AJNR Am J Neuroradiol*. 1990;11:709–712.

Berge JK, Bergman RA. Variations in size and in symmetry of foramina of the human skull. *Clin Anat*. 2001;14:406–413.

Bonneville F, Cattin F, Marsot-Dupuch K, et al. T1 signal hyperintensity in the sella region: Spectrum of findings. *Radiographics*. 2006; 26:93–113.

Bowsher D. Trigeminal neuralgia: An anatomically oriented review. *Clin Anat*. 1997;10:409–415.

Brant-Zawadzki M, Kelly W, Kjos B, et al. MRI and characterization of normal and abnormal intracranial cerebrospinal fluid (CSF) spaces. *Neuroradiology*. 1085;27:3–8.

Cagirankaya LB, Kansu O, Hatipoglu MG. Is torus palatinus a feature of a well-developed maxilla. *Clin Anat*. 2004;17:623–625.

Caldas JGMP, Iffenecker C, Attal P, et al. Anomalous vessel in the middle ear: The role of CT and MR angiography. *Neuroradiology*. 1998;40:748–751.

Cankal F, Ugur HC, Tekdemir I, et al. Fossa navicularis: Anatomic variation at the skull base. *Clin Anat*. 2004;17:118–122.

Casoli V, Dauphin N, Taki C, et al. Anatomy and blood supply of the subgaleal fascia flap. *Clin Anat*. 2004;17:392–399.

Caulo M, Briganti C, Mattei PA, et al. New morphologic variants of the hand motor cortex as seen with MRI in a large study population. *AJNR Am J Neuroradiol*. 2007;28:1480–1485.

Chakeres DW, Whitaker CDS, Dashner RA, et al. High-resolution 8 tesla imaging of the formalin-fixed normal human hippocampus. *Clin Anat*. 2005;18:88–91.

Collignon F, Link M. Paraclinoid and cavernous sinus regions: Measurement of critical structures relevant for surgical procedure. *Clin Anat*. 2005;18:3–9.

Counsell SJ, Maalouf EF, Fletcher AM, et al. MRI assessment of myelination in the very preterm brain. *AJNR Am J Neuroradiol*. 2002;23(5): 872–881.

Cure JJK, Van Tassel P, Smith MT. Normal and variant anatomy of the dural venous sinuses. *Semin Ultrasound CT MR*. 1994;15:499–519.

Currarino G, Votteler TP. Lesions of the accessory parotid gland in children. *Pediatr Radiol*. 2006;36:1–7.

Das CJ, Seith A, Gamanagatti S, et al. On the AJR viewbox. Ectopic pituitary adenoma with an empty sella. *AJR Am J Roentgenol*. 2006;186(5):1468–1469.

Dashner RA, Clark DL, Kangarlu A, et al. Epoxy-resin injection of the cerebral arterial microvasculature: An evaluation of the limits of spatial resolution in 8 tesla MRI. *Clin Anat*. 2005;18:164–170.

Davagnanam I, Chavda SV. Identification of the normal jugular foramen and lower cranial nerve anatomy: Contrast-enhanced 3D fast imaging employing steady-state acquisition MRI. *AJNR Am J Neuroradiol*. 2007, Published online Dec 7.

Doig TN, McDonald SW, McGregor IA. Possible routes of spread of carcinoma of the maxillary sinus to the oral cavity. *Clin Anat*. 1998;11:149–156.

Elazab EEB, Abdel-Hameed FAM. The arterial supply of the temporalis muscle. *Surg Radiol Anat*. 2006;28:241–247.

Fan YF, Chong VF, Tan KP. Subarachnoid spaces in infants and young children. *Ann Acad Med Singapore*. 1993;22:732–735.

Filipovic B, Teofilovski-Parapid G. Linear parameters of normal and abnormal cava septi pellucidi: A post-mortem study. *Clin Anat*. 2004;17:626–630.

Gardner R, Hogan RE. Three-dimensional deformation-based hippocampal surface anatomy, projected on MR images. *Clin Anat*. 2005;18:481–487.

Golzarian J, Baleriaux D, Bank WO, et al. Pineal cyst: Normal or pathological? *Neuroradiology*. 1993;35:251–253.

Goodmurphy CW, Ovalle WK. Morphological study of two human facial muscles: Orbicularis oculi and corrugator supercilii. *Clin Anat*. 1999;12:1–11.

Greyling LM, Grange LE, Meiring JH. Mandibular spine: A case report. *Clin Anat*. 1997;10:416–418.

Gulekon N, Anil A, Poyraz A, et al. Variations in the anatomy of the auriculotemporal nerve. *Clin Anat*. 2005;18:15–22.

Hamamoto M, Murakami G, Kataura A. Topographical relationships among the facial nerve, chorda tympani nerve and round window with special reference to the approach route for cochlear important surgery. *Clin Anat*. 2000;13:251–256.

Hamilton BE, Salzman KL, Osborn AG. Anatomic and pathologic spectrum of pituitary infundibulum lesions. *AJR Am J Roentgenol*. 2007;188:W223–W232.

Harn SD, Durham TM. Anatomical variations and clinical implications of the artery to lingual nerve. *Clin Anat*. 2003;16:294–299.

Honda K, Kawashima S, Kashima M, et al. Relationship between sex, age, and the minimum thickness of the roof of the glenoid fossa in normal temporomandibular joints. *Clin Anat*. 2005;18:23–26.

Isobe M, Murakami G, Katakaura A. Variations of the uncinate process of the lateral nasal wall with clinical implications. *Clin Anat*. 1998;11:295–303.

Jacob CE, Rupa V. Infralabyrinthine approach to the petrous apex. *Clin Anat*. 2005;18:423–427.

Jelacic S, de Regt D, Weinberger E. Interactive digital MR atlas of the pediatric brain. *Radiographics*. 2006;26(2):497–501.

Jergenson MA, Norton NS, Opack JM, et al. Unique origin of the inferior. alveolar artery. *Clin Anat*. 2005;18:597–601.

Kahilogullari G, Ugur HC. Accessory middle cerebral artery originating from callosomarginal artery. *Clin Anat*. 2006;19:694–695.

Kahn JL, Wolfram-Gabel R, Bourjat P. Anatomy and imaging of the deep fat of the face. *Clin Anat*. 2000;13:373–382.

Kakizaki H, Zako M, Nakano T, et al. An anomalous muscle linking superior and inferior rectus muscles in the orbit. *Anat Sci Int*. 2006; 81:197–199.

Kieser JA, Herbison GP. Anatomical knowledge and clinical evaluation of the muscles of mastication. *Clin Anat*. 2000;13:94–96.

Lane JI, Witte RJ, Hensson OW, et al. Imaging microscopy of the middle and inner ear: Part II: MR microscopy. *Clin Anat*. 2005;18:409–415.

Levine D, Cavazos C, Kazan-Tannus JF, et al. Evaluation of real-time single-shot fast spin-echo MRI for visualization of the fetal midline corpus callosum and secondary plate. *AJR Am J Roentgenol*. 2006;187:1505–1511.

Lee HY, Kim C-H, Kim JY, et al. Surgical anatomy of the middle turbinate. *Clin Anat*. 2006;19:493–496.

Lidov MW, Silvers AR, Mosesson RE, et al. Pantopaque simulating thrombosed intracranial aneurysms on MRI. *J Comput Assist Tomogr*. 1996;20(2):225–227.

Lisanti C, Carlin C, Banks KP, et al. Normal MRI appearance and motion-related phenomena of CSF. *AJR Am J Roentgenol*. 2007;188:716–725.

Loukas M, Curry B. Bilateral lateral bipartite levator palpebrae superioris muscles. *Clin Anat*. 2006;19:695–699.

Loukas M, Kapos T, Louis RG Jr, et al. Gross anatomical, CT and MRI analyses of the buccal fat pad with special emphasis on volumetric variations. *Surg Radiol Anat*. 2006;28:254–260.

Loukas M, Louis RG, Childs RS. Anatomical examination of the recurrent artery of Heubner. *Clin Anat*. 2006;19:25–31.

Lukic IK, Gluncic V, Marusic A. Extracranial branches of the middle meningeal artier. *Clin Anat*. 2001;14:292–294.

Madhavi C, Holla SJ. Triplication of the lesser occipital nerve. *Clin Anat*. 2004;17:667–671.

McCardle C, Richardson CJ, Nicholas DA, et al. Developmental features of neonatal brain imaging. Part I. *Radiology*. 1997;162(1):223.

von Ludinghausen M. Bilateral supernumerary rectus muscles of the orbit. *Clin Anat*. 1998;11:271–277.

von Ludinghausen M, Kagayama I, Miura M, et al. Morphological peculiarities of the deep infratemporal fossa in advanced age. *Surg Radiol Anat*. 2006;28:284–292.

Nael K, Ruehm SG, Michaely HJ, et al. Multistation whole-body high-spatial resolution MR angiography using a 32-channel MR system. *AJR Am J Roentgenol*. 2007;188:529–539.

Nael K, Villablanca JP, Pope WB, et al. Supraaortic arteries: Contrast enhanced MR angiography at 2.0 T—highly accelerated parallel acquisition for improved spatial resolution over an extended field of view. *Radiology*. 2007;242:600–609.

Nambiar P, Naidu MDK, Subramaniam K. Anatomical variability of the frontal sinuses and their application in forensic identification. *Clin Anat*. 1999;12:16–19.

NINDS, NIMH, NICHD. *Pediatric Anatomic Neuroimaging Database Initiative*. http://grants.nih.gov/grants/guide/notice-files/not98-072.html, 1998.

Nemeth AJ, Henson JW, Mullins ME, et al. Improved detection of skull metastasis with diffusion-weighted MRI. *AJNR Am J Neuroradiol*. 2007;28:1088–1092.

Peuker ET, Fischer G, Filler TJ. Entrapment of the lingual nerve due to an ossified pterygospinous ligament. *Clin Anat*. 2001;14:282–284.

Penhall B, Townsend G, Tomo S, et al. The pterygoideus proprius muscle revisited. *Clin Anat*. 1998;11:332–337.

Pessa JE, Zadoo VP, Garza PA, et al. Double or bifid zygomaticus major muscle: Anatomy, incidence, and clinical correlation. *Clin Anat*. 1998;11:310–313.

Pinar YA, Bilge O, Govsa F. Anatomic study of the blood supply of perioral region. *Clin Anat*. 2005;18:330–339.

Rao PVVP. Median (third) occipital condyle. *Clin Anat*. 2002;15:148–151.

Ray B, Singh LK, Das CJ, et al. Ectopic supernumerary tooth on the inferior nasal concha. *Clin Anat*. 2006;19:68–74.

Richards AT, Digges N, Norton NS, et al. Surgical anatomy of the parotid duct with emphasis on the major tributaries forming the duct and the relationship of the facial nerve to the duct. *Clin Anat*. 2004;17:463–467.

Sage MR, Blumbergs PC. Primary empty sella turcica: A radiological-anatomical correlation. *Australas Radiol*. 2000;44:341–348.

Sanchis-Gimeno JA, Herrera M, Sanchez-del-Campo F, et al. Differences in ocular dimensions between normal and dry eyes. *Surg Radiol Anat*. 2006;28:267–270.

Stefani MA, Schneider FL, Marrone ACH, et al. Anatomic variations of anterior cerebral artery cortical branches. *Clin Anat*. 2000;13:231–236.

Small S, Fukui MB, Reinmuth OM. What is a 'normal anatomic variant'? Transient left lateral medullary ischemia in a patient with a fenestrated left vertebral artery. *Neurology*. 1994;44:1358–1359.

Smoker WR. Craniovertebral junction: Normal anatomy, craniometry, and congenital anomalies. *Radiographics*. 1994;14(2):255–277.

Solomon LW, Pantera EA, Monaco E, et al. A diagnostic challenge: Anterior variant of mandibular lingual bone depression. *Gen Dent*. 2006;54:336–340.

Stacey RJ, Miles JB. Magnetic resonance tomographic angiography of the arterial circle (of Willis). *Clin Anat*. 1998;11:338–341.

Steen RG, Hamer RM, Lieberman JA. Measuring brain volume by MRI: Impact of measurement precision and natural variation on sample size requirements. *AJNR Am J Neuroradiol*. 2007;28:1119–1125.

Stuckey SL, Goh TD, Heffernan T, et al. Hyperintensity in the subarachnoid space on FLAIR MRI. *AJR Am J Roentgenol*. 2007;189(4):913–921.

Suganthy J, Raghuram L, Antonisamy B, et al. Gender- and age-related differences in the morphology of the corpus callosum. *Clin Anat*. 2003;16:396–403.

Sumi M, Van Cauteren M, Takagi Y, et al. Balanced turbo field-echo sequence for MRI of parotid gland disease. *AJR Am J Roentgenol*. 2007;188:228–232.

Taccone A, Oddone M, Occhi M, et al. MRI "road-map" of normal age-related bone marrow. I. Cranial bone and spine. *Pediatr Radiol*. 1995;25(8):588–595.

Taitz C. Bony observations of some morphological variations and anomalies of the craniovertebral region. *Clin Anat*. 2000;13:354–360.

Tarroun A, Bonnefoy M, Bouffard-Vercelli J, et al. Could linear MRI measurements of hippocampus differentiate normal brain aging in elderly persons from Alzheimer's disease? *Surg Radiol Anat*. 2007;29:77–81.

Tubbs RS, Salter EG, Oakes WJ. Duplication of the occipital condyles. *Clin Anat*. 2005;18:92–95.

Tubbs RS, Tyler-Kabara EC, Salter EG, et al. Unusual finding of the craniocervical junction. *Clin Anat*. 2005;18:449–451.

Tubbs RS, Kelly DR, Lott R, et al. Complete ossification of the human falx cerebri. *Clin Anat*. 2006;19:147–150.

Tubbs RS, Loukas M. Duplication of the superior sagittal sinus. *Clin Anat*. 2006;19:728.

Tubbs RS, Salter EG, Oakes WJ. Bony anomaly of Meckel's cave. *Clin Anat*. 2006;19:75–77.

Tuccar E, Tekdemir I, Aslan A, et al. Radiological anatomy of the intratemporal course of facial nerve. *Clin Anat*. 2000;13:83–87.

Ullah M, Khan T. Anomalous muscle adjacent to temporalis. *Clin Anat*. 2006;19:648–650.

Ustun C. Galen and his anatomic eponym: Vein of Galen. *Clin Anat*. 2004;17:454–457.

Ward SC, Ahuja A, Ma HT. Case report: Asymmetrical development of the gyri recti presenting as a suprasellar mass: Case report and description of six further cases. *Br J Radiol*. 1994;67:1268–1269.

Watanabe A, Nagaseki Y, Ohkubo S, et al. Anatomical variations of the ten triangles around the cavernous sinus. *Clin Anat*. 2003;16:9–14.

Wei W, Xin-Ya S, Cai-Dong L, et al. Relationship between extracellular matrix both in choroid plexus and the wall of lateral ventricles. *Clin Anat*. 2000;13:422–428.

Weir P, Suttner NJ, Flynn P, et al. Normal skull suture variant mimicking intentional injury. *Br Med J*. 2006;332:1020–1021.

Weninger WJ, Prokop M. *In vivo* 3D analysis of the adipose tissue in the orbital apex and the compartments of the parasellar region. *Clin Anat*. 2004;17:112–117.

Wiles CCR, Wrigley B, Greene JRT. Re-examination of the medullary rootlets of the accessory and vagus nerves. *Clin Anat*. 2007;20:19–22.

Wolfram-Gabel R, Kahn JL. Adipose body of the orbit. *Clin Anat*. 2002;15:186–192.

Wolpert SM. The circle of Willis. *AJNR Am J Neuroradiol*. 1997;18:1033–1034.

Yasutaka S, Kominami R, Taniguchi Y, et al. Relative positions of the arteries and veins on the dorsolateral surface of the human cerebrum. *Clin Anat*. 2002;18:112–115.

Yigit O, Cinar U, Uslu B, et al. Giant concha bullosa: A case report. *Kulak Burun Bogaz Ihtis Derg*. 2004;13:77–79.

Yilmazlar S, Rocaeli H, Aydiner F, et al. Medial portion of the cavernous sinus: Quantitative analysis of the medial wall. *Clin Anat*. 2005;18:416–422.

Chapter 2

The Neck

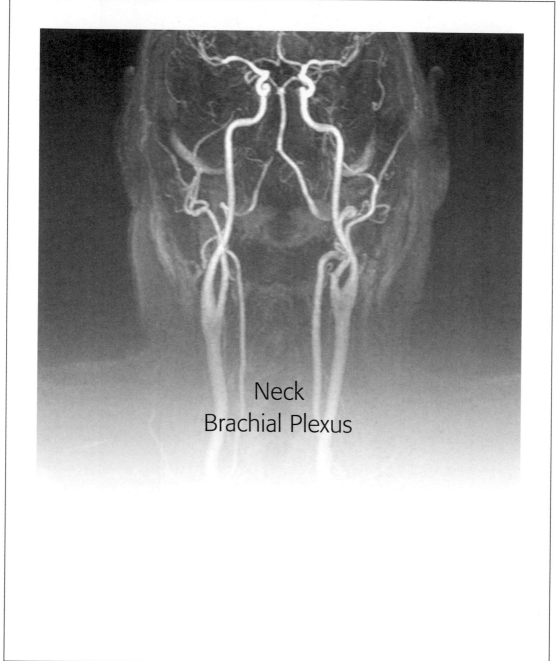

Neck

Brachial Plexus

David A. Miller, Robert A. Pooley, and Laura W. Bancroft

■ Neck

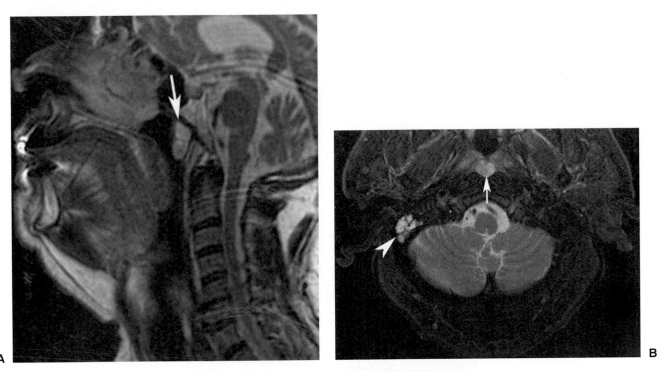

A   **B**

FIGURE 2-1   Nasopharyngeal cyst. A: Sagittal T1-weighted and **(B)** axial T2-weighted images show a hyperintense focus (*arrows*) in the posterior nasopharynx, consistent with a nasopharyngeal cyst. Note the changes from right-sided mastoiditis (*arrowhead*).

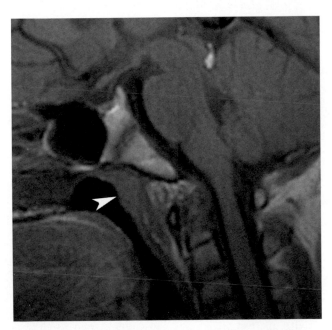

FIGURE 2-2   Adenoidal tissue in a child. Sagittal T1-weighted image shows adenoidal tissue (*arrowhead*) in this 8-year-old child, which is within normal limits for age.

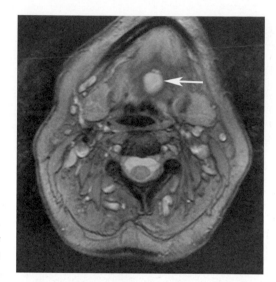

FIGURE 2-3 **Thyroglossal duct cyst.** Axial T2-weighted image shows a fluid-intensity structure (*arrow*) within the central base of the tongue, consistent with thyroglossal duct cyst.

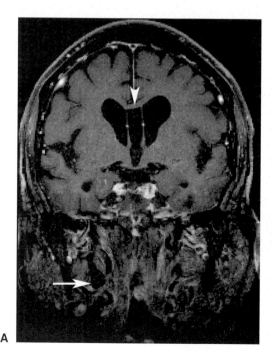

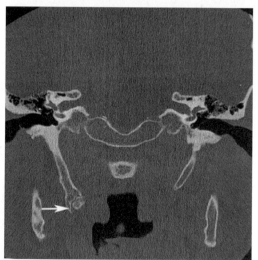

FIGURE 2-4 **Prominent styloid processes.** **A:** Coronal image shows a hypointense linear structure (*arrows*) paralleling the oropharynx (*Cavum septum pellucidum* = *arrowhead*). **B** and **C:** Coronal projection of CT images demonstrate two elongated, articulating right styloid processes (*arrows*).

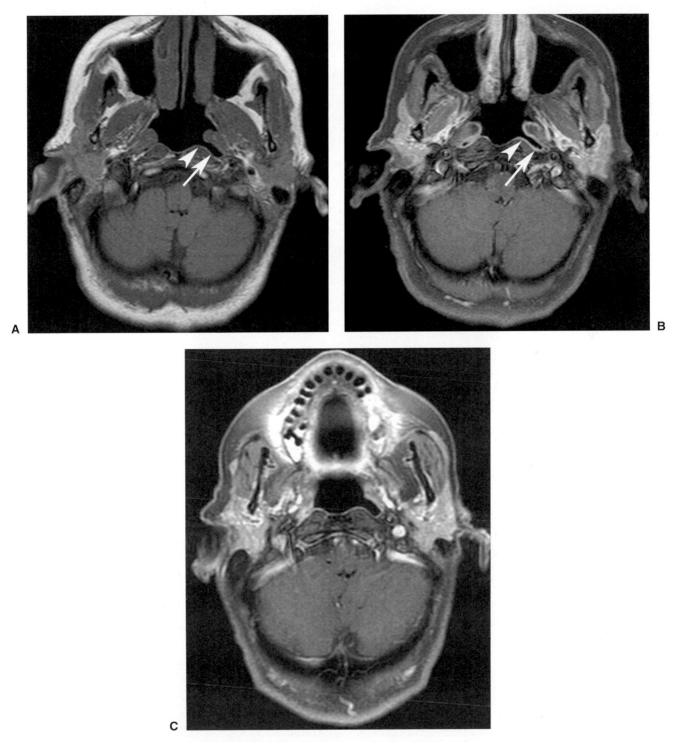

FIGURE 2-5 Asymmetric fossa of Rosenmuller and Eustachian tube orifice. Axial T1-weighted images **(A)** before and **(B)** after contrast administration show asymmetry of the fossa of Rosenmuller (*arrowhead*) and the Eustachian tube orifice (*arrow*). **C:** There was no underlying lesion and adjacent image confirmed this appearance was not due to obliquity in the axial acquisition.

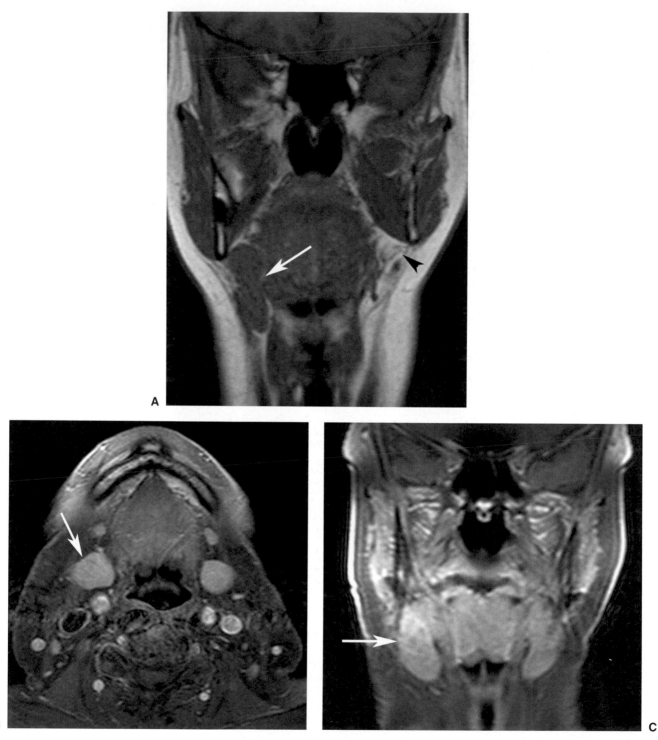

FIGURE 2-6 Asymmetric submandibular glands. A: Coronal T1-weighted enhanced image shows the right submandibular gland (*arrow*) but absence of the left gland (*arrowhead*). T1-weighted enhanced **(B)** coronal and **(C)** axial images show normal variant enlargement of the right submandibular glands (*arrows*) in two different patients.

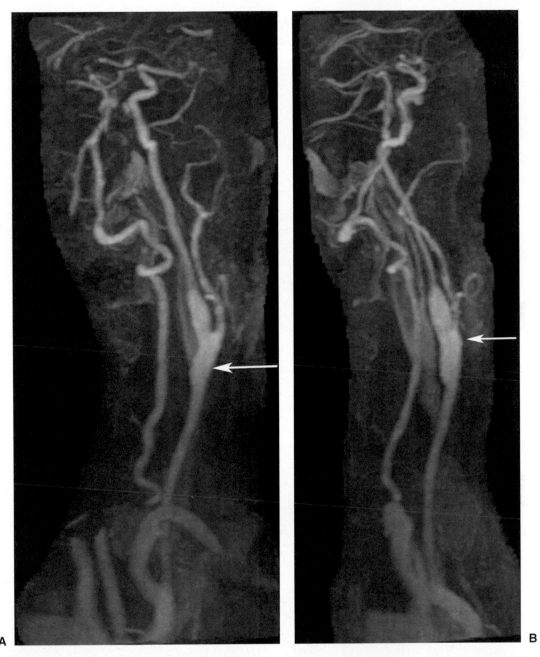

A

B

FIGURE 2-7 **Carotid endarterectomy and patch graft. (A** and **B)** Coronal oblique projections of MRAs in two patients demonstrate the expected deformity of the carotid bulb (*arrows*) after endarterectomy and patch graft.

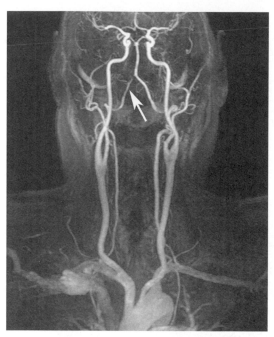

FIGURE 2-8   Narrowed right vertebral artery. Coronal MRA shows narrowing of the right vertebral artery (*arrow*).

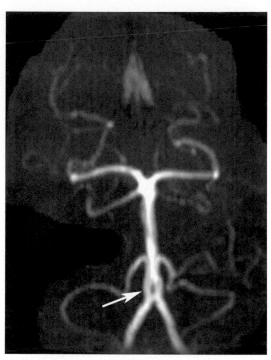

FIGURE 2-9   Fenestrated basilar artery. Coronal projection from MRA shows focal fenestration (*arrow*) of the proximal basilar artery.

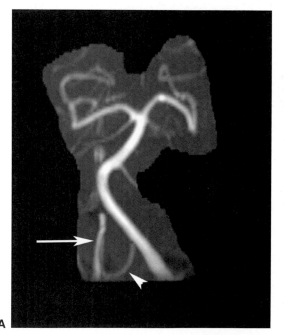

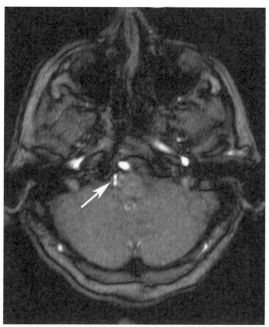

FIGURE 2-10   Nondominant right vertebral artery ends in the posterior inferior cerebellar artery. A: Posterior cranial fossa in maximum intensity projection (MIP) and **(B)** axial source images show the nondominant right vertebral artery (*arrow*) ending in the posterior inferior cerebellar artery (*arrowhead*).

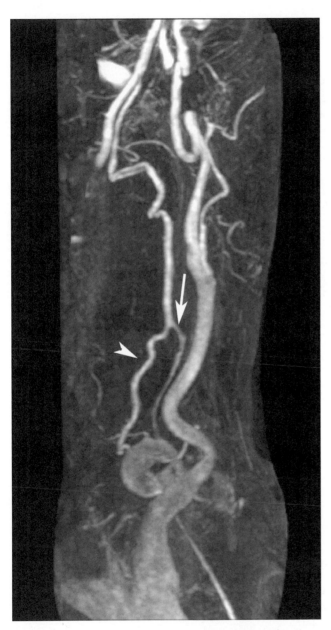

FIGURE 2-11 Anomalous vessel (*arrow*) from right thyro-cervical trunk to right vertebral artery (*arrowhead*).

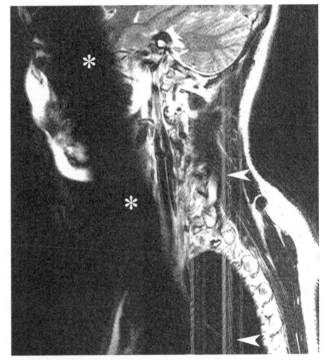

FIGURE 2-12 **Zipper artifact.** The zipper artifact (*arrow-heads*) shown in this sagittal image is likely due to collapsed signal located inferiorly from tissue in the fall-off region of the gradient magnetic field. The dark band (*asterisk*) is the normal result of a saturation band placed to null signal.

Brachial Plexus

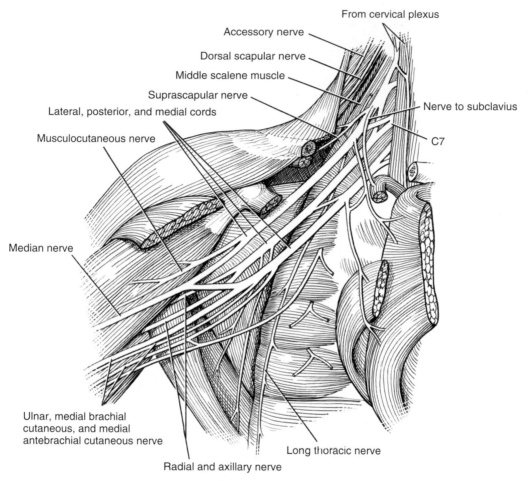

From cervical plexus

Accessory nerve

Dorsal scapular nerve

Middle scalene muscle

Suprascapular nerve

Lateral, posterior, and medial cords

Musculocutaneous nerve

Nerve to subclavius

C7

Median nerve

Ulnar, medial brachial cutaneous, and medial antebrachial cutaneous nerve

Radial and axillary nerve

Long thoracic nerve

FIGURE 2-13 Illustration of brachial plexus. Typical brachial plexus is depicted, although over 38 variations of the brachial plexus have been described in the literature. (From Berquist TH. *MRI of the musculoskeletal system*, 5th ed. Lippincott Williams & Wilkins; 2006.)

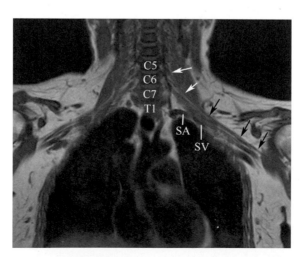

C5
C6
C7
T1

SA
SV

FIGURE 2-14 Normal brachial plexus in coronal plane. Coronal T1-weighted images through the brachial plexus show the left exiting C5-T1 nerve roots, trunks, divisions, cords and branches (arrows) (SA = subclavian artery, SV = subclavian vein).

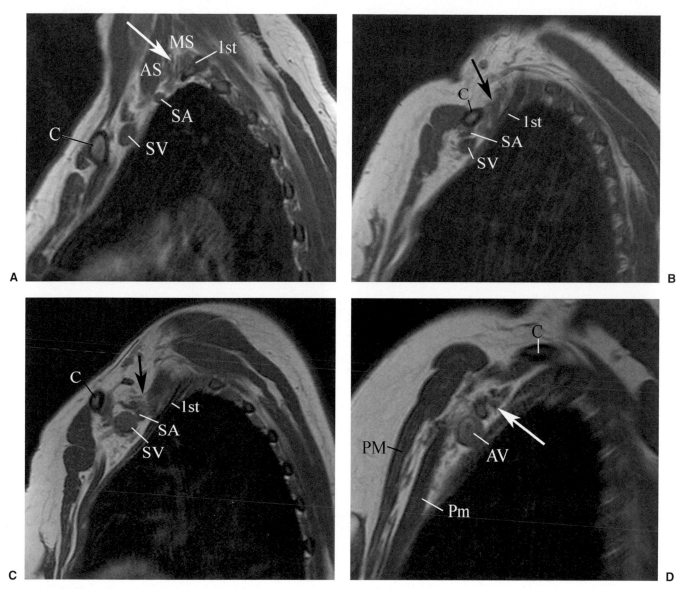

FIGURE 2-15 Normal brachial plexus and surrounding structures vary in sagittal plane, depending upon arm positioning.
A: Imaging of the plexus at the level of the interscalene triangle, arm down (Trunks of brachial plexus = arrow, MS = middle scalene, AS = anterior scalene, 1st = 1st rib, SA = subclavian artery, SV = subclavian vein, C = clavicle). **B:** Imaging of the plexus at the level of the costoclavicular space, arm up (Cords of brachial plexus = arrow, SA = subclavian artery, SV = subclavian vein, C = clavicle). **C:** Imaging of the plexus at the level of the costoclavicular space, arm down (Cords of brachial plexus = arrow, SA = subclavian artery, SV = subclavian vein, C = clavicle, 1st = 1st rib). **D:** Imaging of the plexus at the level of the retropectoralis minor space, arm down (Cords of brachial plexus = arrow, PM = pectoralis major, Pm = pectoralis minor, AV = axillary vein, C = clavicle).

Suggested Readings

Neck

Al-Khateeb TH, Al Zoubi F. Congenital neck masses: A descriptive retrospective study of 252 cases. *J Oral Maxillofac Surg*. 2007;65(11):2242–2247.

Bergman RA, Thompson SA, Afifi AK, et al., ed. *Compendium of human anatomic variation*. Baltimore: Urban & Schwarzenberg; 1988.

Celik HH, Ozdemir B, Aksit MD. Abnormal digastric muscle with unilateral quadrification of the anterior belly. *Clin Anat*. 2002;15:32–34.

Cushing KE, Ramesh V, Gardner-Medwin D, et al. Tethering of the vertebral artery in the congenital arcuate foramen of the atlas vertebra: A possible cause of vertebral artery dissection in children. *Dev Med Child Neurol*. 2001;43:491–496.

Elliott JM, Jull GA, Noteboom JT, et al. Magnetic resonance imaging study of cross-sectional area of the cervical extensor musculature in an asymptomatic cohort. *Clin Anat*. 2007;20:35–40.

Fitzgerald T. Sternomastoid paradox. *Clin Anat*. 2001;14:330–331.

Gardiner KJ, Irvine BW, Murray A. Anomalous relationship of the spinal accessory nerve to the internal jugular vein. *Clin Anat*. 2002;15:62–63.

Gluncic V, Ivkic G, Marin D, et al. Anomalous origin of both vertebral arteries. *Clin Anat*. 1999;12:281–284.

Khaki AA, Shokouhi G, Shoja MM, et al. Ansa cervicalis as a variant of spinal accessory nerve plexus: A case report. *Clin Anat*. 2006;19:540–543.

Larsson SG, Lufkin RB. Anomalies of digastric muscles: CT and MR demonstration. *J Comput Assist Tomogr*. 1987;11:422–425.

Liu D, Kitajima M, Awai K, et al. Ectopic cervical thymus in an infant. *Radiat Med*. 2006;19:554–557.

Mahne A, El-Haddad G, Alavi A, et al. Assessment of age-related morphological and functional changes of selected structures of the head and neck by computed tomography, magnetic resonance imaging, and positron emission tomography. *Semin Nucl Med*. 2007;37(2):88–102.

Nael K, Ruehm SG, Michaely HJ, et al. Multistation whole-body high-spatial resolution MR angiography using a 32-channel MR system. *AJR Am J Roentgenol*. 2007;188:529–539.

Nael K, Villablanca JP, Popoe WB, et al. Supraaortic arteries: Contrast-enhanced MR angiography at 3.0 T—highly accelerated parallel acquisition for improved spatial resolution over an extended field of view. *Radiology*. 2007;242:600–609.

Nayak BS. Surgically important variations of the jugular veins. *Clin Anat*. 2006;19:544–546.

Rosenheimer JL, Lowey J, Lozanoff S. Levator claviculae muscle discovered during physical examination for cervical lymphadenopathy. *Clin Anat*. 2000;13:298–301.

Rubinstein D, Escott EJ, Hendrick LL. The prevalence and CT appearance of the levator claviculae muscle: A normal variant not to be mistaken for an abnormality. *AJNR Am J Neuroradiol*. 1999;20:583–586.

Ruiz Santiago F, Lopez Milena G, Chamorro Santos C, et al. Levator claviculae muscle presenting as a hard clavicular mass: Imaging study. *Eur Radiol*. 2001;111:2561–2563.

Saadeh FA, El-Sabban M, Hawi JS. Rare variations of the mylohyoid muscle: Case study. *Clin Anat*. 2001;14:285–287.

Siclari F, Burger IM, Fasel JHD, et al. Developmental anatomy of the distal vertebral artery in relationship to variants of the posterior and lateral spinal arterial systems. *AJNR Am J Neuroradiol*. 2007;28:1185–1190.

Simic P, Borovecki F, Jelic M, et al. Anomalous branch of the left common carotid artery. *Clin Anat*. 2004;17:409–412.

Tagil SM, Ozcakar L, Bozkurt MC. Insight into understanding the anatomical and clinical aspects of supernumerary rectus capitis posterior muscles. *Clin Anat*. 2005;18:373–375.

Tubbs RS, Salter EG, Oakes WJ. Unusual origin of the omohyoid muscle. *Clin Anat*. 2004;17:578–582.

Turan-Ozdemir S, Coskun H, Balban M. Phlebectasia of the external jugular vein associated with duplication of the internal jugular vein. *Clin Anat*. 2004;17:522–525.

Turan-Ozdemir S, Oygucu IH, Kafa IM. Bilateral abnormal anterior bellies of digastric muscles. *Anat Sci Int*. 2004;79:95–97.

Walsh DW, Ho VB, Borke RC, et al. Anomalous course of the common carotid arteries: CT and MRA illustration—a case report. *Angiology*. 1998;49:235–238.

Weiglein AH, Moriggl B, Schalk C, et al. Arteries in the posterior cervical triangle in man. *Clin Anat*. 2005;18:553–557.

White DK, Davidson HC, Harnsberger HR, et al. Accessory salivary tissue in the mylohyoid boutonniere: A clinical and radiologic pseudolesion of the oral cavity. *AJNR Am J Neuroradiol*. 2001;22:4006–4412.

Yamamoto S, Watanabe M. Novel collateral connecting the external and internal carotid arteries. *Clin Anat*. 2004;17:70–72.

Zumpano MP, Hartwell S, Jagos CS. Soft tissue connection between rectus capitus posterior minor and the posterior atlanto-occipital membrane: A cadaveric study. *Clin Anat*. 2006;19:522–527.

Brachial Plexus

Bergman RA, Thompson SA, Afifi AK, et al. In: Bergman RA, ed. *Compendium of human anatomic variation*. Urban & Schwarzenberg; Baltimore. 1988.

Cagli K, Ozcazar L, Beyazit M, et al. Thoracic outlet syndrome in an adolescent with bilateral bifid ribs. *Clin Anat*. 2006;19:558–560.

Castillo M. Imaging the anatomy of the brachial plexus: Review and self-assessment module. *AJR Am J Roentgenol*. 2005;185:S196–S204.

Crocker MJN, Odutoye TA. The importance of structures adjacent to the first rib. *Clin Anat*. 2006;19:368–369.

Demondion X, Herbinet P, Van Sint Jan S, et al. Imaging assessment of the thoracic outlet syndrome. *RadioGraphics*. 2006;26:1735–1750.

Hirasawa K. *Arbeiten aus der dritten abteilung des anatomischein Institutes der Kaiserlichen Universitat Kyoto. Series A: Undtersuchungen uber das periphere nervensstem. Book 2: Plexus brachialis und die nerven des peripheren nervensystems*. Kyoto: 1931.

Hug U, Burg D, Meyer VE. Cervical outlet syndrome due to an accessory part of the trapezius muscle in the posterior triangle of the neck. *J Hand Surg [Br]*. 2000;25:311–313.

Loukas M, Hullett J, Louis RG Jr, et al. The gross anatomy of the extrathoracic course of the intercostobrachial nerve. *Clin Anat*. 2006;19:106–111.

Paraskevas G, Ioannidis O, Papaziogas B, et al. An accessory middle scalene muscle causing thoracic outlet syndrome. *Folia Morphol (Praha)*. 2007;66(3):194–197.

Vilensky JA. "C3, C4, C5 keep you alive," or do they? *Clin Anat*. 2006;19:130–131.

Chapter 3

Cervical Spine

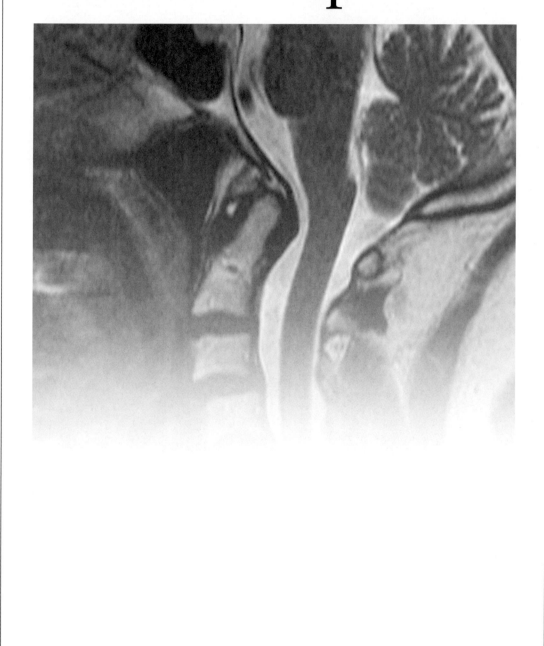

David A. Miller and Laura W. Bancroft

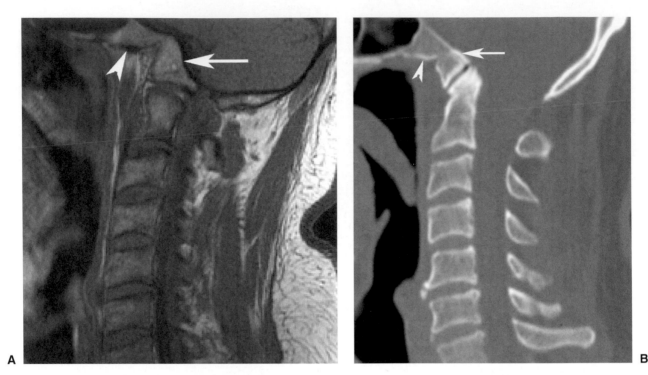

FIGURE 3-1 **Atlantooccipital assimilation. A:** Sagittal T1-weighted image and **(B)** sagittal CT reconstruction show fusion of C1 (*arrow*) and the occiput (*arrowhead*).

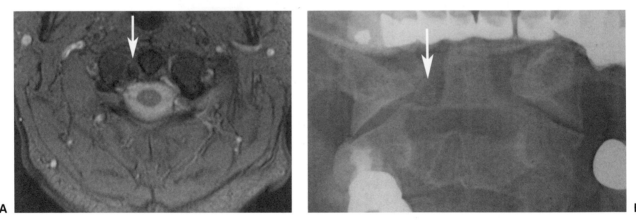

FIGURE 3-2 **Ununited ossification center lateral mass of C1. A:** Axial T2-weighted image demonstrates an ununited ossification center of the right lateral mass of C1 (*arrow*). **B:** Odontoid view radiograph confirms the ununited ossification center (*arrow*).

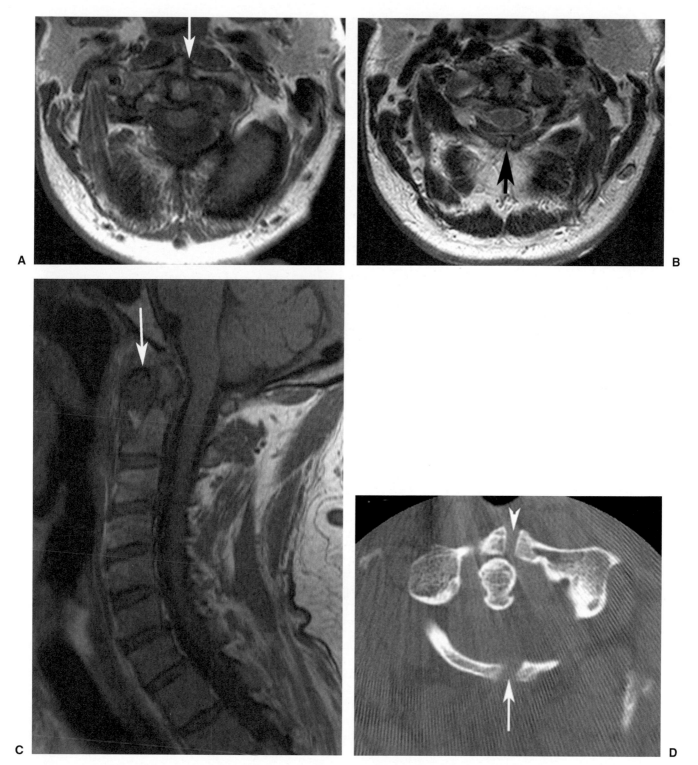

FIGURE 3-3 Unfused anterior and posterior arches of C1. Axial images show ununited **(A)** anterior (*arrow*) and **(B)** posterior (*arrow*) arches of C1. **C:** Sagittal T1-weighted image through the anterior cleft (*arrow*) may be confusing. **D:** Axial CT nicely demonstrates both anterior (*arrowhead*) and posterior (*arrow*) clefts on the same image.

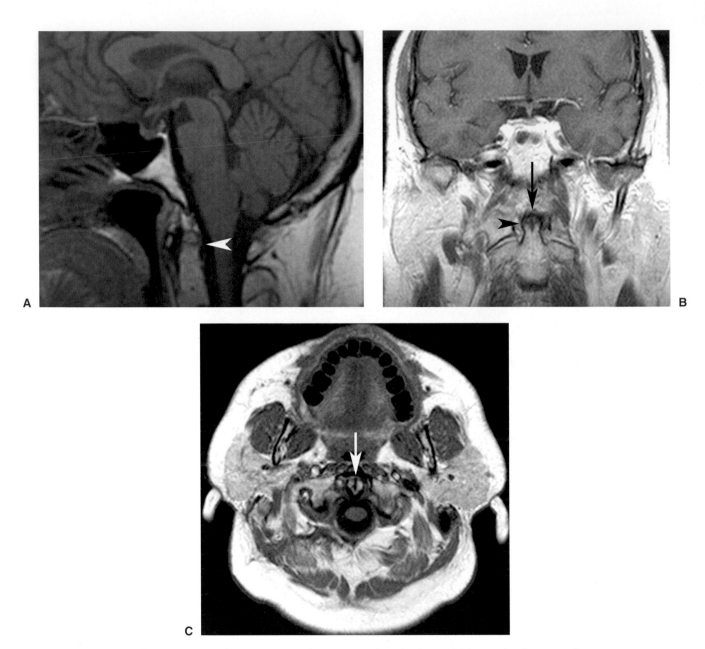

FIGURE 3-4 **C2 ossification center lines. A:** Sagittal, **(B)** coronal, and **(C)** axial T1-weighted images demonstrate transverse (*arrowhead*) and longitudinal (*arrows*) hypointense lines through the dens, consistent with sites of prior synchondroses.

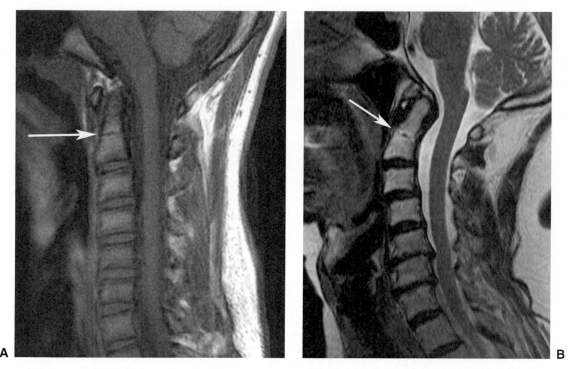

FIGURE 3-5 **Odontoid cleft. A:** Coronal and **(B)** axial T1-weighted images show a cleft (*arrows*) through the dens, consistent with normal variant.

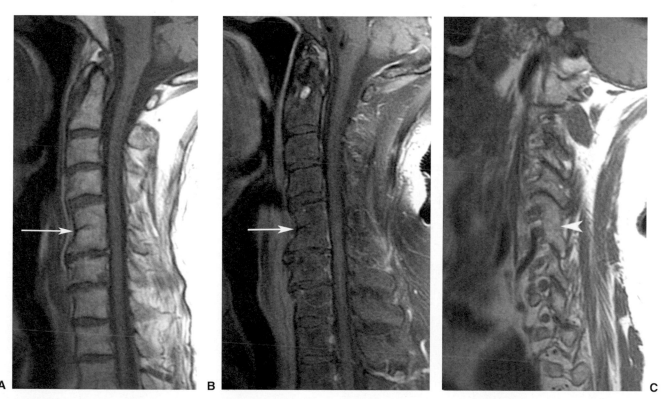

FIGURE 3-6 **Congenital fusion C5-6 bodies and facet joints.** Sagittal T1-weighted images **(A)** pre- and **(B)** post enhancement demonstrate a small portion of residual disc material (*arrows*) at site of C5-6 vertebral body fusion. Note the decreased anterior-to-posterior body width, consistent with congenital fusion from segmentation failure. **C:** Parasagittal image demonstrates fusion of the C5-6 facet joints (*arrowhead*).

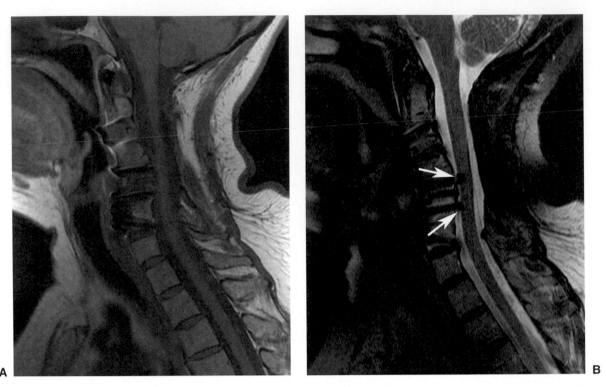

FIGURE 3-7 **Multiple ACDF artifact. A:** Sagittal T1-weighted image shows artifact from prior anterior corpectomy, discectomy and fusion. **B:** Artifact on sagittal T2-weighted image causes some artifact (*arrows*), limiting evaluation of portions of the spinal cord.

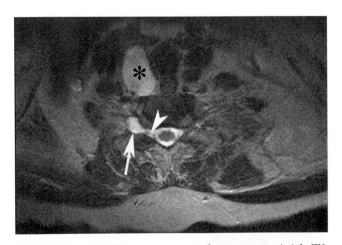

FIGURE 3-8 **C7-T1 nerve root sleeve cyst.** Axial T2-weighted image demonstrates a right C7-T1 nerve root sleeve cyst (*arrow*) with intact nerve root (*arrowhead*). Note the thyroid nodule (*asterisk*).

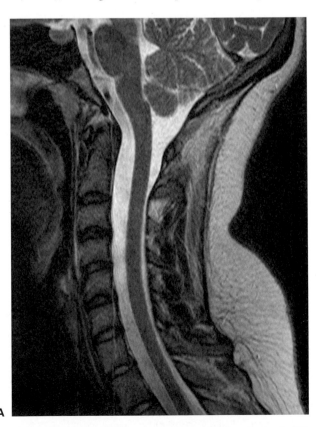

FIGURE 3-9 **Prominent central canal. A:** Sagittal T2-weighted images demonstrate relative prominence of the central spinal canal relative to the size of the spinal cord.

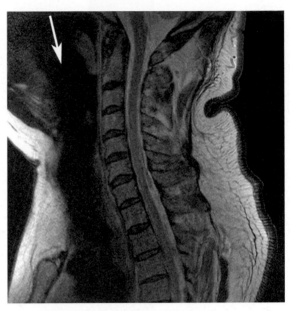

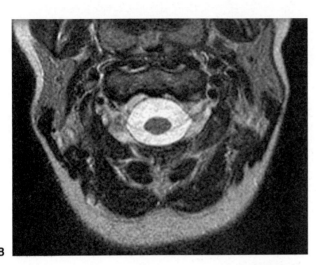

FIGURE 3-9 Prominent central canal. (*continued*) **B:** Axial T2-weighted images demonstrate relative prominence of the central spinal canal relative to the size of the spinal cord.

FIGURE 3-10 Saturation band artifact. Linear band of signal void (*arrow*) anterior to the cervical spine is attributed to intentional placement of saturation band, which limits pulsation artifact from the neck vessels and swallowing.

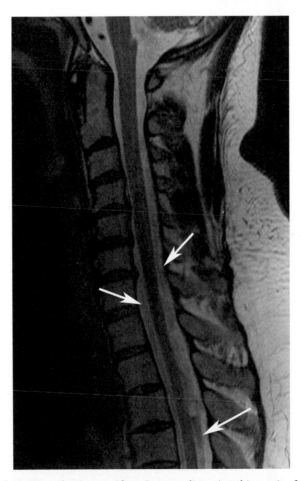

FIGURE 3-11 Cerebrospinal fluid (CSF) pulsation artifact. Intermediate signal intensity foci anterior and posterior to the cord (*arrows*) is due to CSF pulsation artifact. Intense CSF pulsation results in the inflow of CSF and protons into the imaging plane. This artifact can be reduced by reordering K-space and increasing the number of interleaving acquisitions.

Suggested Readings

Bergman RA, Thompson SA, Afifi AK, et al. *Compendium of human anatomic variation*. Baltimore: Urban & Schwarzenberg; 1988.

Chen JJ, Branstetter BF IV, Welch WC. Multiple posterior vertebral fusion abnormalities: A case report and review of the literature. *AJR Am J Roentgenol*. 2006;186:1256–1259.

Dean NA, Mitchell BS. Anatomic relation between the nuchal ligament (ligamentum nuchae) and the spinal dura mater in the craniocervical region. *Clin Anat*. 2002;15:182–185.

Harrison DE, Harrison DD, Haas JW, et al. Do sagittal plane anatomical variations (angulation) of the cervical facets and C2 odontoid affect the geometrical configuration of the cervical lordosis? *Clin Anat*. 2005;18:104–111.

Humphreys BK, Kenin S, Hubbard BB, et al. Investigation of connective tissue attachments to the cervical spinal dura mater. *Clin Anat*. 2004;16:152–159.

Kazan S, Yildirim F, Sindel M, et al. Anatomical evaluation of the groove for the vertebral artery in the axis vertebrae for atlanto-axial transarticular screw fixation technique. *Clin Anat*. 2000;13:237–243.

Kiray A, Arman C, Naderi S, et al. Surgical anatomy of the cervical sympathetic trunk. *Clin Anat*. 2005;18:179–185.

von Ludinghausen M, Fahr M, Prescher A, et al. Accessory joints between basiocciput and atlas/axis in the median plane. *Clin Anat*. 2005;18:558–571.

Lustrin ES, Karakas SP, Ortiz AO, et al. Pediatric cervical spine: Normal anatomy, variants, and trauma. *Radiographics*. 2003;23:539–560.

Massengill AD, Huynh SL, Harris JH Jr. C2-3 facet joint "pseudofusion": Anatomic basis of a normal variant. *Skeletal Radiol*. 1997;26:27–30.

Mercer SR, Bogduk N. Clinical anatomy of ligamentum nuchae. *Clin Anat*. 2003; 16(6):484–493.

Oh CS, Chung IH, Koh KS, et al. Intradural anastomoses between the accessory nerve and the posterior roots of the cervical nerves: Their clinical significance. *Clin Anat*. 2001;14:424–427.

Oh CS, Chung IH, Koh KS, et al. Morphologic study of the connections between the accessory nerve and the posterior root of the first cervical nerve. *Clin Anat*. 2002;15:267–270.

Pfirmann CWA, Binkert CA, Zanetti M, et al. MR morphology of alar ligaments and occipitoatlantoaxial joints: Study in 50 asymptomatic subjects. *Radiology*. 2001;218:133–137.

Smoker WR. Craniovertebral junction: Normal anatomy, craniometry, and congenital anomalies. *Radiographics*. 1994;14(2):255–277.

Section II

THE UPPER EXTREMITY

Chapter 4

Shoulder/Arm

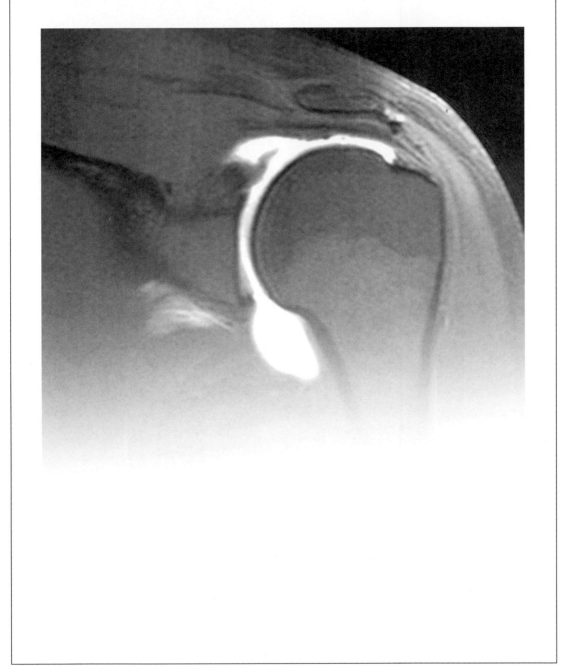

Laura W. Bancroft, Jeffrey J. Peterson, and John E. Kirsch

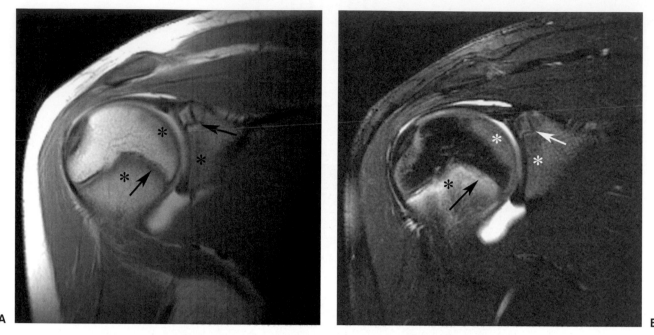

FIGURE 4-1 **Normal pediatric shoulder.** Coronal oblique FSE **(A)** proton density and **(B)** T2-weighted fat-suppressed MR arthrographic images demonstrate the normal physes (*arrows*) and signal intensities of the shoulder in a child. Note the relatively greater proportion of red marrow (*asterisk*) in children compared with adults.

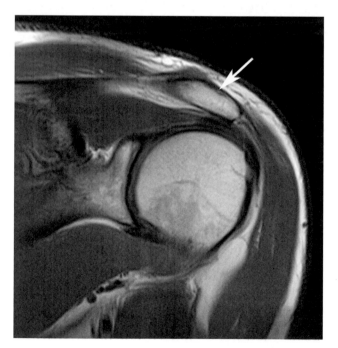

FIGURE 4-2 **Downsloping acromion.** Coronal oblique FSE proton density image shows a laterally downsloping acromion (*arrow*), which can be associated with rotator cuff pathology. Acromia can also downslope anteriorly in the sagittal projection. The shape of the acromia can be flat, curved, or hooked.

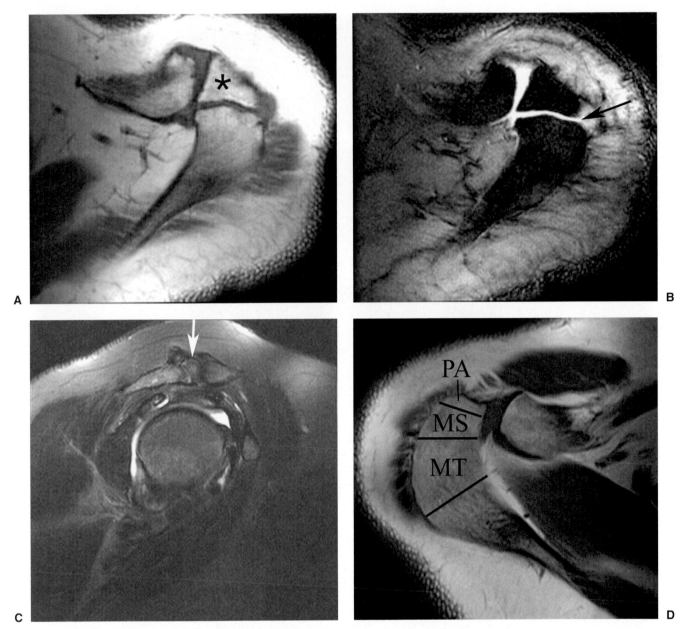

FIGURE 4-3 **Os acromiale.** **A:** The axial plane is the best orientation to identify an os acromiale (*asterisk*), which is the unfused distal acromion. **B:** Axial double echo steady state (DESS) image shows high signal (*arrow*) between the os acromiale and remaining acromion. This indicates lack of fibrous or cartilaginous union, and potential for mobility and impingement upon the rotator cuff. **C:** An os acromiale (*arrow*) can easily be missed in the sagittal plane. **D:** Various sites of os acromiale (*Preacromion = PA, Mesoacromion = MS, Meta-acromion = MT*).

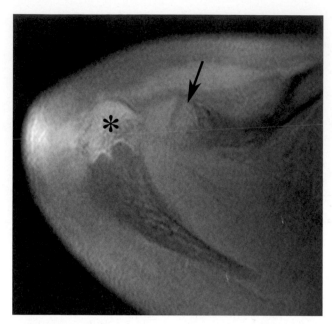

FIGURE 4-4 Unfused acromial ossification center. Axial T1-weighted fat-suppressed image in skeletally immature patient demonstrates the normally unfused acromial ossification center (*asterisk*), which should not be confused with an os acromiale. Also note the unfused distal clavicle (*arrow*).

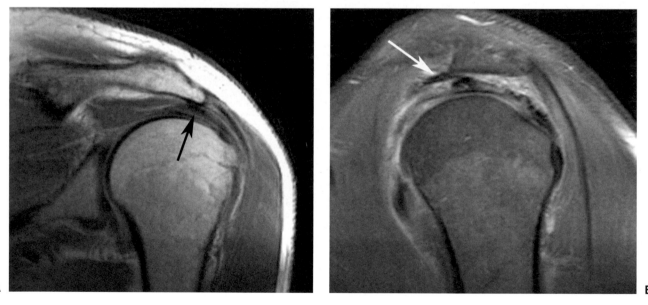

FIGURE 4-5 Acromial pseudospur. A: Coronal oblique image shows a small hypointense focus (*arrow*) inferior to the distal acromion. This is the normal coracoacromial ligament, which should not be confused with an osseous spur. **B:** Sagittal FSE proton density fat-suppressed image shows the coracoacromial ligament (*arrow*) as it attaches onto the acromion.

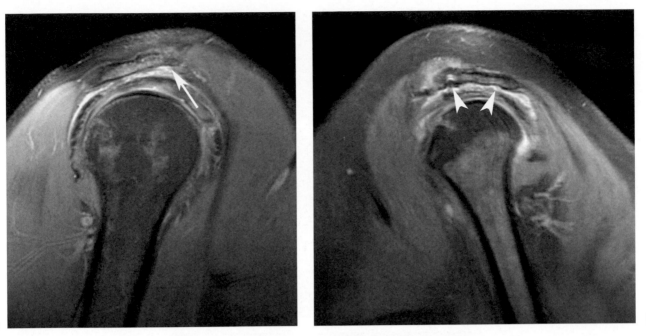

FIGURE 4-6 **Acromioplasty.** Postoperative imaging after acromioplasty can demonstrate **(A)** subtle undersurface concavity (*arrow*), **(B)** more obvious changes with susceptibility artifact (*arrowheads*), or even larger defects.

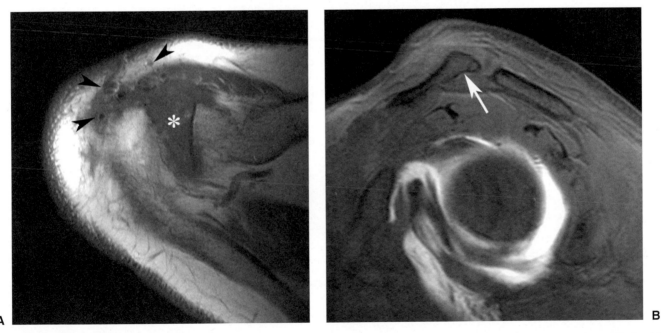

FIGURE 4-7 **Distal clavicular resection. A:** Expected appearance of the shoulder after distal clavicular resection (*asterisk*) should not be confused with an erosive process. Note the sharp, well-corticated osseous margins, lack of any subchondral signal changes, and postsurgical susceptibility artifact (*arrowheads*) on this axial T1-weighted image. **B:** Smooth undersurface defect (*arrow*) in a different patient after distal clavicular resection.

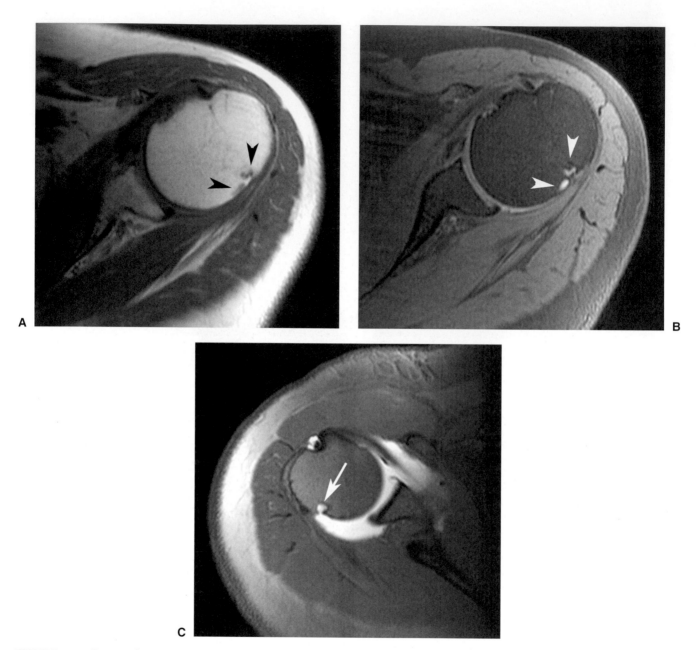

FIGURE 4-8 **Cystic changes in the bare area of the humeral head.** Normal cystic changes (*arrowheads*) are present in the posterior humeral head on axial **(A)** T1-weighted and **(B)** double echo steady state (DESS) images. There is no cartilage overlying the posterior aspect of the humeral head, hence the term *bare area*. **C:** More defined, single cyst (*arrow*) is filled with contrast on this MR arthrogram.

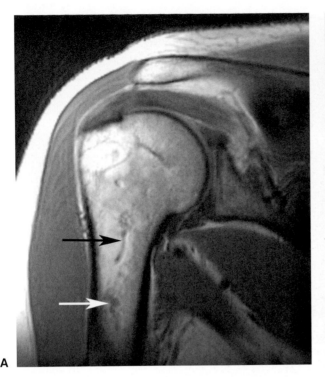
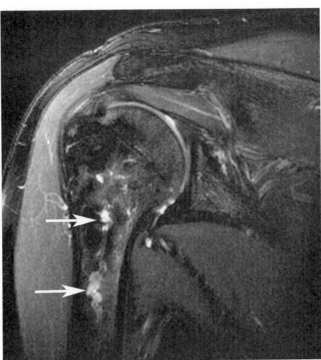

FIGURE 4-9 Prominent intraosseous vessels. Coronal oblique **(A)** T1-weighted and **(B)** FSE T2-weighted fat-suppressed images show prominent intramedullary vessels (*arrows*) within the proximal humerus, of no clinical consequence.

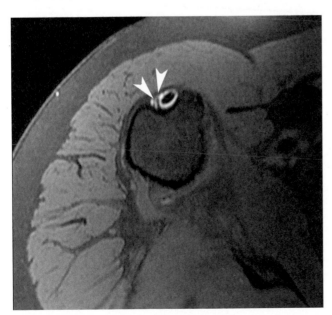

FIGURE 4-10 Vincular biceps. Axial MR arthrogram shows thin synovial bands (*arrowheads*) within the superior portion of the biceps tendon sheath, which are normal variants.

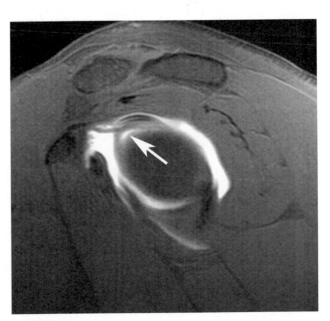

FIGURE 4-11 Sublabral foramen. Sagittal MR arthrogram demonstrates contrast extending through the normal variant sublabral foramen (*arrow*), where the anterosuperior labrum is not attached.

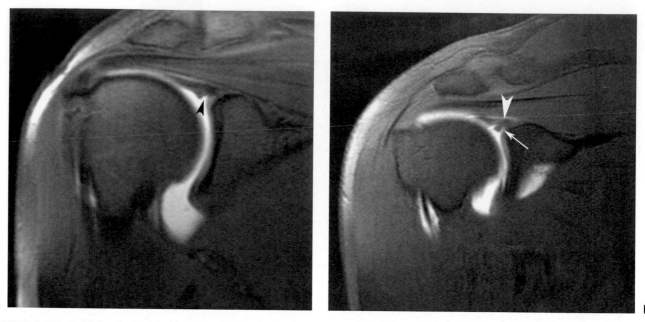

FIGURE 4-12 Sublabral recess. A: Coronal oblique MR arthrogram demonstrates a thin, smooth sublabral recess (*arrowhead*) that is oriented from an inferolateral to a superomedial. This normal variant should not be confused with a superior labral tear, which would be irregular, wide, and oriented into the substance of the labrum. **B:** Sublabral recess (*arrow*) in a different patient extends beneath the biceps-labral complex (*arrowhead*).

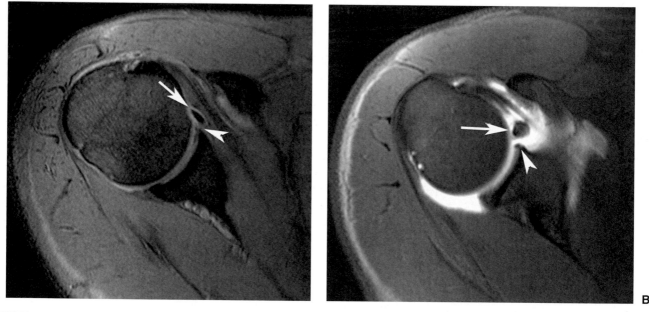

FIGURE 4-13 Buford complex. A: Axial double echo steady state (DESS) image shows absence of the anterior labrum (*arrowhead*) and a prominent middle glenohumeral ligament (*arrow*), consistent with normal variant Buford complex. **B:** Axial images demonstrate an absent anterosuperior labrum (*arrowhead*) and a thickened middle glenohumeral ligament (*arrow*) in different patients, representing the normal variant Buford complex. This is found in 1.5% of the population and should not be mistaken for an avulsed, thickened labrum.

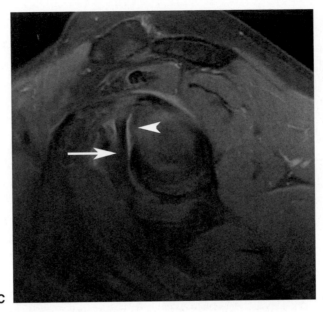

FIGURE 4-13 **Buford complex.** (*continued*) **C:** sagittal images demonstrate an absent anterosuperior labrum (*arrowhead*) and a thickened middle glenohumeral ligament (*arrow*) in different patients, representing the normal variant Buford complex. This is found in 1.5% of the population and should not be mistaken for an avulsed, thickened labrum.

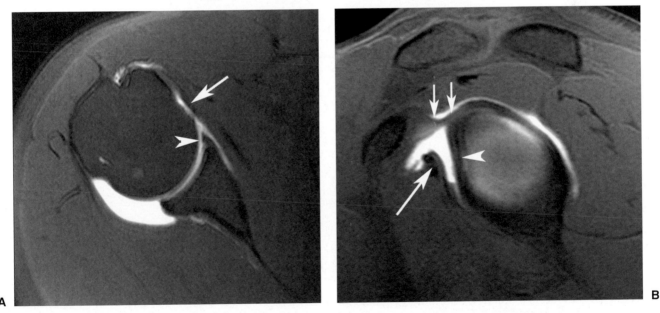

FIGURE 4-14 **Absent middle glenohumeral ligament (MGHL). A:** Axial and **(B)** sagittal MR arthrographic images show absence of the MGHL, which is normally situated between the anterior labrum (*arrowhead*) and the subscapularis (*arrow*). Note the presence of the superior glenohumeral ligament (*double arrows*).

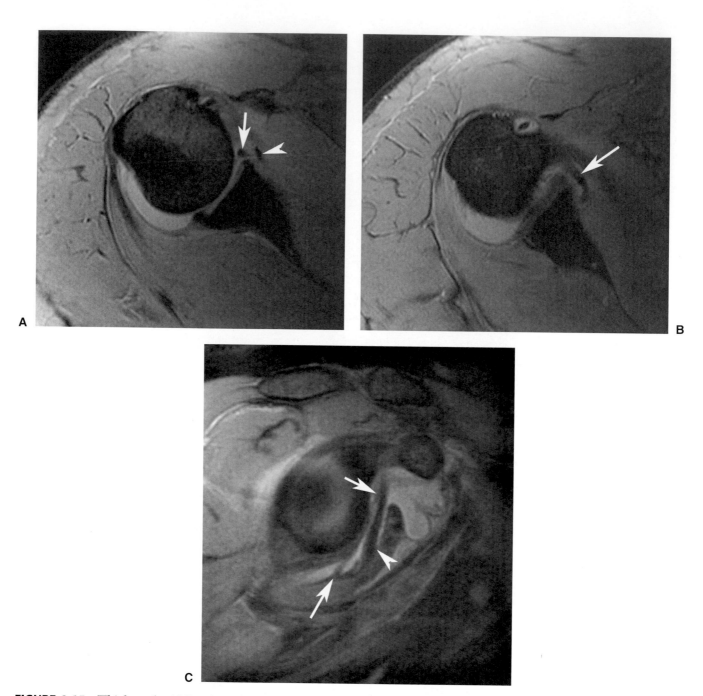

FIGURE 4-15 Thickened middle glenohumeral ligament (MGHL) and superior attachment of anterior band of inferior glenohumeral ligament (IGHL). Axial imaging through the **(A)** superior and **(B)** inferior joint demonstrate a superior origin of the anterior band of the inferior glenohumeral ligament (*arrow*), above the midpoint of the glenohumeral joint. The MGHL (*arrowhead*) is thickened. **C:** Sagittal image shows the high origin of the anterior band of the IGHL (*arrows*) and the thickened MGHL (*arrowhead*), both normal variants and confirmed with arthroscopy.

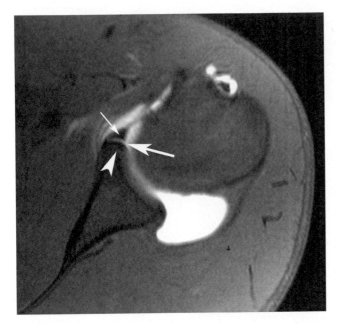

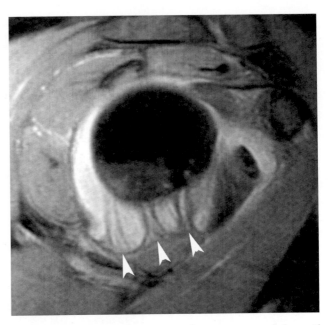

FIGURE 4-16 Normal recess between labrum and anterior band of inferior glenohumeral ligament (IGHL). Axial MR arthrogram shows normal extension of contrast (*large arrow*) between the anterior labrum (*arrowhead*) and a thickened anterior band of the inferior glenohumeral ligament (*small arrow*). Findings were confirmed with arthroscopy. This should not be confused with pathology, since both the labrum and glenohumeral ligament are firmly attached.

FIGURE 4-17 Normal corrugated appearance of the axillary recess. Sagittal FSE proton density (PD) fat-suppressed image shows prominent corrugation (*arrowheads*) of the axillary recess, which is a normal variation of this portion of the inferior glenohumeral ligament.

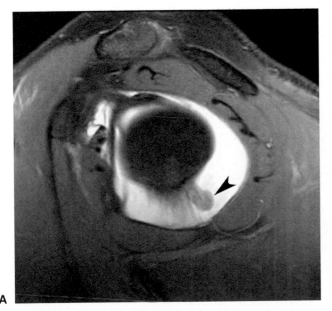

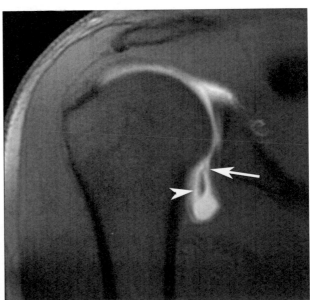

FIGURE 4-18 Synovial frond. A: Sagittal and **(B)** coronal oblique images through the glenohumeral joint shows a single, prominent synovial frond (*arrowhead*) extending from the capsule (*arrow*).

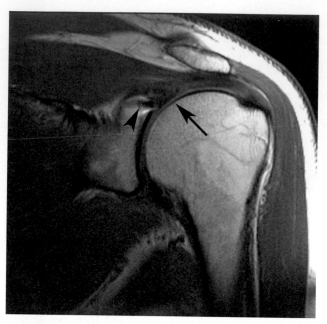

FIGURE 4-19 Healed labral repair. Coronal oblique proton density image demonstrates some artifact around the intact superior labral anchor (*arrowhead*) and low signal intensity within the reattached labrum (*arrow*). No fluid equivalent signal extended within or subjacent to the labrum on any sequence and second look arthroscopy confirmed a healed, intact labrum.

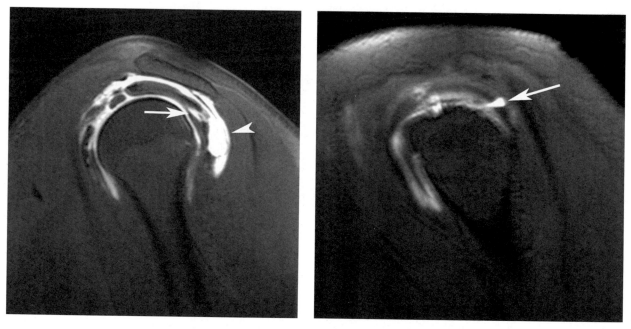

FIGURE 4-20 Portal holes after arthroscopy. A and **B:** Sagittal oblique MR arthrograms in two different patients show extension of intra-articular contrast through linear defects (*arrow*) in the infraspinatus tendons at site of prior posterior arthroscopy portal. Note communication of the defect into the subacromial/subdeltoid bursa (*arrowhead*) in patient (**A**).

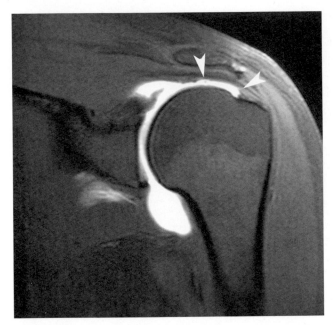

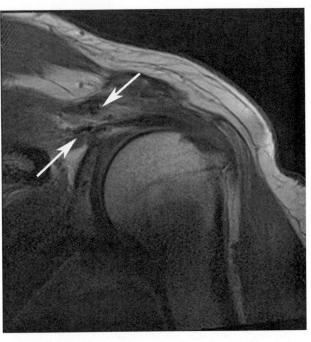

FIGURE 4-21 **Postoperative debridement of partial thickness rotator cuff tear.** Coronal oblique MR arthrogram shows a smooth, shallow defect (*arrowheads*) in the articular side of the supraspinatus tendon following debridement of low-grade partial thickness tear. This "longer than deep" appearance of the normal postdebridement cuff is in contradistinction to a rotator cuff retear, in which the defect is deeper than its medial-to-lateral extent.

FIGURE 4-22 **Postoperative repair of myotendinous junction tear.** Focal contour alteration of the supraspinatus myotendinous junction (*arrows*) and susceptibility artifact at site of intact repair.

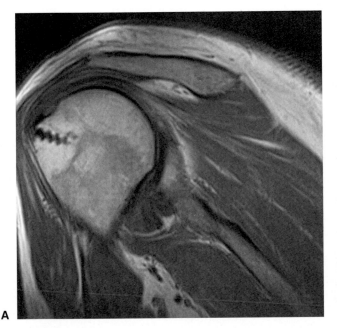

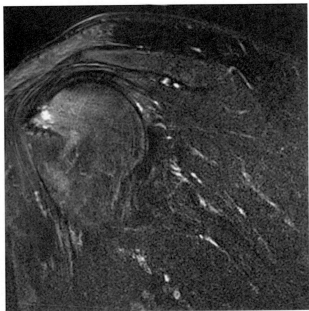

A

B

FIGURE 4-23 **Postoperative rotator cuff repair.** Normal, expected appearance of an intact supraspinatus tendon repair with bioabsorbable screw on coronal oblique **(A)** proton density and **(B)** FSE T2-weighted fat-suppressed images.

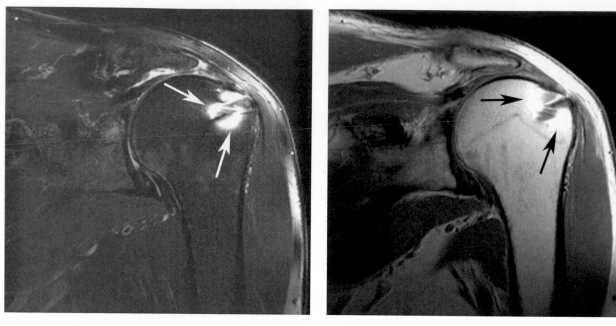

FIGURE 4-24   Metallic suture anchor artifact. Hyperintense signal (*arrows*) around the rotator cuff suture anchor on both **(A)** FSE T2-weighted fat-suppressed and **(B)** proton density images is due to metallic susceptibility artifact. This artifact would be lessened by utilizing short tau inversion recovery (STIR) (as opposed to chemical sat suppression) technique.

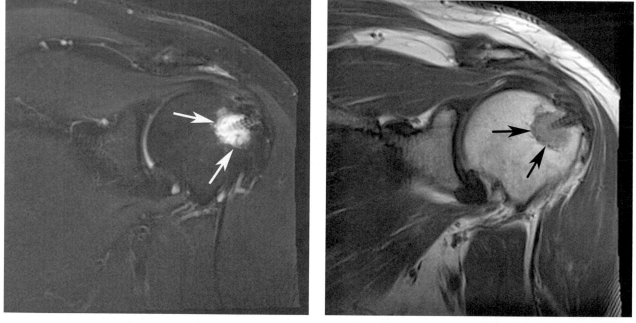

FIGURE 4-25   Osteolysis around bioabsorbable suture anchor. A: The hyperintense T2-weighted signal (*arrows*) around the suture anchor is fairly similar in appearance to Figure 4-24A. **B:** However, note the abnormal low signal intensity marrow signal in the humeral head on the proton density image. This is due to reactive cystic change about the anchor, not merely from misregistration artifact, as in Figure 4-21.

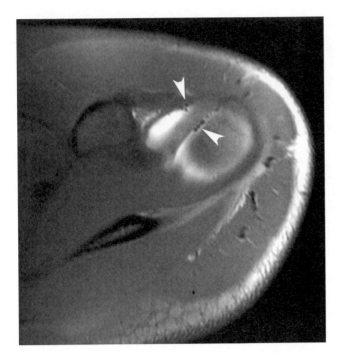

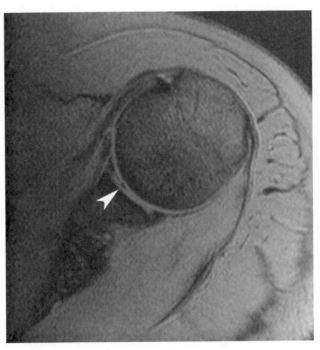

FIGURE 4-26 Gas bubble artifact on MR arthrogram. Tiny hypointense foci (*arrowheads*) are aligned in a linear manner posterior to the superior glenohumeral ligament and long head of the biceps tendon, consistent with inadvertently injected gas bubbles during arthrogram. Their nondependent location and uniformity should not be misinterpreted as loose bodies.

FIGURE 4-27 Vacuum phenomenon in glenohumeral joint. Axial double echo steady state (DESS) image shows blooming effect of a small amount of gas (*arrowhead*) in the shoulder joint, due to vacuum phenomenon.

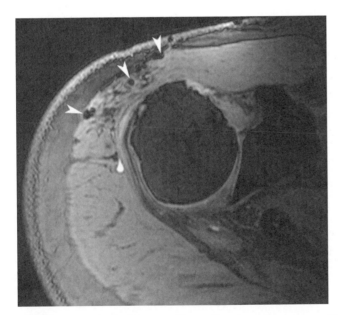

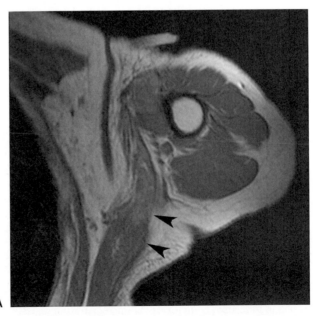

FIGURE 4-28 Soft tissue artifact after open rotator cuff repair. Axial DESS (double echo steady state, volumetric gradient echo) image shows small foci of susceptibility artifact (*arrowheads*) along incision for open rotator cuff repair.

FIGURE 4-29 Latissimus dorsi myocutaneous flap. A: Altered muscle location may be iatrogenic, as in this case of latissimus dorsi myocutaneous flap placement (*arrowheads*).

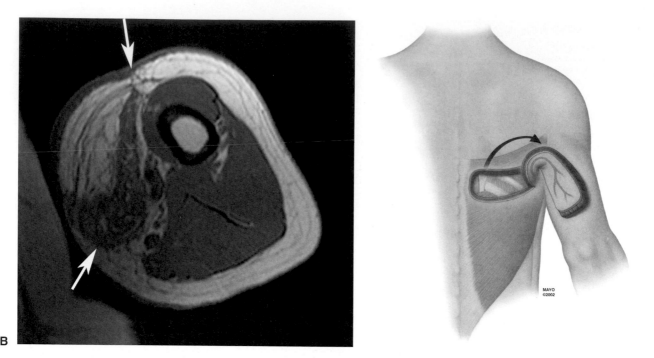

FIGURE 4-29   Latissimus dorsi myocutaneous flap. (*continued*) **B:** Flap placement into the medial arm (*arrows*) shows muscular fibers with striations of fat as well as subcutaneous fat. This should not be mistaken for a soft tissue mass. **C:** Illustration of rotated latissimus dorsi flap.

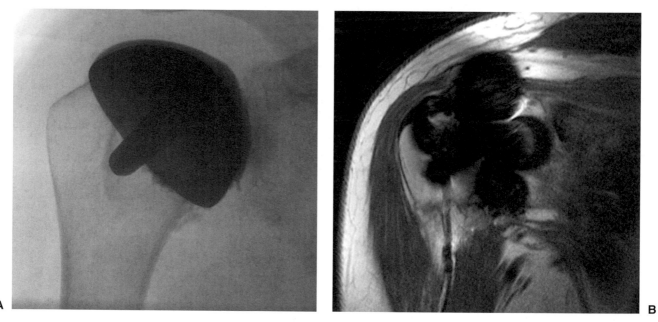

FIGURE 4-30   Humeral resurfacing artifact. A and **B:** The rounded configuration of the humeral head resurfacing arthroplasty results in lobulated, complex signal misregistration on **(B)** MRI.

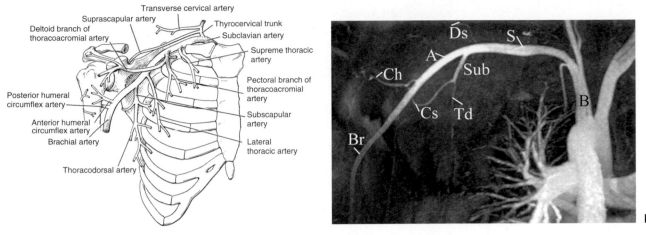

A

B

FIGURE 4-31 **Shoulder MRA.** Although vascular anatomy can be variant, the usual arterial supply to the shoulder comes from the brachiocephalic (*B*), subclavian (*S*), axillary (*A*), dorsal (descending) scapular (*Ds*), subscapularis (*Sub*), thoracodorsal (*Td*), circumflex scapular (*Cs*), circumflex humeral (*Ch*) and brachial (*Br*) arteries.

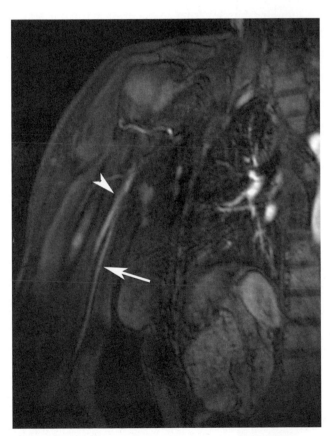

FIGURE 4-32 **Persistent superficial brachial artery.** The persistent superficial brachial artery (*arrow*) arises from brachial artery (*arrowhead*) in the upper arm, and continues distally as the radial artery.

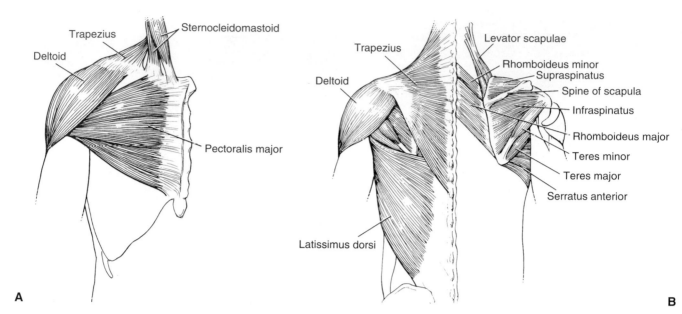

FIGURE 4-33 ■ **Illustrations of the shoulder muscles from (A) anterior and (B) posterior.** (From Berquist TH. *MRI of the musculoskeletal system*, 5th ed. Philadelphia: Lippincott Williams & Wilkins; 2006.)

Table 4-1 Muscles of the shoulder and upper arm

Muscles	Origin	Insertion	Action	Innervation
Intrinsic				
Deltoid	Lateral clavicle, acromion, scapular spine	Deltoid tuberosity humerus	Abductor of humerus	Axillary nerve (C5, C6)
Supraspinatus	Supraspinous fossa of scapula	Greater tuberosity superiorly	Abductor of humerus	Suprascapular nerve (C5, C6)
Infraspinatus	Infraspinous fossa of scapula	Posterior inferior greater tuberosity	Lateral rotation humerus	Suprascapular nerve (C5, C6)
Teres minor	Lateral midscapular border	Lateral inferior facet, greater tuberosity	External rotator of humerus	Axillary nerve (C5, C6)
Subscapularis	Suprascapular fossa	Lesser tuberosity	Internal rotator of humerus	Subscapular nerves (C5-7)
Teres major	Inferior lateral scapula	Medial intertubercular groove	Internal rotation, adduction, extensor of humerus	Subscapular nerve (C5-6)
Extrinsic				
Trapezius	Ligamentum nuchae, thoracic spinous processes	Distal clavicle, acromion, scapular spine	Retractor and elevator of scapula	Spinal accessory and C2, C3
Latissimus dorsi	Spinous processes T6-12, lumbar, upper sacrum	Medial intertubercular groove	Adductor, internal rotator, and extensor of humerus	Thoracodorsal nerve (C6-8)
Levator scapulae	Posterior tubercles, C1-4 transverse processes	Upper medial scapula	Elevates medial scapula	Cervical plexus (C3-4)

Table 4-1 Muscles of the shoulder and upper arm (*continued*)

Muscles	Origin	Insertion	Action	Innervation
Rhomboidei				
Major	C2-T5 spinous processes	Posterior medial scapula	Retractor of scapula	Dorsal scapular nerve (C5)
Minor	Ligamentum nuchae C7 and T1 spinous processes	Posterior medial scapula at base of scapular spine	Retractor of scapula	Dorsal scapular nerve (C5)
Serratus anterior	Anterior ribs 1–9	Anterior medial scapula	Protractor, anterior drawing of scapula	Long thoracic nerve (C5-7)
Pectoral region				
Pectoralis major	Inferomedial clavicle, sternum, and costochondral junctions	Lateral intertubercular groove	Adductor of humerus	Medial and lateral anterior thoracic nerves (C5-T1)
Pectoralis minor	Anterior ribs 2–5	Coracoid of scapula	Depress angle of scapula	Medial pectoral nerve (C8-T1)
Subclavius	Anteromedial rib 1	Midinferior clavicle	Stabilize sternoclavicular joint	Subclavian nerve

(From Carter BL, Morehead J, Walpert JM, et al. *Cross-sectional anatomy: computed tomography and ultrasound correlation.* New York: Appleton-Century Crofts; 1977; Iannotti JP, Gabriel JP, Schneck SL, et al. The normal glenohumeral relationship. *J Bone Joint Surg.* 1992;74A:491–500; and Rosse C, Rosse PG. *Hollinsheads textbook of anatomy.* Philadelphia: Lippincott-Raven; 1997.)

Table 4-2 Variant muscular anatomy of the pectoral region

Pectoralis major (accessory head inferior to abdominal head, attach at lateral biceps groove, absent abdominal slip, absent sternocostal head, fibers cross midline)

Pectoralis minor (aplasia—partial/complete)

Accessory muscles (sternalis, sternoclavicularis, sternoscapularis, sternocoracoideus, sternohumeralis, sternochondrocarcoideus, pectoralis quartus, subclavius, costoepitrochlearis, chondroepitrochelaris, chondrohumeralis)

Table 4-3 Muscle variations of the rotator cuff

Supraspinatus (two muscle bellies, accessory slips, attachment to pectoralis major/minor)

Infraspinatus (infraspinatus superficialis = fascicle extending onto greater tuberosity of humerus)

Subscapularis (accessory = subscapularis minor or secundus)

Teres minor (absent, teres minusus scapulae = partial separation, can fuse with infraspinatus)

(Compiled from Berman RA, Thompson SA, Afiti AK, et al. Compendium of human anatomic variation. Munchen, Baltimore: Urban and Schwartzenberg; 1988.)

Suggested Readings

Alegre MLS, Marin C, Mardones GG. Duplication of the scapula. *Skeletal Radiol*. 2003;32:728–730.

Berman RA, Thompson SA, Afiti AK, Saadeh FA. *Compendium of human anatomic variation*. Munchen, Baltimore: Urban and Schwartzenberg; 1988.

Cavdar S, Zeybek A, Bayramicli M. Rare variation of the axillary artery. *Clin Anat*. 2000;13:66–68.

Chang EY, Moses DA, Babb JS, Schweitzer ME. Shoulder impingement: Objective 3D shape analysis of acromial morphologic features. *Radiology*. 2006;239:497–505.

Cogswell LK, Giele H. Anatomical study to investigate the feasibility of pedicled nerve, free vessel gastrocnemius muscle transfer for restoration of biceps function. *Clin Anat*. 2001;14:242–245.

De Maeseneer M, Van Roy F, Lenchik L, et al. CT and MR arthrography of the normal and pathologic anterosuperior labrum and labral-bicipital complex. *RadioGraphics*. 2000;20:S67–S81.

Del Sol M, Olave E. Elevator muscle of the tendon of latissimus dorsi muscle. *Clin Anat*. 2005;18:112–114.

Demirkan AF, Sargon MF, Erkula G, et al. The spinoglenoid ligament: An anatomic study. *Clin Anat*. 2003;16:511–513.

El-Naggar MM, Zahir FL. Two bellies of the coracobrachialis muscle associated with a third head of the biceps brachii muscle. *Clin Anat*. 2001;14:379–382.

Gelber PE, Reina F, Monllau JC, et al. Innervation patterns of the inferior glenohumeral ligament: Anatomical and biomechanical relevance. *Clin Anat*. 2006;19:304–311.

Graichen H, Bonel H, Stammberger T, et al. Three-dimensional analysis of the width of the subacromial space in healthy subjects and patients with impingement syndrome. *AJR Am J Roentgenol*. 1999;172:1081–1096.

Grainfer AJ, Tirman PFJ, Elliott JM, et al. MR anatomy of the subcoracoid bursa and the association of subcoracoid effusion with tears of the anterior rotator cuff and the rotator interval. *AJR Am J Roentgenol*. 2000;174:1377–1380.

Heers G, Gotz J, Schubert T, et al. MRI of the intraarticular disk of the acromioclavicular joint: A comparison with anatomical, histological and in-vivo findings. *Skeletal Radiol*. 2007;36:23–28.

Jin W, Ryu KN, Kwon SH, et al. MR arthrography in the differential diagnosis of type II superior labral anteroposterior lesion and sublabral recess. *AJR Am J Roentgenol*. 2006;187:887–893.

Jin W, Ryu KN, Park YK, et al. Cystic lesions in the posterosuperior portion of the humeral head on MR arthrography: Correlations with gross and histologic findings in cadavers. *AJR Am J Roentgenol*. 2005;184:1211–1215.

Mahakkanukrah P, Somsarp V. Dual innervation of the brachialis muscle. *Clin Anat*. 2002;15:206–209.

Malcic-Gurbuz J, Gurunuoglu R, Ozdogmus O, et al. Unique case of trifurcation of the brachial artery: Its clinical significance. *Clin Anat*. 2002;15:224–227.

Melling M, Wilde J, Schnallinger M, et al. Rare variant of the brachial artery: Superficial lateral inferior type VII EAB. *Clin Anat*. 2000;13:216–222.

Merida-Velasco JR, Rosriguez Vasquez JF, Merida Velasco JA, et al. Axillary arch: Potential cause of neurovascular compression syndrome. *Clin Anat*. 2003;16:514–529.

Monk AO, Berry E, Limb D, et al. Laser morphometric analysis of the glenoid fossa of the scapula. *Clin Anat*. 2001;14:320–323.

Nakatani T, Tanaka S, Mizukami S. Bilateral four-headed biceps brachii muscles: The median nerve and brachial artery passing through a tunnel formed by a muscle slip from the accessory head. *Clin Anat*. 1998;11:209–212.

Olsen OE, Lie RT, Lachman RS, et al. Ossification sequence in infants who die during the perinatal period: Population-based references. *Radiology*. 2002;225:240–244.

Pouliart N, Gagey O. Significance of the latisimmus dorsi for shoulder instability. I. Variations in its anatomy around the humerus and scapula. *Clin Anat*. 2005;18:493–499.

Pouliart N, Gagey O. Significance of the latissimus dorsi for shoulder instability. II. Its influence on dislocation behavior in a sequential cutting protocol of the glenohumeral capsule. *Clin Anat*. 2005;18:500–509.

Rodriquez-Niedenfuhr, Vazquez T, Choi D. Supernumerary humeral heads of the biceps brachii muscle revisited. *Clin Anat*. 2003;16:197–203.

Rose SC, Kadir S. Arterial anatomy of the upper extremities. In: Kadir S, ed. *Atlas of normal and variant angiographic anatomy*. Philadelphia: WB Saunders; 1991:55–95.

Saeed M, Rufai AA. Median and musculocutaneous nerves: Variant formation and distribution. *Clin Anat*. 2003;16:453–457.

Tubbs RS, Salter EG, Oakes WJ. Anomaly of the suprascapular nerve: Case report and review of the literature. *Clin Anat*. 2006;19:599–601.

Turgut HB, Peker T, Gulekon N, et al. Axillopectoral muscle (Langer's muscle). *Clin Anat*. 2005;18:220–223.

Williams MM, Snyder SJ, Buford D Jr. The Buford complex—the "cord-like" middle glenohumeral ligament and absent anterosuperior labrum complex: A normal anatomic capsulolabral variant. *Arthroscopy*. 1994;10:241.

Chapter 5

Elbow

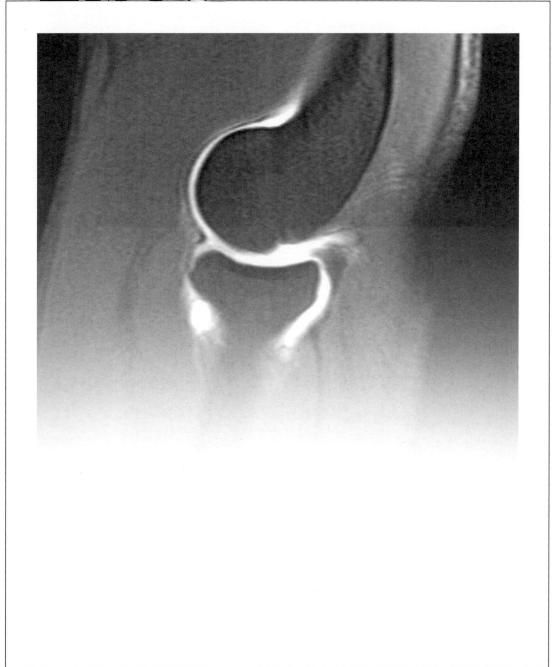

Laura W. Bancroft, Thomas H. Berquist, and Debbie J. Merinbaum

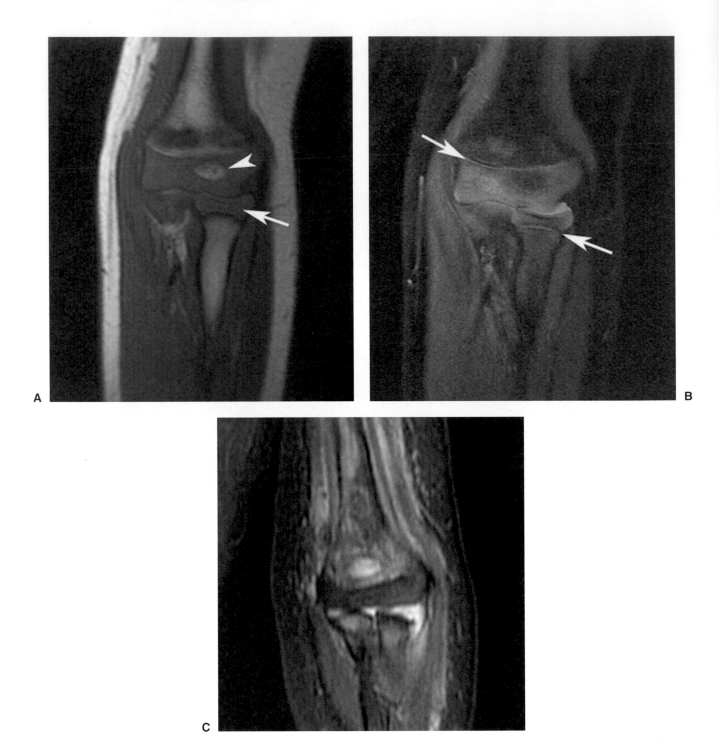

FIGURE 5-1 Normal elbow in a two-and-a-half-year-old child. A: Coronal T1-weighted image shows the capitellar ossification center (*arrowhead*) in a two-and-a-half-year-old child that has fatty marrow signal intensity. The developing radial head ossification center (*arrow*) is discrete from the radial head cartilage on T1-weighted image, but not yet ossified. **B:** Coronal FSE proton density fat-suppressed image shows hyperintense signal within the physes (*arrows*) that is more intense than the adjacent cartilaginous epiphyses. **C:** Compared to **(B)**, coronal short tau inversion recovery (STIR) sequence shows greater and more heterogeneous signal intensity throughout the bones in this normal child.

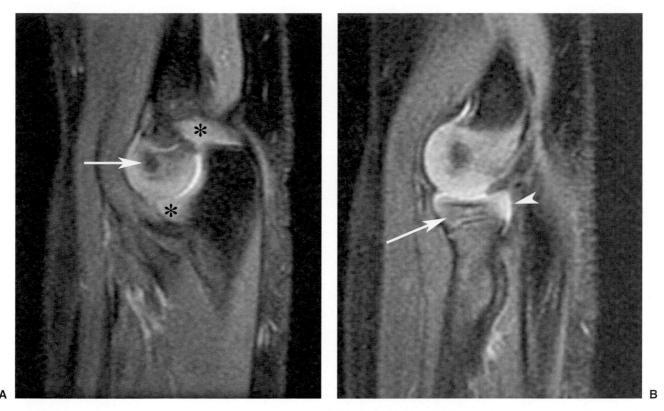

A   B

FIGURE 5-2   Normal elbow in a two-and-a-half-year-old child. A: Sagittal FSE T2-weighted fat-suppressed image shows the unmineralized portions (*asterisk*) of the olecranon that are isointense to the articular cartilage. Note the trochlear ossification center (*arrow*). **B:** Sagittal image through the radiocapitellar joint shows the maturing radial head ossification center (*arrow*) and cartilaginous portion (*arrowhead*) of the radial head.

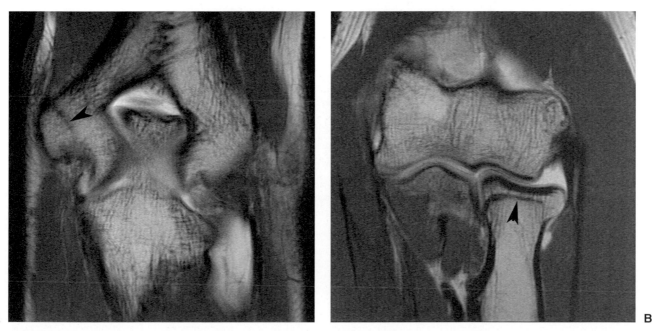

A   B

FIGURE 5-3   Prominent physeal scars. A and **B:** Coronal T1-weighted images from arthrogram show normal, linear low signal intensity physeal scars (*arrowheads*) that should not be confused with nondisplaced fractures.

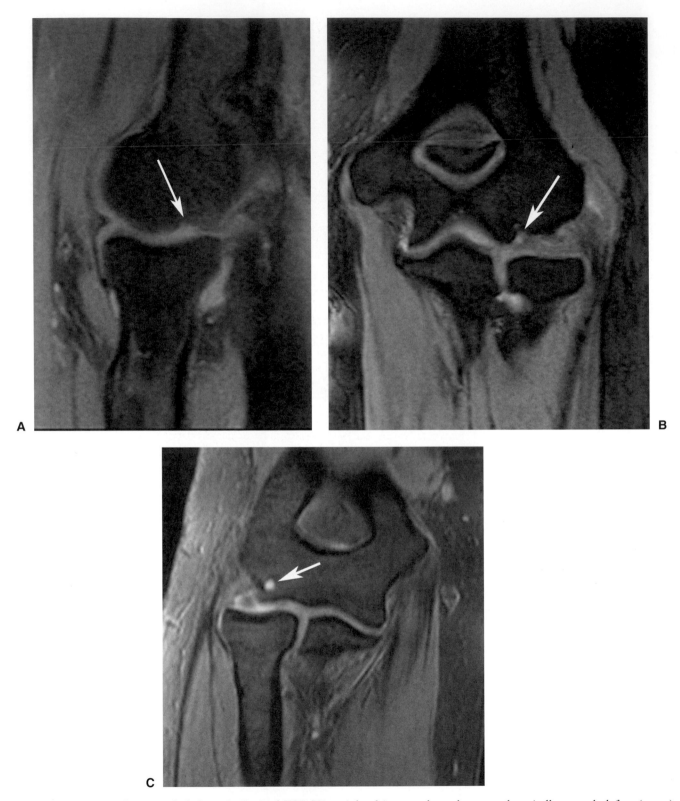

FIGURE 5-4   Capitellar pseudodefect. A: Sagittal FSE T2-weighted images show the normal capitellar pseudodefect (*arrow*), which is normally devoid of cartilage and should not be misinterpreted as an impaction injury. **B** and **C:** Coronal double echo steady state (DESS) images show the normal structures at the site of prior synchondrosis.

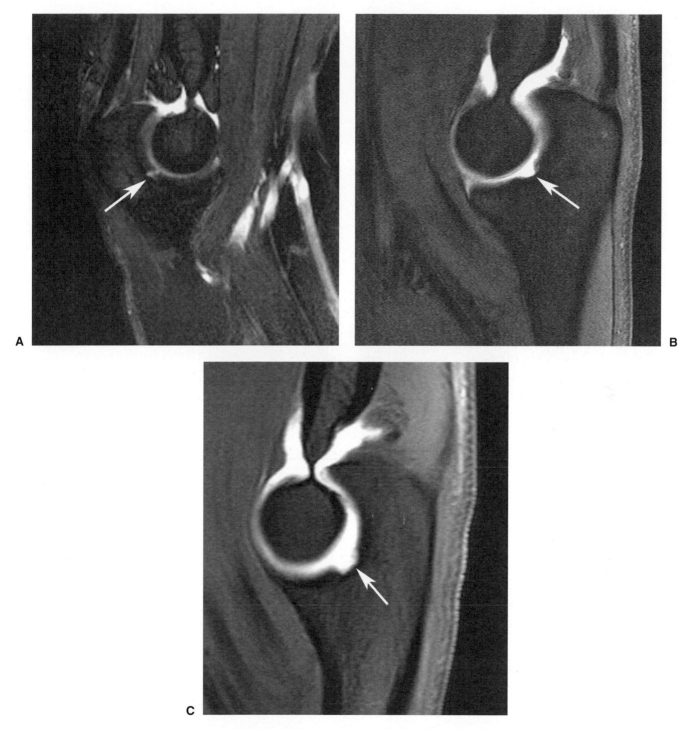

FIGURE 5-5   Olecranon pseudodefect. Sagittal **(A)** T2-weighted and **(B)** MR arthrographic images show normal olecranon pseudodefects (*arrows*) that should not be misinterpreted as osteochondral defects. **C:** Prominent olecranon pseudodefect (*arrow*) in a different patient.

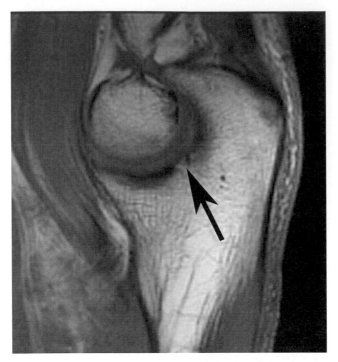

FIGURE 5-6   Transverse trochlear ridge. The normal transverse trochlear ridge of the olecranon (*arrow*) provides further stabilization to the elbow.

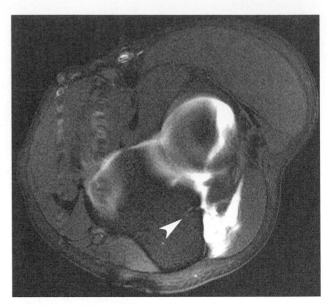

FIGURE 5-7   Olecranon nutrient vessel. Axial MR arthrogram shows contrast within an olecranon nutrient vessel (*arrowhead*).

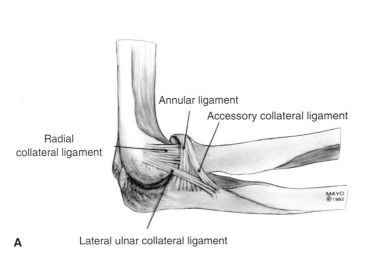

Radial collateral ligament

Annular ligament

Accessory collateral ligament

Lateral ulnar collateral ligament

MAYO © 1982

A

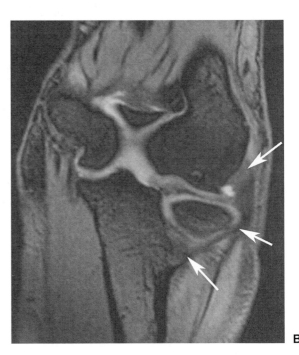

B

FIGURE 5-8   Lateral collateral ligament. A: Illustration of the lateral collateral ligament of the elbow. This traditional description occurs in only one quarter of dissected specimens. **B:** Coronal double echo steady state (DESS) show the lateral ulnar collateral ligament (*arrows*), which is the strongest elbow stabilizer and variably present.

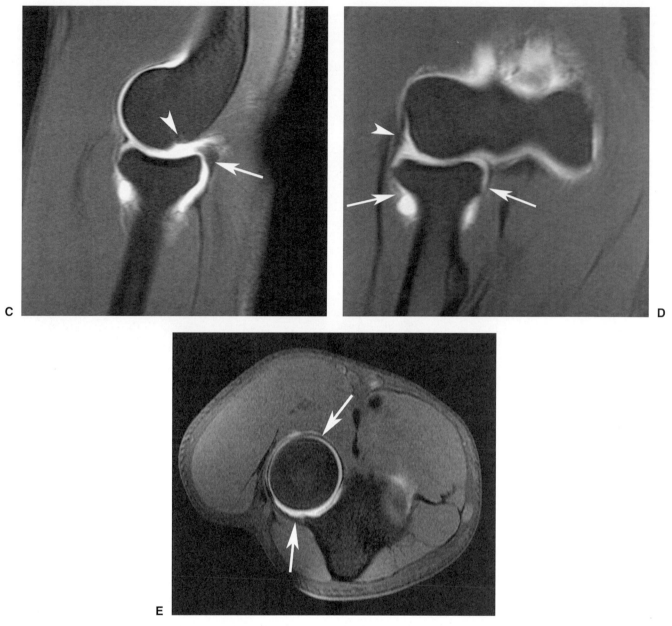

FIGURE 5-8 Lateral collateral ligament. (*continued*) **C:** sagittal MR arthrograms show the lateral ulnar collateral ligament (*arrows*), which is the strongest elbow stabilizer and variably present. **D:** Coronal and **(E)** axial MR arthrographic images show the radial collateral ligament proper (*arrowhead*) and the annular ligament (*arrows*).

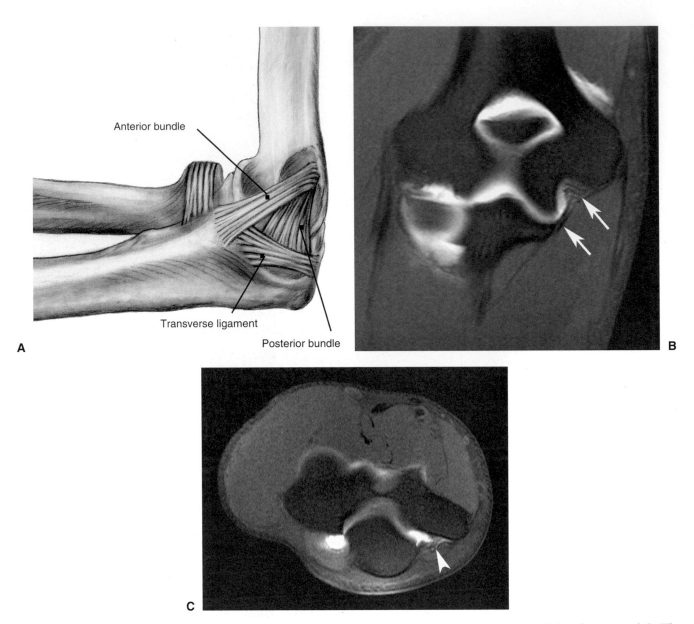

FIGURE 5-9 **Medial collateral ligament. A:** Illustration of the medial (or ulnar) collateral ligament of the elbow. **B** and **C:** The anterior (*arrows*) and posterior (*arrowhead*) bands of the medial collateral ligament are usually present, although the transverse (or oblique) band is only present in approximately a quarter of cases.

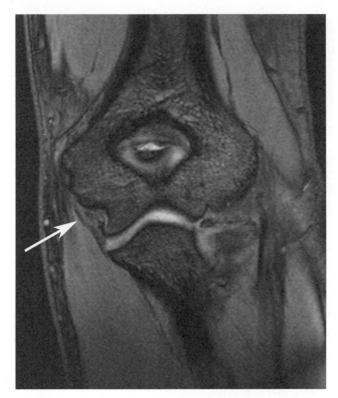

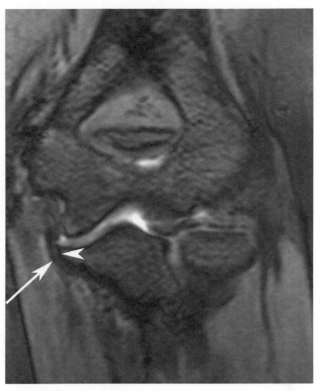

FIGURE 5-10 Heterogeneous signal in the proximal anterior band of the ulnar collateral ligament. Coronal double echo steady state (DESS) image shows the normal fan-shaped proximal aspect of the anterior band of the ulnar collateral ligament (*arrow*), with increased and slightly heterogeneous signal intensity. The distal attachment onto the sublime tubercle is smaller and lower in signal intensity.

FIGURE 5-11 Anterior band ulnar collateral ligament (UCL) attachment distal to sublime tubercle. Although the anterior band of the UCL usually attaches directly onto the sublime tubercle, normal variation includes a more distal attachment (*arrow*) a few millimeters distal to the tubercle. The fluid (*arrowhead*) in the recess should not be mistaken for a partial thickness ligamentous tear.

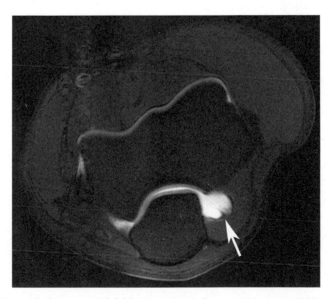

FIGURE 5-12 Synovial folds. Normal, thin synovial folds (*arrow*) may be conspicuous on MR arthrography of the elbow.

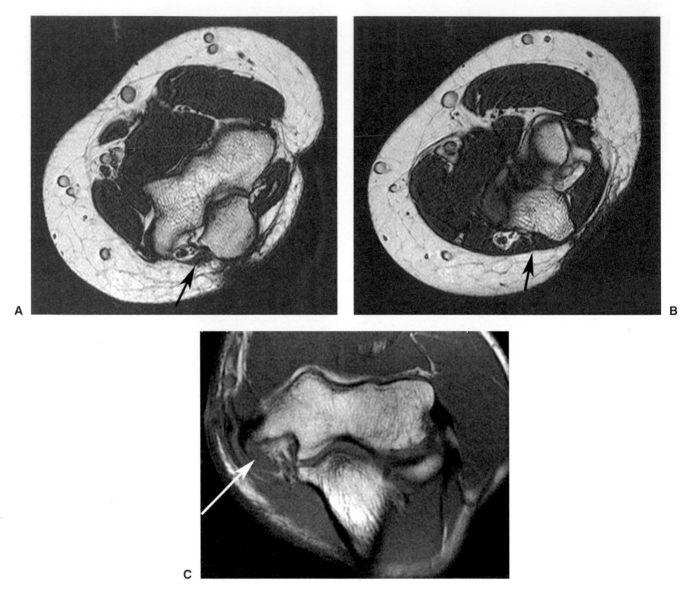

FIGURE 5-13 Anconeus epitrochlearis. A–C: Axial and coronal images demonstrate an anconeus epitrochlearis (*arrows*), which is also called the *accessory anconeus*. The medial head of the triceps can extend distally to form an arch across the ulnar groove in this variation, and has the potential to create mass effect and impinge upon the ulnar nerve.

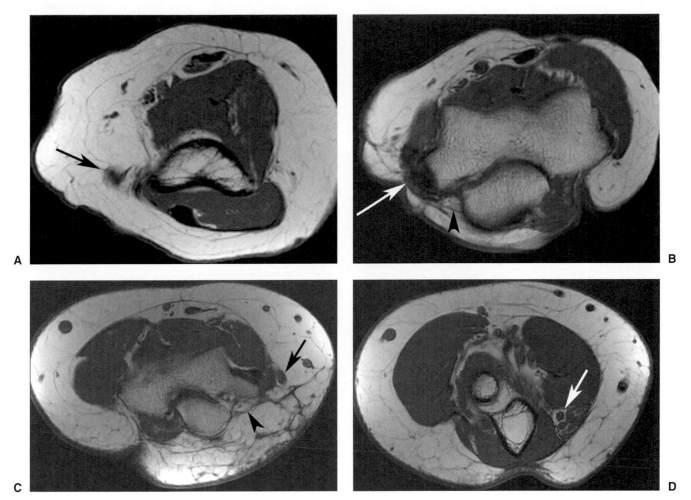

FIGURE 5-14 **Ulnar transposition. A:** Axial T1-weighted image superior to the elbow joint shows the transposed ulnar nerve (*arrow*), which could be mistaken for a subcutaneous vein on this single image. **B:** However, imaging distally shows an empty cubital tunnel (*arrowhead*) and anteromedial displacement of the ulnar nerve (*arrow*). **C:** Ulnar transposition in a different patient shows anteromedial displacement of the ulnar nerve (*arrow*) out of the cubital tunnel (*arrowhead*). **D:** More distal imaging shows return of the ulnar nerve (*arrow*) to its normal location.

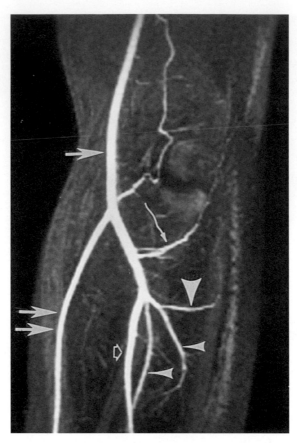

FIGURE 5-15 MRA of elbow and proximal forearm. Although arterial anatomy can be variant, the usual configuration is presented. The distal brachial artery (*large arrow*), proximal radial (*double arrow*), and ulnar (*open arrow*) arteries are demonstrated. The proximal portions of the anterior and posterior ulnar recurrent arteries (*curved arrow*), anterior and posterior interosseous arteries (*small arrowheads*) and posterior interosseous recurrent artery (*large arrowhead*) are well visualized. (From Berquist TH. MRI of the Musculoskeletal System, 5th ed. Philadelphia: Lippincott Williams & Wilkins, 2006.)

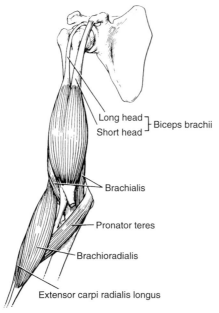

FIGURE 5-16 Illustration of superficial flexors of elbow. (From Berquist TH. *MRI of the musculoskeletal system*, 5th ed. Philadelphia: Lippincott Williams & Wilkins, 2006.)

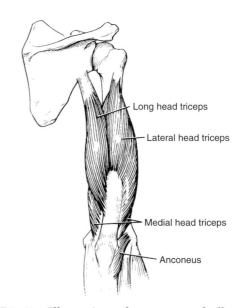

FIGURE 5-17 Illustration of extensors of elbow. (From Berquist TH. *MRI of the musculoskeletal system*, 5th ed. Philadelphia: Lippincott Williams & Wilkins, 2006.)

Table 5-1 Muscles of the elbow

Muscle	Origin	Insertion	Action	Blood Supply	Innervation
Biceps brachii	Two heads 1. Supraglenoid tubercle 2. Coracoid	1. Radial tuberosity (bursa separates tendon from tuberosity) 2. Aponeurosis to forearm flexors	Elbow flexor supinator	Brachial branches	Musculocutaneous C5-6
Brachialis	Low 2/3 anterior humerus	Coronoid and ulnar tuberosity	Elbow flexor	Brachial branches	Musculocutaneous C5-6
Brachioradialis	Supracondylar ridge lateral humerus	Distal lateral radius	Elbow flexor	Radial and radial recurrent arteries	Radial C5-6
Pronator teres	Two heads 1. Medial supracondylar ridge and interosseous membrane 2. Coronoid of ulna	Midlateral radius	Pronation accessory elbow flexor	Ulnar and recurrent ulnar arteries	Median C5-7
Triceps brachii	Three heads 1. Infraglenoid tubercle 2. Posterior humerus above radial groove 3. Lower 2/3	Olecranon	Elbow extensor	Profunda brachii	Radial
Anconeus	Posterolateral epicondyle	Lateral olecranon and proximal ulna	Elbow extensor	Recurrent radial artery	Radial
Supinator	Lateral epicondyle, radial ligament, annular ligament, ulna	Upper lateral radius	Supination	Radial artery	Median

(From Berquist TH. *MRI of the musculoskeletal system*, 4th ed. Philadelphia: Lippincott Williams & Wilkins, 2001; Rosse C, Rosse PC. *Hollinshead's textbook of anatomy*. Philadelphia: Lippincott–Raven, 1997; Morrey BF. *The elbow and its disorders*, 3rd ed. Philadelphia: WB Saunders, 2000.)

Suggested Readings

Abu-Hijleh MF. Three-headed biceps brachii muscle associated with duplicated musculocutaneous nerve. *Clin Anat*. 2005;18:376–379.

Beckett KS, McConnell P, Lagopoulos M, et al. Variations in the normal anatomy of the collateral ligaments of the human elbow joint. *J Anat*. 2000;197:507–511.

Bozkurt MC, Tagil SM, Ersoy M, et al. Muscle variations and abnormal branching and course of the ulnar nerve in the forearm and hand. *Clin Anat*. 2004;17:64–66.

Chow JCY, Papachristos AA. An aberrant anatomic variation along the course of the unar nerve about the elbow with coexistent cubital tunnel syndrome. *Clin Anat*. 2006;19:661–664.

Contreras MG, Warner MA, Charboneau WJ, et al. Anatomy of the ulnar nerve at the elbow: Potential relationship of acute ulnar neuropathy of gender differences. *Clin Anat*. 1998;11:372–378.

El-Naggar MM, Al-Saggaf S. Variant of the coracobrachialis muscle with a tunnel for the median nerve and brachial artery. *Clin Anat*. 2004;17:139–143.

Fuss FK. The ulnar collateral ligament of the human elbow joint: Anatomy, function and biomechanics. *J Anat*. 1991;175:203–212.

Gormus G, Ozcelik M, Celik HH, et al. Variant origin of the ulnar artery. *Clin Anat*. 1998;11:62–64.

Hennerbicler A, Etzer C, Gruber S, et al. Lateral arm flap: Analysis of its anatomy and modification using a vascularized fragment of the distal humerus. *Clin Anat*. 2003;16:204–214.

Jeon IH, Fairbain KJ, Neumann L, et al. MRI of edematous anconeus epitrochlearis: Another cause of medial elbow pain? *Skeletal Radiol*. 2005;24:103–107.

Kim YS, Yeh LR, Trudell D, et al. MRI of the major nerves about the elbow: Cadaveric study examining the effect of flexion and extension of the elbow and pronation and supination of the forearm. *Skeletal Radiol*. 1998;27:419–426.

Konjengbam M, Elangbam J. Radial nerve in the radial tunnel: Anatomic sites of entrapment neuropathy. *Clin Anat*. 2004;17:21–25.

Kumar MR. Multiple arterial variations in the upper limb of a south Indian female cadaver. *Clin Anat*. 2004;17:233–235.

Latev MD, Dalley AF. Nerve supply of the brachioradialis muscle: Surgically relevant variations of the extramuscular branches of the radial nerve. *Clin Anat*. 2005;18:488–492.

Lordan J, Rauh P, Spinner RJ. The clinical anatomy of the supracondylar spur and the ligament of Struthers. *Clin Anat*. 2005;18:548–551.

Loukas M, Curry B. A case of an atypical radial artery. *Clin Anat*. 2006;19:706–707.

Loukas M, Louis RG, South G, et al. A case of an accessory brachialis muscle. *Clin Anat*. 2006;19:550–553.

Mannan A, Sarikcioglu L, Ghani S, et al. Superficial ulnar artery terminating in a normal ulnar artery. *Clin Anat*. 2005;18:602–605.

Mitsuyasu H, Yoshida R, Shah M, et al. Unusual variant of the extensor carpi radialis brevis muscle: A case report. *Clin Anat*. 2004;17:61–63.

Morrey BF, An KN. Functional anatomy of the ligaments of the elbow. *Clin Orthop Rel Res*. 1985;201:85–89.

Nael K, Ruehm SG, Michaely HJ, et al. Multistation whole-body high-spatial resolution MR angiography using a 32-channel MR system. *AJR Am J Roentgenol*. 2007;188:529–539.

Oh CS, Chung IH, Koh KS. Anatomical study of the accessory head of the flexor pollicis longus and the anterior interosseous nerve in Asians. *Clin Anat*. 2000;13:434–438.

Ozan H, Atasever A, Sinav C, et al. An unusual insertion of accessory biceps brachii muscle. *Kaibogaku Zasshi*. 1997;72:515–529.

Ray B, Rai AL, Roy TS. Unusual insertion of the coracobrachialis muscle to the brachial fascia associated with high division of brachial artery. *Clin Anat*. 2004;17:672–676.

Rose SC, Kadir S. Arterial anatomy of the upper extremities. In: Kadir S, ed. *Atlas of normal and variant angiographic anatomy*. Philadelphia: WB Saunders; 1991:55–95.

Rosenberg ZS, Beltran J, Cheung Y, et al. MRI of the elbow: Normal variant and potential diagnostic pitfalls of the trochlear groove and cubital tunnel. *AJR Am J Roentgenol*. 1995;164:415–418.

Sarikcioglu L, Yildirim FB, Chiba S. Unilateral occurrence of a chondroepitrochlearis muscle. *Clin Anat*. 2004;17:272–275.

Tiengo C, Macchi V, Porzionato A, et al. Anatomical study of perforator arteries in the distally based radial forearm fasciosubcutaneous flap. *Clin Anat*. 2004;17:636–642.

Tubbs RS, Salter EG, Oakes WJ. Triceps brachii muscle demonstrating a fourth head. *Clin Anat*. 2006;19:657–660.

Vicente DP, Calvet PF, Burgaya AC, et al. Innervation of biceps brachii and brachialis: Anatomical and surgical approach. *Clin Anat*. 2005;18:186–194.

Chapter 6

Forearm

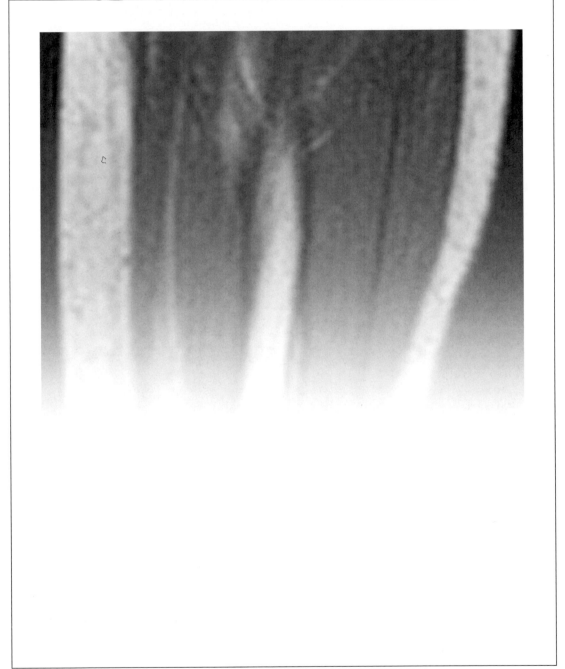

Laura W. Bancroft, Thomas H. Berquist, and Debbie J. Merinbaum

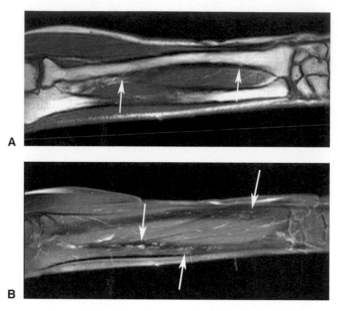

FIGURE 6-1 **Aggressive osteopenia.** Long axis imaging through the forearm demonstrates multiple small, mottled foci (*arrows*) of fat-equivalent signal in the radial and ulnar cortices on (**A**) T1-weighted images and higher signal on (**B**) FSE T2-weighted images. Findings are caused by cortical tunneling from osteopenia and should not be mistaken for malignancy.

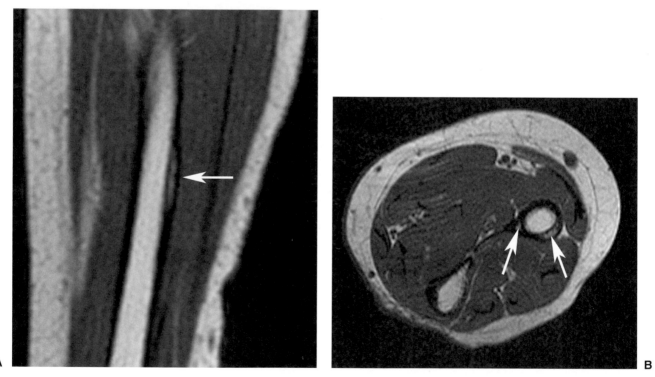

FIGURE 6-2 **Normal contour of mid-radius.** T1-weighted (**A**) long axis and (**B**) axial imaging through the mid-forearm demonstrates apparent cortical thickening (*arrows*) of the mid radius, which is merely the normal contour.

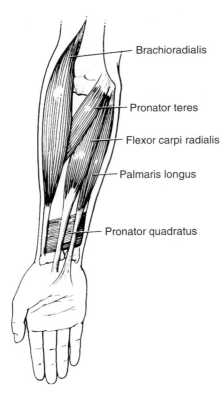

FIGURE 6-3 **Illustration of pronators of forearm.** (From Berquist TH. *MRI of the musculoskeletal system*, 5th ed. Lippincott Williams & Wilkins; 2006.)

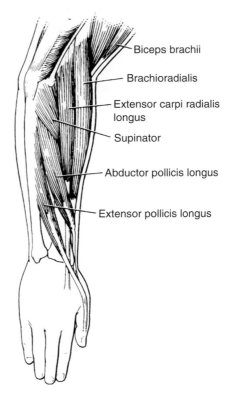

FIGURE 6-4 **Illustration of supinators of forearm.** (From Berquist TH. *MRI of the musculoskeletal system*, 5th ed. Lippincott Williams & Wilkins; 2006.)

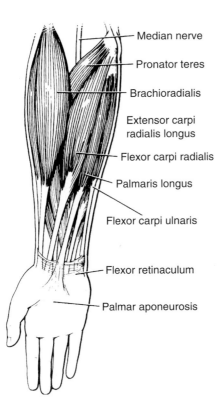

FIGURE 6-5 **Illustration of superficial flexor and extensors of forearm.** (From Berquist TH. *MRI of the musculoskeletal system*, 5th ed. Lippincott Williams & Wilkins; 2006.)

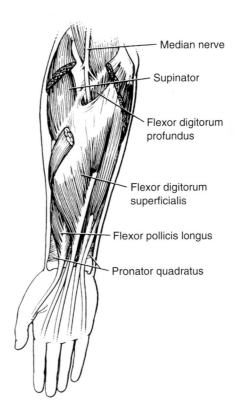

FIGURE 6-6 **Illustration of intermediate flexors of forearm.** (From Berquist TH. *MRI of the musculoskeletal system*, 5th ed. Lippincott Williams & Wilkins; 2006.)

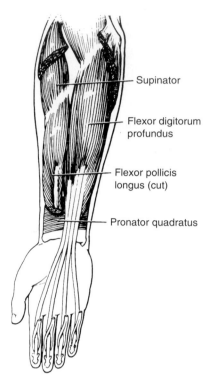

FIGURE 6-7 **Illustration of deep flexors of forearm.** (From Berquist TH. *MRI of the musculoskeletal system*, 5th ed. Lippincott Williams & Wilkins; 2006.)

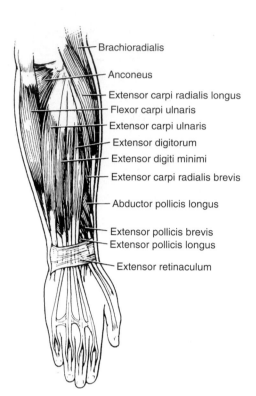

FIGURE 6-8 **Illustration of extensors of forearm.** (From Berquist TH. *MRI of the musculoskeletal system*, 5th ed. Lippincott Williams & Wilkins; 2006.)

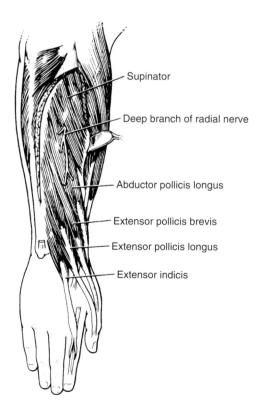

FIGURE 6-9 **Illustration of deep extensors of forearm.** (From Berquist TH. *MRI of the musculoskeletal system*, 5th ed. Lippincott Williams & Wilkins; 2006.)

Table 6-1 Muscles of the forearm

Muscles	Origin	Insertion	Action	Innervation
Flexors				
Superficial group				
Pronator teres	Two heads 1. Medial supracondylar ridge and interosseous membrane 2. Coronoid of ulna	Midlateral radius	Pronator, elbow flexor	Median C5-7
Flexor carpi radialis	Common flexor tendon (medial epicondyle)	Second metacarpal base	Wrist flexor	Median
Palmaris longus	Common flexor tendon (medial epicondyle)	Palmar aponeurosis	Wrist flexor	Median
Flexor carpi ulnaris	Two heads 1. Common flexor tendon 2. Upper radius and distal to tubercle	Hamate hook and fifth metacarpal base	Wrist flexor	Ulnar nerve
Intermediate group				
Flexor digitorum superficialis	Two heads 1. Common flexor tendon 2. Upper radius and distal to tubercle	Base 2–5 middle phalanx	Flexion proximal interphalangeal joints	Median
Deep group				
Flexor digitorum profundus	Anterior 2/3 ulna and interosseous membrane	Distal phalanges 2–5	Flexion of fingers	Median and ulnar
Flexor pollicis longus	Middle 1/3 radius and interosseous membrane	Distal phalanx thumb	Thumb flexor	Median
Pronator quadratus	Distal 1/4 anterior ulna	Distal 1/4 anterior radius	Pronation	Median
Extensors				
Superficial group				
Brachioradialis	Low 2/3 anterior humerus	Coronoid and ulnar tuberosity	Elbow flexor	Radial C5-6
Extensor carpi radialis longus	Low 1/3 supracondylar ridge humerus	Radial dorsal base second metacarpal	Extend wrist	Radial
Extensor carpi radialis brevis	Common extensor tendon lateral epicondyle	Base third metacarpal	Extend wrist	Radial
Extensor digitorum	Common extensor tendon lateral epicondyle	Distal 2–5 phalanges	Common extensor fingers	Radial
Extensor digiti minimi	Extensor digitorum	Distal small finger	Extensor fifth finger	Radial
Extensor carpi ulnaris	Two heads 1. Common extensor tendon 2. Posterior ulnar border	Medial side base fifth metacarpal	Wrist extensor, ulnar abduction	Radial

(continued)

Table 6-1 Muscles of the forearm *(continued)*

Muscles	Origin	Insertion	Action	Innervation
Deep group				
Abductor pollicis longus	Posterior ulna, interosseous membrane, middle posterior radius	Lateral base first metacarpal	Long abduction thumb	Radial
Extensor pollicis brevis	Midposterior radius	Base proximal phalanx of thumb	Extensor thumb	Radial
Extensor pollicis longus	Mid 1/3 posterior radius	Base distal phalanx of thumb	Extends phalanges of thumb	Radial
Extensor indicis	Posterior radius and interosseous membrane	Proximal phalanx index finger	Extensor index finger	Radial

(From Berquist TH. *MRI of the musculoskeletal system*, 4th ed. Philadelphia: Lippincott Williams & Wilkins; 2001; Rosse C, Rosse PC. *Hollinshead's textbook of anatomy*. Philadelphia: Lippincott–Raven; 1997; Morrey BF. *The elbow and its disorders*, 3rd ed. Philadelphia: WB Saunders; 2000.)

Suggested Readings

Canovas F, Mouilleron P, Bonnel F. Biometry of the muscular branches of the median nerve to the forearm. *Clin Anat*. 1998;11:239–245.

Lopez Milena G, Ruiz Santiago F, Chamorro Santos C, et al. Forearm soft tissue mass caused by an accessory muscle. *Skeletal Radiol*. 2001;11:1487–1489.

Nael K, Ruehm SG, Michaely HJ, et al. Multistation whole-body high-spatial resolution MR angiography using a 32-channel MR system. *AJR Am J Roentgenol*. 2007;188:529–539.

Rose SC, Kadir S. Arterial anatomy of the upper extremities. In: Kadir S, ed. *Atlas of normal and variant angiographic anatomy*. Philadelphia: WB Saunders; 1991:55–95.

Tao KZ, Chen EY, Ji RM, et al. Anatomical study on arteries of fasciae in the forearm fasciocutaneous flap. *Clin Anat*. 2000;13:1–5.

Tiengo C, Macchi V, Stecco C. Epifascial accessory palmaris longus muscle. *Clin Anat*. 2006;19:554–557.

Van Riet RP, Van Glabeek FV, Neale PG, et al. Anatomical considerations of the radius. *Clin Anat*. 2004;17:564–569.

Chapter 7

Wrist/Hand

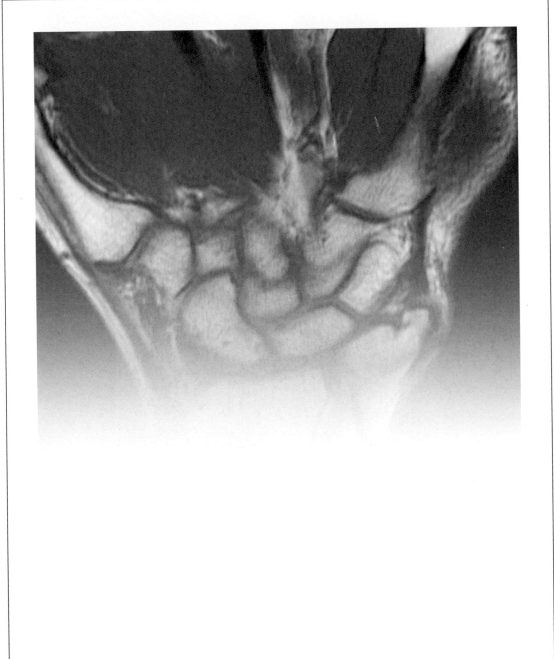

Laura W. Bancroft, Mark J. Kransdorf, and Thomas H. Berquist

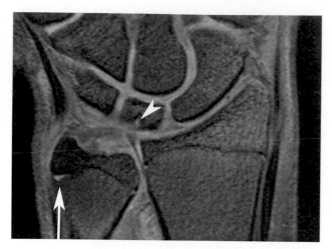

FIGURE 7-1   Pediatric wrist. Coronal double echo steady state (DESS) image shows high signal cartilage (*arrow*) within unfused portion of the ulnar physis. Note the nutrient foramen in the lunate (*arrowhead)* and mild ulnar negative variance.

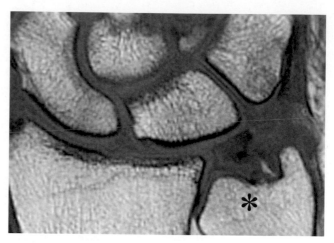

FIGURE 7-2   Ulnar negative variance. Coronal T1-weighted image shows mild ulnar negative variance (*asterisk*), which can be asymptomatic or potentially associated with Keinbock disease (ostechondrosis of the lunate).

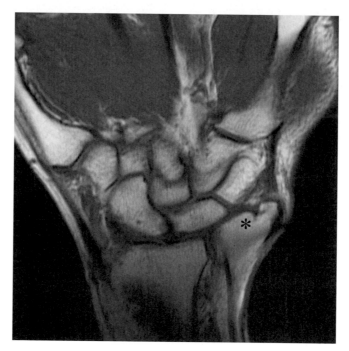

FIGURE 7-3   Ulnar positive variance and warp. Ulnar positive variance (*asterisk*) in this case is accentuated by warping artifact. Ulnar positive variance may be an incidental finding, associated with Madelung deformity or ulnolunate impaction syndrome.

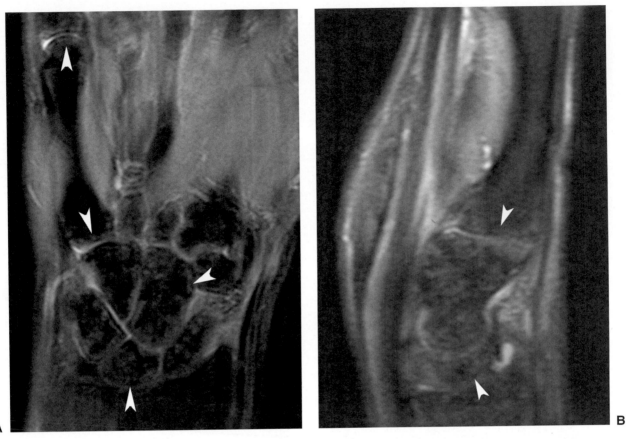

FIGURE 7-4 **Osteopenia. A** and **B:** Diffuse subcortical and intracortical mottling (*arrowheads*) on FSE T2-weighted fat-suppressed imaging is present in this patient with osteopenia. Signal changes may be due to hyperemia. The overlying cartilage is preserved and there is no underlying marrow edema-like signal. Therefore, findings should not be confused with erosions.

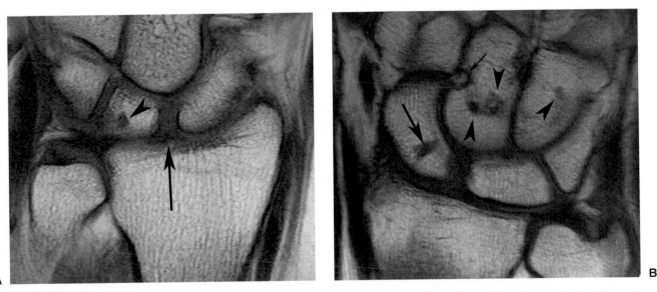

FIGURE 7-5 **Nutrient foramina. A:** Dorsal and volar lunate nutrient foramina (*arrowhead*) should not be confused with erosions. Note the prominent scapholunate interval (*arrow*) with intact ligament. **B:** Coronal T1-weighted images show normal nutrient foramina (*arrowheads*) in the capitate and triquetrum. Note the scaphoid bone island (*large arrow*) and normal deep groove in the lateral capitate at site of ligamentous attachment (*small arrow*).

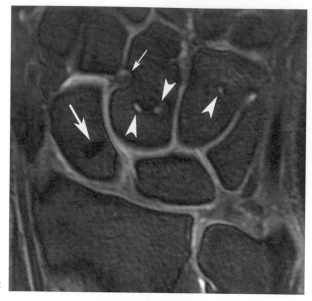

C

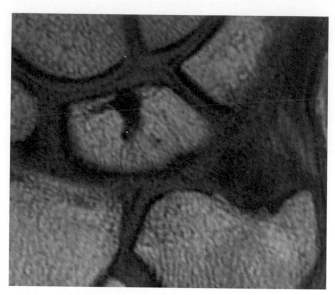

FIGURE 7-5 **Nutrient foramina.** (*continued*) **C:** Coronal double echo steady state (DESS) images show normal nutrient foramina (*arrowheads*) in the capitate and triquetrum. Note the scaphoid bone island (*large arrow*) and normal deep groove in the lateral capitate at site of ligamentous attachment (*small arrow*).

FIGURE 7-6 ■ **Bone island.** Classic appearance of a lunate bone island (enostosis) shows a spiculated signal void which blends with the normal trabeculae.

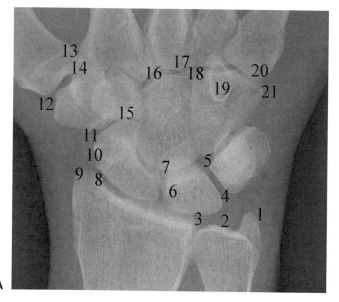

A

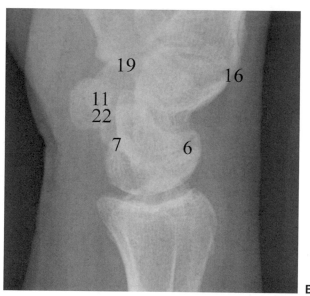

B

FIGURE 7-7 **Accessory ossicles and sesamoids.** Illustrations of accessory ossicles and sesamoids in the **(A)** frontal and **(B)** lateral projections (*1 = lunula* [*unfused ossification center of ulnar styloid process*], *2 = triangulare, 3 = ossicle at radioulnar articulation, 4 = accessory ossicle between lunate and triquetrum, 5 = epipyramis, 6 = epilunate, 7 = hypolunate, 8 = os para naviculare, 9 = unfused ossification center of radial styloid process, 10 = os vesalianum, 11 = epitrapezium, 12 = paratrapezium, 13 = secondary trapezium, 14 = secondary trapezoid, 15 = os centrale carpi, 16 = os styloideum, 17 = Gruber ossicle, 18 = secondary capitate, 19 = os hamuli proprium, 20 = os vesalianum, 21 = os ulnare externum, 22 = radial externum*).

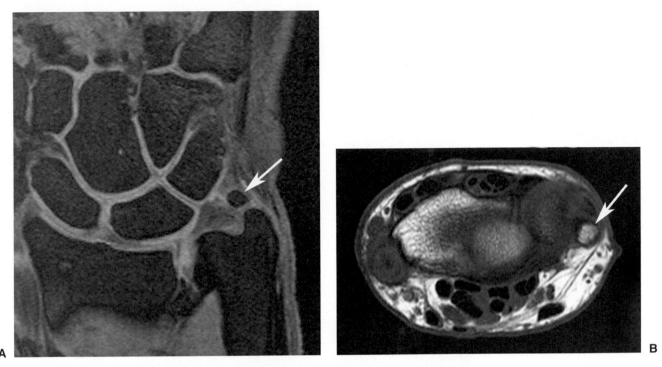

FIGURE 7-8 **Lunula. A** and **B:** Accessory ossicle distal to the ulnar styloid (*arrow*) is commonly present. Note that the ulnar styloid is normal in length and overlying cartilage; therefore, this normal variant should not be mistaken for an old avulsion fracture.

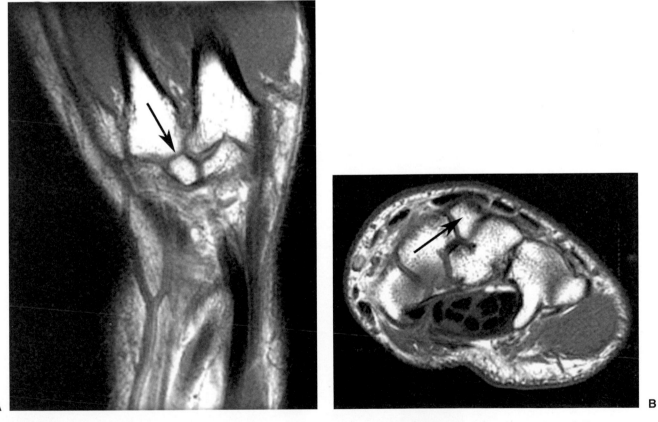

FIGURE 7-9 **Os styloideum. A** and **B:** Normal variant ossicle (*arrows*) dorsal to the capitate is known as an *os styloideum*.

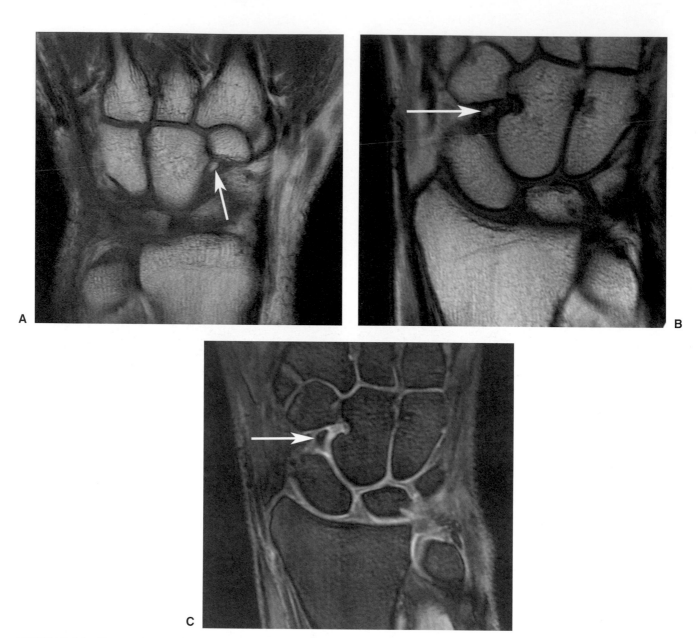

FIGURE 7-10 Os carpi centrale. A and **B:** Coronal T1-weighted images in two different patients show small accessory ossicles (*arrows*) between the scaphoid, capitate and trapezoid. This can develop in the deep fossa in the radial side of the capitate. **C:** Double echo steady state (DESS) image in the same patient as (**B**) shows low signal intensity within the os carpi centrale (*arrow*), due to blooming of the trabeculae.

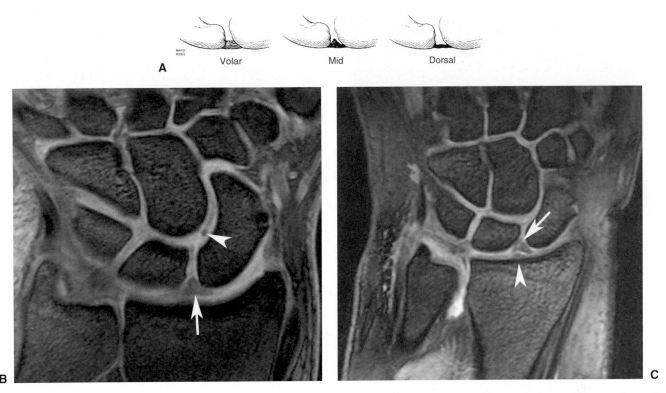

FIGURE 7-11 **Normal scapholunate ligament. A:** Illustration of the normal configuration of the scapholunate ligament depending on its location. (From Berquist TH. *MRI of the musculoskeletal system*, 5th ed. Philadelphia: Lippincott Williams & Wilkins; 2006). **B:** Normal triangular appearance of the mid scapholunate ligament (*arrow*) on double echo steady state (DESS) image (*Vacuum phenomenon = arrowhead*). **C:** Coronal DESS image shows a thin linear cleft (*arrow*) through the scapholunate ligament, which can be a normal variant, as in this case with arthroscopically intact ligament. Notice the relative prominence of the radial articular cartilage (*arrowhead*) between the scaphoid and lunate fossae.

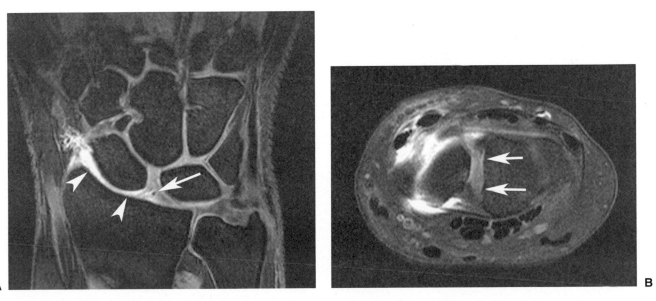

FIGURE 7-12 **Intact scapholunate ligament repair. A:** Mild heterogeneity of the scapholunate ligament (*arrow*) is present after primary ligamentous repair. Injected radiocarpal contrast (*arrowheads*) does not communicate with midcarpal joint, consistent with intact ligament. Scar tissue in the surgical bed prevents contrast extension into the ulnar aspect of the radiocarpal joint. **B:** Axial MR arthrogram shows integrity of the entire repaired scapholunate ligament (*arrows*).

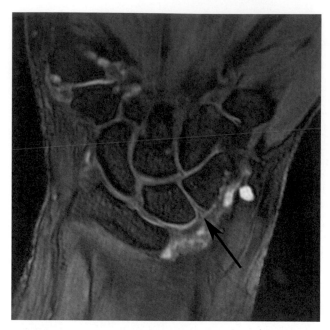

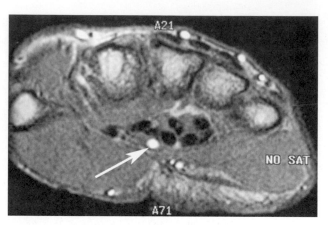

FIGURE 7-14 Persistent median artery. Axial FSE T2-weighted image shows a persistent median artery (*arrow*) in a patient who presented with "three pulses" in the wrist. A persistent median artery typically arises from the interosseous artery and supplies some of the palmar digital arteries that are normally supplied by the superficial palmar arch.

FIGURE 7-13 Lunatotriquetral ligament cleft. Coronal double echo steady state (DESS) sequence shows a thin, linear cleft (*arrow*) within the proximal aspect of the lunatotriquetral ligament. Arthroscopy demonstrated an intact ligament.

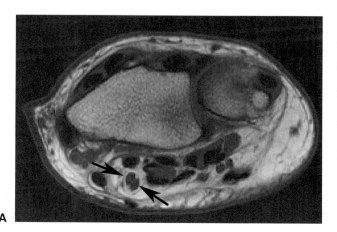

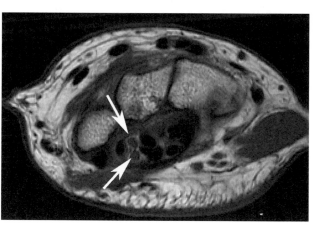

FIGURE 7-15 Bifid median nerve. A and **B:** The median nerve has prematurely bifurcated (*arrows*) proximal to the carpal tunnel. This is a normal variant of no clinical consequence.

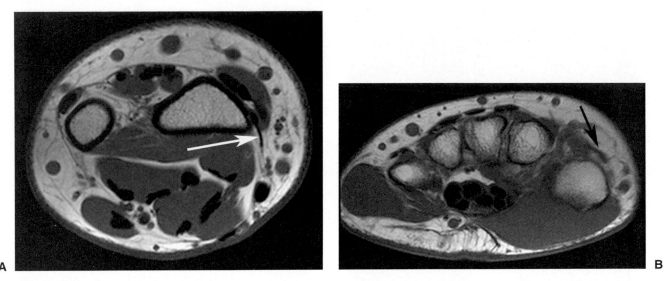

FIGURE 7-16 **Accessory first dorsal extensor muscle. A** and **B:** Axial T1-weighted images demonstrate an accessory first dorsal extensor muscle (*arrows*), normal variant.

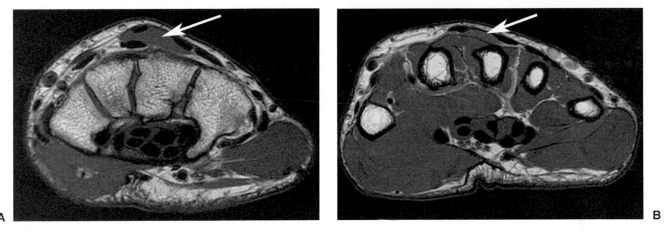

FIGURE 7-17 **Extensor digitorum brevis manus muscle. A** and **B:** Axial T1-weighted images demonstrate an extensor digitorum brevis manus muscle (*arrows*), normal variant.

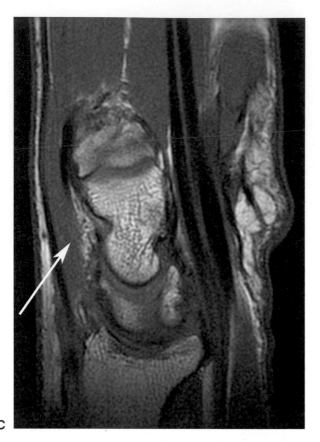

C

FIGURE 7-17 Extensor digitorum brevis manus muscle. (*continued*) **C:** sagittal T1-weighted images demonstrate an extensor digitorum brevis manus muscle (*arrows*), normal variant.

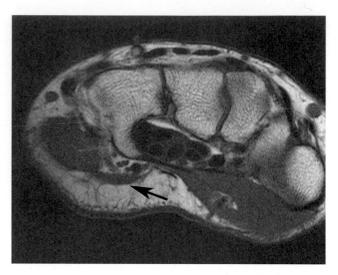

FIGURE 7-18 Accessory abductor digiti minimi muscle. Most accessory muscles within the Guyon canal are accessory abductor minimi muscles (*arrow*), which are located along the volar side of the neurovascular bundle and fuse with the abductor digiti minimi distally. These accessory slips of muscle may be asymptomatic or can cause ulnar nerve compression symptoms.

Table 7-1 Muscles of the hand

Muscles	Origin	Insertion	Action	Innervation
Lumbricals (four)	Tendons of flexor digitorum profundus	Extensor aponeurosis	Extensors of interphalangeal joints	Radial or first and second lumbricals—median nerve, third and fourth ulnar nerve
Flexor pollicis longus	Anterior middle one-third radius and interosseous membrane	Distal phalanx thumb	Flexor of thumb	Median nerve (anterior interosseous branch)
Interossei palmar (three)	Second, fourth, and fifth metacarpal diaphysis	Extensor aponeurosis	Abduction and adduction of fingers	Deep branch of ulnar nerve
Dorsal (four)	First to fifth metacarpal diaphyses	Proximal phalanges	Abduction and adduction of fingers	Deep branch of ulnar nerve
Abductor pollicis brevis	Flexor retinaculum, trapezium	Radial side proximal phalanx thumb	Abductor of thumb	Median nerve
Flexor pollicis brevis	Flexor retinaculum, trapezium, and trapezoid	Radial flexor aspect proximal phalanx thumb	Flexes and rotates thumb	Median nerve
Opponens pollicis	Flexor retinaculum, trapezium	Radial diaphysis first metacarpal	Stabilize and opposition of thumb	Median nerve

Table 7-1 Muscles of the hand (*continued*)

Muscles	Origin	Insertion	Action	Innervation
Adductor pollicis	Third metacarpal, trapezium, trapezoid, capitate	Base proximal phalanx thumb	Adduction of thumb	Median nerve
Palmaris brevis	Palmar aponeurosis (ulnar side)	Medial skin palm	Draws skin laterally	Deep branch ulnar nerve
Abductor digiti minimi	Pisiform	Ulnar base fifth proximal phalanx	Abductor fifth finger	Deep branch ulnar nerve
Flexor digiti minimi brevis	Hamate hook, flexor retinaculum	Ulnar base fifth proximal phalanx	Flexor fifth metacarpophalangeal (MCP) joint	Deep branch ulnar nerve
Opponens digiti minimi	Flexor retinaculum, distal hamate hook	Fifth metacarpal diaphysis	Draws fifth metacarpal anteriorly	Deep branch ulnar nerve

(From Berquist TH. Magnetic resonance imaging of the elbow and wrists. *Top Magn Reson Imaging*. 1989;1:15–27; Rosse C, Rosse PC. *Hollinshead's textbook of anatomy*. Philadelphia: Lippincott–Raven; 1997; Bishop AT, Gabel G, Carmichael SW. Flexor carpi radialis tendinitis. Part I: Operative anatomy. *J Bone Joint Surg Am*. 1994;76A:1009–1014.)

Table 7-2 Muscle variation in the hand/wrist

Lumbricals (absent, bifid distally, accessory slips, aberrant attachments)

Palmaris brevis (absent, vary in size, may join flexor digiti minimi brevis, insert onto pisiform)

Abductor digit minimi (absent, two or three slips, accessory heads [accessorius ad abductorem digiti minimi manus, pisimetacarpeus, pisiunicinatus, pisiannularis])

Flexor digiti minimi brevis (joined or replaced by abductor or opponens digiti minimi, absent)

Extensor digiti minimi (proprius, manus)

Extensor indicis proprius

Interosseous (doubled, second muscle may have three heads, absent)

(Compiled from Berman RA, Thompson SA, Afiti AK. Compendium of human anatomic variation. Baltimore: Urban and Schwartzenberg;1988.)

Suggested Readings

Beatty JD, Remedios D, McCullough CJ. An accessory extensor tendon of the thumb as a cause of dorsal wrist pain. *J Hand Surg Br*. 2000;25:110–111.

Bilge O, Pinar Y, Ozer MA, et al. A morphometric study on the superficial palmar arch of the hand. *Surg Radiol Anat*. 2006;28:343–350.

Clavert P, Dosch JC, Wolfram-Gabel R, et al. New findings on intermetacarpal fat pads: Anatomy and imaging. *Surg Radiol Anat*. 2006;28:351–354.

D'Costa S, Jiji PJ, Nayak SR, et al. Anomalous muscle belly to the index finger. *Ann Anat*. 2006;188:473–475.

De Ary-Pires B, Francisca Valdez C, Perin Shecaira A, et al. Cleland's and Grayson's ligaments of the hand: A morphometrical investigation. *Clin Anat*. 2007;20:68–76.

Dodds SD. A flexor carpi radialis brevis muscle with an anomalous origin on the distal radius. *J Hand Surg Am*. 2006;31:1507–1510.

Gassner EM, Schocke M, Peer S, et al. Persistent median artery in the carpal tunnel: Color Doppler ultrasonographic findings. *J Ultrasound Med*. 2002;21:455–461.

Johnson RK, Shrewsbury MM. Neural pattern in the human pollical distal phalanx. *Clin Anat*. 2005;18:428–433.

Jones DP. Bilateral palmaris profundus in association with bifid median nerve as a cause of failed carpal tunnel release. *J Hand Surg [Am]*. 2006;31:741–743.

Kang L, Carter T, Wolge SW. The flexor carpi radialis brevis muscle: An anomalous flexor of the wrist and hand. A case report. *J Hand Surg Am*. 2006;31:1511–1513.

Lamas C, Carrera A, Proubasta I, et al. The anatomy and vascularity of the lunate: Considerations applied to Kienböck's disease. *Chir Main*. 2007;26(1):13–20.

McQueen F, Ostergaard M, Peterfly C, et al. Pitfalls in scoring MR images of rheumatoid arthritis wrist and metacarpophalangeal joints. *Ann Rheum Dis*. 2005;64:48–55.

Malloy MA, Finger DR. Clinical image: Carpal tunnel syndrome from accessory lumbrical muscles. *Arthritis Rheum*. 2000;43:707.

Oettle AC, van Niekerk A, Boon JM, et al. Evaluation of Allen's test in both arms and arteries of left and right-handed people. *Surg Radiol Anat*. 2006;28:3–6.

Rose SC, Kadir S. Arterial anatomy of the upper extremities. In: Kadir S, ed. *Atlas of normal and variant angiographic anatomy*. Philadelphia: WB Saunders; 1991:55–95.

Tubbs RS, Salter EG, Oakes WJ. Contrahentes digitorum muscle. *Clin Anat*. 2005;18:606–608.

Tubbs RS, Loukas M. An unusual formation of the deep palmar arch. *Clin Anat*. 2006;19:708–709.

Varley I, Wales CJ, Carter LM. The median artery: Its potential implications for the radial forearm flap. *J Plast Reconstr Aesthet Surg*. 2007; Epub ahead of print.

Yalcin B, Kutoglu T, Ozan H, et al. The extensor indicis et medii communis. *Clin Anat*. 2006;19:112–114.

Section III

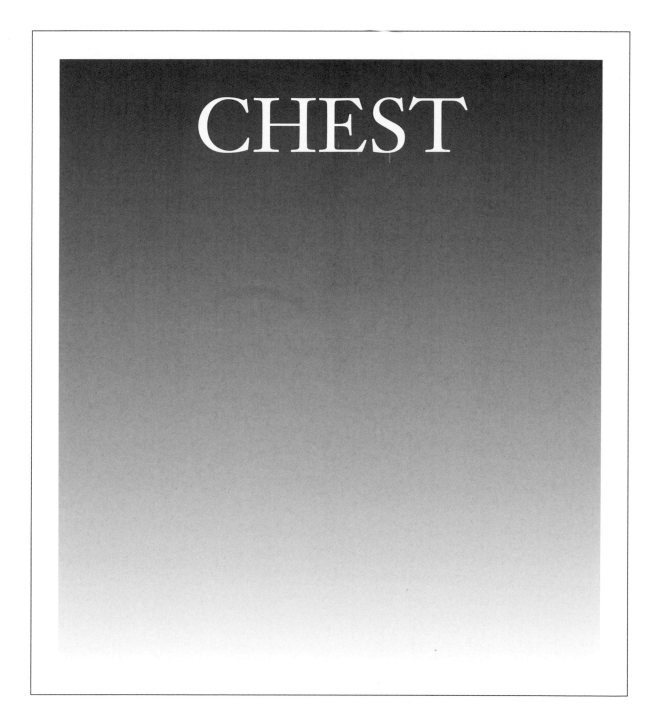

CHEST

Chapter 8

Breast

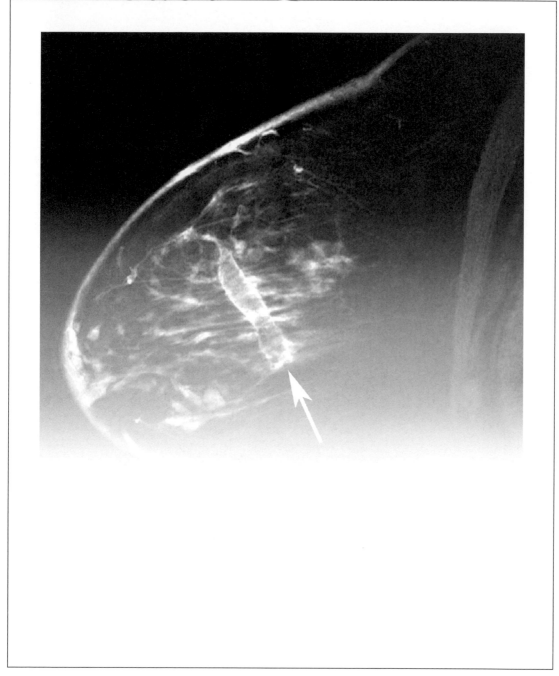

Elizabeth R. DePeri

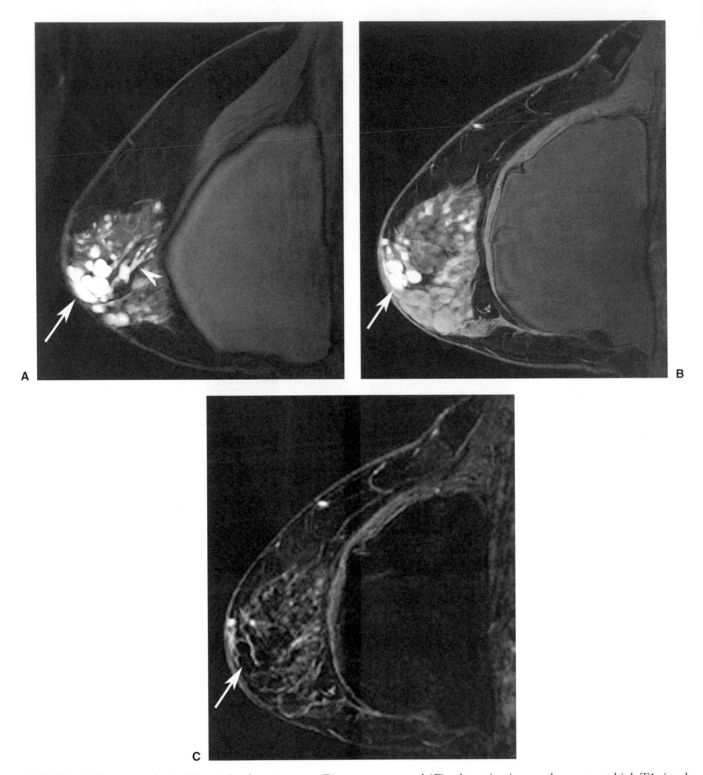

FIGURE 8-1 **Duct ectasia. A:** T1-weighted precontrast, **(B)** postcontrast and **(C)** subtraction images demonstrate high T1 signal and no enhancement. In the retroareolar region, ectasia takes a more cystic form (*long arrow*), while it appears more linear centrally (*arrowhead*).

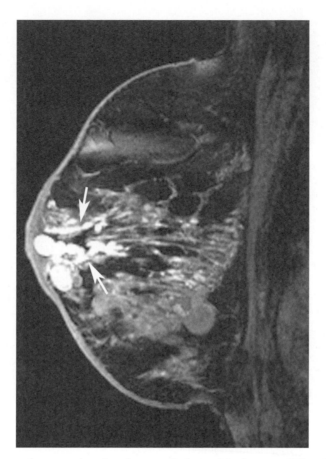

FIGURE 8-2 **Duct ectasia.** Retroareolar nonenhancing duct ectasia (*arrows*) is shown on T1-weighted sagittal image.

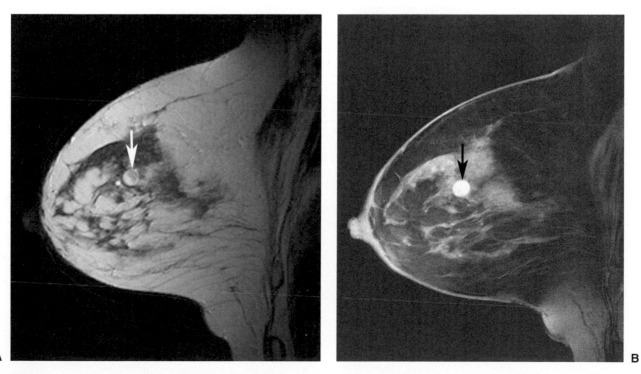

FIGURE 8-3 **Cyst. A:** T2-weighted, **(B)** T1-weighted precontrast enhanced sagittal images demonstrate hyperintense T1- and T2 signal, and thin uniform wall enhancement of a cyst (*arrows*). Precontrast cyst contents may be hypointense, intermediate signal, or hyperintense. Cyst walls may variably enhance.

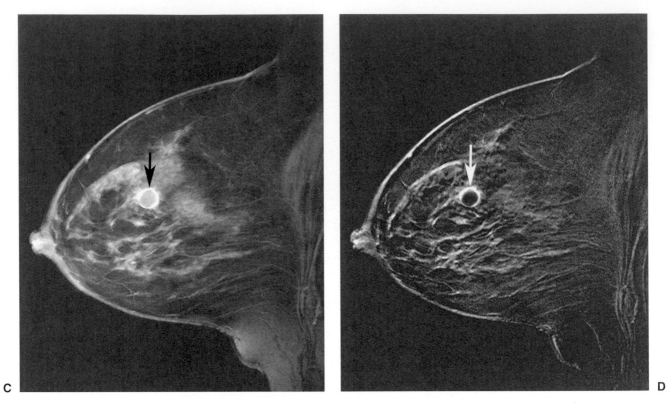

FIGURE 8-3   Cyst. (*continued*) **C:** T1-weighted postcontrast and (**D**) subtracted T1-weighted enhanced sagittal images demonstrate hyperintense T1- and T2 signal, and thin uniform wall enhancement of a cyst (*arrows*). Precontrast cyst contents may be hypointense, intermediate signal, or hyperintense. Cyst walls may variably enhance.

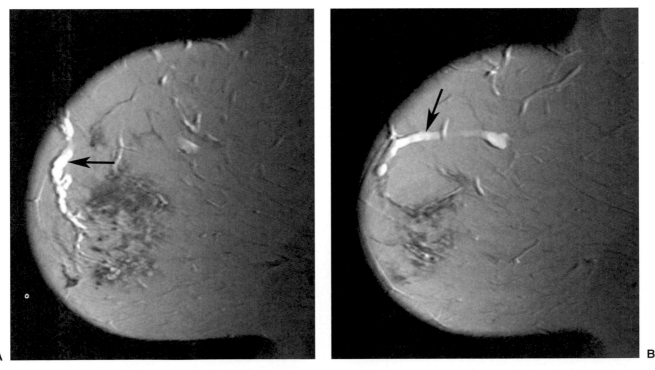

FIGURE 8-4   Ecstatic intramammary vessels. A and **B:** T2-weighted images demonstrate ecstatic, enlarged veins (*arrows*) anteriorly in the breast with hyperintense signal due to slow flow.

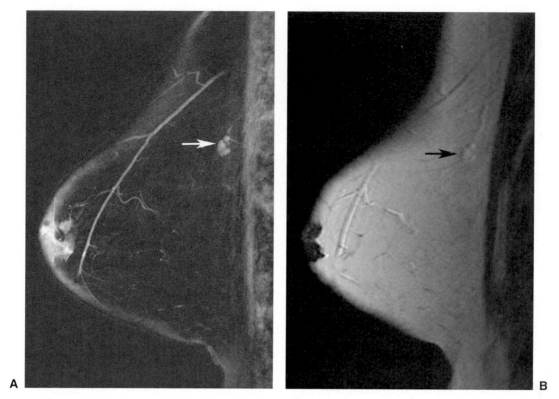

FIGURE 8-5 **Normal lymph node. A:** T1-weighted enhanced sagittal image demonstrates moderate enhancement of an architecturally normal posterosuperior lymph node (*arrow*). **B:** T2-weighted image demonstrates chemical shift artifact caused by fat and nodal soft tissue (*arrow*) misregistration in the frequency-encoding direction. Incidental note is made of artifact from suture in the subareolar region.

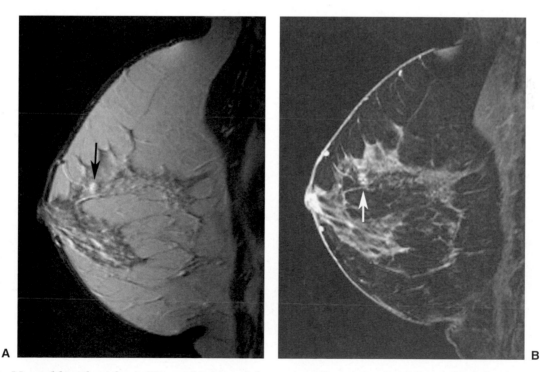

FIGURE 8-6 **Normal lymph node. A:** T2-weighted image demonstrates hyperintense signal and **(B)** T1-weighted postcontrast image demonstrates moderate enhancement in an ovoid lobulated nodule (*arrow*).

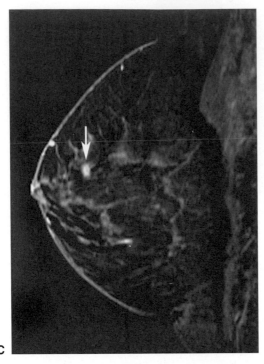

C

FIGURE 8-6 **Normal lymph node.** (*continued*) **C:** Subtracted image confirming moderate enhancement in the nodule (*arrow*), consistent in signal and architecturally with a normal lymph node.

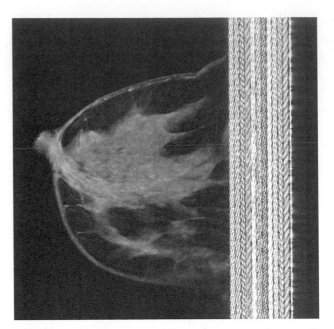

FIGURE 8-7 **Radiofrequency interference artifact.** Radiofrequency (RF) interference from a second nearby MR scanner. RF lines occur parallel to the phase direction (superior–inferior direction) at distinct frequencies along the frequency-encoding axis (anterior–posterior direction) in the image. Line artifacts are observed at several frequencies due to multiple frequencies in the transmitted RF during multislice acquisition.

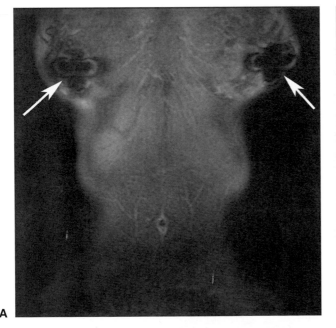

A

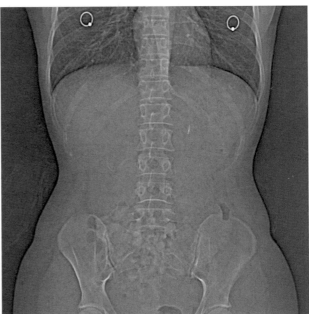

B

FIGURE 8-8 **Metal artifact from nipple rings. A:** Coronal MRI shows metal artifact (*arrows*) obscuring the breast tissue. Spatial distortion and spin dephasing are observed due to differences in magnetic susceptibility of the metal rings compared to that of air and tissue. **B:** CT topogram shows nipple rings.

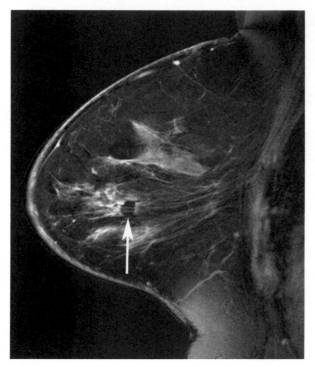

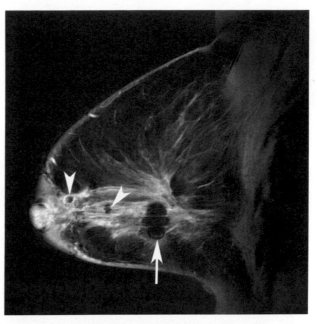

FIGURE 8-9 Artifact from biopsy marker. Sagittal T1-weighted enhanced image demonstrates a small central metallic signal void (*arrow*), consistent with site of radiopaque marker placed at the time of percutaneous needle biopsy.

FIGURE 8-10 Artifacts from biopsy marker and surgical sutures. Large central breast signal void (*arrow*) is consistent with metal artifact at site of radiopaque marker placed at the time of percutaneous needle biopsy. Small signal voids (*arrowheads*) more anteriorly are round and linear, consistent with postsurgical changes after periareolar incision.

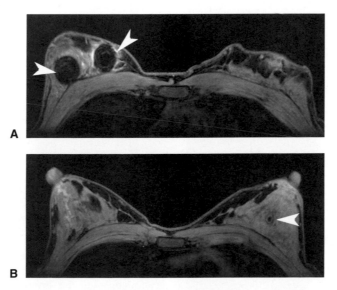

FIGURE 8-11 Artifact from biopsy marker. A and B: Axial T1-weighted images demonstrate round artifacts (*arrowheads*) of varying sizes produced by different types of metallic percutaneous biopsy tissue markers.

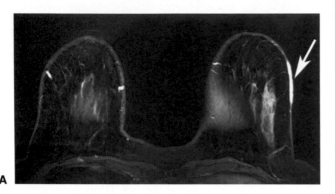

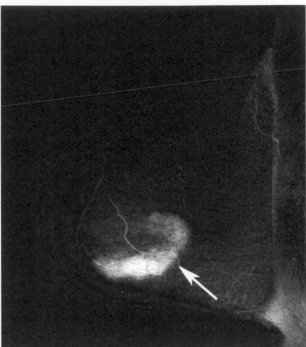

FIGURE 8-12 **Keloid. A:** Axial and **(B)** sagittal contrast-enhanced T1-weighted images through the skin of the lateral aspect of the left breast demonstrate localized thickening and mild enhancement (*arrows*) in region of known keloid scar.

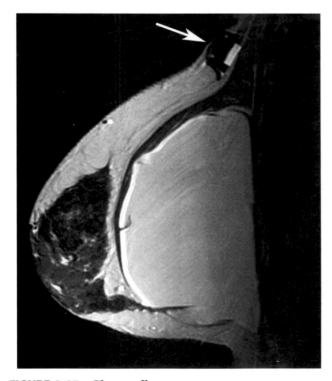

FIGURE 8-13 **Chest wall port.**

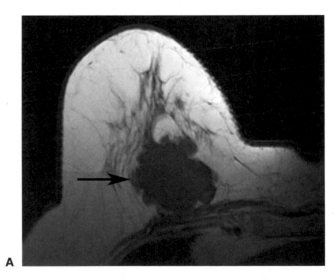

FIGURE 8-14 **Intraparenchymal hemangioma. A:** T1-weighted enhanced image demonstrates a lobulated T2 hypointense and T1 intermediate signal posterior breast mass (*arrow*), with linear streaks of enhancement, and an atypical appearance for breast cancer.

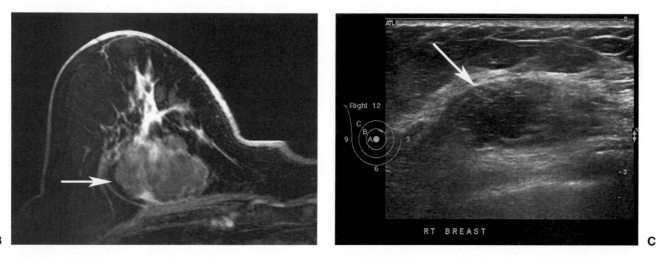

B   C

FIGURE 8-14 **Intraparenchymal hemangioma.** (*continued*) **B:** T2-weighted axial image demonstrates a lobulated T2 hypointense and T1 intermediate signal posterior breast mass (*arrow*), with linear streaks of enhancement, and an atypical appearance for breast cancer. **C:** Ultrasound image demonstrates a heterogeneous hypoechoic macrolobulated mass (*arrow*) without acoustic edge shadowing.

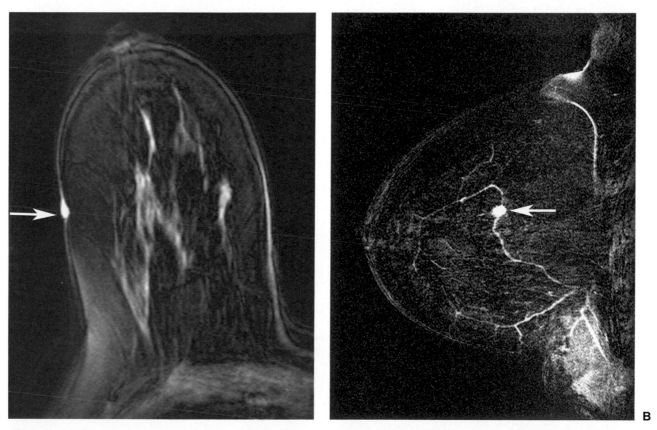

A   B

FIGURE 8-15 **Skin hemangioma. A:** Axial and **(B)** sagittal contrast-enhanced T1-weighted images through the skin of the lateral aspect of the right breast demonstrate localized enhancement in region of visible cherry angioma (*arrows*).

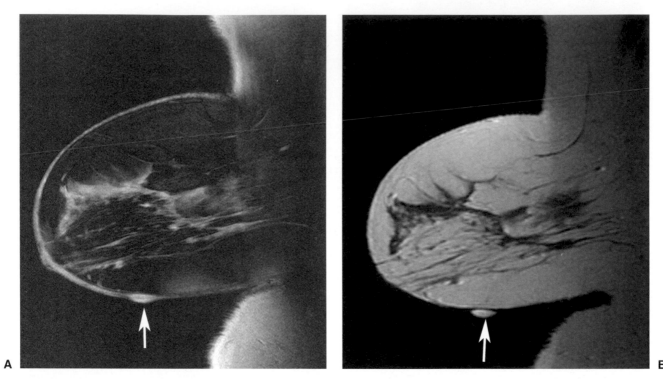

FIGURE 8-16   Skin lipoma. A: T1-weighted precontrast and **(B)** T2-weighted sagittal images show a skin lipoma (*arrows*) in the inferior aspect of the breast. Lipoma is a similar signal to fat on the T2-weighted image, although more difficult to delineate on T1-weighted image where skin elevation is apparent.

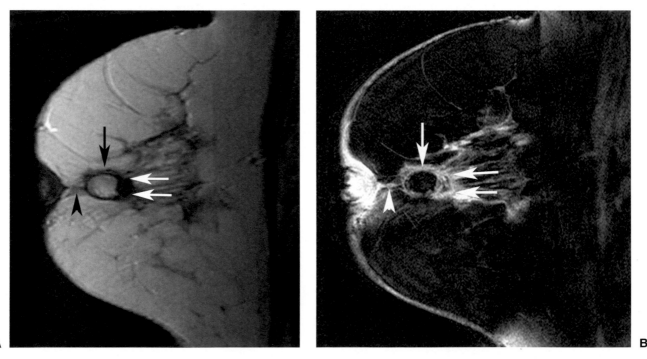

FIGURE 8-17   Fat necrosis after lumpectomy. A: T1-weighted enhanced and **(B)** T2-weighted sagittal images demonstrate an ovoid mass (*arrow*) with a central signal isointense to fat. The nonenhancing margin is T2-hypointense and the posterior rim is focally thickened (*double arrows*). However, T1 signal is mixed without enhancement, eliminating concern for residual or recurrent tumor. There is associated nipple retraction with a fibrous connection (*arrowhead*) to postsurgical change.

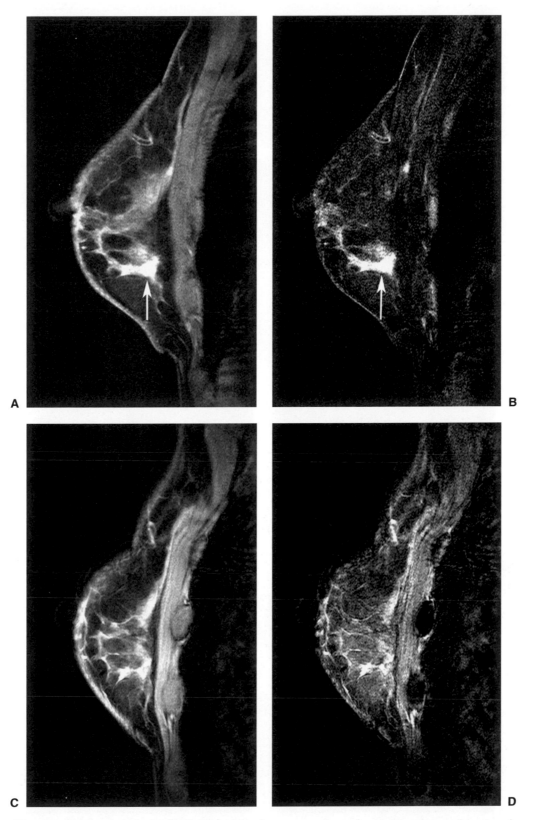

FIGURE 8-18 Hormonal influence. Sagittal **(A)** T1-weighted contrast-enhanced and **(B)** subtracted images through the right lower inner quadrant performed on day 46 of the menstrual cycle in a perimenopausal patient demonstrates a concerning, irregular mass inferiorly (*arrows*). **C–D:** Similar images performed 14 days later on day 8 of the next menstrual cycle demonstrate resolution of all concerning enhancement.

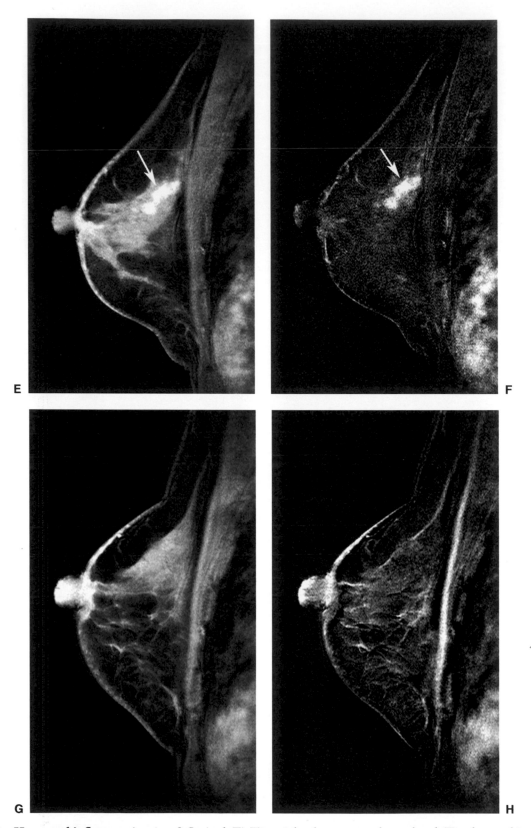

FIGURE 8-18 **Hormonal influence.** (*continued*) Sagittal (**E**) T1-weighted contrast-enhanced and (**F**) subtracted images through the left upper outer quadrant performed on day 46 of the menstrual cycle in a perimenopausal patient demonstrate a focal area of abnormal signal (*arrows*). **G–H:** Similar images performed 14 days later on day 8 of the next menstrual cycle, demonstrate resolution of all concerning enhancement.

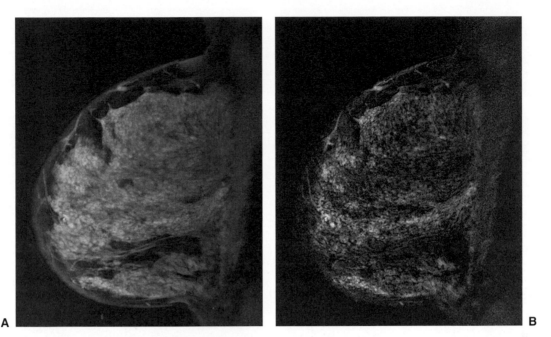

FIGURE 8-19 Benign stippled parenchymal enhancement. A: Sagittal enhanced T1-weighted and **(B)** subtracted images demonstrate uniform, diffuse stippled breast enhancement. This is frequently seen in benign tissue, either in multiple regions or diffusely. Focal or segmental stippled enhancement should be considered suspicious.

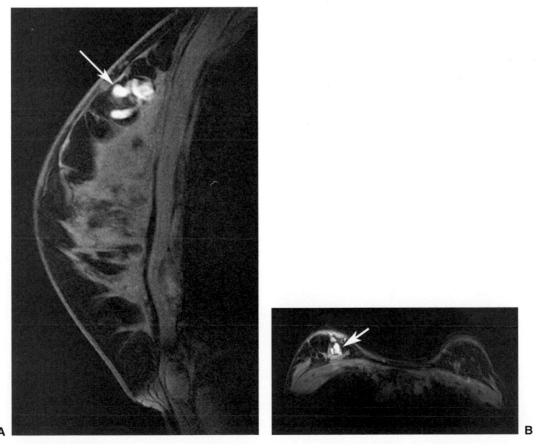

FIGURE 8-20 Hematoma after fine needle aspiration (FNA). A: Sagittal and **(B)** axial noncontrast images demonstrate hyperintense T1-weighted signal in a lobulated superior breast mass, correlating with the site of recent FNA.

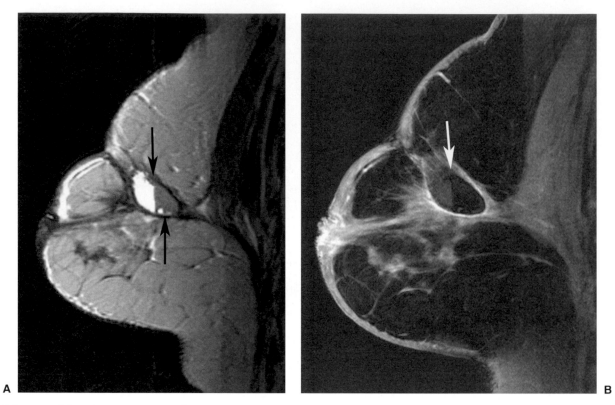

FIGURE 8-21   Chronic postoperative hematoma. A: Sagittal T2-weighted image demonstrates an ovoid mixed signal mass with fluid–fluid levels from layering blood products (*arrows*). The advancing edge of each signal (*arrows*) into the opposite chamber of the mass is due to slow movement of these differing hematocrit layers with the patient in the prone position. Incidental note is made of fibrous connections to the scar superiorly with skin retraction, and to the nipple, explaining the patient's heme-positive nipple discharge. **B:** Sagittal T1-weighted postcontrast image demonstrates a thin rim of enhancement of the cavity wall and low T1-weighted signal in the region of the protein and blood elements in this old hematoma.

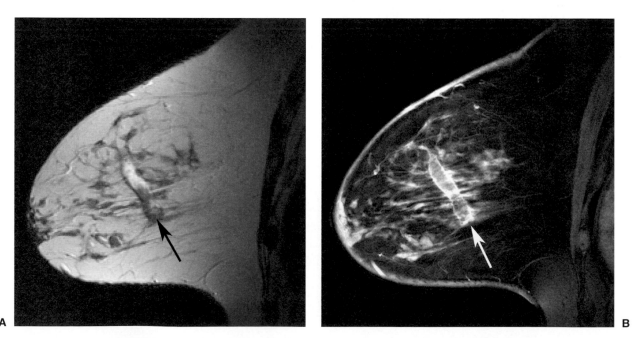

FIGURE 8-22   Post core biopsy changes. A: T2-weighted and **(B)** T1-weighted enhanced sagittal images demonstrate a linear cavity (*arrows*) after stereotactic core biopsy with a 9-gauge vacuum-assisted biopsy device. Mixed T2-weighted signal is consistent with subacute blood, and there is thin uniform enhancement of the cavity wall.

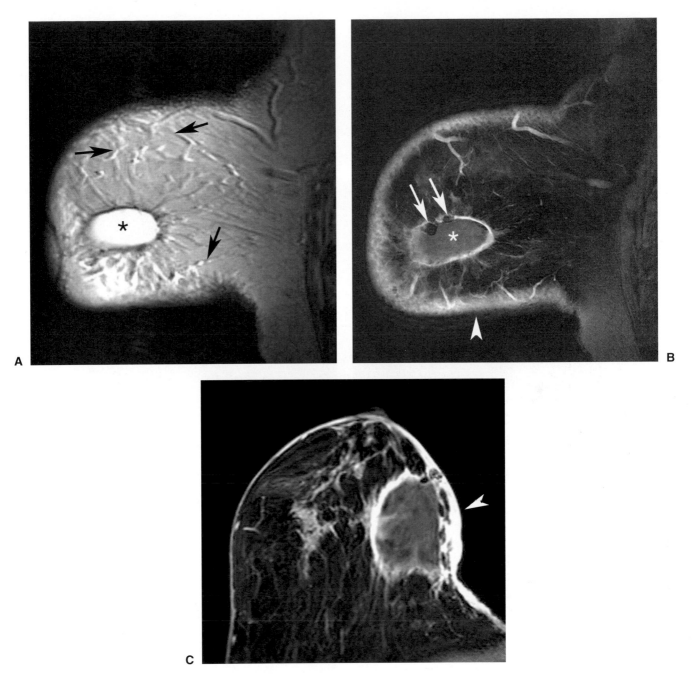

FIGURE 8-23 **Post breast conservation treatment changes. A:** Sagittal T2-weighted image demonstrates an ovoid high signal seroma (*asterisk*) in the surgical bed and diffuse, linear paraligamentous and subdermal high signal edema (*arrows*) after whole breast radiation. This edema is analogous to trabecular thickening on mammography. **B:** Sagittal T1-weighted contrast-enhanced image demonstrates thin uniform enhancement of the wall of the surgical cavity (*asterisk*) (best noted posteriorly) and low signal hemosiderin superiorly (*arrows*). The inferior skin is more thickened, edematous and enhancing, which is typical after breast conservation. **C:** Axial T1-weighted contrast-enhanced image demonstrates the medial surgical cavity with thickening and enhancement of the overlying skin (*arrowhead*).

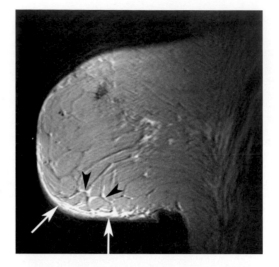

FIGURE 8-24 Post radiation therapy change. Subdermal (*arrows*) and paraligamentous (*arrowheads*) hyperintense T2-weighted signal is consistent with edema or effusion, and is analogous to trabecular thickening.

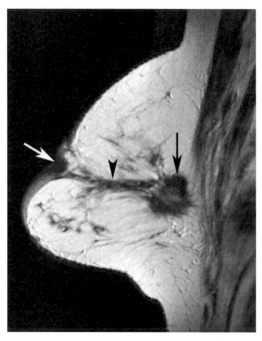

A

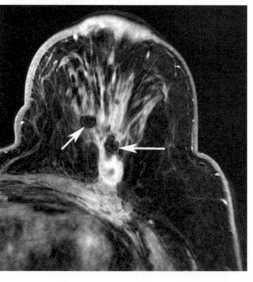

B

C

FIGURE 8-25 Post surgical change at 12 months. **A:** Sagittal T2-weighted image demonstrates mixed signal in the posterior tumor bed (*black arrow*), consistent with fibrotic scar and central fat necrosis. Linear low signal scarring extends anteriorly into the central aspect of the breast (*arrowhead*) and there is nipple retraction (*white arrow*). **B:** Sagittal T1-weighted enhanced image shows signal voids (*arrow*) from surgical clips and mild enhancement of the postoperative changes. There is no focal or intense enhancement to suggest residual or recurrent tumor. Skin is diffusely thickened with mild enhancement, slightly greater inferiorly (*arrowheads*). **C:** Axial enhanced T1-weighted image shows skin and trabecular thickening and mild enhancement. Note delayed enhancement more focally in the tumor bed, consistent with granulation tissue. Signal voids (*arrows*) are from surgical clips.

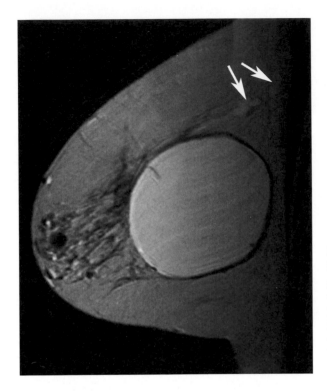

FIGURE 8-26 Silicone in lymph nodes. Sagittal T2-weighted image depicts subglandular silicone implant, which appears encapsulated and without evidence of implant rupture on this image. Increased signal in two lymph nodes (*arrows*) in the axillary tail of the breast and linear high signal band between the lymph nodes and the implant are suggestive of previous rupture.

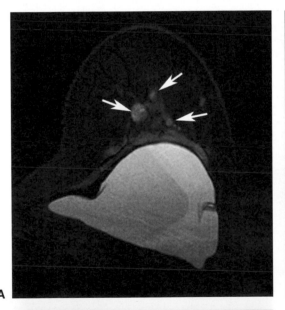

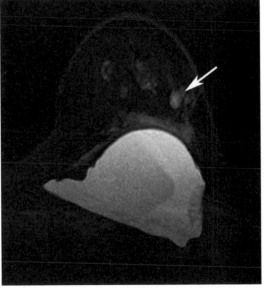

A

B

C

FIGURE 8-27 Silicone granuloma. A–C: Axial T2-weighted water-suppressed images demonstrate an intact silicone implant and multiple T2-hyperintense round masses within the breast parenchyma (*arrows*). These are consistent with granulomas and residual silicone after previous implant rupture. Previous implants have been replaced.

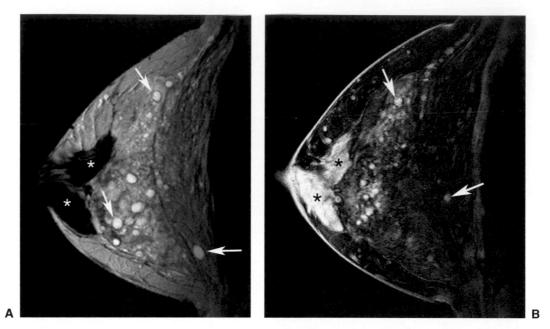

FIGURE 8-28 **Silicone injections. A:** Sagittal T2-weighted and **(B)** T1-weighted enhanced images show hyperintense signal and enhancement in innumerable silicone granulomata (*arrows*) after silicone injections for augmentation. Breast tissue anteriorly (*asterisk*) is low on T2-weighted imaging, diffusely enhances, and stable on sequential imaging: findings may be due to chronic inflammation or fibrotic reaction.

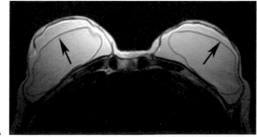

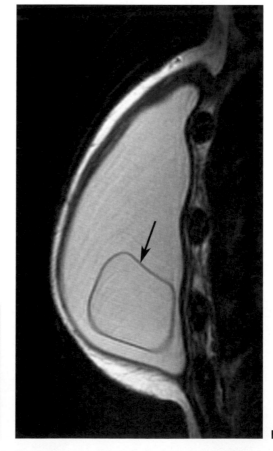

FIGURE 8-29 **Implant variants, intact gel–gel dual lumen. A:** Bilateral axial and **(B)** sagittal T2-weighted images demonstrate intact dual-chamber silicone gel implants. The linear outlines of the inner gel chambers (*arrows*) are hypointense and uninterrupted.

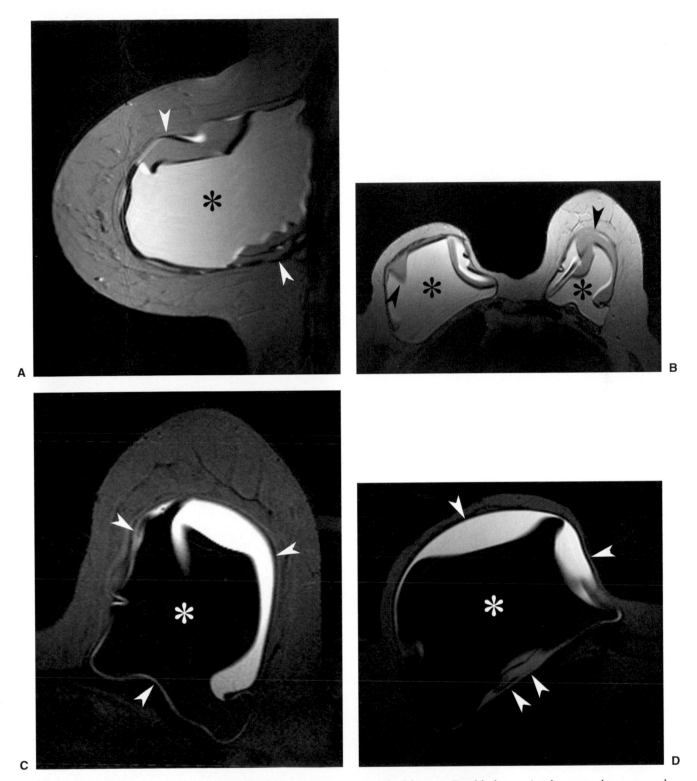

FIGURE 8-30 Implant variants, intact saline inner–silicone outer dual lumen. Double lumen implants are demonstrated on **(A)** sagittal T2-weighted, **(B)** axial T2-weighted, **(C)** axial left T2-weighted image with water suppression and **(D)** axial right T2-weighted image with water suppression (*Central saline chamber = asterisk, Thinner outer silicone chamber = arrowheads, Normal radial folds = double arrowheads*).

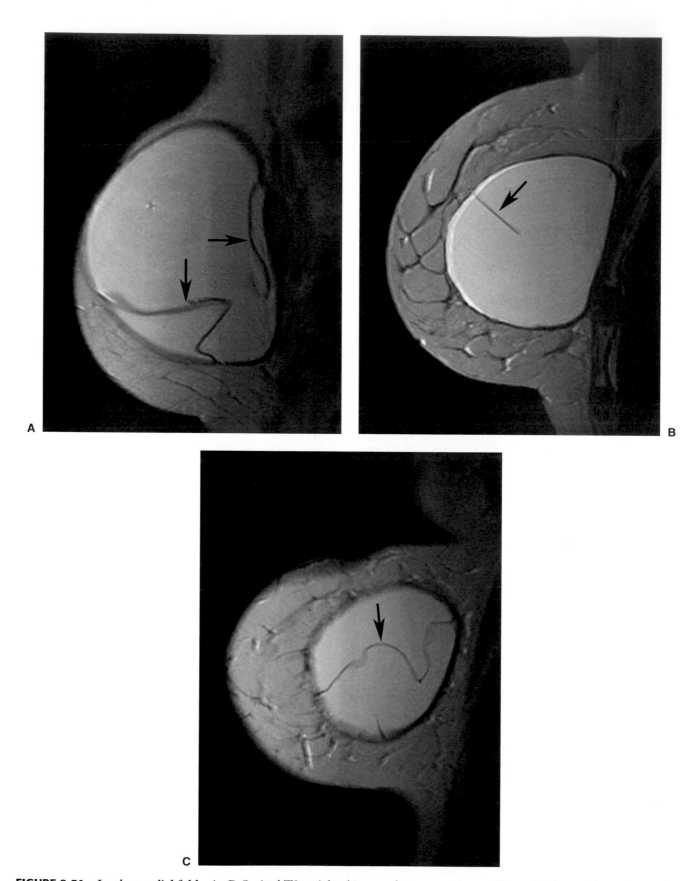

FIGURE 8-31 Implant radial folds. A–C: Sagittal T2-weighted images demonstrate intact silicone implants with contiguous low signal lines (*arrows*). Radial folds must extend to the implant capsule.

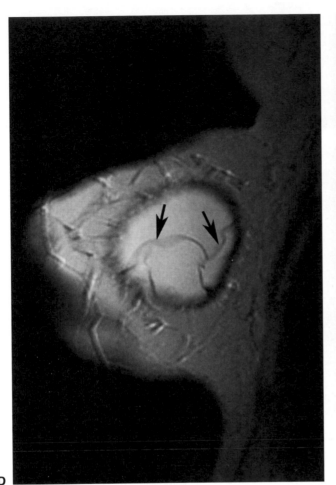

D

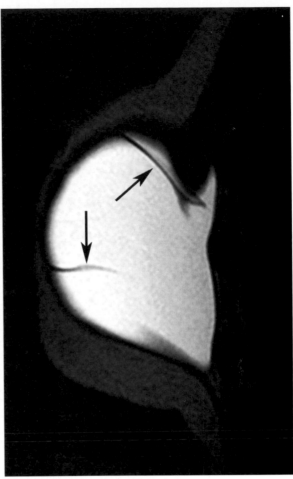

E

FIGURE 8-31 **Implant radial folds.** (*continued*) **D** and **E:** Sagittal T2-weighted images demonstrate intact silicone implants with contiguous low signal lines (*arrows*). Radial folds must extend to the implant capsule.

Suggested Readings

Amano Y, Aoki R, Kumita S, et al. Silicone-selective multishot echo-planar imaging for rapid MRI survey of breast implants. *Eur Radiol.* 2007;17(7):1875–1878.

Delille JP, Slanetz PJ, Yeh ED, et al. Physiologic changes in breast magnetic resonance imaging during the menstrual cycle: Perfusion imaging, signal enhancement, and influence of the T1 relaxation time of breast tissue. *Breast J.* 2005;11(4):236–241.

Gallardo X, Sentís M, Castañer E, et al. Enhancement of intramammary lymph nodes with lymphoid hyperplasia: A potential pitfall in breast MRI. *Eur Radiol.* 1998;8(9):1662–1665.

Genson CC, Blane CE, Helvie MA, et al. Effects on breast MRI of artifacts caused by metallic tissue marker clips. *AJR Am J Roentgenol.* 2007;188:372–376.

Harvey JA, Hendrick RE, Coll JM, et al. Breast MR imaging artifacts: How to recognize and fix them. *Radiographics.* 2007;27:S131–S145.

Hirose M, Otsuki N, Hayano D, et al. Multi-volume fusion imaging of MR ductography and MR mammography for patients with nipple discharge. *Magn Reson Med Sci.* 2006;5(2):105–112.

Kawahara S, Hyakusoku H, Ogawa R, et al. Clinical imaging diagnosis of implant materials for breast augmentation. *Ann Plast Surg.* 2006;57(1):6–12.

Kim SM, Kim HH, Shin HJ, et al. Cavernous haemangioma of the breast. *Br J Radiol.* 2006;79(947):e177–e180.

Kuhl CK. Current status of breast MR imaging. Part 2. Clinical applications. *Radiology.* 2007;244(3):672–691.

Macura KJ, Ouwerkerk R, Jacobs MA, et al. Patterns of enhancement on breast MR images: Interpretation and imaging pitfalls. *Radiographics.* 2006;26:1719–1734.

Müller-Schimpfle M, Ohmenhaüser K, Stoll P, et al. Menstrual cycle and age: Influence on parenchymal contrast medium enhancement in MR imaging of the breast. *Radiology.* 1997;203(1):145–149.

Ojeda-Fournier H, Choe KA, Mahoney MC. Recognizing and interpreting artifacts and pitfalls in MR imaging of the breast. *Radiographics.* 2007;27:S147–S164.

Chapter 9

Thoracic Spine

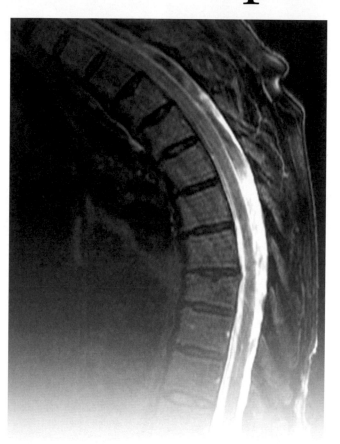

Laura W. Bancroft and Debbie J. Merinbaum

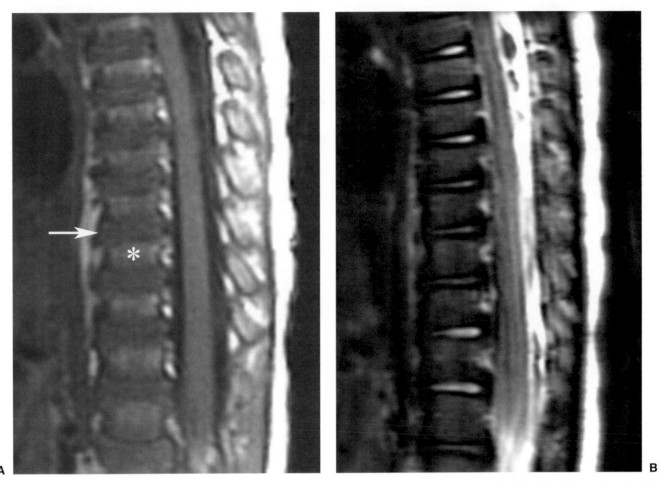

FIGURE 9-1 **Pediatric spine.** **A:** Normal sagittal T1-weighted thoracic spine MRIs in a 9-month-old child. Notice that the T1 signal intensities make the intervertebral discs (*arrow*) appear almost as tall as the vertebral bodies (*asterisk*). **B:** Correlating sagittal FSE T2-weighted image delineates the true dimensions of the spinal elements.

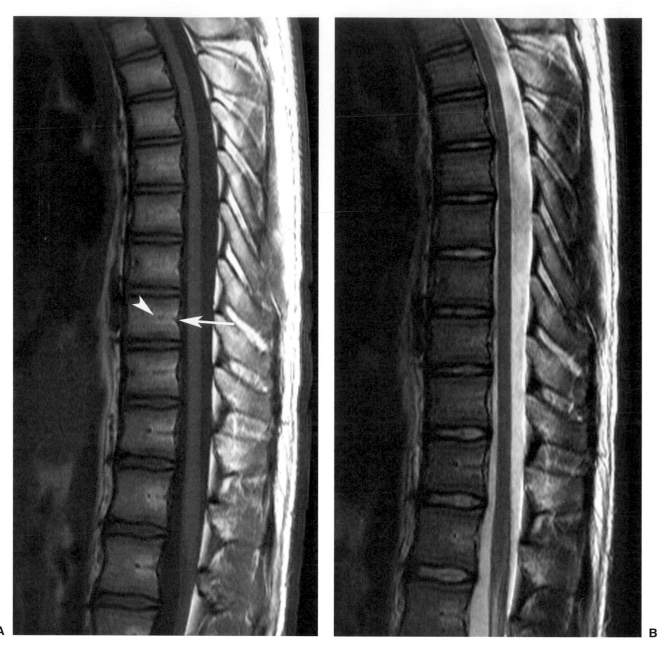

FIGURE 9-2   Adolescent spine. Normal sagittal thoracic spine MRIs in a 17-year-old adolescent on **(A)** T1- and **(B)** FSE T2-weighted images. Notice the yellow marrow (*arrowhead*) around the basivertebral veins (*arrow*) on **(A)** T1-weighted image.

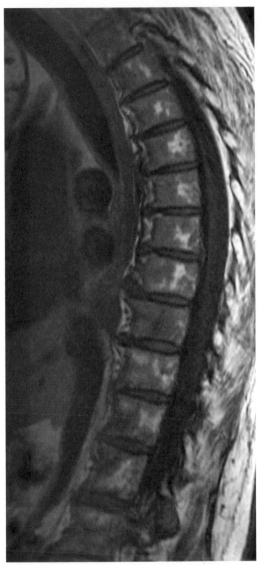

FIGURE 9-3 Heterogeneous marrow. Sagittal T1-weighted image shows a normal heterogeneous pattern of red and yellow marrow in an adult.

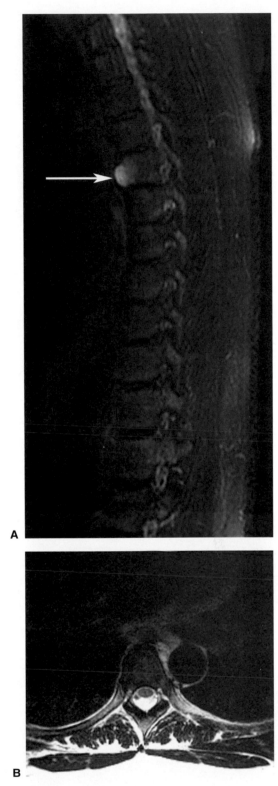

A

B

FIGURE 9-4 Artifact anterior to T5. Sagittal enhanced FSE T2-weighted fat-suppressed image **(A)** demonstrates a hyperintense focus (*arrow*) anterior and to the left of the T5 vertebra. This was not confirmed on **(B)** axial imaging or on CT scan of the chest performed the same day, consistent with an artifact likely from esophageal contents.

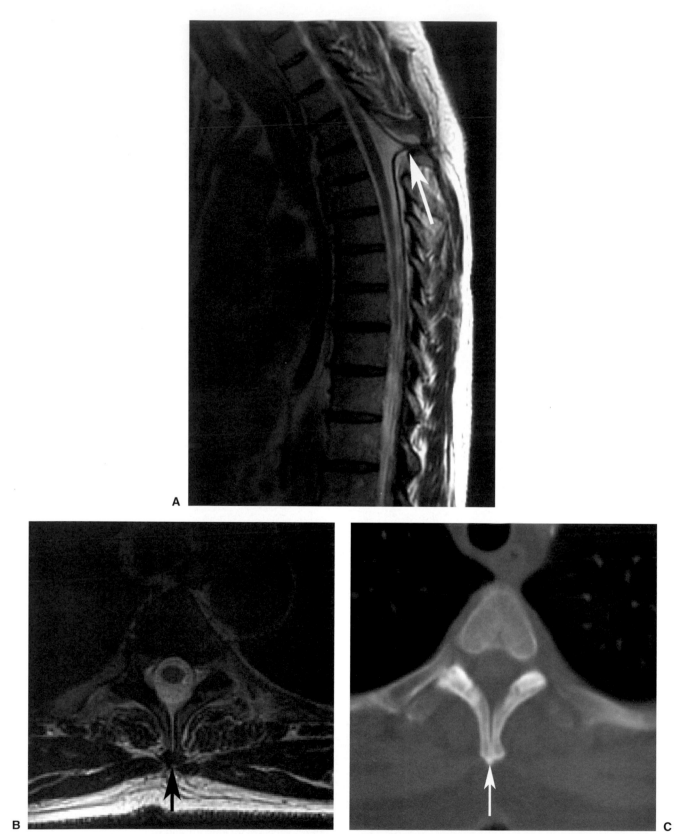

FIGURE 9-5 Bifid T5 spinous process. Sagittal FSE T2-weighted image **(A)** of the thoracic spine demonstrates deformity of the posterior elements of T5, with posterior displacement and tenting of the dural sac, and a fibrous connection (*arrow*) between the skin and thecal sac. **B:** Axial FSE T2-weighted and **(C)** CT images better delineate the bifid spinous process (*arrows*).

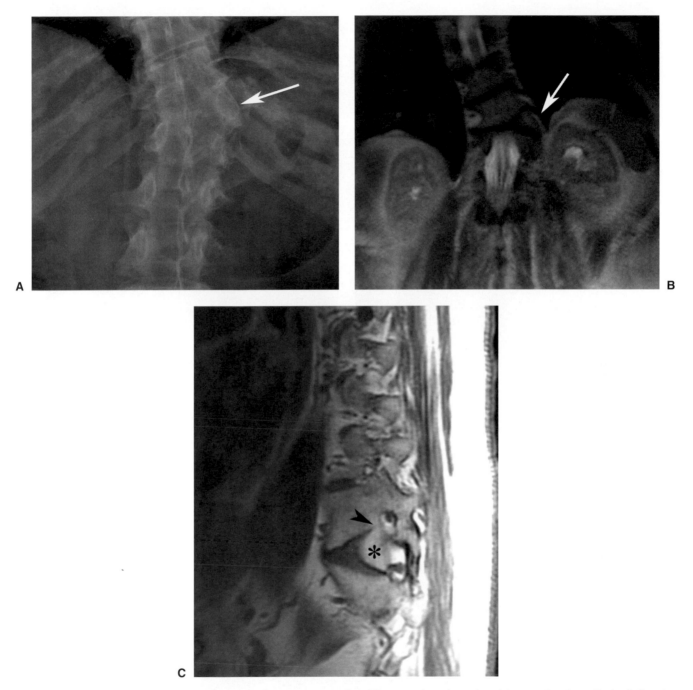

FIGURE 9-6 **Hemivertebra.** **A:** Radiograph demonstrates a left T11 vertebra (*arrow*), with associated scoliotic deformity. **B:** Coronal T2-weighted image shows the classic appearance of a wedge-shaped hemivertebra (*arrow*). These variants also have a half arch with a transverse process, superior and inferior articular processes, and half a spinous process. **C:** Sagittal T1-weighted image shows fusion (*arrowhead*) of the hemivertebra (*asterisk*) to T10.

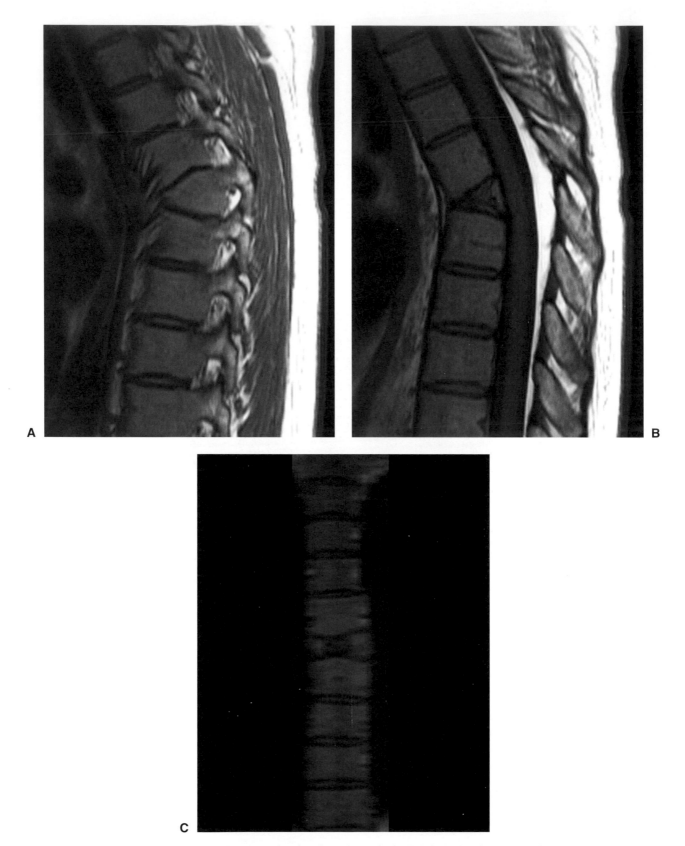

FIGURE 9-7   Butterfly vertebra. Sagittal T1-weighted images through the **(A)** lateral and **(B)** central aspects of the spine show a variable degree of vertebral body wedging and a kyphotic deformity. **C:** Coronal reconstruction in this patient shows a classic butterfly vertebra.

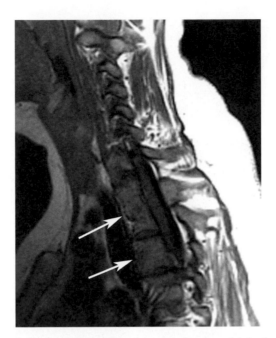

FIGURE 9-8 **Multiple fused segments.** Sagittal T1-weighted image shows multiple fused cervicothoracic segments (*arrows*), which can be incidental or associated with Klippel-Feil syndrome.

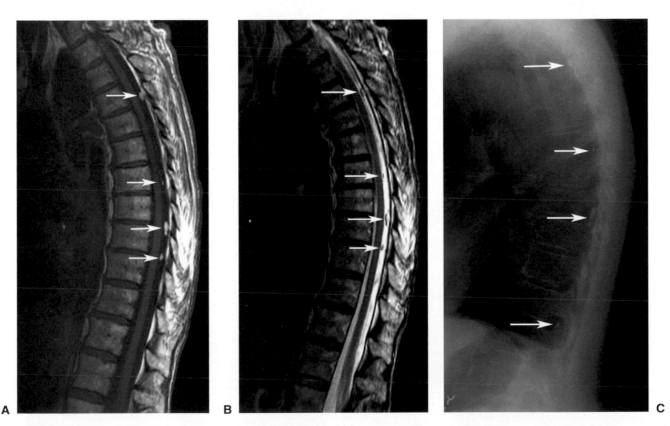

FIGURE 9-9 **Pantopaque. A:** Sagittal T1- and **(B)** T2-weighted fat-suppressed images of the thoracic spine demonstrate several globular foci (*arrows*) of signal within the posterior cerebrospinal fluid (CSF) that approximates fat signal on both sequences. The oil-based contrast material is most conspicuous on T1-weighted imaging. **C:** Correlative thoracic spine radiograph confirms the dense residual Pantopaque (*arrows*) within the thoracic canal.

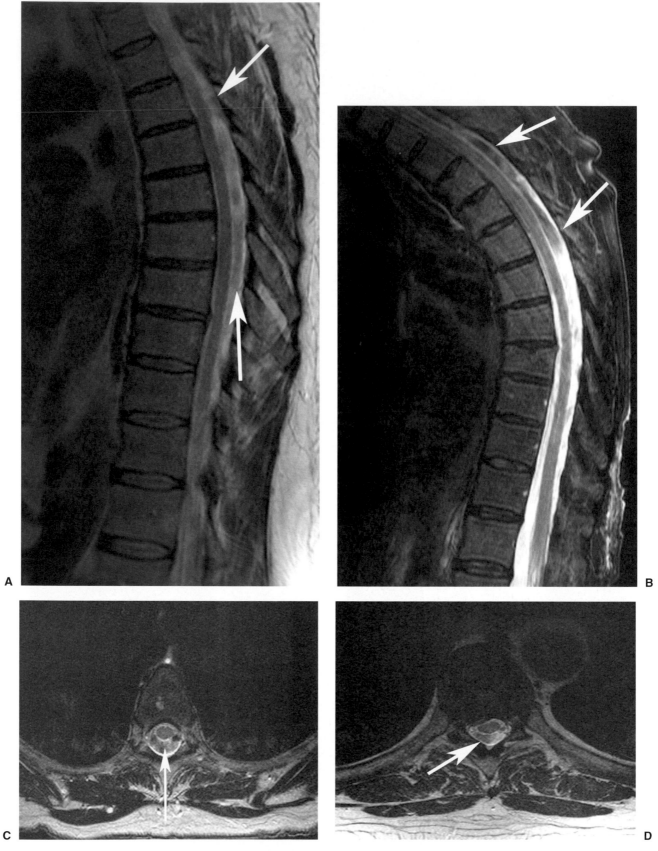

FIGURE 9-10 Cerebrospinal fluid (CSF) flow artifact. A and **B:** Sagittal FSE T2-weighted images in different patients show flow artifact (*arrows*) within the CSF space **C** and **D:** Axial images display the flow phenomenon (*arrows*) relative to the cord.

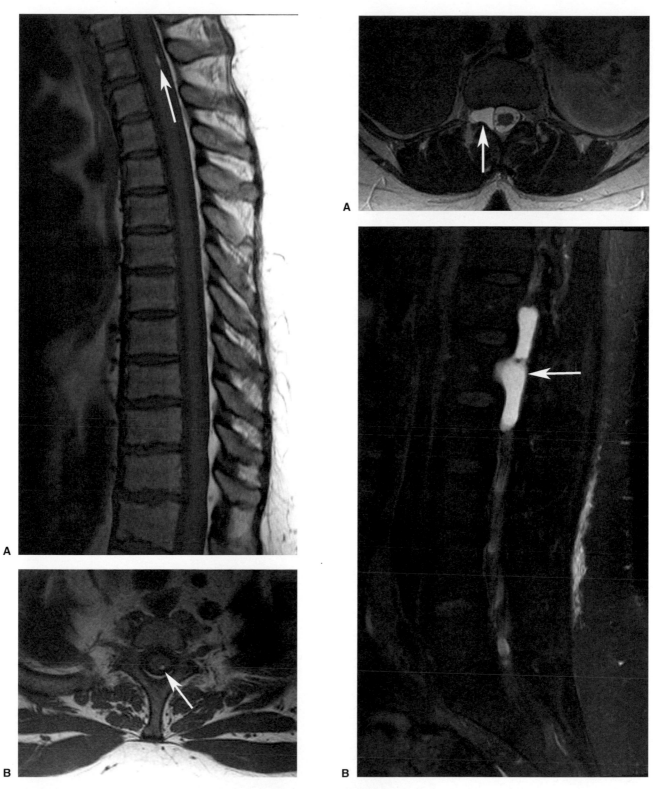

FIGURE 9-11 Intradural lipoma. A: Sagittal and **(B)** axial T1-weighted images demonstrate a small intradural lipoma (*arrows*), which can be similar in appearance to Pantopaque. Subtraction images may be helpful to differentiate this lipoma from intrathecal hemorrhage.

FIGURE 9-12 Extradural arachnoid cyst. A: Axial and **(B)** sagittal T2-weighted images show a right-sided extradural arachnoid cyst (*arrows*) extending from T12 to L1. Notice the mild expansile remodeling of the adjacent osseous structures.

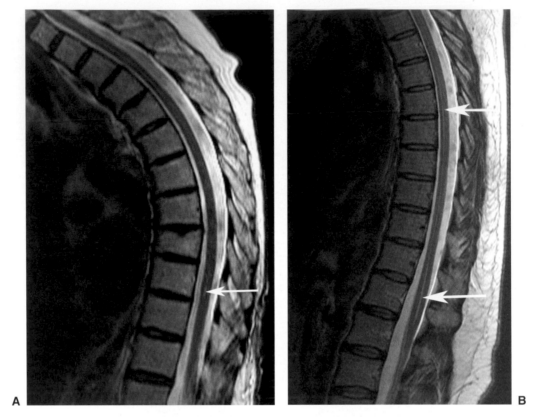

FIGURE 9-13 **Central canal of the spinal cord. A** and **B:** Sagittal FSE T2-weighted images in two different patients delineate the normal central canal (*arrows*) of the spinal cord that can be visualized at multiple levels.

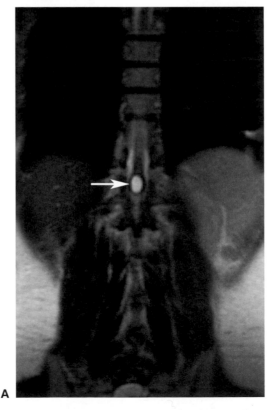

FIGURE 9-14 **Spinal cord terminal ventricle. A:** Coronal FSE T2-weighted image shows a focally prominent distal central canal (*arrow*), termed a *terminal ventricle* or *fifth ventricle*.

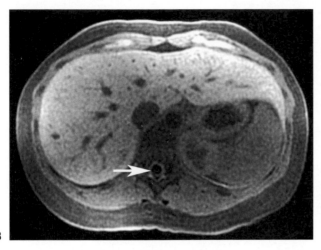

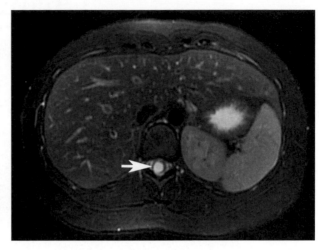

B

C

FIGURE 9-14 **Spinal cord terminal ventricle.** (*continued*) Axial **(B)** T1- and **(C)** T2-weighted images show a focally prominent distal central canal (*arrows*), termed a *terminal ventricle* or *fifth ventricle*.

Suggested Readings

Belmont PJ Jr, Kuklo TR, Taylor KF, et al. Intraspinal anomalies associated with isolated congenital hemivertebra: The role of routine magnetic resonance imaging. *J Bone Joint Surg Am*. 2004;86-A(8): 1704–1710.

Bergman RA, Thompson SA, Afifi AK, et al. In: Bergman RA, Thomson SA, Afifi AK. et al. ed. *Compendium of human anatomic variation*. Baltimore: Urban & Schwarzenberg;1988.

Chandraraj S, Briggs CA, Opeskin K. Disc herniations in young and end-plate vascularity. *Clin Anat*. 1998;11:171–176.

Christodoulou AG, Apostolou T, Ploumis A, et al. Pedicle dimensions of the thoracic and lumbar vertebrae in the Greek population. *Clin Anat*. 2005;18:404–408.

Duvoisin B, Landry M. Pantopaque droplets: Another cause of hyperintensity on unenhanced T1-weighted MR images of the brain. *AJR Am J Roentgenol*. 1997;168(2):569.

Griffith JF, Yeung DWK, Antonio GE, et al. Vertebral marrow fat content and diffusion and perfusion indexes in women with varying bone density: MR evaluation. *Radiology*. 2006;241:831–839.

Hatipoglu HG, Selvi A, Ciliz D, et al. Quantitative and diffusion MR imaging as a new method to assess osteoporosis. *AJNR Am J Neuroradiol*. 2007;28:1934–1937.

Hauger O, Cotten A, Chateil JF, et al. Giant cystic Schmorl's nodes: Imaging findings in six patients. *AJR Am J Roentgenol*. 2001;176(4): 969–972.

Krueger EC, Perry JO, Wu Y, et al. Changes in T2 relaxation times associated with maturation of the human intervertebral disk. *AJNR Am J Neuroradiol*. 2007;28:1237–1241.

Lee RA, van Zundert AA, Breedveld P, et al. The anatomy of the thoracic spinal canal investigated with magnetic resonance imaging (MRI). *Acta Anaesthesiol Belg* 2007;58(3):163–167.

Lisanti C, Carlin C, Banks KP, et al. Normal MRI appearance and motion-related phenomena of CSF. *AJR Am J Roentgenol*. 2007;188: 716–725.

Loughenbury PR, Wadhwani S, Soames RW. The posterior longitudinal ligament and peridural (epidural) membrane. *Clin Anat*. 2006;19: 487–492.

Montazei JL, Divine M, Lepage E, et al. Normal spinal bone marrow in adults: Dynamic gadolinium-enhanced MR imaging. *Radiology*. 2003; 229:703–709.

Newell RLM. The spinal epidural space. *Clin Anat*. 1999;12:375–379.

Pfirrmann CWA, Resnick D. Schmorl nodes of the thoracic and lumbar spine: Radiographic-pathologic study of prevalence, characterization, and correlation with degenerative changes of 1,650 spinal levels in 100 cadavers. *Radiology*. 2001;219:368.

Sonel B, Yalçin P, Oztürk EA, et al. Butterfly vertebra: A case report. *Clin Imaging*. 2001;25(3):206–208.

Suojanen J, Wang AM, Winston KR. Pantopaque mimicking spinal lipoma: MR pitfall. *J Comput Assist Tomogr*. 1988;12(2):346–348.

Wu HTH, Morrison WB, Schweitzer ME. Edematous Schmorl's nodes on thoracolumbar MR imaging: Characteristics patterns and changes over time. *Skeletal Radiol*. 2006;35:21.

Chapter 10

Intrathoracic

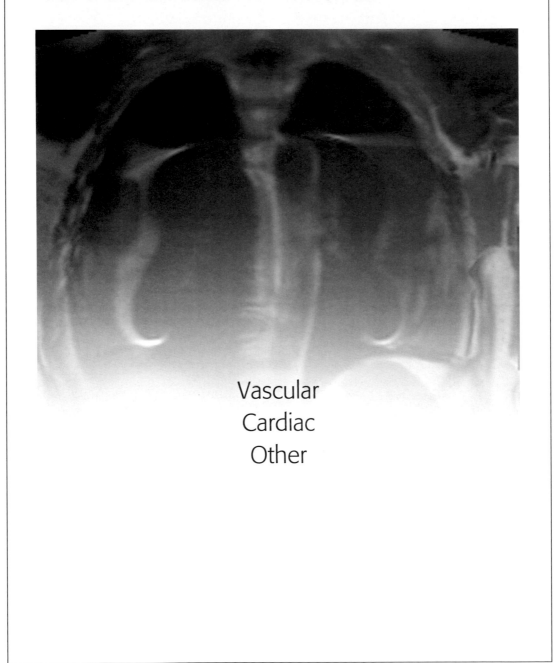

Vascular

Cardiac

Other

Laura W. Bancroft, Ronald S. Kuzo, and J. Mark McKinney

▣ Vascular

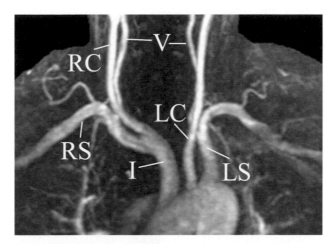

FIGURE 10-1 MRA of aortic arch. Conventional aortic arch anatomy occurs in approximately 75% of the population, in which the first branch is the innominate artery (*I*), followed by the left common carotid artery (*LC*), and then the left subclavian artery (*LS*). The vertebral arteries (*V*) originate from the respective subclavian arteries (*Right subclavian artery = RS, right common carotid artery = RC*).

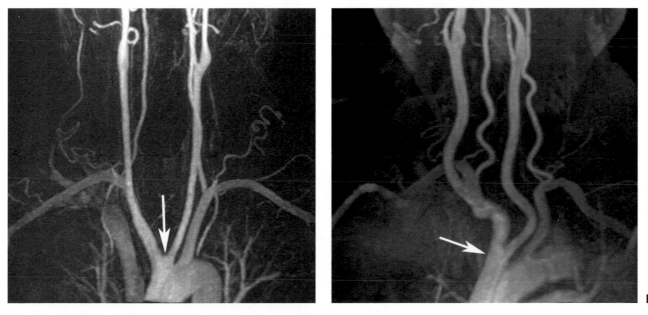

FIGURE 10-2 Bovine arch. A and **B:** MRAs in two different patients show a bovine arch (*arrows*), in which the innominate and left carotid arteries have a common origin from the aortic arch. This is the most common variant of the aortic arch and occurs in approximately 20% of the population.

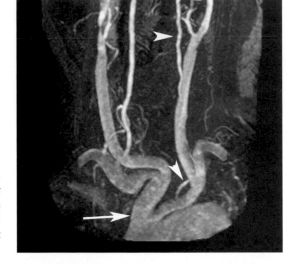

FIGURE 10-3 Single brachiocephalic trunk. Rare MRA of all of the great vessels originating from a single brachiocephalic trunk (*arrow*). This differs from a bovine arch, because the left vertebral artery (*arrowheads*) originates from this trunk, not the aorta.

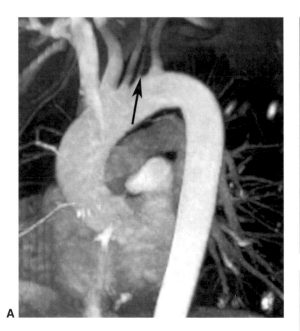

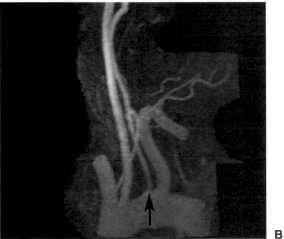

FIGURE 10-4 Left vertebral artery originates from aorta. A–C: Coronal oblique MRAs show variant anatomy in which the left vertebral artery (*arrow*) originates from the aorta, as opposed to the left subclavian artery. This variant occurs in approximately 6% of the population.

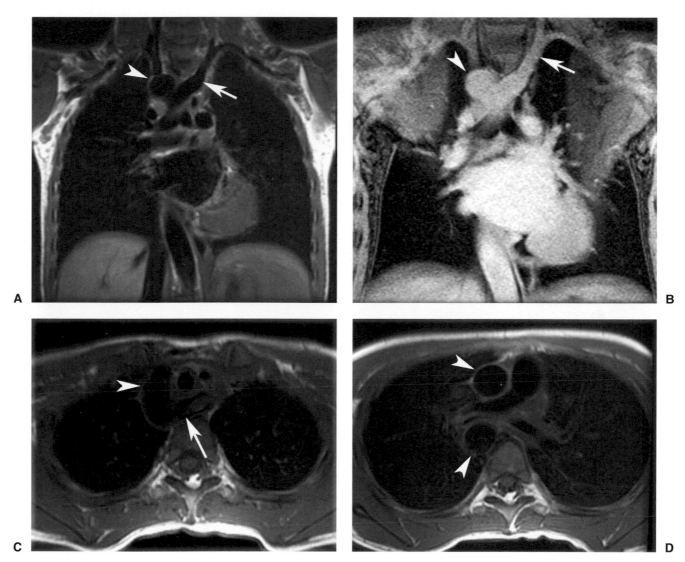

FIGURE 10-5   Right aortic arch and aberrant left subclavian artery. A and **B:** Coronal imaging shows a right aortic arch (*arrowhead*) occurs due to persistence of the right fourth branchial arch, and is most commonly associated with an aberrant left subclavian artery (*arrow*). **C** and **D:** Right aortic arch (*arrowhead*) is rarely associated with congenital heart defects if the arteries branch in the following order (as in this case)—left common carotid, right common carotid, right subclavian, then the left subclavian (*arrow*).

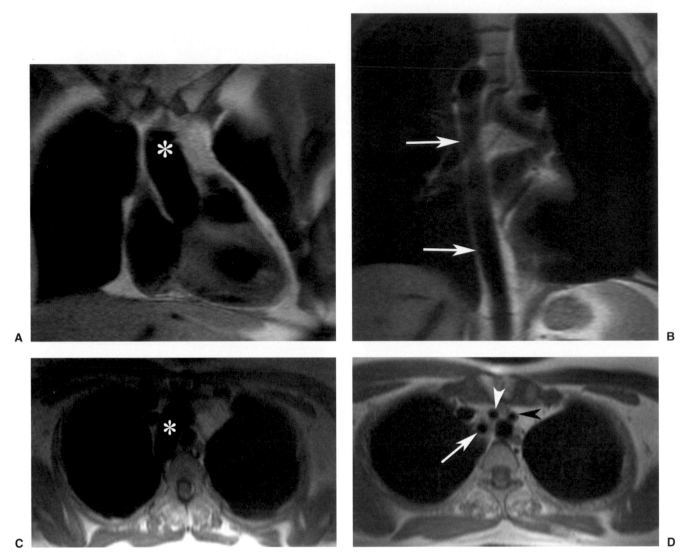

FIGURE 10-6 Right aortic arch with mirror imaging vessels. A and **B:** Coronal images demonstrate a right aortic arch (*asterisk*) and descending aorta (*arrows*). **C** and **D:** Axial images show the right-sided arch (*asterisk*) and mirror image vessels—left brachiocephalic trunk (*black arrowhead*), right common carotid (*white arrowhead*) and right subclavian (*arrow*) arteries. Congenital heart disease is common in these individuals with reverse order vessels.

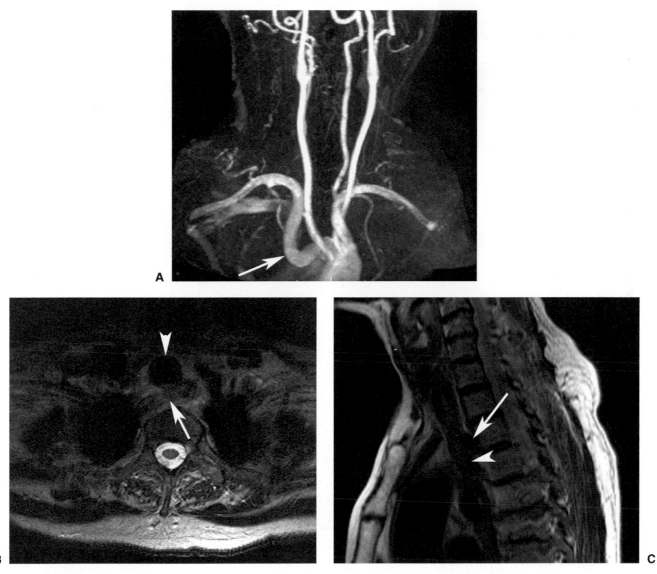

FIGURE 10-7   Aberrant right subclavian artery. A: MRA shows acute angulation of the aberrant right subclavian artery (*arrow*), which arises from the descending aorta distal to the origin of the left subclavian artery. This variant occurs in approximately 1% of individuals. **B:** Axial T2-weighted image shows extension of the aberrant vessel (*arrow*) posterior to the trachea (*arrowhead*) and esophagus. **C:** Sagittal T1-weighted image shows the aberrant right subclavian artery (*arrow*) posterior to the esophagus (*arrowhead*).

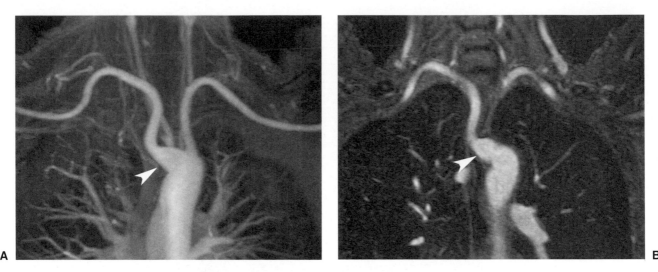

FIGURE 10-8 Diverticulum of Kommerel. A and **B:** Coronal MRAs in different patients show focal dilatation (*arrowheads*) of the origin of the aberrant right subclavian artery, known as a *diverticulum of Kommerel*.

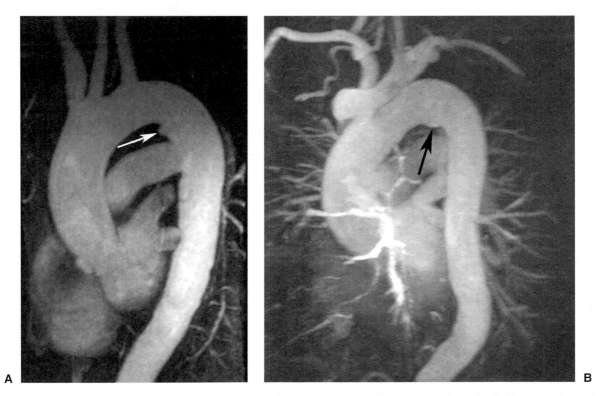

FIGURE 10-9 Ductus diverticulum. A and **B:** Coronal oblique projections from MRAs show focal dilatation (*arrows*) of the anteromedial portion of the proximal descending aorta. This is termed *ductus diverticulum*, which is due to the most distal segment of the embryonic right arch.

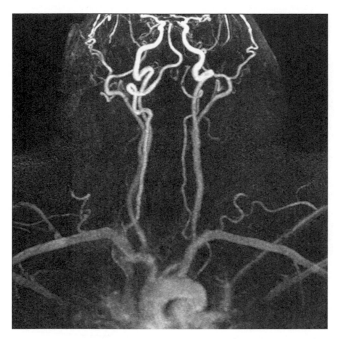

FIGURE 10-10 Poor bolus timing. Decreased signal is observed inferiorly due to poor bolus timing. Signal wrap (aliasing) of the subclavian arteries is also observed due to insufficient oversampling in the left-right direction.

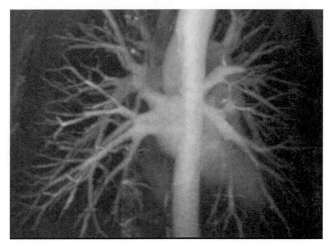

FIGURE 10-11 Normal pulmonary vascularity. MR angiography can be useful to evaluate the pulmonary vascularity in patients with iodinated contrast allergies.

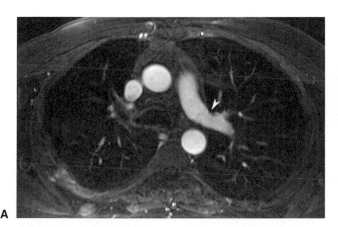

A

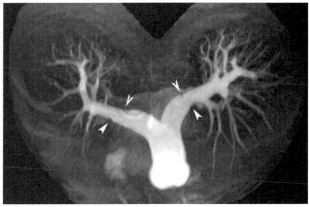

B

FIGURE 10-12 MRA after double lung transplant. A: Axial and **(B)** maximum intensity projection (MIP) images of the pulmonary arteries show slight contour alterations at the anastomoses (*arrowheads*) between native and recipient vessels.

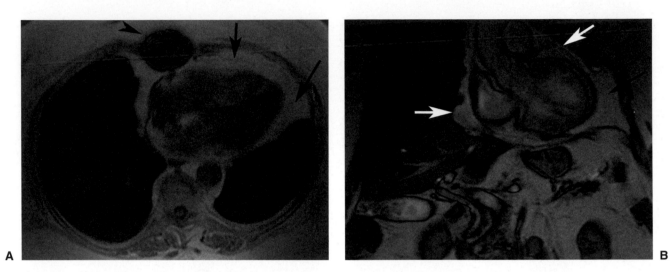

FIGURE 10-13 **Mediastinal lipomatosis. A** and **B:** Prominent mediastinal fat (*arrows*) is usually commensurate with the amount of overall body fat (*Sternotomy artifact = arrowhead*).

▣ Cardiac

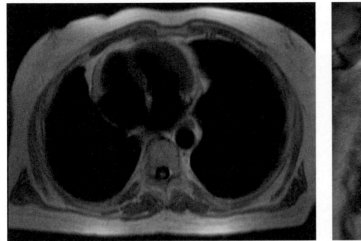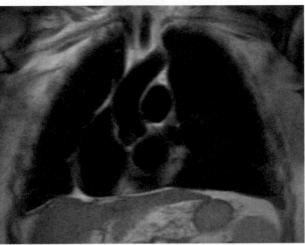

A   B

FIGURE 10-14 **Dextrocardia.** Axial **(A)** and coronal **(B)** T1-weighted images show a case of dextrocardia. Dextrocardia refers to the heart being situated on the right side of the body and occurs in less than 1% of the population. This should not be confused with dextrocardia situs inversus, which refers to the heart being a mirror image situated on the right side.

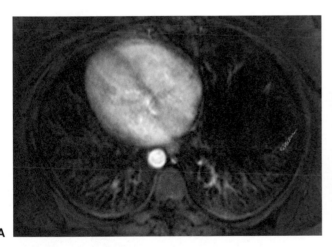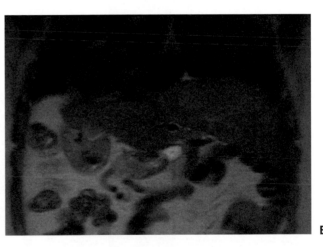

A   B

FIGURE 10-15 **Dextrocardia situs inversus totalis. A:** Axial and **(B)** coronal volumetric interpolated breath-hold examination (VIBE) images after gadolinium administration show dextrocardia in the presence of situs inversus. All of the major visceral organs are reversed from their normal positions, and less than 1 in 10,000 people are affected.

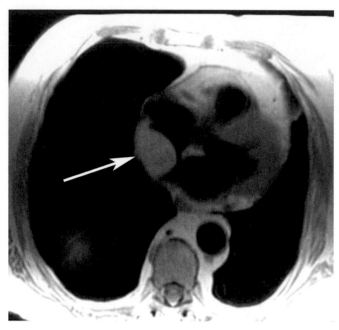

FIGURE 10-16   Lipomatous hypertrophy of interatrial septum. Axial T1-weighted image shows focal lipomatous hypertrophy (*arrow*) of the interatrial septum. This is a relatively uncommon disorder in which fat is deposited between the myocardial fibers, but can produce a mass-like bulge on imaging.

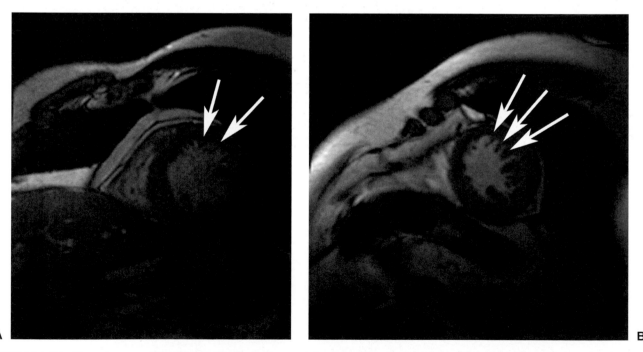

FIGURE 10-17   Prominent trabeculation in the left ventricle. A and **B:** Short axis imaging through the left ventricle shows prominent trabeculation (*arrows*) of the wall, which is a normal finding.

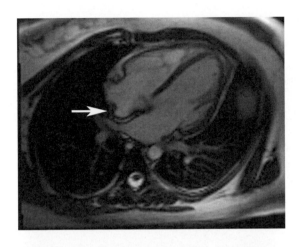

FIGURE 10-18 Prominent crista terminalis. Axial true fast imaging with steady state precision (FISP) image shows a prominent crista terminalis (*arrow*), which is the line of union between the right atrium and right auricle.

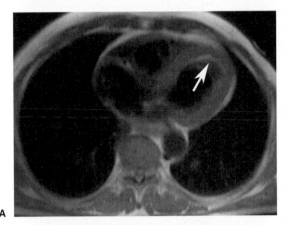

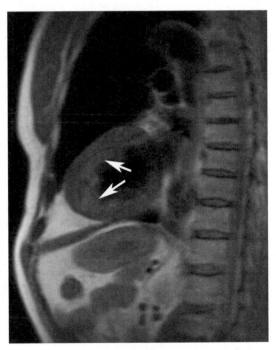

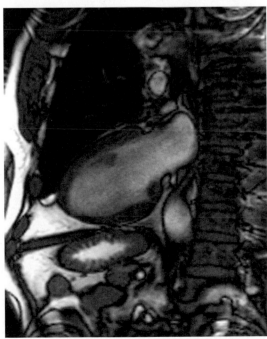

FIGURE 10-19 Artifactual hyperintense subendocardial signal around the left ventricle on HASTE imaging. A and **B:** Artifactual hyperintense subendocardial signal (*arrows*) can exist on half-Fourier acquisition single shot turbo spin-echo (HASTE) imaging, for indeterminate reasons. **C:** This artifact is not reproducible on true fast imaging with steady state precision (FISP) imaging. Lack of abnormal signal on true FISP imaging supports artifact and mitigates against subendocardial hemorrhage from infarction.

■ Other

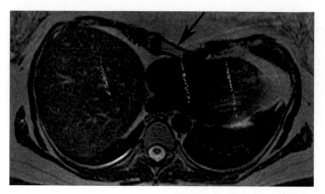

FIGURE 10-20 Sternal tilt. Axial T2-weighted image shows tilt of the sternum (*arrow*) which, if extreme as in this case, can result in mass effect upon the heart.

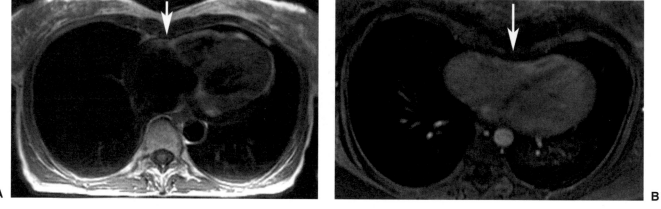

FIGURE 10-21 Pectus excavatum. A: Mild and **(B)** more marked cases of pectus excavatum (*arrows*) due to variations in the sternum.

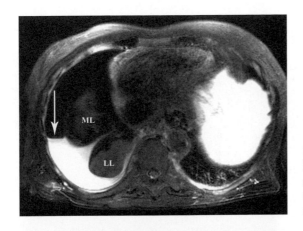

FIGURE 10-22 Hydropneumothorax with mass-like consolidation. Axial T2-weighted image shows mass-like consolidation of the right lower lobe (*LL*) in this patient with a large hydropneumothorax (*arrow*) (*Right middle lobe = ML*).

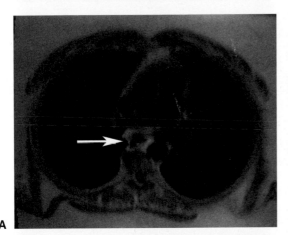

A

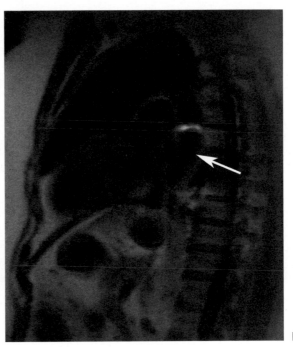

B

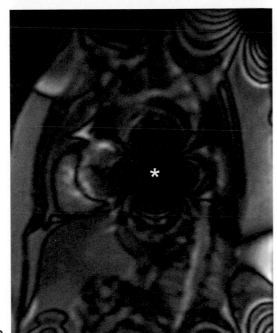

C

FIGURE 10-23 Metal artifact obscuring heart from esophageal probe. A and **B:** Spin dephasing (*arrows*) is observed due to differences in magnetic susceptibility of a metallic esophageal pH probe compared to that of tissue. **C:** Artifact (*asterisk*) is quite extensive on true fast imaging with steady state precision (FISP) imaging and characteristic constructive/destructive interference patterns are also observed due to fall-off of the magnetic field at the edges.

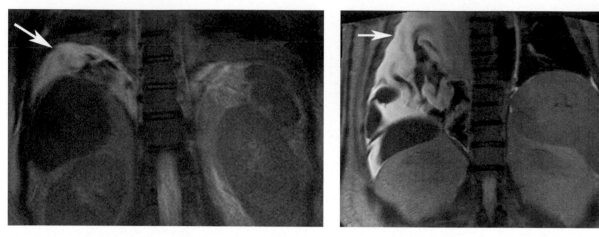

FIGURE 10-24 **Pleural effusion artifact.** Coronal T2-weighted images demonstrate **(A)** small and **(B)** massive right pleural effusions, with motion artifact within the fluid (*arrows*) and compression of the adjacent lung.

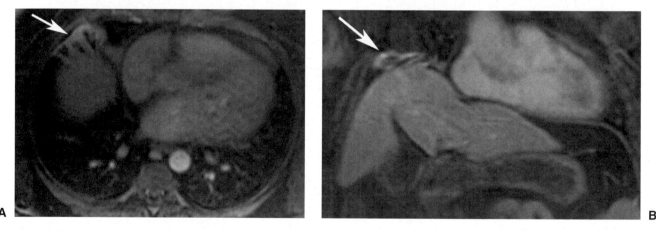

FIGURE 10-25 **Eventration with atelectasis. A:** Axial and **(B)** coronal T2-weighted images show partial eventration of the right hemidiaphragm with atelectasis of the right lung base (*arrows*).

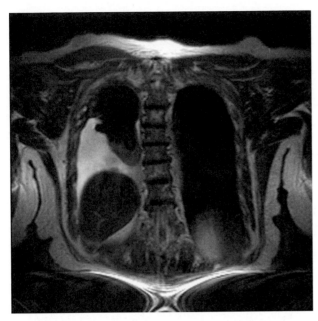

FIGURE 10-26 Poor patient positioning. The patient was positioned too far in the inferior direction of the scanner bore. Severe fall-off of the main magnetic and gradient field is observed at the bottom of this image.

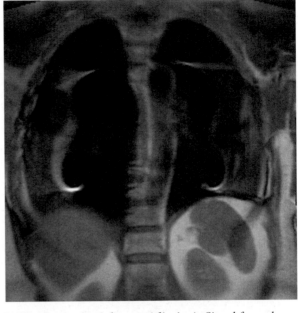

FIGURE 10-27 Signal wrap (aliasing). Signal from the arms has been aliasing (wrapped) into the image due to insufficient oversampling in the left-right direction. The shape of the artifact is likely modified due to geometric distortion from the outer parts of the arms being located in a region of fall-out of the magnetic field.

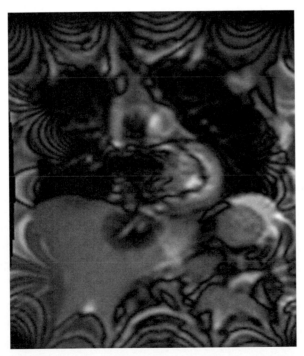

FIGURE 10-28 Magnetic field inhomogeneity. Characteristic constructive/destructive interference patterns due to fall-off of the magnetic field at the edges.

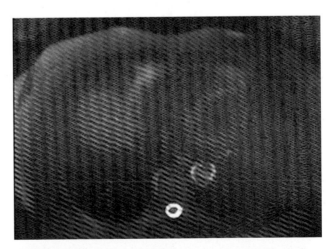

FIGURE 10-29 Reconstruction error. Interference pattern of lines at various spatial frequencies and angles, incorrectly reconstructed into the image, possibly due to receiver-induced error, spikes in the raw data (k-space) or poor receiver coil connection.

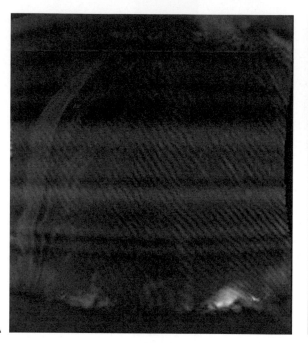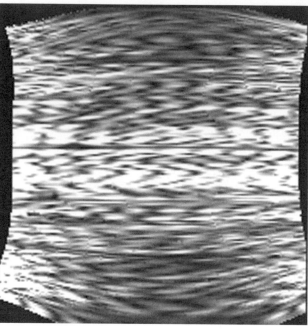

FIGURE 10-30 **Reconstruction error. A** and **B:** Artifact consistent with receiver-induced error in two different patients. The curvature at the edges is due to gradient linearity correction.

Suggested Readings

Anderson RH, Webb S, Brown NA. Clinical anatomy of the atrial septum with reference to its developmental components. *Clin Anat.* 1999;12:362–374.

Aquino SL, Duncan GR, Hayman LA. Nerves of the thorax: Atlas of normal and pathologic findings. *Radiographics.* 2001;21:1275–1281.

Bales GS. Great cardiac vein variations. *Clin Anat.* 2004;17:436–443.

Bansmann PM, Priest AN, Mueller leile K, et al. MRI of the coronary vessel wall at 3 T: Comparison of radial and Cartesian k-space sampling. *AJR Am J Roentgenol.* 2007;188:70–74.

Barbaix E, Kerckaert I, D'Herde K, et al. Simultaneous occurrence of a thyromediastnal muscle, a truncus bicaroticobrachialis, and a left superior vena cava. *Clin Anat.* 2003;16:176–181.

Becmeur F, Horta P, Donato L, et al. Accessory diaphragm—review of 31 cases in the literature. *Eur J Pediatr Surg.* 1995;5:43–47.

Bergman RA, Thompson SA, Afifi AK, et al. ed. *Compendium of human anatomic variation.* Baltimore: Urban & Schwarzenberg; 1988.

Boll DT, Bossert AS, Aschoff AJ, et al. Synergy of MDCT and cine MRI for the evaluation of cardiac motility. *AJR Am J Roentgenol.* 2006;186:S379–S386.

Castaner E, Gallardo X, Rimola J, et al. Congenital and acquired pulmonary artery anomalies in the adult: Radiologic overview. *Radiographics.* 2006;26:349–371.

Cherian SB, Ramesh BR, Madhyastha S. Persistent left superior vena cava. *Clin Anat.* 2006;19:561–565.

Donnelly LF, Frusg DP, Foss JN, et al. Anterior chest wall: Frequency of anatomic variations in children. *Radiology.* 1999;212:837–840.

Fabrizio PA, Clemente FR. Approach to dissection of the anterior thoracic wall and the entrance to the thoracic cavity. *Clin Anat.* 1998; 11:246–249.

Furlong J, Morrison WB, Carrino JA. Imaging of the talus. *Foot Ankle Clin.* 2004;9(4):685–701.

Gaudio C, Di Michele S, Cera M, et al. Prominent crista terminalis mimicking a right atrial myxoma: Cardiac magnetic resonance aspects. *Eur Rev Med Pharmacol Sci.* 2004;8:165–168.

Gerlis LM, Anderson RH. Anatomical conundrum: Unusual position of the aortic arch. *Clin Anat.* 1998;11:278–281.

Gerlis LM, Anderson RH. Unusual origin and course of the left pulmonary artery. *Clin Anat.* 2001;14:373–378.

Groves EM, Bireley W, Dill K, et al. Quantitative analysis of ECG-gated high-resolution contrast-enhanced MR angiography of the thoracic aorta. *AJR Am J Roentgenol.* 2007;188:522–528.

Guttentag AR, Salwen JK. Keep your eyes on the ribs: The spectrum of normal variants and diseases that involve the ribs. *Radiographics.* 1999;19:1125–1142.

Ho VB, Foo TKF. Impact of "cine MR imaging: Potential for the evaluation of cardiovascular function." *AJR Am J Roentgenol.* 2006;187: 605–608.

Kadir S. Regional anatomy of the thoracic aorta. In: Kadir S, ed. *Atlas of normal and variant angiographic anatomy.* Philadelphia: WB Saunders; 1991:19–54.

Kadir S. Superior vena cava and thoracic veins. In: Kadir S, ed. *Atlas of normal and variant angiographic anatomy.* Philadelphia: WB Saunders; 1991:163–175.

Katoh M, Spuentrup E, Buecker A, et al. MRI of coronary vessel walls using radial k-space sampling and steady-state free precession imaging. *AJR Am J Roentgenol.* 2006;186:S401–S406.

Kellenberger CJ, Yoo SJ, Buchel ERV. Cardiovascular MR imaging in neonates and infants with congenital heart disease. *Radiographics.* 2007;27:5–18.

Kervancioglu M, Ozbag D, Kervancioglu P, et al. Echocardiographic and morphologic examination of left ventricular false tendons in human and animal hearts. *Clin Anat.* 2003;16:389–395.

Konuskan B, Bozjurt MC, Tagil SM, et al. Cadaveric observation of an aberrant left subclavian artery: A possible cause of thoracic outlet syndrome. *Clin Anat.* 2005;18:215–216.

Lal M, Ho SY, Anderson RH. Is there such a thing as the "tendon of the infundibulum" in the heart? *Clin Anat.* 1997;10:307–312.

Layton KF, Kallmes DF, Cloft HJ, et al. Bovine aortic arch variant in humans: Clarification of a common misnomer. *AJNR Am J Neuroradiol.* 2006;27:1541–1542.

Mawatari T, Murakami G, Koshino T, et al. Posterior pulmonary lobe: Segmental and vascular anatomy in human specimens. *Clin Anat.* 2000;13:257–262.

Morrison JJ, Codispoti M, Campanella C. Surgically relevant structure on the ascending aorta. *Clin Anat.* 2003;16:253–255.

Nakatani T, Tanaka S, Mizokami S. Anomalous triad of a left-sided inferior vena cava, a retroesopageal right subclavian artery, and bilateral superficial brachial arteries in one individual. *Clin Anat.* 1998;11:112–117.

Nael K, Ruehm SG, Michaely HJ, et al. Multistation whole-body high-spatial resolution MR angiography using a 32-channel MR system. *AJR Am J Roentgenol.* 2007;188:529–539.

Ohno Y, Hatabu H, Murase Km, et al. Primary pulmonary hypertension: 3D dynamic perfusion MRI for quantitative analysis of regional pulmonary perfusion. *AJR Am J Roentgenol.* 2007;188:48–56.

Piegger J, Kovacs P, Ambach E. Extremely high origin of the right coronary artery from the ascending aorta. *Clin Anat.* 2001;14:369–372.

Pietrasik K, Bakon L, Zdunek P, et al. Clinical anatomy of internal thoracic artery branches. *Clin Anat.* 1999;12:307–314.

Porzionato A, Macchi V, Parenti A, et al. Unusual fibrous band on the left aspect of the aortic arch. *Clin Anat.* 2005;18:137–140.

Reig J, Petit M. Main trunk of the left coronary artery: Anatomic study of the parameters of clinical interest. *Clin Anat.* 2004;17:6–13.

Sarna A, Hayman LA, Laine FJ, et al. Coronal imaging of the ostiomeatal unit: Anatomy of 24 variants. *J Comput Assist Tomogr.* 2002;26:153–157.

Shah AS, Kukar A, Chaudhry FA, et al. Unusual anomalous single papillary muscle causing symptomatic mid-left ventricular cavity obstruction: Octopus papillary muscle. *J Am Soc Echocardiogr.* 2006;19:939.

Shapiro LB, Watt-Smith SR, Milosevic AM, et al. Cross-sectional imaging of a cadaveric human heart. *Clin Anat.* 1998;11:75–80.

Singh B, Ramsaroop L, Maharaj J, et al. Case of double superior vena cava. *Clin Anat.* 2005;18:366–369.

Subotich D, Mandarich D, Katchar V, et al. Lung resection for primary bronchial carcinoma in a patient with complete sinus inversus. *Clin Anat.* 2006;19:358–362.

Szpinda M. A new variant of aberrant left brachiocephalic trunk in man: Case report and literature review. *Folia Morphol (Praha).* 2005;64:47–50.

Vogel-Claussen J, Pannu H, Spevak PJ, et al. Cardiac valve assessment with MR imaging and 64-section multidetector row CT. *Radiographics.* 2006;26:1769–1784.

Von Ludinghausen M, Ohmachi N. Right superior septal artery with "normal" right coronary and extopic "early" aortic origin: A contribution to the vascular supply of the interventricular septum of the human heart. *Clin Anat.* 2001;14:312–319.

Vorster W, De Plooy PT, Meiring JH. Abnormal origin of internal thoracic and vertebral arteries. *Clin Anat.* 1998;11:33–37.

Yildiz H, Ugurel S, Soylu K, Accessory cardiac bronchus and tracheal bronchus anomalies. *Surg Radiol Anat.* 2006;28:646–649.

Yuksel M, Yuksel E. Anomalous branching order of the superior and lateral thoracic arteries. *Clin Anat.* 1997;10:394–396.

www.anatomyatlases.org.

Zajick DC Jr, Morrison WB, Schweitzer ME, et al. Benign and malignant processes: Normal values and differentiation with chemical shift MR imaging in vertebral marrow. *Radiology.* 2005;237(2):590–596.

Section IV

ABDOMEN

Chapter 11

Liver and Biliary System

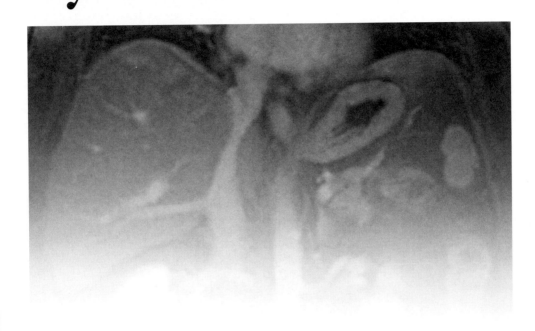

Liver

Biliary

Mellena D. Bridges

■ Liver

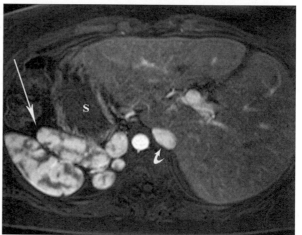

FIGURE 11-1   Bare area of the liver. Ascites (*A*) outlines the lateral and lateral upper surfaces of the liver, but is prevented by peritoneal reflections from dissecting into the bare area (*arrows*).

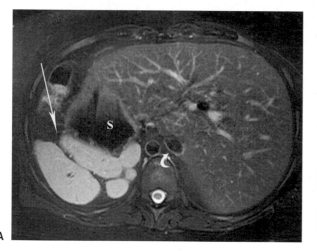

A

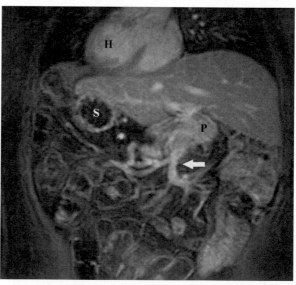

FIGURE 11-2   Situs inversus totalis. Axial fat-suppressed **(A)** T2-weighted and **(B)** enhanced T1-weighted images localize the liver to the left upper quadrant, and multiple splenic nodules to the right upper quadrant (*arrow*). Positions of the aorta and inferior vena cava (*curved arrow*) are reversed. **C:** Coronal enhanced T1-weighted image shows displacement of pancreatic head (*P*) and superior mesenteric vein (*arrow*) to the left. Stomach (*S*) and heart (*H*) on the right.

C

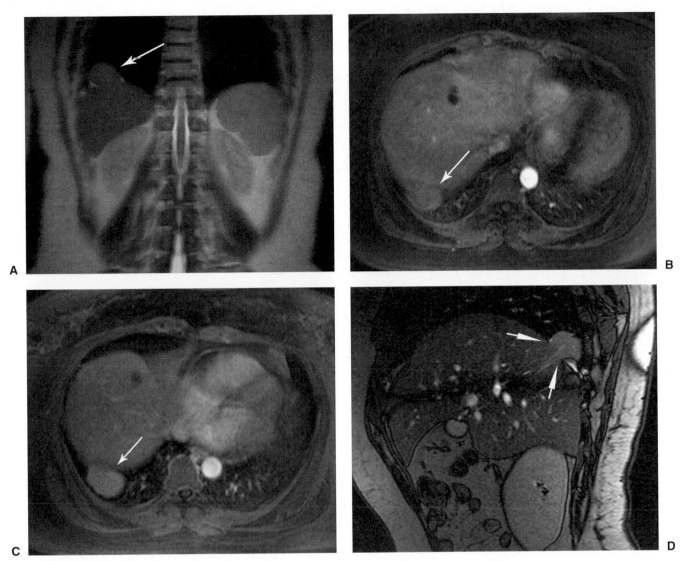

FIGURE 11-3 **Liver-containing Bochdalek hernia simulates a pleural mass. A:** A homogeneous mass projects into the right hemithorax (*arrow*) on coronal T2-weighted single-shot image. Axial enhanced T1-weighted images in **(B)** arterial and **(C)** portal dominant phases demonstrate progressive enhancement of the mass, presumably due to venous outflow impairment. **D:** Sagittal steady state free precession (SSFP) image shows continuity of mass with liver, as well as some traversing vessels (*Margins of hernia = short arrows*).

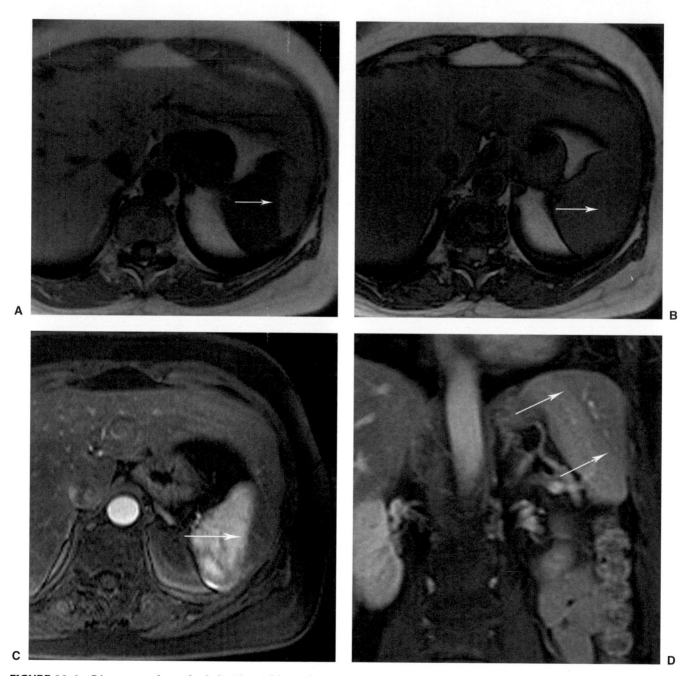

FIGURE 11-4 **Liver extends to the left side and lateral to spleen, a potential pitfall. A:** In-phase gradient echo image shows typical T1 intensity difference between liver (*arrow*) and spleen. **B:** Fatty liver loses signal intensity on opposed phase image, becoming isointense to spleen. **C:** Axial arterial phase T1-weighted image brings out the differences between the two tissues, whereas a (**D**) later coronal image shows near isointensity.

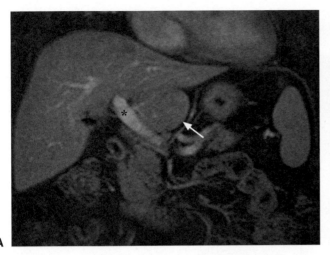

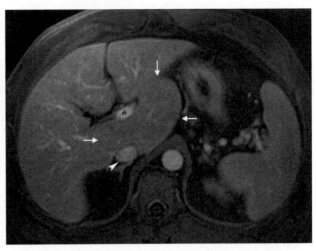

FIGURE 11-5 Large caudate lobe simulates an abdominal mass. A: Coronal enhanced T1-weighted image demonstrates a mass (*arrow*) medial to the portal vein (*asterisk*). **B:** Axial enhanced image clearly shows the mass to be liver tissue. Notice the wide separation of portal vein (*asterisk*) and inferior vena cava (*arrowhead*) (*Caudate = arrows*).

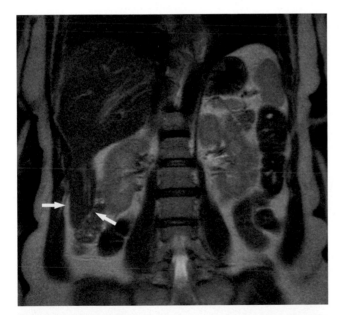

FIGURE 11-6 Riedel lobe simulates hepatomegaly. The Riedel lobe is a long tongue of liver tissue (*arrows*) that projects inferiorly from the right hepatic lobe, and is a normal variant.

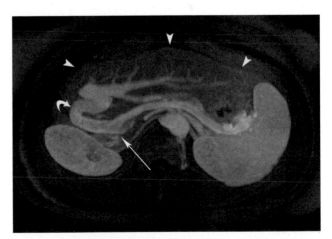

FIGURE 11-7 Hypertrophied lateral hepatic segment following trisegmentectomy. Axial subvolume maximum intensity projection (MIP) image from an enhanced T1-weighted data set demonstrates a very large lateral segment (*arrowheads*) and lays out the similarly hypertrophied portal vasculature (*Portosplenic confluence = long arrow, Left portal vein = curved arrow*).

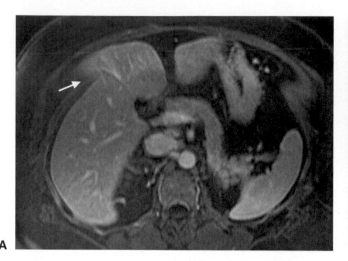
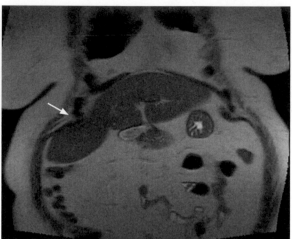

FIGURE 11-8 **Prominent ribcage indentation simulates herniated liver. A:** Axial enhanced T1-weighted image shows the left hepatic lobe displaced anteriorly (*arrow*). **B:** Coronal T2-weighted image demonstrates that accumulated visceral fat has pushed the soft liver upward and outward, creating an impression from the ribcage (*arrow*) on its upper and anterior surfaces.

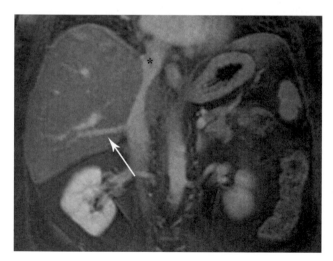

FIGURE 11-9 **Accessory hepatic vein, a common variant,** drains the lower right hepatic lobe (*Accessory vein = arrow, IVC at level of usual venous confluence = asterisk*). IVC, inferior vena cava.

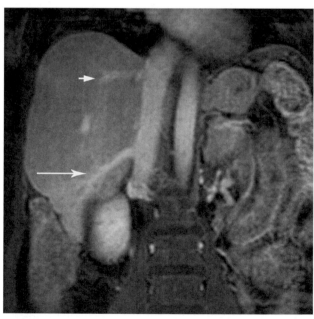

FIGURE 11-10 **Accessory right hepatic vein, a common variant.** Enhanced coronal T1-weighted image shows a sizable accessory right hepatic vein (*arrow*) draining the inferior portion of the right hepatic lobe into the inferior vena cava (*Normal position of hepatic vein = short arrow*).

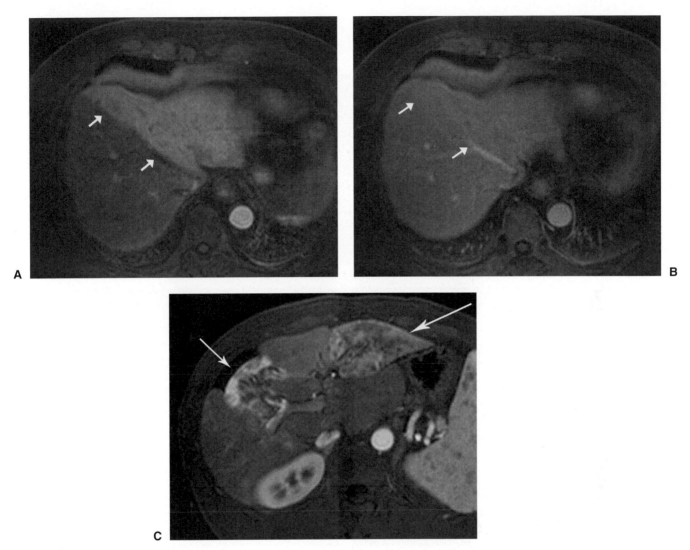

FIGURE 11-11 **Regional hyperenhancement in the arterial phase due to left portal venous thrombosis. A:** Transient left lobar arterial phase hyperenhancement (*short arrows*) is no longer visible on (**B**) portal venous phase T1-weighted image. **C:** Arterial phase image in another patient reveals several areas of peripheral atrophy (*arrows*) due to chronic subsegmental portal venous occlusion.

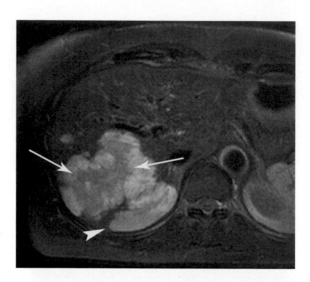

FIGURE 11-12 Internal fibrosis in large hemangioma. Fat-suppressed T2-weighted image in same patient as Fig. 11-13 shows the internal fibrosis or hyalinization as area of decreased signal intensity (*arrows*), a common feature of larger hemangiomas. Striking lobulation (*arrowhead*) is also appreciated.

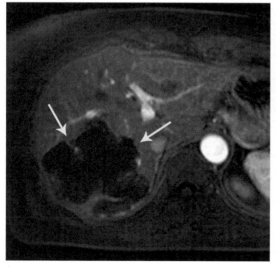

A

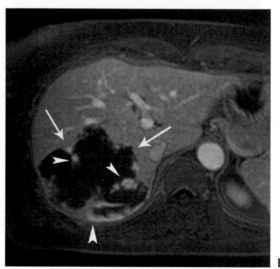

B

FIGURE 11-13 Slow enhancement of large hemangioma. A: Hemangioma (*arrows*) reveals very little nodularity on arterial dominant enhanced T-weighted image. **B:** By portal phase, characteristic discontinuous peripheral nodules (*arrowheads*) are visible within the hemangioma (*arrows*). **C:** Fifteen minutes later, much of lesion (*arrows*) is isointense with the blood pool, but there is a significant area of central hyalinization (*curved arrow*).

C

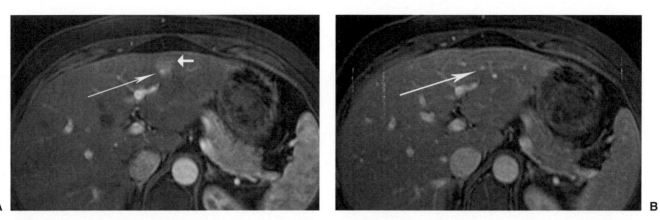

FIGURE 11-14 **Arterial hyperenhancement around a subcentimeter hemangioma. A:** T1-weighted image obtained early after contrast injection demonstrates a geographic area of increased parenchymal enhancement (*short arrow*) around a small, flash-filling hemangioma (*long arrow*). **B:** By portal phase, perilesional enhancement about the hemangioma (*arrow*) has resolved.

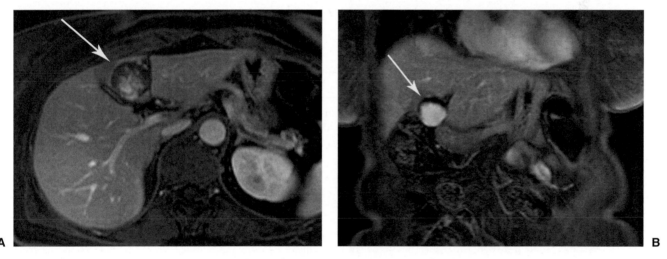

FIGURE 11-15 **Exophytic hemangioma mistaken for gallbladder mass. A:** Enhanced T1-weighted image shows a round, apparently heterogeneous lesion (*arrow*) under the medial segment of the liver. **B:** Orthogonal image proves this to be the top of a large peripheral puddle of contrast (*arrow*), consistent with hemangioma. Patterns like this are often responsible for a so-called inside-outside pattern of hemangioma enhancement.

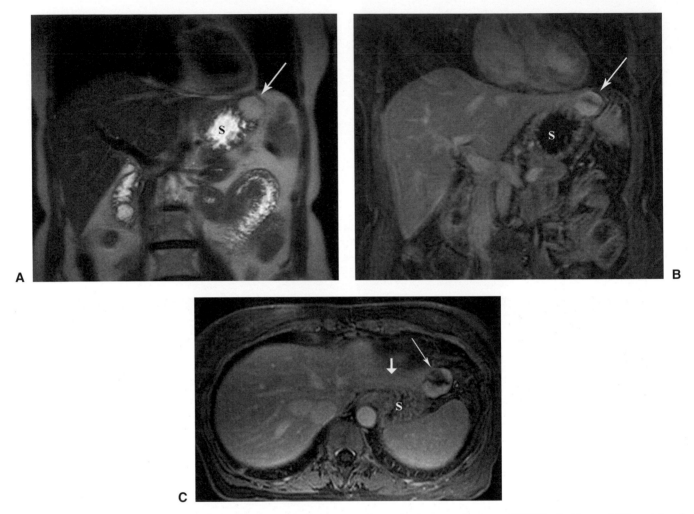

FIGURE 11-16 Exophytic hepatic hemangioma mimics a gastrointestinal stromal tumor (GIST). A: Coronal T2-weighted image demonstrates moderately hyperintense lesion in the left upper quadrant (*arrow*), seemingly arising from the outer gastric wall. **B:** Coronal enhanced T1-weighted image shows strong enhancement (*arrow*) (*Stomach = S*). **C:** Axial enhanced image shows the relationship of the lesion (*long arrow*) to a slender tongue of lateral segment liver tissue (*short arrow*) (*Stomach = S*).

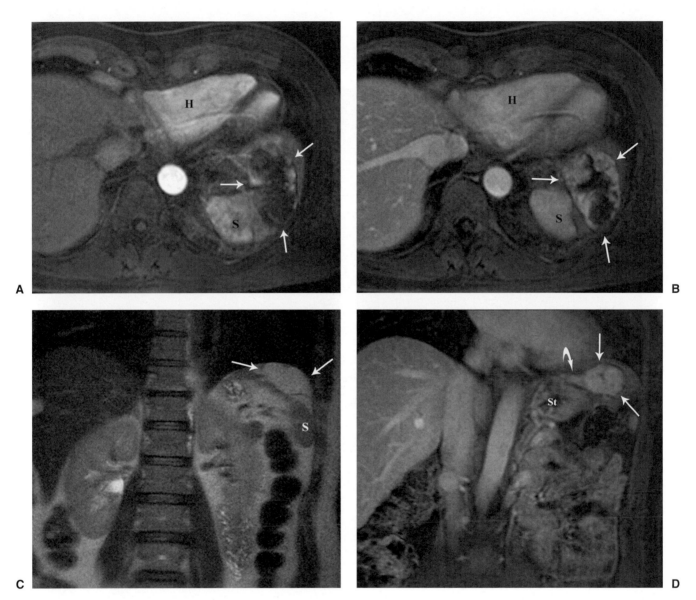

FIGURE 11-17   Pedunculated hemangioma appears as a left upper quadrant mass. Axial **(A)** arterial and **(B)** portal phase T1-weighted images include a posterior left upper quadrant mass (*arrows*). Enhancement occurs in a discontinuous, peripheral, progressive manner, typical of hemangioma (*Heart = H, Spleen = S*). **C:** Mass (*arrows*) is isointense to fat on coronal T2-weighted image (*Spleen = S*). **D:** Delayed coronal enhanced image shows further enhancement of the hemangioma (*arrows*) as well as attachment to a tongue of liver tissue (*curved arrow*) (*Stomach = St*).

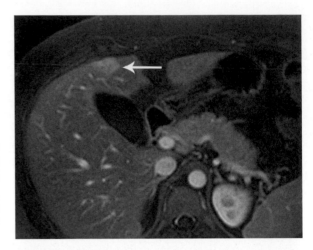

FIGURE 11-18 **Focal nodular hyperplasia (FNH) simulates hemangioma** on portal phase imaging. Focal nodular hyperplasia (*arrow*) is normally subtle on portal phase imaging unless the background liver is abnormal. Here the combination of a fatty liver and a fat-suppressed technique results in signal loss for the liver tissue, but not for the FNH.

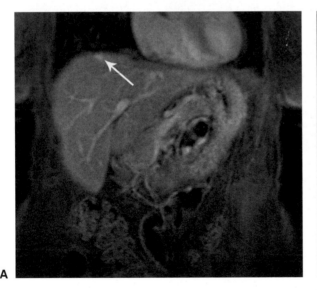

A

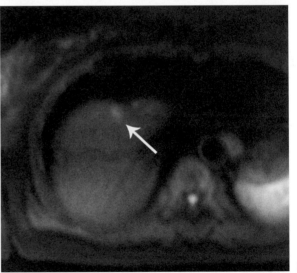

B

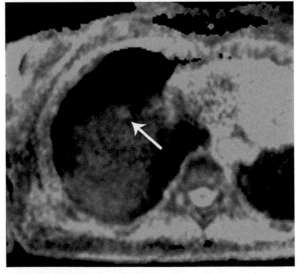

C

FIGURE 11-19 **Unrestricted diffusion in cavernous hemangioma.** Hemangiomas can be quite variable on diffusion-weighted imaging (DWI). **A:** Coronal enhanced T1-weighted image demonstrates small contrast-filled hemangioma (*arrow*) at the liver dome. **B:** Diffusion-weighted echoplanar image with b = 50 shows hyperintensity (*arrow*) at this site. **C:** Apparent diffusion coefficient (ADC) map also shows hyperintensity, consistent with unrestricted water diffusion.

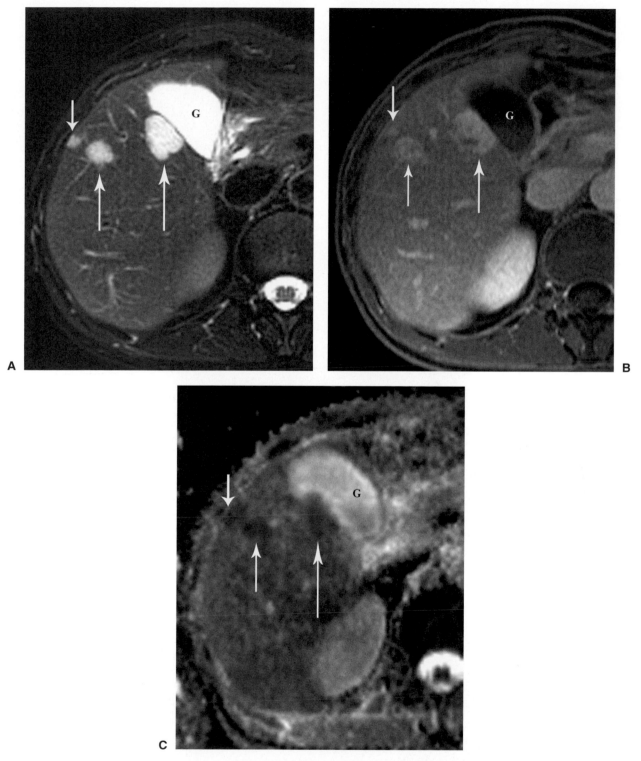

FIGURE 11-20 Diffusion restriction in hemangioma mimics tumor. A: Axial T2-weighted image shows three lobulated hyperintense lesions (*arrows*), consistent with hemangiomas (*G*). **B:** Lesions (*arrows*) are isointense to blood pool on delayed postcontrast image, as expected (*G*). **C:** Apparent diffusion coefficient (ADC) map from diffusion-weighted imaging (DWI) demonstrates restricted diffusivity in the lateral two lesions (*shorter arrows*) (*Long arrow = third hemangioma, Gallbladder = G*).

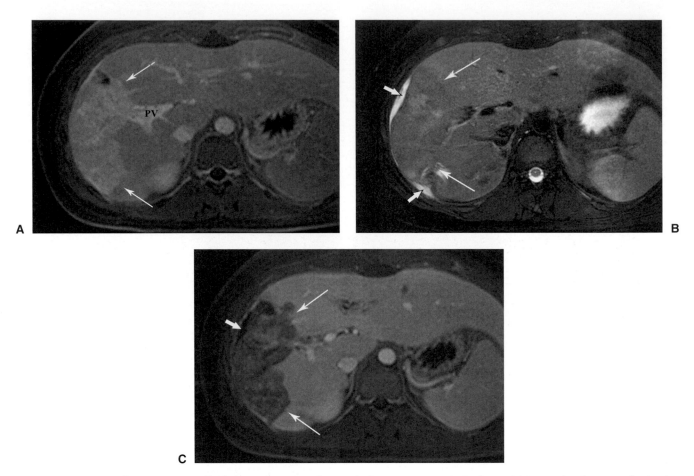

FIGURE 11-21 **"Fill in" is not sufficient evidence to diagnosis hemangioma. A:** Enhanced T1-weighted image obtained at 10 minutes demonstrates a lobulated, peripheral mass (*arrows*) that is isointense with blood vessels, and had been interpreted as a *hemangioma* at previous imaging (*Right portal vein = PV*). **B:** T2-isointensity (*long arrows*) and capsular retraction (*short arrows*) are features inconsistent with hemangioma. **C:** On image obtained earlier postcontrast, this biopsy-proven hemangioendothelioma (*long arrows*) shows neither appropriate nodular nor discontinuous peripheral enhancement (*Capsular retraction = short arrow*).

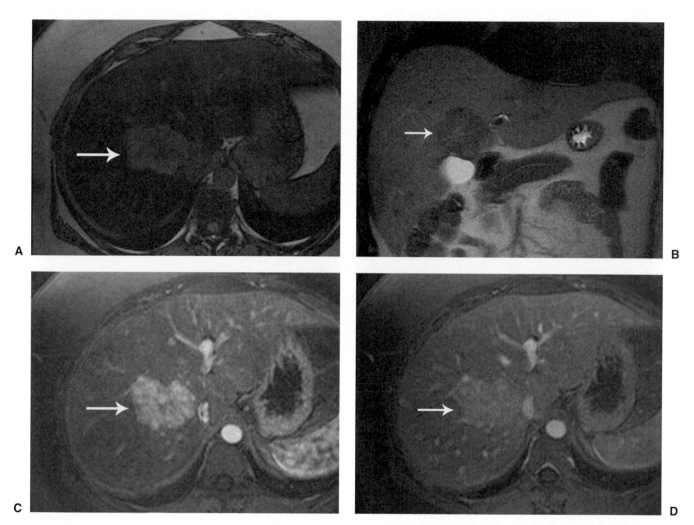

FIGURE 11-22   Focal nodular hyperplasia (FNH) more conspicuous than usual because of background steatosis. A: FNH (*arrow*) is hyperintense on opposed phase T1-weighted imaging because of signal drop-out in the background liver. **B:** In contrast, the lesion (*arrow*) appears hypointense on a coronal T2-weighted image because of the increased signal from adjacent fatty in liver tissue. With application of fat suppression, the FNH (*arrow*) is atypically visible on both **(C)** arterial dominant and **(D)** portal phase T1-weighted imaging. Typically this benign lesion would be inconspicuous on all pulse sequences except the arterial phase acquisition.

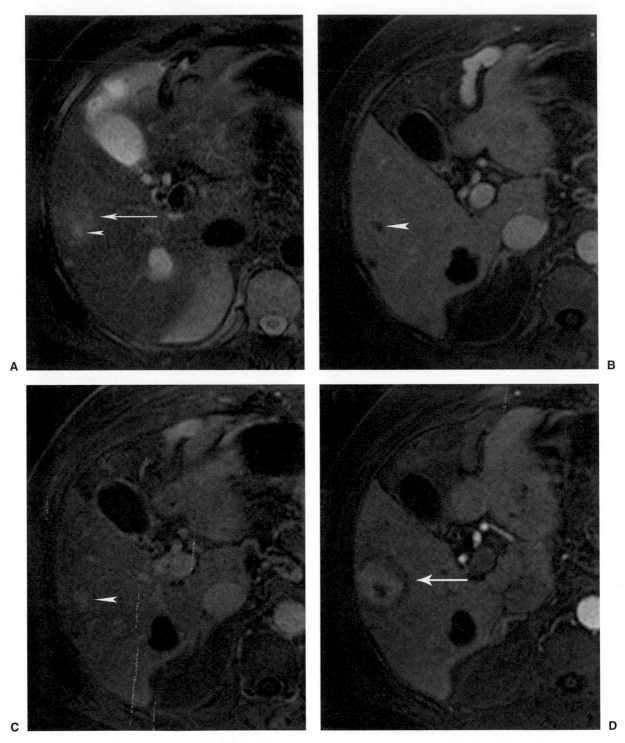

FIGURE 11-23 **Hepatocellular carcinoma (HCC) simulates focal nodular hyperplasia (FNH). A:** Subtle lesion on T2-weighted image is mildly hyperintense (*arrow*), with a central focus of stronger signal (*arrowhead*). Central focus (*arrowhead*) enhances poorly on **(B)** portal phase imaging, but eventually accumulates contrast on **(C)** delayed imaging, as might be seen with a central scar in FNH. **D:** However, lesion (*arrow*) has a malignant target appearance on arterial phase imaging and is a surgically proven HCC.

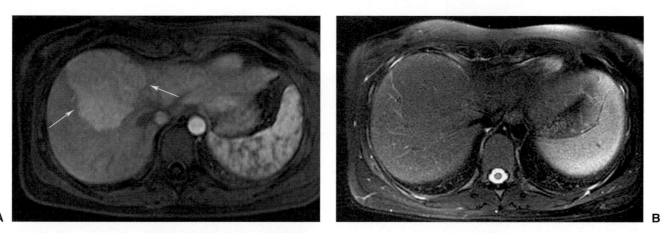

FIGURE 11-24 **Atypical large focal nodular hyperplasia (FNH) lacks a central scar. A:** T1-weighted arterial phase image shows intense, diffuse enhancement of this mass (*arrows*), but without obvious central organization around a "scar." **B:** T2-weighted image confirms the lack of internal features, more commonly a feature of small FNH.

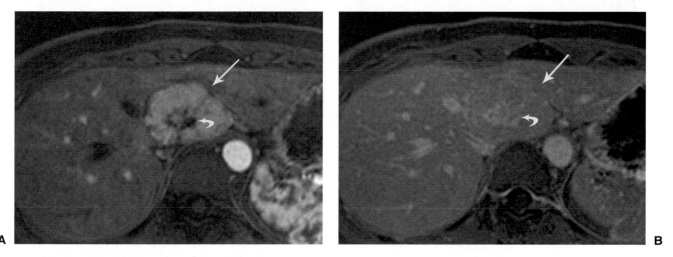

FIGURE 11-25 **Typical central scar in focal nodular hyperplasia (FNH). A:** Lobulated, arterially hyperenhancing mass (*arrow*) on enhanced T1-weighted image has a central area of diminished enhancement (*curved arrow*). **B:** Scar within the FNH becomes hyperintense on delayed enhanced imaging.

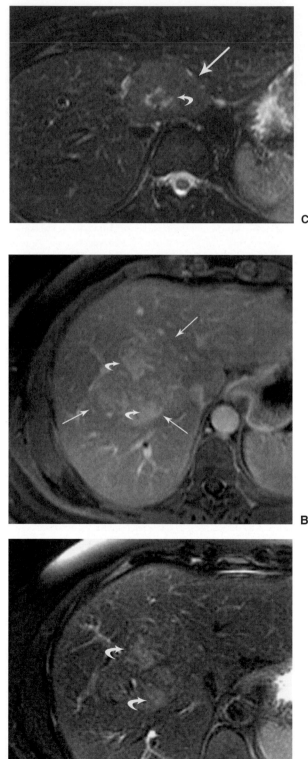

FIGURE 11-25 **Typical central scar in focal nodular hyperplasia.** (*continued*) **C:** Scar in the interior of the FNH (*arrow*) is hyperintense on T2-weighted image.

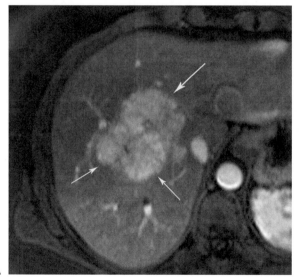

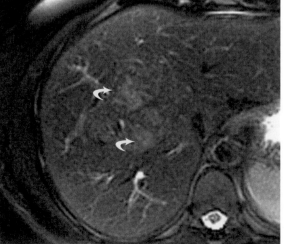

FIGURE 11-26 **Atypical scar in focal nodular hyperplasia (FNH). A:** Typical intense arterial enhancement in large, lobulated FNH (*arrows*). **B:** Portal phase image shows accumulation of contrast in two polygonal areas (*curved arrows*) within the lesion (*arrows*), one of which is quite peripheral. **C:** Areas (*curved arrows*) are also hyperintense on T2-weighted images, consistent with intralesional vascular scar.

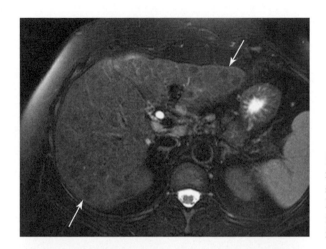

FIGURE 11-27 Multifocal hepatic steatosis as mass-like T2-hypointense lesions. Axial fat-suppressed T2-weighted image demonstrates multiple hypointense nodules (*arrows*). This appearance is due to focal steatosis that is sufficiently severe to lose signal intensity with frequency-selective fat suppression.

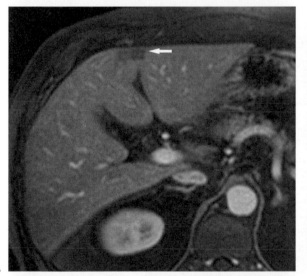

A

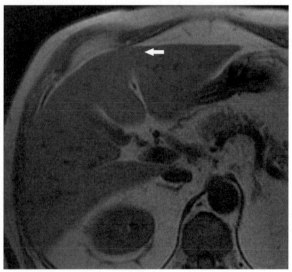

B

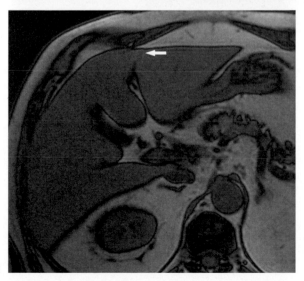

C

FIGURE 11-28 Focal perfusion alteration, a common normal variant, simulates hypovascular mass. **A:** Axial enhanced T1-weighted image shows a small, peripheral area of diminished enhancement (*arrow*) along the fissure for the falciform ligament. **B:** In-phase and **(C)** opposed-phase gradient echo images demonstrate no correlative signal alterations (*arrow*), excluding the other common variant in this location, focal steatosis.

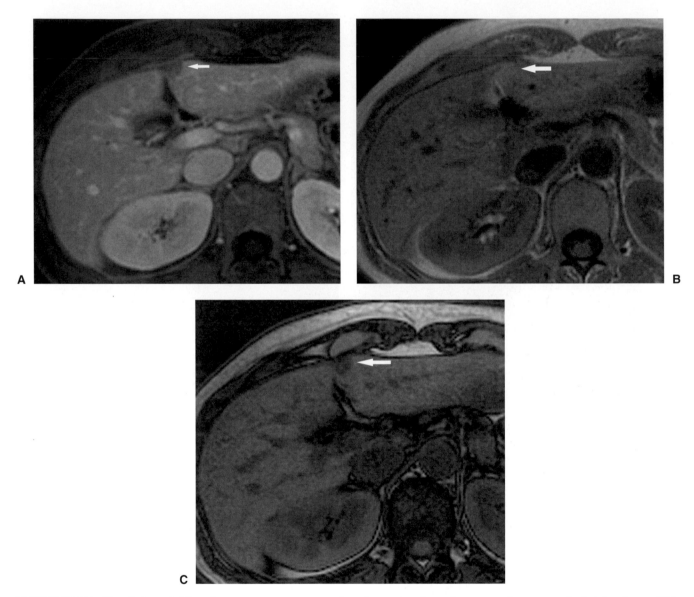

FIGURE 11-29 **Focal fatty infiltration, a common normal variant, simulates hypovascular mass. A:** Axial enhanced T1-weighted image demonstrates a small, peripheral area of apparently diminished enhancement (*arrow*) along the fissure for the falciform ligament. There is increased signal in this region (*arrow*) on (**B**) in-phase gradient echo image, and decreased signal on (**C**) opposed-phase image. Imaging behavior is diagnostic of intracellular lipid.

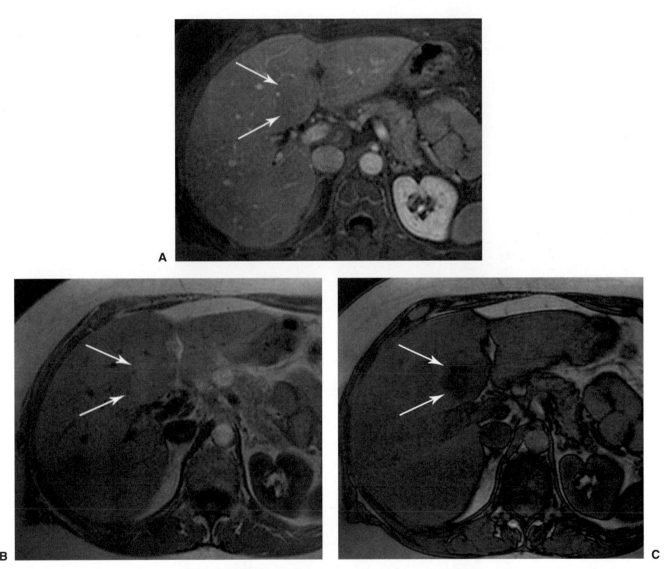

FIGURE 11-30 **Focal fatty infiltration in the perihilar aspect of segment IV simulates a hypovascular mass lesion. A:** Axial T1-weighted image demonstrates apparently reduced enhancement (*arrows*). The combination of increased signal on **(B)** in-phase and decreased signal on **(C)** opposed-phase gradient echo images is consistent with fatty infiltration. This location is a common site of steatosis, as is the liver adjacent to the gallbladder fossa.

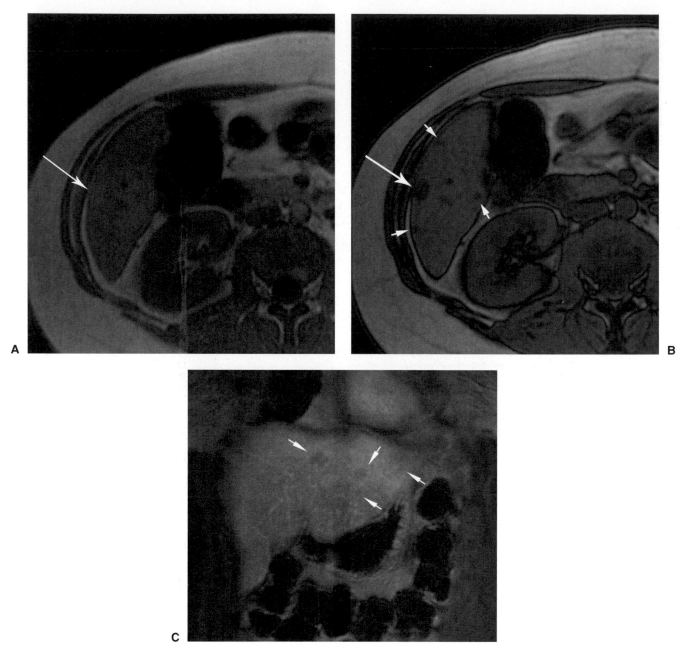

FIGURE 11-31 Multifocal fatty infiltration simulates metastases in breast cancer patient. A: Axial in-phase T1-weighted gradient echo image is unremarkable except for a subtle area of higher signal intensity laterally (*arrow*). **B:** Opposed-phase image at same level shows profound signal drop here (*long arrow*) and elsewhere (*short arrows*). **C:** Coronal enhanced T1-weighted image reveals further foci of steatosis (*arrows*).

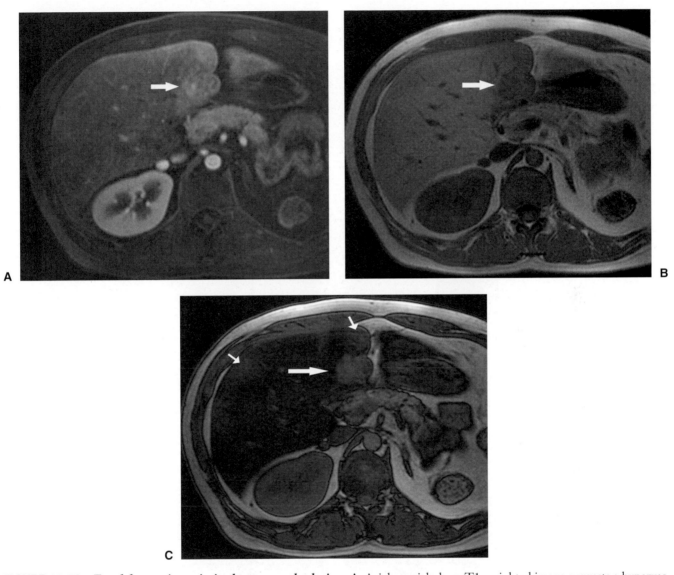

FIGURE 11-32   Focal fat sparing mimics hypervascular lesion. A: Axial arterial phase T1-weighted image suggests a hypervascular nodule (*arrow*) in segment IV along the fissure for the falciform ligament. **B:** This focus (*arrow*) is slightly hypointense to surrounding liver on in-phase gradient sequence. **C:** Opposed-phase image proves the real abnormality to be the rest of the liver, which is quite fatty. This (*long arrow*) and other areas of fat sparing are now also clearly demonstrated (*small arrows*).

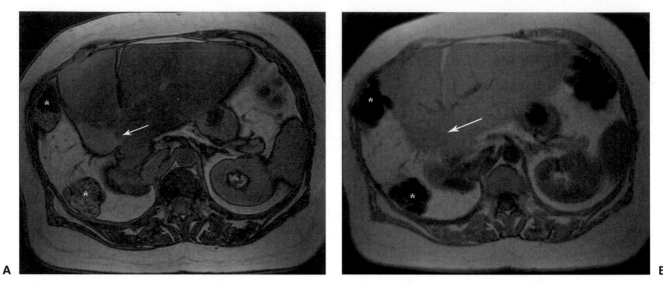

FIGURE 11-33 **Fat sparing** along surgical margin, **a potential pitfall. A:** In-phase and **(B)** opposed-phase gradient echo images show absence of right liver lobe, hypertrophy and steatosis of the liver remnant, along with a mass-like focus of fat sparing (*arrow*) at the resection margin. Notice the movement of the hepatic flexure (*asterisk*) into the surgical defect.

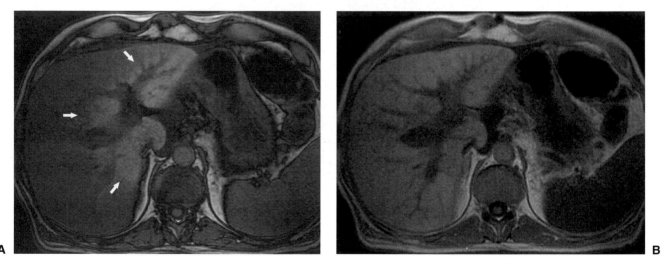

FIGURE 11-34 **Focal fat sparing in radiation field. A:** Opposed-phase gradient echo T1-weighted image demonstrates higher signal intensity in the treated part of the liver (*arrows*) in this patient with pancreatic cancer. **B:** Parenchymal changes are more subtle on in-phase image. Normal liver has a much greater capacity than abnormal liver to accumulate intracellular lipid.

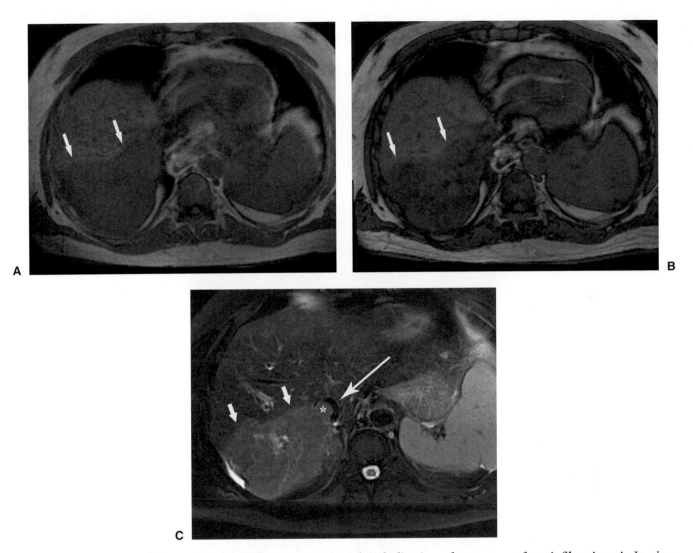

FIGURE 11-35 **Opposed-phase signal loss due to transarterial embolization of tumor, not fatty infiltration. A:** In-phase and **(B)** opposed-phase T1-weighted images show segmental heterogeneous signal loss (*arrows*) due to prior arterial embolization rather than focal fat. Polyvinyl alcohol and LC Beads (N-fil Hydrogel microspheres) were utilized. **C:** Retracting tumor thrombus (*asterisk*) in the inferior vena cava (*long arrow*) is demonstrated on axial T2-weighted image.

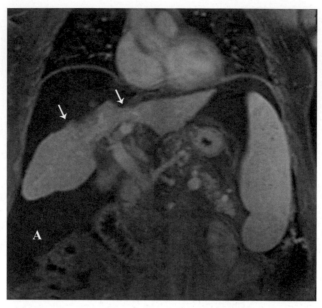

FIGURE 11-36   Nonuniform liver fibrosis. Coronal enhanced T1-weighted image in a cirrhotic patient demonstrates profound volume loss and surface retraction (*arrows*) primarily involving segments IV and VIII (*Ascites = A*).

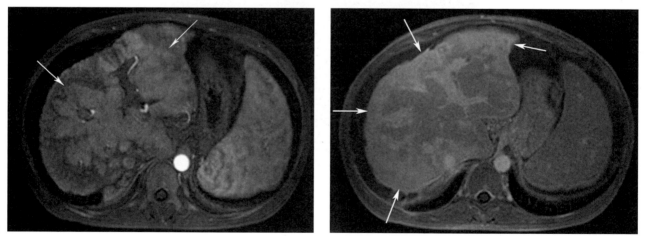

FIGURE 11-37   Regenerative liver hypertrophy simulates hypervascular mass. A: Axial T1-weighted image in the arterial dominant phase of contrast enhancement suggests a large, lobulated, hypervascular central liver tumor (*arrows*). **B:** Signal intensities reverse on delayed phase imaging, as peripheral fibrosis (*arrows*) becomes obvious in this patient with central liver regeneration in the setting of primary sclerosing cholangitis (PSC).

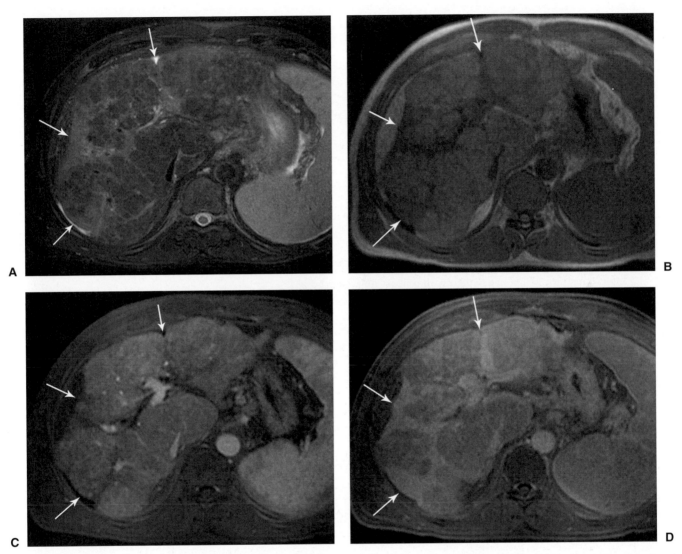

FIGURE 11-38 Focal fibrosis mimics infiltrative masses on T2 and delayed enhanced imaging. **A:** Axial fat-suppressed T2-weighted image demonstrates confluent bands of high signal intensity (*arrows*). **B:** On T1-weighted image, these areas (*arrows*) are low in signal intensity relative to background liver. **C:** Early portal and **(D)** delayed phase enhanced T1-weighted images show slow, but finally very strong, accumulation of contrast in the fibrosis (*arrows*).

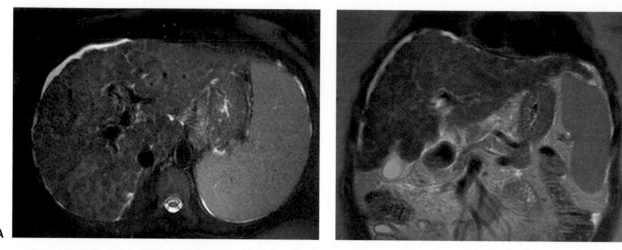

FIGURE 11-39 **Reticular high T2 signal due to fibrosis. A:** Axial fat-suppressed and **(B)** coronal T2-weighted images show reticular high signal throughout in a patient with primary biliary cirrhosis.

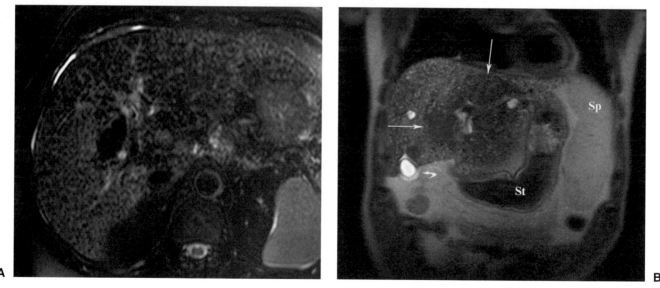

FIGURE 11-40 **Fibrosis appears as fine network of T2-hyperintense nodules. A:** Axial fat-suppressed and **(B)** coronal T2-weighted images demonstrate what appears to be a diffuse pattern of tiny hyperintense nodules. Liver fibrosis is related to polycystic renal disease (*Area of regeneration/sparing = arrows, Edematous gallbladder wall = curved arrow, Enlarged spleen = Sp, Stomach = St*).

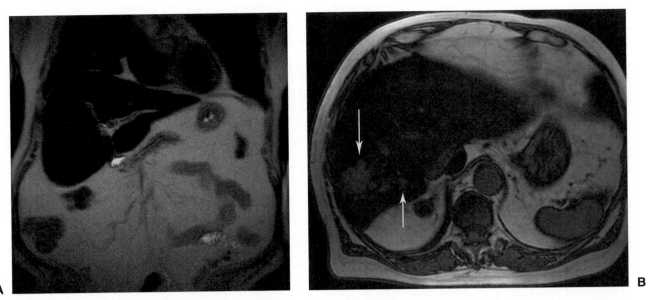

FIGURE 11-41 Profound signal loss in hepatic hemochromatosis. A: Coronal T2-weighted image shows striking loss of hepatic signal intensity due to diffuse parenchymal iron deposition. **B:** Conspicuity of multifocal hepatocellular carcinoma (*arrows*) is increased by the liver's intense background hypointensity on this T1-weighted axial image.

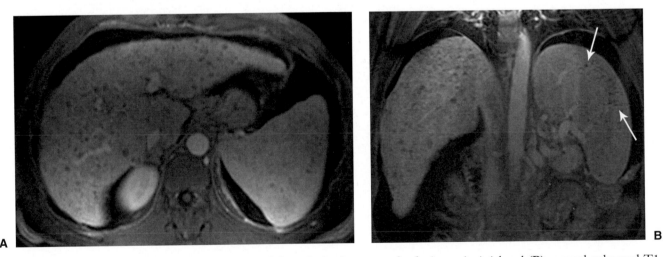

FIGURE 11-42 Iron content in regenerative nodules mimics hypovascular lesions. A: Axial and **(B)** coronal enhanced T1-weighted images demonstrate multiple hypointense foci in a cirrhotic liver, compatible with siderotic nodules (*Splenic Gamna-Gandy bodies = arrows*).

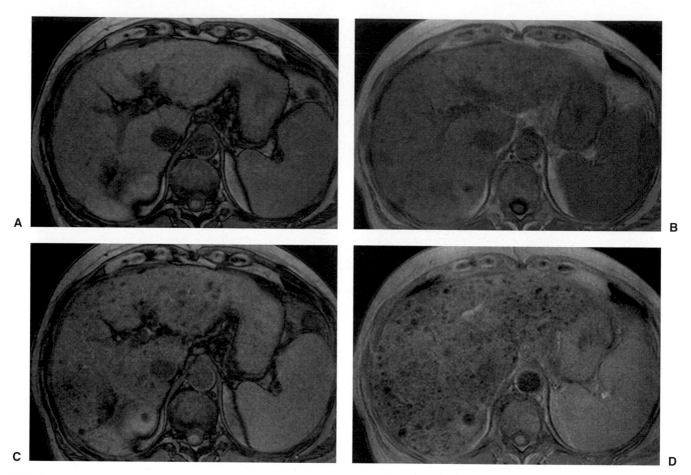

FIGURE 11-43 **Conspicuity of iron-containing liver nodules** on gradient echo imaging increases with echo time (TE). **A:** TE = 2.3 msec (opposed phase). **B:** TE = 4.6 (in-phase). **C:** TE = 7.0 (opposed phase). **D:** TE = 9.2 (in-phase).

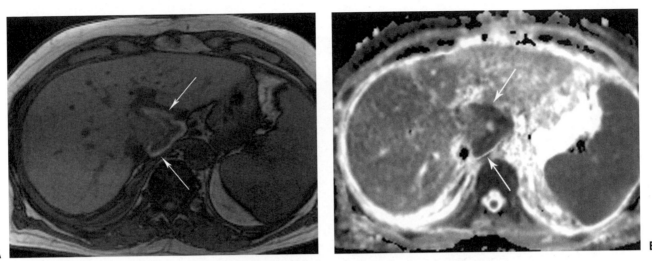

FIGURE 11-44 Typical peripheral hyperintensity and restricted diffusion in postoperative hematoma can mimic malignancy or infection. **A:** Small hematoma (*arrows*) outlines the caudate lobe of a transplanted liver on axial T1-weighted gradient echo image. Hyperintense rim does not enhance following contrast administration. **B:** Marked lesion hypointensity in an apparent diffusion coefficient (ADC) map reflects profound restriction of water motion within the clot (*arrows*).

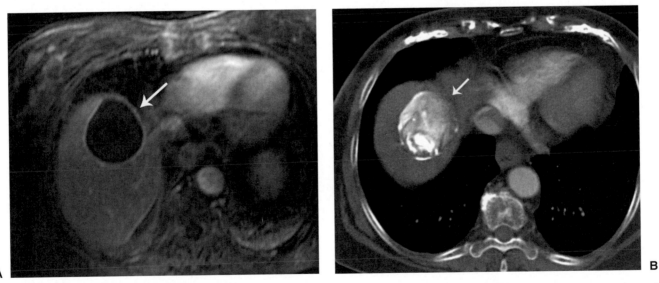

FIGURE 11-45 Due to lack of mobile protons, calcium can be a significant pitfall for MRI. **A:** Axial contrast-enhanced T1-weighted image through the liver dome demonstrates a homogeneous-appearing, nonenhancing mass (*arrow*). **B:** Correlative CT shows a densely calcified echinococcal cyst (*arrow*).

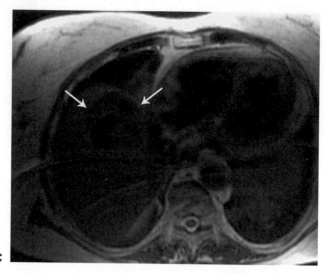

C

FIGURE 11-45 Due to lack of mobile protons, calcium can be a significant pitfall for MRI. (*continued*) **C:** Precontrast T1-weighted image represents the cyst (*arrow*) as composed of swirling low signal.

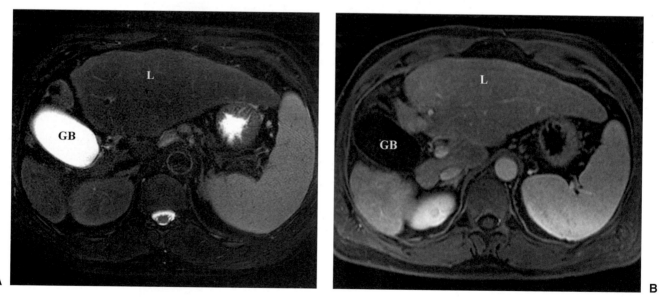

A

B

FIGURE 11-46 Empty gallbladder sign of cirrhosis. Axial **(A)** fat-suppressed T2 and **(B)** enhanced T1-weighted images demonstrate enlargement of the lateral segment (*L*) and profound atrophy of the liver tissue surrounding the gallbladder (*GB*), a clue to the diagnosis of cirrhosis.

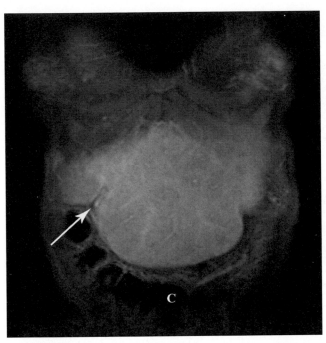

FIGURE 11-47   Enlarged left lateral segment a clue to cirrhosis. Coronal enhanced T1-weighted image through the anterior abdomen shows an apron of lateral segment tissue that displaces the transverse colon (*C*) inferiorly. Falciform ligament fissure (*arrow*) marks the boundary between the medial and lateral hepatic segments.

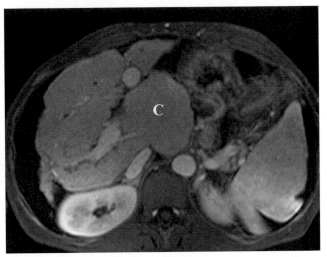

FIGURE 11-48   Enlarged caudate lobe, very common sign of cirrhosis. Axial image shows a severely distorted, cirrhotic liver with a very large caudate lobe (*C*).

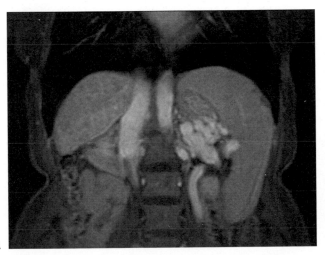

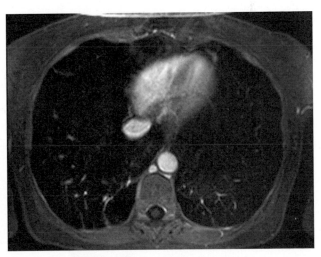

FIGURE 11-49   Liver cirrhosis and emphysema in α-1 antitrypsin deficiency. A: Coronal and **(B)** axial enhanced T1-weighted images demonstrate massive hyperinflation of lung bases as well as cirrhosis, varices, and splenomegaly. Although imaged during expiration, the diaphragms appear flattened and the heart small.

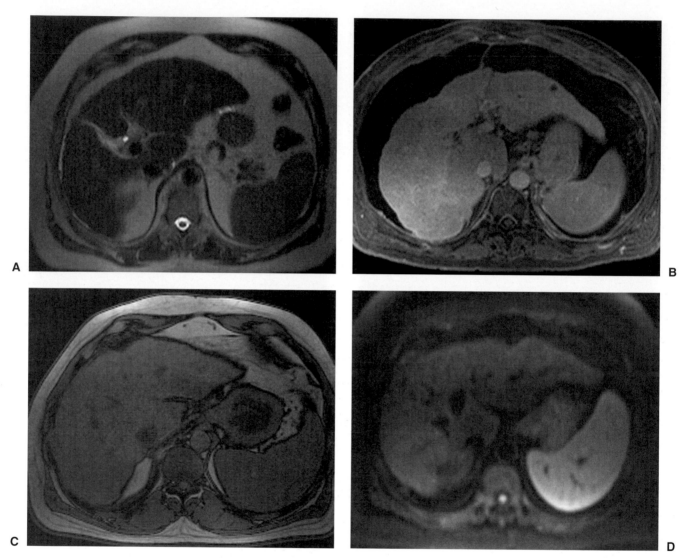

FIGURE 11-50 Author's favorite animal signs in cirrhosis. **A:** Manatee morphology due to lateral segment and caudate enlargement, with atrophy elsewhere. **B:** Anteater sign. **C:** Shark sign. **D:** Baby bird birthing sign.

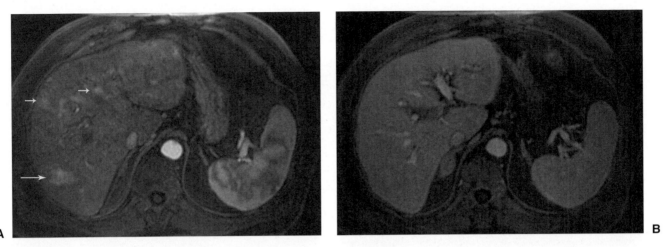

FIGURE 11-51 **Arterioportal shunting complicates imaging of cirrhosis, mimicking early hepatocellular carcinoma.** **A:** Enhanced arterial phase T1-weighted image shows scattered small hypervascular foci (*arrows*). **B:** Tiny vascular shunts, common in cirrhotic liver, tend to be occult on all other imaging sequences, including the portal phase.

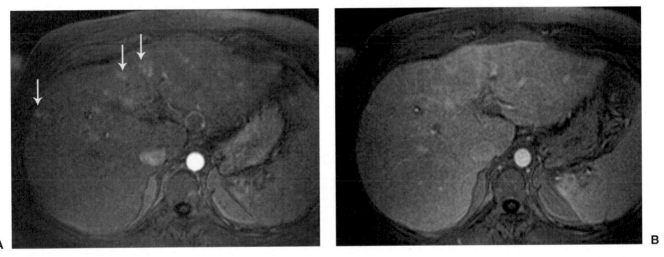

FIGURE 11-52 **Vascular shunting in another cirrhotic patient. A:** Enhanced arterial phase fat-suppressed T1-weighted image shows a number of hypervascular lesions (*arrows*). **B:** No corresponding lesions are visible on the portal phase image. Arterioportal and arteriovenous shunting can lead to false-positive diagnoses of hepatocellular carcinoma.

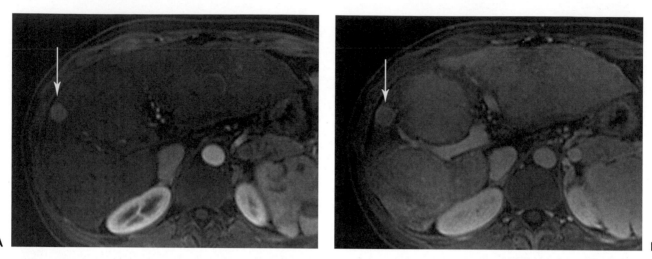

FIGURE 11-53 **Hyperenhancing regenerative nodule simulates tumor. A:** Arterial and **(B)** portal phase T1-weighted images in a patient with chronic Budd-Chiari syndrome depict a round, uniformly enhancing, peripheral mass (*arrow*). Notice lack of suspicious washout or pseudocapsule.

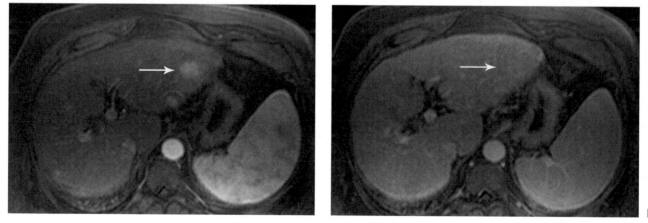

FIGURE 11-54 **Hepatocellular carcinoma (HCC) seen only on arterial phase T1-weighted imaging. A:** Uniformly enhancing nodule (*arrow*) is imaged during arterial dominant phase. **B:** Lesion (*arrow*) rapidly becomes isointense to liver. More typically, these small HCC will show washout on later phases of imaging.

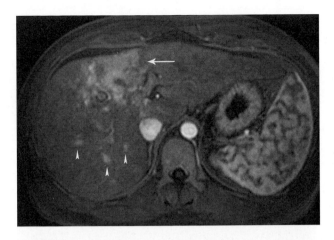

FIGURE 11-55 Focal hepatitis simulates hepatocellular carcinoma. Fat-suppressed T1-weighted image obtained during arterial dominant phase shows confluent enhancement in segment IV (*arrow*) along with several additional small foci (*arrowheads*) in the right lobe. This patient had markedly elevated α-fetoprotein levels and was diagnosed with hepatitis associated with INH (isoniazid) therapy.

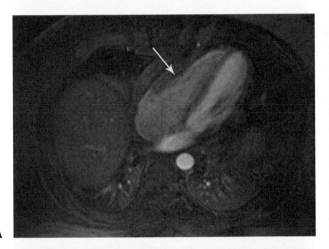

A

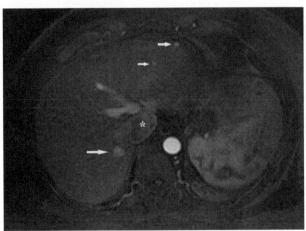

B

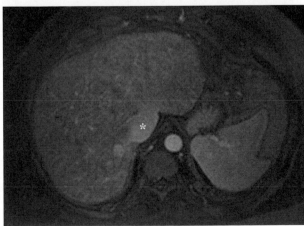

C

FIGURE 11-56 Hypervascular nodules mimic malignancy in a patient with constrictive pericarditis. A: Axial enhanced arterial phase T1-weighted image through the lower chest demonstrates reduced right ventricle size and an abnormally straightened wall (*arrow*), consistent with constrictive pericarditis. **B:** At least three hyperintense liver nodules (*arrows*) are seen, similar to the hyperplastic nodules or vascular shunts commonly seen in cirrhotics. **C:** Later phase of contrast enhancement reveals liver enlargement and congestion (*IVC = asterisk*). IVC, inferior vena cava.

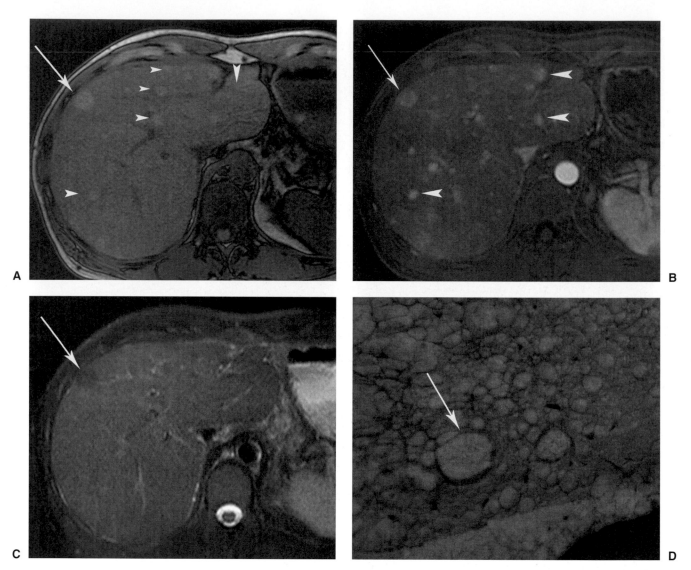

FIGURE 11-57 **Hyperplastic regenerative nodules in cirrhotic liver simulate multifocal hepatocellular carcinoma. A:** In-phase T1-weighted image reveals multiple small hyperintense nodules (*arrowheads*) as well as a larger dominant nodule (*arrow*). **B:** Enhanced image obtained in the arterial dominant phase demonstrates unusual hyperenhancement in many of the nodules. **C:** The dominant nodule (*arrow*) is hypointense on T2-weighted imaging. **D:** Cut liver surface shows these benign hyperplastic lesions (*arrow*) in a sea of fibrosis and regenerative nodules.

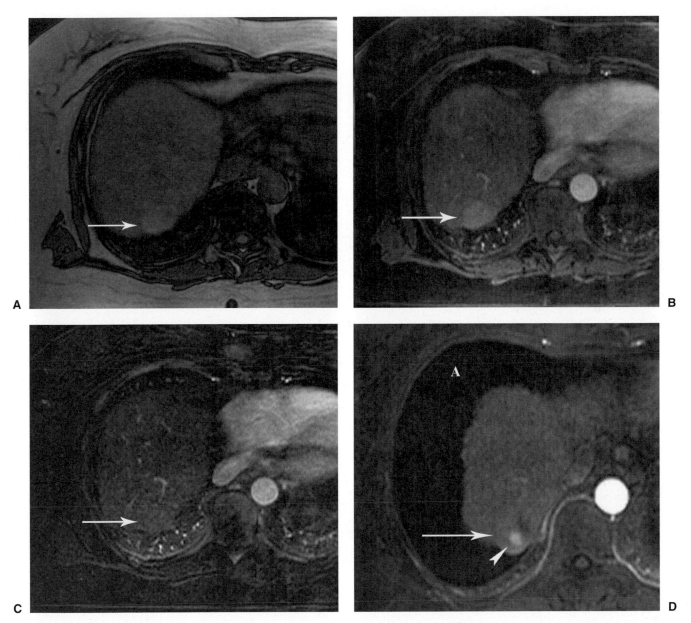

FIGURE 11-58 **Nodule enhancement or just the preexisting high T1 signal? Subtraction technique answers the question.**
A: Opposed-phase T1-weighted image through the dome of a cirrhotic liver shows multiple hyperintense nodules, with a dominant nodule posteriorly (*arrow*). **B:** Enhancement is suggested on arterial phase image, but is excluded by **(C)** subtraction technique. **D:** Two years later, the nodule (*arrow*) persists, but now contains a focus of hepatocellular carcinoma, demonstrating true enhancement (*arrowhead*) (*Ascites = A*).

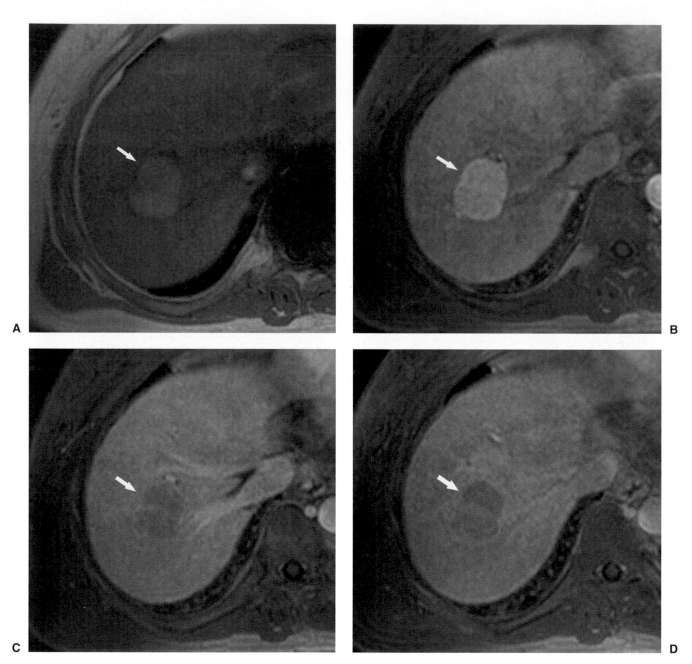

FIGURE 11-59 Typical enhancement pattern of well-differentiated hepatocellular carcinoma (HCC). **A:** Axial unenhanced T1-weighted image reveals 3-cm, well-circumscribed, high signal intensity mass (*arrow*). **B:** The lesion (*arrow*) becomes even more conspicuous during arterial phase imaging due to intense enhancement. **C:** Portal and (**D**) delayed phase images demonstrate "washout" of the HCC (*arrows*) relative to the background cirrhotic liver.

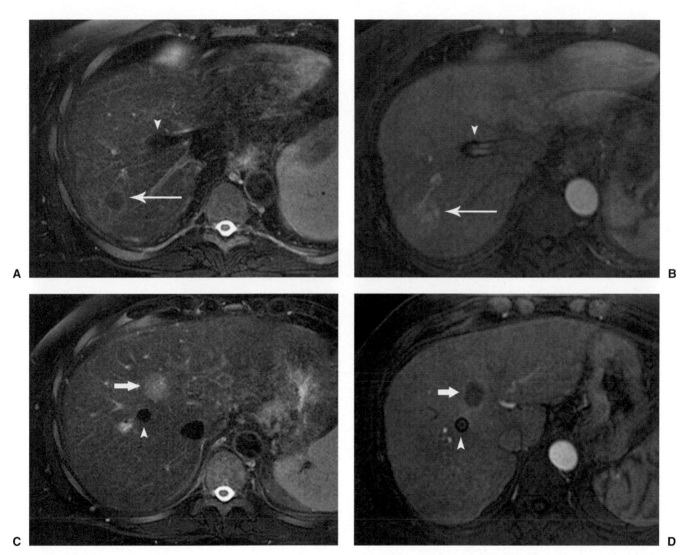

FIGURE 11-60 **Widely variable T2 appearance of hepatocellular carcinoma (HCC) demonstrated in the same liver.** Small nodule (*arrow*) demonstrates low signal on **(A)** T2-weighted imaging as well as brisk arterial enhancement on **(B)** T1-weighted enhanced image, a common appearance for small HCC (*TIPS = arrowhead*). **C** and **D**: In contrast, another nodule (*short arrow*) in the same patient demonstrates high T2-weighted signal intensity and poor arterial enhancement, consistent with hypovascular HCC (*TIPS = arrowhead*).

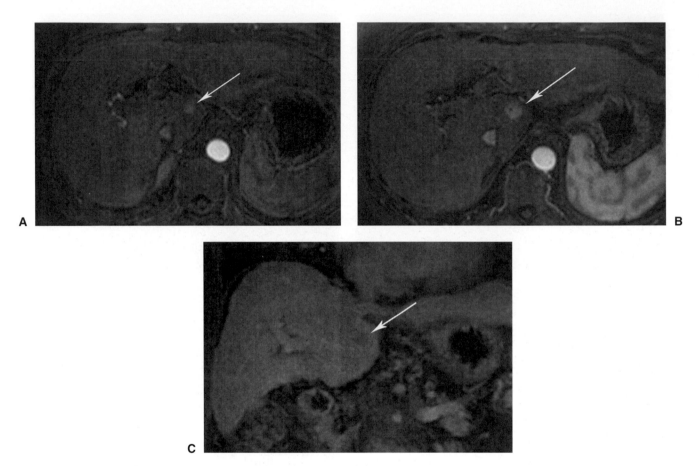

FIGURE 11-61 Rapid growth of hepatocellular carcinoma. Although 6- to 12-month follow-up is usually adequate for small hypervascular lesions, a subset of these will grow rapidly. **A:** Arterial phase T1-weighted image shows tiny focus of enhancement (*arrow*) in the caudate, which is occult on all other sequences. **B** and **C:** Two months later, the lesion (*arrow*) has grown significantly and shows washout on **(C)** delayed phases.

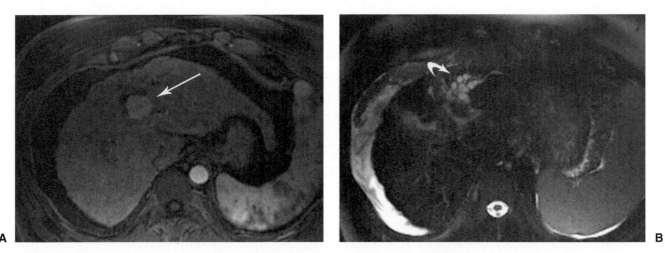

FIGURE 11-62 **Unusual intrahepatic biliary obstruction by hepatocellular carcinoma (HCC). A:** Well-defined hypervascular HCC (*arrow*) is shown on arterial phase T1-weighted image. **B:** There is marked segmental biliary dilatation (*curved arrow*) on a level just cephalad. Biliary obstruction is more typically a feature of cholangiocarcinoma, but is occasionally seen with HCC.

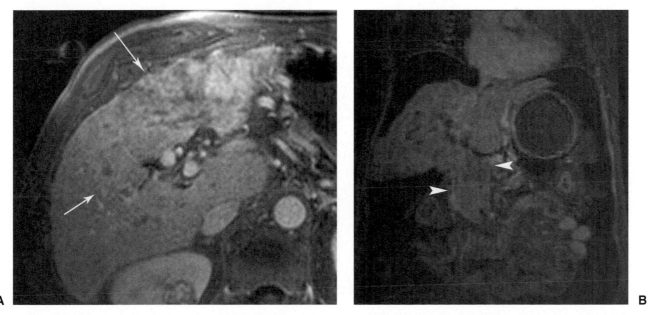

FIGURE 11-63 **Tumor recognition and measurement can be difficult in infiltrative hepatocellular carcinoma (HCC). A:** Notice how difficult it is to delineate tumor margins (*arrows*) on this enhanced T1-weighted image. **B:** In another patient, diffuse hypovascular HCC occupies nearly the entire liver. Tumor invades and distends the portal vein (*arrowheads*).

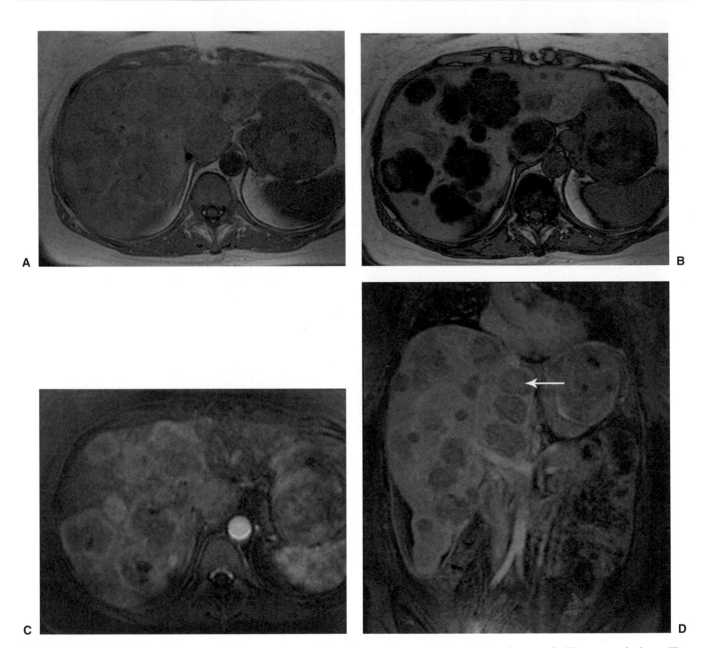

FIGURE 11-64 Multifocal hepatocellular carcinoma simulates adenomatosis. A: In-phase and **(B)** opposed-phase T1-weighted images show striking signal loss in multiple lesions, compatible with internal lipid or glycogen. Both hepatocellular adenoma and carcinoma can show this behavior. **C:** Axial arterial dominant T1-weighted image shows early, peripheral enhancement. **D:** Coronal image shows tumor burden to better advantage, as well as the interval central accumulation of contrast (*arrow*), behavior suggestive of malignancy.

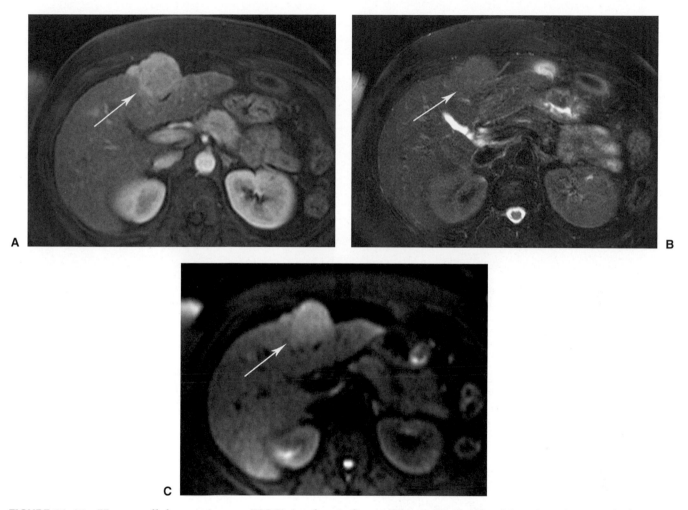

FIGURE 11-65 **Hepatocellular carcinoma (HCC) is often indiscernible on T2-weighted imaging. A:** Arterial phase T1-weighted image demonstrates large, well-circumscribed HCC (*arrow*). **B:** Lesion (*arrow*) is isointense on fat-suppressed T2-weighted image, as is often the case with well-differentiated hepatocellular tumors. **C:** The HCC (*arrow*) is more conspicuous on echoplanar diffusion-weighted image (b = 50) in this case.

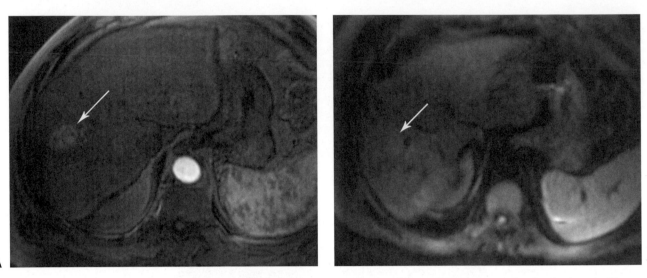

FIGURE 11-66 **Hepatocellular carcinoma (HCC) is commonly indiscernible on diffusion weighted imaging. A:** Hypervascular HCC (*arrow*) is conspicuous on arterial phase T1-weighted image. **B:** Echoplanar diffusion-weighted image (DWI) at same level fails to detect the tumor. Although often very sensitive for liver metastases, DWI can be quite insensitive to HCC, especially when small.

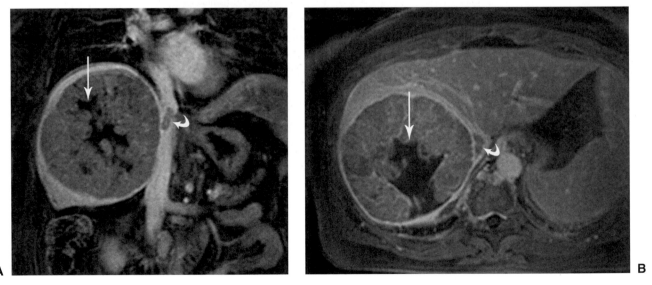

FIGURE 11-67 **Conventional hepatocellular carcinoma (HCC) simulates fibrolamellar carcinoma. A:** Coronal and (**B**) axial enhanced T1-weighted images show large, circumscribed mass with a stellate central scar (*arrow*) that extends to the posterior capsule, suggesting fibrolamellar HCC in this noncirrhotic liver. However, the inferior vena cava (IVC) tumor thrombus (*curved arrow*) is more consistent with the true diagnosis, conventional HCC.

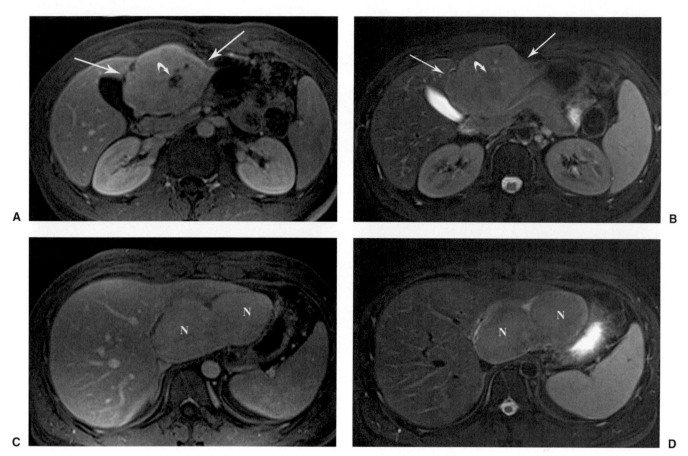

FIGURE 11-68 **Fibrolamellar hepatocellular carcinoma simulates focal nodular hyperplasia (FNH). A:** Large, circumscribed, exophytic liver mass (*arrows*) is uniformly isointense to liver, except for a possible small central scar (*curved arrow*). **B:** However, the "scar" is not hyperintense on correlative T2-weighted image. FNH is excluded by large metastatic nodes (*N*), which are almost isointense to liver on **(C)** enhanced and **(D)** T2-weighted images, consistent with the hepatocellular origin of the tumor.

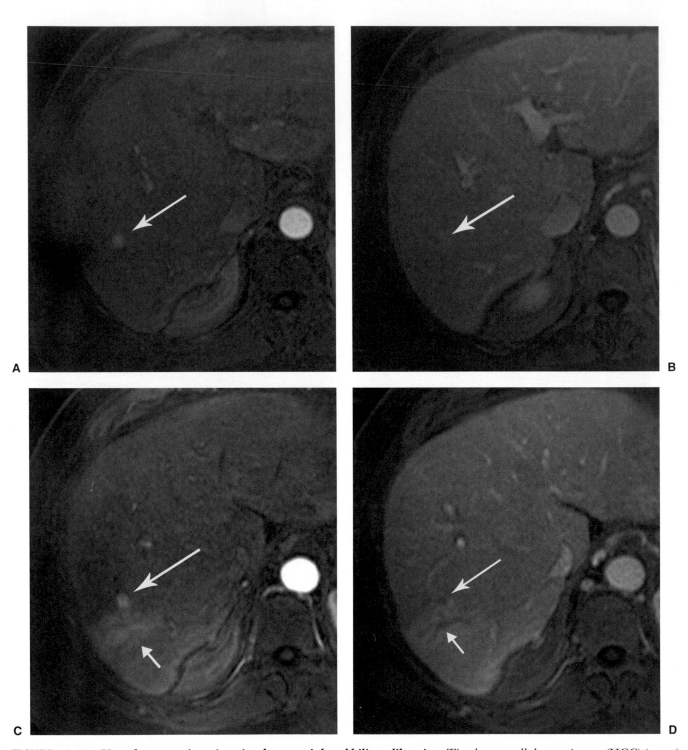

FIGURE 11-69 Vascular tumor invasion simulates peripheral biliary dilatation. Tiny hepatocellular carcinoma (HCC) (*arrow*) on **(A)** arterial and **(B)** portal phase imaging, with typical early hyperenhancement followed by washout. **C** and **D**: Two months later, new regional enhancement has appeared around branching hypointense material (*short arrow*), representing portal venous tumor invasion, proved at explant (*HCC = long arrows*).

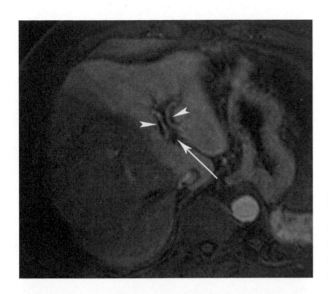

FIGURE 11-70 Increased lobar enhancement associated with left portal vein occlusion. Axial T1-weighted image obtained immediately following contrast injection demonstrates left lobar hyperenhancement from increased arterial blood flow due to occlusion of the left portal vein (*arrow*) (*Left hepatic arteries = arrowheads*).

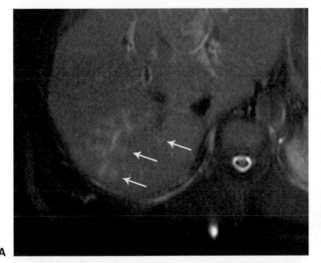

A

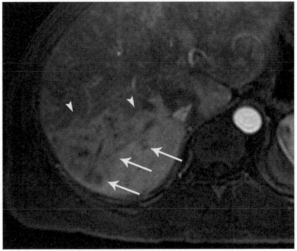

B

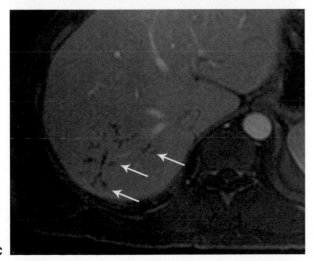

C

FIGURE 11-71 Benign peripheral portal venous thrombosis simulates biliary abnormality. **A:** Branching hyperintensity (*arrows*) is identified on axial T2-weighted image. **B:** Hyperenhancement of segment VII (*arrowheads*) on arterial dominant enhanced T1-weighted image (*Portal venous thrombosis = arrows*). **C:** The responsible portal venous thrombus (*arrows*) is more obvious when enhancement normalizes on portal phase imaging. Etiology was never determined.

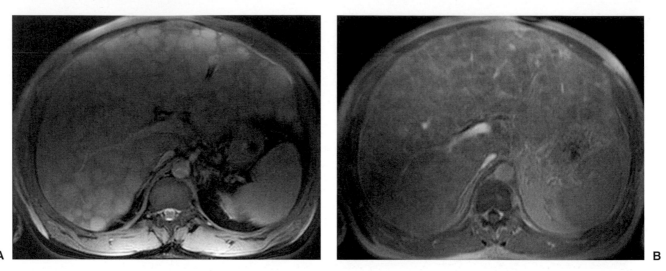

FIGURE 11-72 Multinodular hepatic lymphoma mimics cirrhotic nodules. Axial **(A)** steady state free precession (SSFP) and **(B)** in-phase T1-weighted images demonstrate enlargement of the liver by innumerable well-defined lymphomatous nodules.

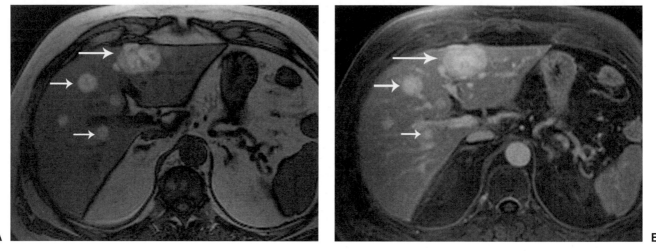

FIGURE 11-73 Melanoma metastases with very high T1 signal intensity. A: Axial opposed-phase image shows a number of T1-hyperintense lesions (*arrows*). **B:** High signal becomes even more intense following contrast administration in these hypervascular tumors (*arrows*). Differential for T1-hyperintense lesions includes hematoma/proteinaceous fluid, fat, and melanin, as well as dysplastic nodules and early hepatocellular carcinoma (HCC).

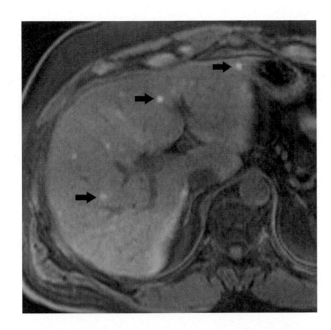

FIGURE 11-74 Melanoma metastases. Increased signal intensity within these hepatic metastases (*arrows*) is presumably due to intralesional melanin on this unenhanced, fat-suppressed, T1-weighted gradient echo sequence. Caveat: not all melanoma metastases will be T1-hyperintense.

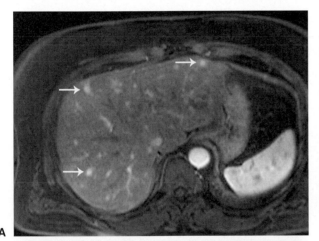

A

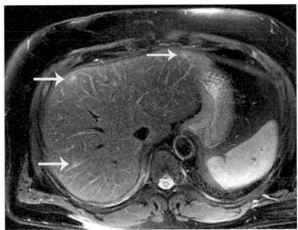

B

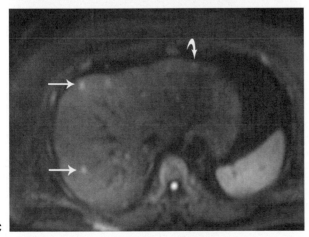

C

FIGURE 11-75 Small hypervascular metastases, subtle on T2-weighted imaging. A: Arterial dominant enhanced T1-weighted image demonstrates multiple tiny hyperenhancing liver nodules (*arrows*). **B:** Poor conspicuity of these lesions (*arrows*) on fat-suppressed T2-weighted image is common with both hypervascular metastases and with primary liver neoplasia. **C:** There is improved conspicuity of these lesions (*arrows*) on diffusion-weighted imaging (b = 50). Notice decreased lesional signal (*curved arrow*) in the superior left hepatic lobe, near the heart.

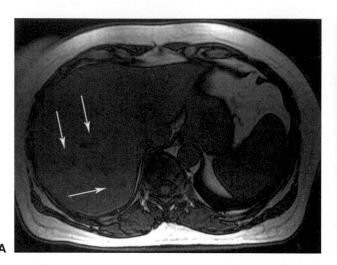
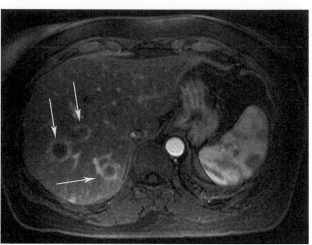

FIGURE 11-76 Focal fat sparing around metastases from colon cancer. A: Opposed-phase T1-weighted axial image shows a rim of higher signal around three mildly hypointense metastases (*arrows*) in a fatty liver. The perilesional fat sparing is common with both benign and malignant lesions. **B:** Axial portal phase T1-weighted image shows the underlying metastases (*arrows*) as ring-enhancing lesions.

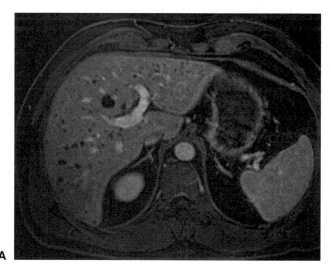
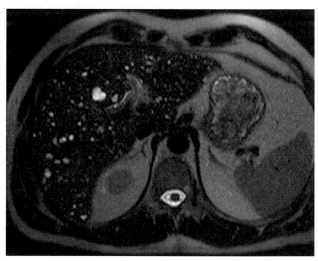

FIGURE 11-77 Biliary hamartomas simulate metastases in cancer patient. A: Axial enhanced T1-weighted image demonstrates multiple, very small, avascular foci that were previously mistaken for metastases in this patient with history of renal cell carcinoma. **B:** Axial T2-weighted image confirms the cystic nature of these biopsy-proven benign lesions.

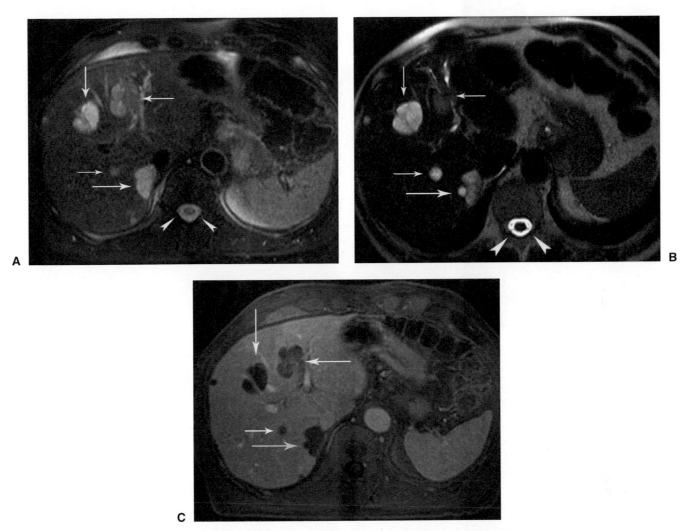

FIGURE 11-78 **Cystic gastrointestinal stromal tumor (GIST) liver metastases, unusual in untreated malignancy. A:** Axial fat-suppressed, moderately T2-weighted image reveals a variety of well-circumscribed lesions (*arrows*), some of which are quite cystic (*CSF = arrowheads*). **B:** However, a more heavily T2-weighted image shows that none of these lesions (*arrows*) is isointense to cerebrospinal fluid (CSF) (*arrowheads*). **C:** Enhanced T1-weighted imaging demonstrates a range of low-level enhancement (*arrows*). Notice lack of peripheral enhancement.

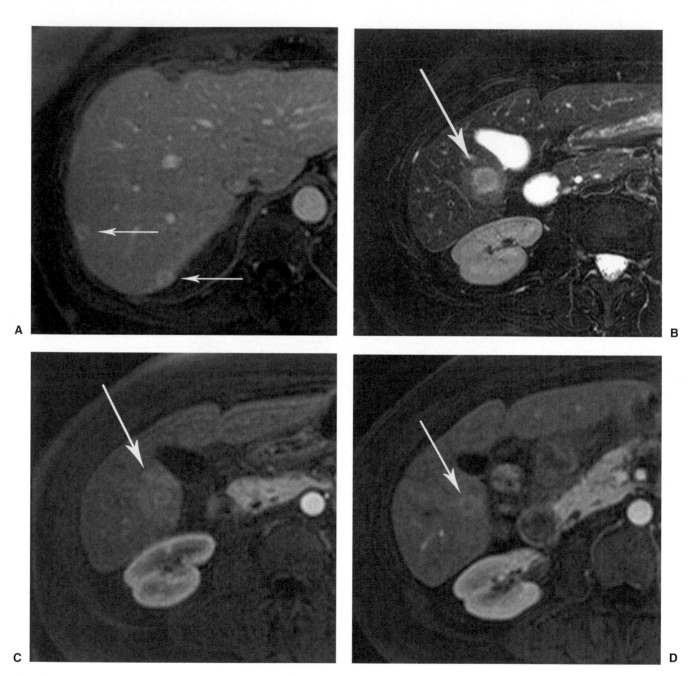

FIGURE 11-79 **Focal hepatitis mimics metastatic disease. A:** Portal phase T1-weighted imaging reveals small, ring-enhancing lesions (*arrows*). At another level, axial **(B)** T2-weighted and **(C)** arterial phase T1-weighted enhanced images show an ill-defined, hyperintense lesion (*arrow*) in segment V. Patient had recently undergone colonoscopy and transverse colonic polypectomy. **D:** After 3 weeks of treatment, this arterial phase ring (*arrow*) was the only evidence remaining of previous abnormalities.

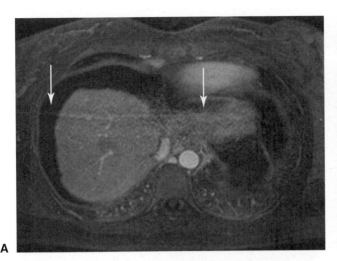
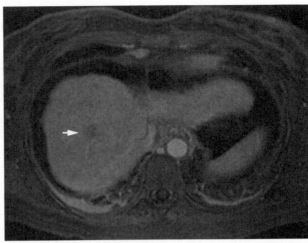

A **B**

FIGURE 11-80 **Parallel imaging artifact reduces conspicuity of liver metastasis. A:** Reduced diagnostic quality due to a band of noise (*arrows*) running horizontally through this enhanced T1-weighted image is caused by parallel imaging technique. Artifact distracts attention from a metastasis. **B:** Sequence repeated without parallel imaging clearly demonstrates the metastasis (*arrow*).

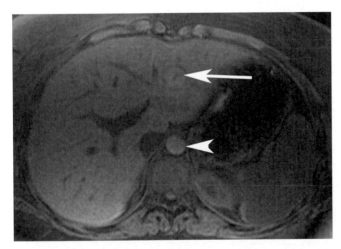
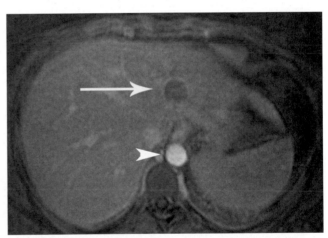

FIGURE 11-81 **Pulsation artifact.** Pulsatile flow in the aorta (*arrowhead*) has produced a ghost image of the aorta (*arrow*) in the phase encoding direction.

FIGURE 11-82 **Pulsation artifact.** On this enhanced T1-weighted image, pulsatile flow in the aorta (*arrowhead*) produces hypointense ghosting (*arrow*) in the phase encoding direction.

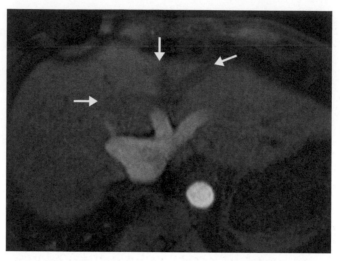

FIGURE 11-83 **Pulsation artifact from inferior vena cava-hepatic venous confluence.** Seen more commonly with arteries than with veins, vascular pulsation, in this case transmitted from the right heart, ghosts across the liver in the phase encode direction.

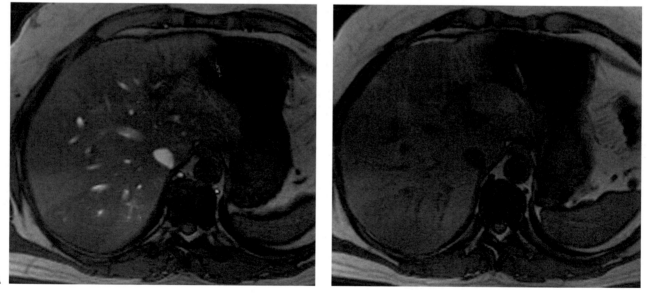

A
B

FIGURE 11-84 **In-flow enhancement. A:** The first of a stack of gradient echo images show intense signal in the hepatic vessels, potentially obscuring actual liver lesions. **B:** This signal did not persist in the remaining images and represents entry phenomenon artifact. The fresh, optimally magnetized blood flowing into the first slice appears very bright in contrast with the stationary tissue because the tissue has already been exposed to multiple radiofrequency (RF) pulses. Thus the stationary tissue (along with the blood in subsequent slices) has not fully regained its longitudinal magnetization and so demonstrates comparatively reduced T1 signal. Other terms used for this appearance are *entry slice phenomenon* and *flow-related enhancement*.

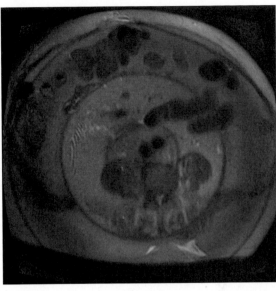

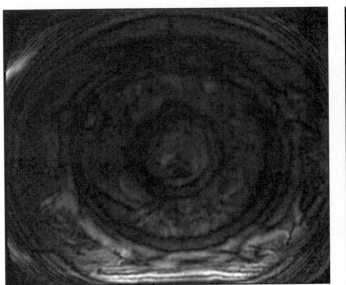

FIGURE 11-85   Field fall-off. A and **B:** Dark bands related to scanning tissue in regions of fall-off of the main magnetic field. This is more prevalent with short-bore systems, in which the magnetic field falls off very rapidly beyond the recommended scanning range in the Z direction. The obscuring concentric circles are even worse due to a very large body habitus (420 lb) in this patient.

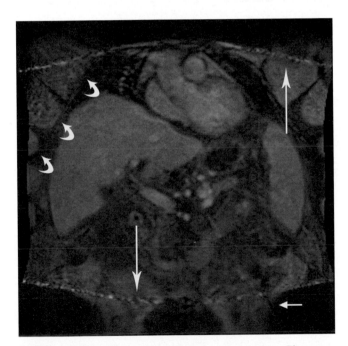

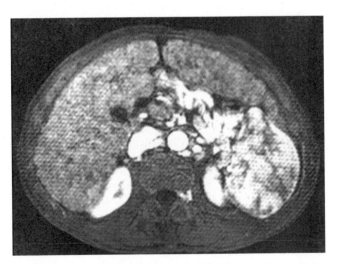

FIGURE 11-87   Spikes in k-space. The lines and cross-hatch pattern in this image are the result of multiple spikes in k-space, caused by system or environmental errors. K-space contains the raw MR data before Fourier reconstruction.

FIGURE 11-86   Magnetic field inhomogeneity. Characteristic constructive/destructive interference patterns due to fall-off of the magnetic field at the edges.

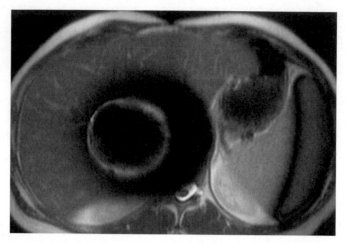

FIGURE 11-88 Metal embolization coils in a surgically created portocaval shunt results in "blowout," a form of susceptibility artifact. Spin echo technique, as here, is less severely affected than gradient echo–based sequences.

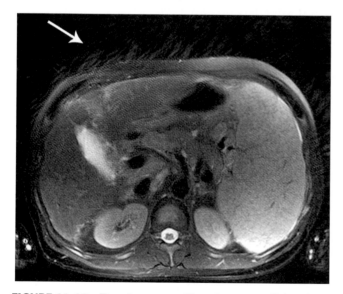

FIGURE 11-89 Respiratory artifact in nontraditional acquisition (Propeller or Blade) sequences. Motion artifact tends to be represented as "shivers" of noise, rather than as discrete parallel bands.

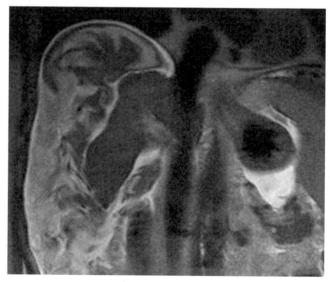

FIGURE 11-90 Motion artifact from ascites in cirrhotic. Complex patterns of signal loss are present in the swirling ascites on T2-weighted single-shot image.

▪ Biliary

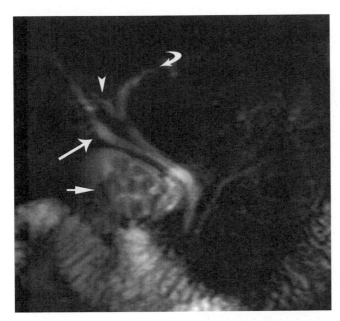

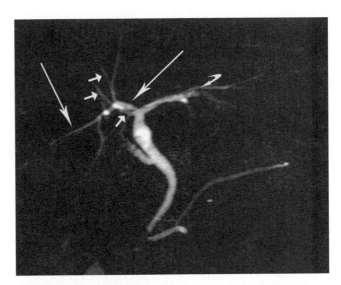

FIGURE 11-92 Posterior right hepatic duct (RHD) crosses and joins left hepatic duct (LHD) just above biliary hilum. This very common normal variant becomes important when planning living donor liver transplant (*Posterior RHD = long arrows, Anterior RHD = short arrows, LHD = curved arrow*).

FIGURE 11-91 Very low insertion of right anterior hepatic duct into the common hepatic duct (CHD). Conventional projectional MRCP image shows anterior right branch merging with the CHD several centimeters below the expected hilum (*arrow*). This is one of a number of anatomic biliary variations (*Gallstones = small arrow, Posterior right hepatic duct = arrowhead, Left hepatic duct = curved arrow*).

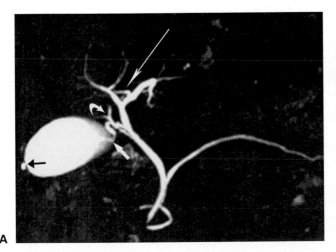

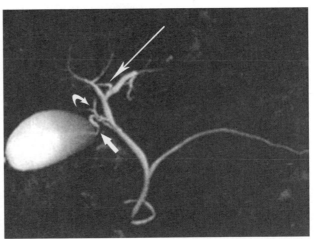

FIGURE 11-93 Accessory right hepatic duct joins the common hepatic duct (CHD) very low, close to the cystic duct confluence. **A:** Maximum intensity projection (MIP) reconstruction of a 3-D T2-weighted acquisition (*Accessory RHD = curved arrow, Cystic duct = short arrow, Small fundal gallbladder adenomyoma = black arrow*). **B:** Conventional projectional thick-slab MRCP. The posterior right hepatic duct (RHD) also joins with the left hepatic duct (*long arrow*), a second variant in this patient.

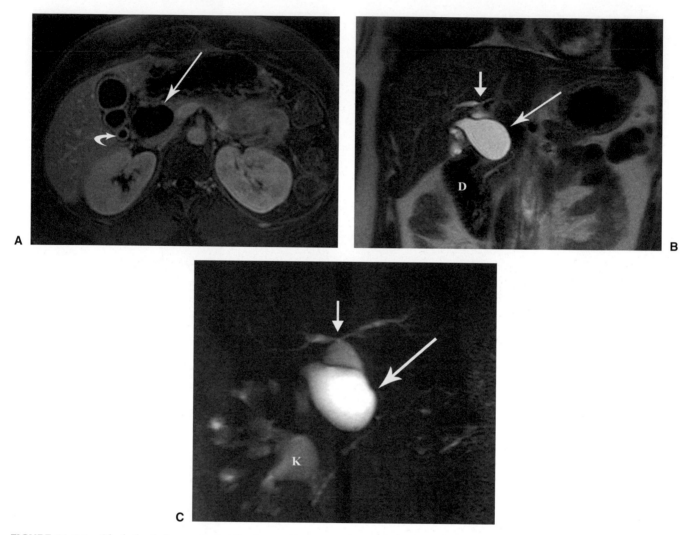

FIGURE 11-94 **Choledochal cyst. A:** Axial enhanced T1-weighted image demonstrates a large cyst in the normal position of the common duct (*arrow*), a previously unrecognized congenital anomaly (*Gallbladder neck = curved arrow*). **B:** Thin slice coronal MRCP shows the choledochal cyst (*long arrow*) to better advantage. Incompletely imaged biliary hilum (*short arrow*) is normal (*Duodenum = D*). **C:** Thick-slab MRCP image confirms the abrupt hilar change (*short arrow*) to normal duct caliber (*Choledochal cyst = long arrow, Right renal collecting system = K*).

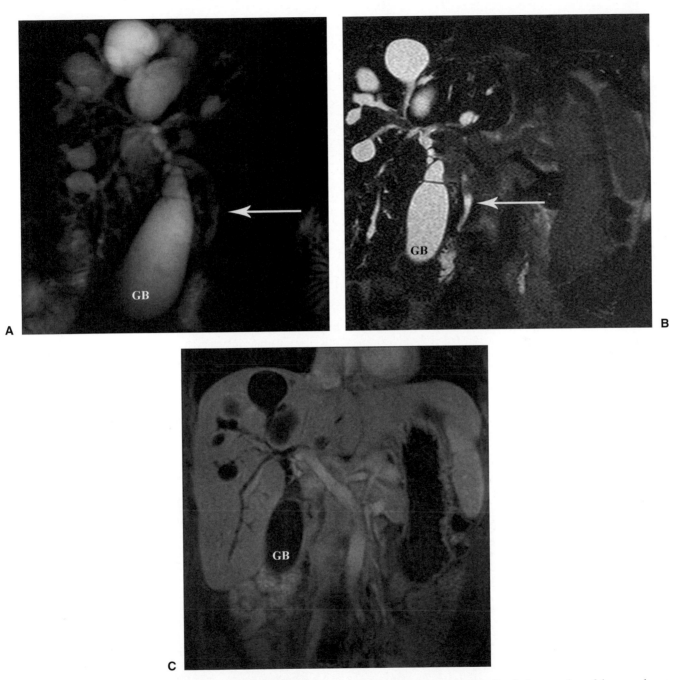

FIGURE 11-95 **Caroli's disease, a rare congenital disorder of intrahepatic bile ducts. A:** Confusing overlay of ducts and cysts on conventional MRCP image (*Gallbladder = GB, Common bile duct = arrow*). **B:** Thin-slice approach reduces overlap and confirms cyst continuity with ducts (*Gallbladder = GB, Common bile duct = arrow*). **C:** Correlative enhanced T1-weighted image also shows continuity of intrahepatic ducts and cysts, a *sine qua non* for Caroli's disease (*Gallbladder = GB*).

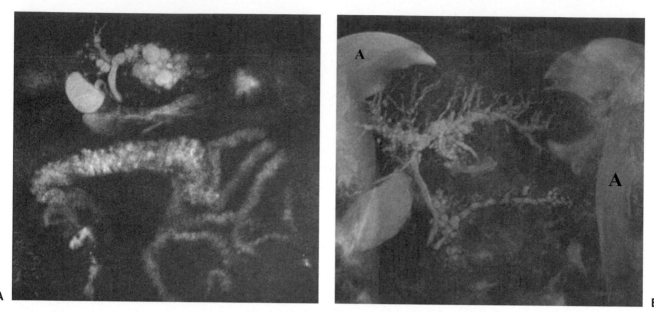

FIGURE 11-96 **Peribiliary cysts can mimic Caroli's disease, but do not communicate with the duct. A:** Coronal projectional MRCP image demonstrates clusters of cysts around the intrahepatic ducts, particularly the left hepatic duct (LHD). **B:** Maximum intensity projection (MIP) reconstruction in another patient shows more diffuse pattern of very small cysts (*Wraparound artifact from ascites = A*).

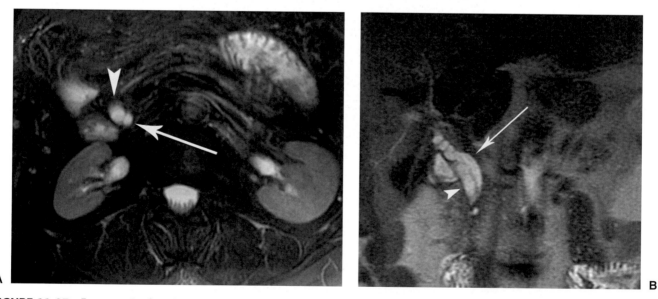

FIGURE 11-97 **Low cystic duct insertion** results in apparent dilatation of the extrahepatic duct. **A:** Axial fat-suppressed T2-weighted and **(B)** coronal thin-slice MRCP images show the cystic duct (*arrows*) crossing medially to descend deep into the pancreas with the common bile duct (*arrowheads*).

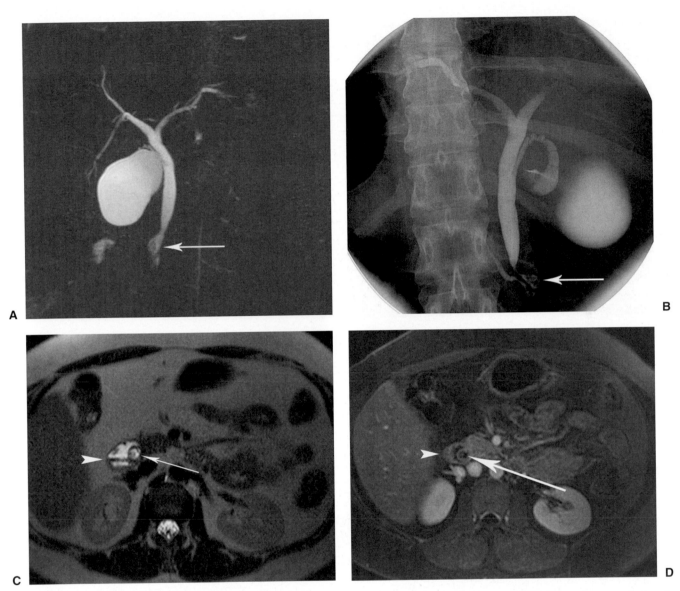

FIGURE 11-98 **Choledochocele simulates duodenal mass. A:** Maximum intensity projection (MIP) image from a volumetric, heavily T2-weighted acquisition shows bulge at end of the common bile duct (*arrow*). **B:** Correlative endoscopic retrograde cholangiopancreatography (ERCP) image (*Distal CBD = arrow*). Axial (**C**) T2 and (**D**) enhanced T1-weighted images show choledochocele (*arrows*) bulging into duodenal lumen (*arrowheads*).

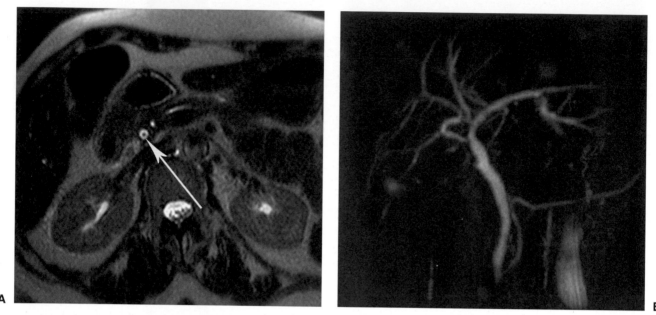

FIGURE 11-99 **Flow artifact in the center of the common bile duct, a common pitfall. A:** The best method of avoiding false-positive diagnoses of choledocholithiasis is to treat central and floating defects (*arrow*) with suspicion and to confirm findings on other imaging planes. **B:** Correlative coronal projectional MRCP.

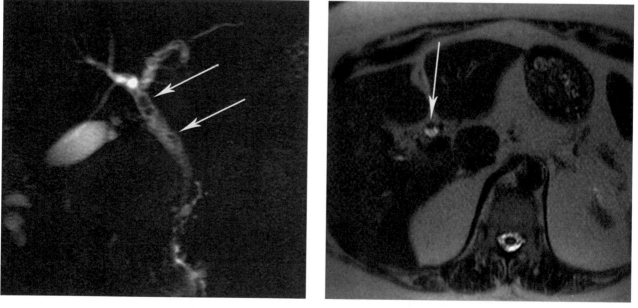

FIGURE 11-100 **Filling defects throughout the ducts are air bubbles** due to sphincterotomy. **A:** High signal intensity bile column interrupted by multiple filling defects (*arrows*). **B:** Axial thin-slice MRCP shows hypointense material (*arrow*) floating anteriorly.

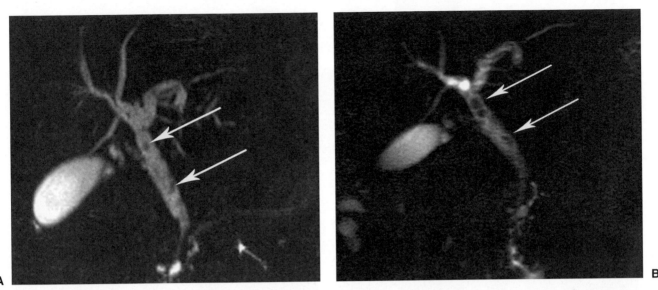

FIGURE 11-101 **Conspicuity of filling defects artifactually reduced on maximum intensity projection (MIP) image.** **A:** MIP reconstruction of a 3-D T2 coronal slab shows effect of compression of a stack of images into a single image representation. **B:** Conventional thick-slab MRCP. The ductal air bubbles, seen as filling defects (*arrows*), will generally be more conpicuous on the projectional image than on the MIP. Best practice is to examine the source images, where conspicuity of stones, bubbles and intraductal masses should be optimal.

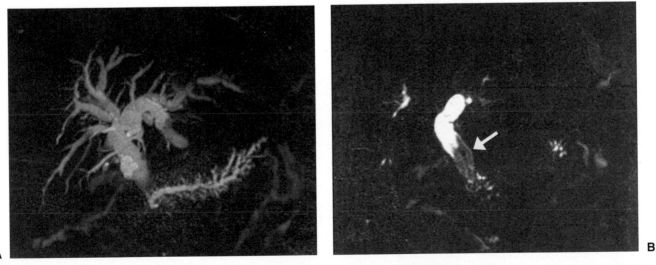

FIGURE 11-102 **Reduction of conspicuity on maximum intensity projection (MIP) reconstruction. A:** MIP image effectively demonstrates dilated common hepatic duct (CHD) and intrahepatic ducts, but the obstructing CBD sludge is quite subtle. **B:** A 1.5-mm thick source image reveals a CBD filled with obstructing, hypointense biliary sludge (*arrow*).

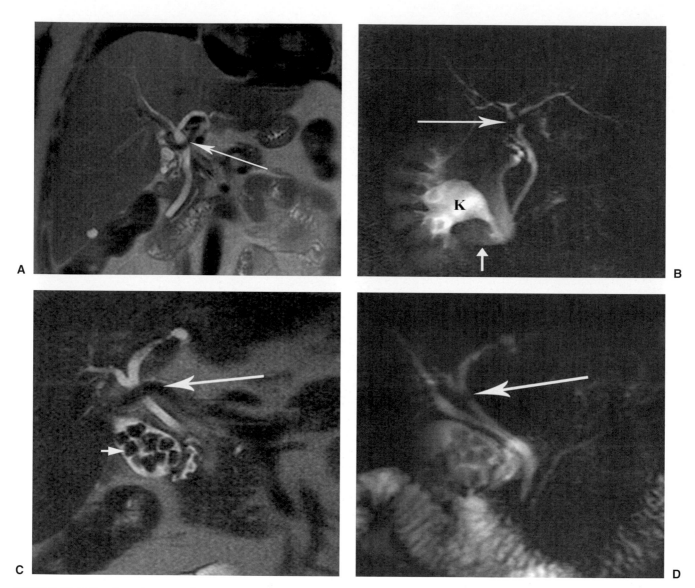

FIGURE 11-103 **Crossing vessel, a common MRCP pitfall. A:** Signal void of the hepatic artery (*arrow*) traverses the common hepatic duct (CHD). Pressure or dephasing from the pulsating vessel can simulate strictures and stones. **B:** Exemplary MRCP in another patient (*Pseudostricture = long arrow, Right renal collecting system = K, Gallbladder = short arrow*). **C** and **D:** Examples in a third patient (*Pseudostricture = long arrows, Cholelithiasis = short arrow*).

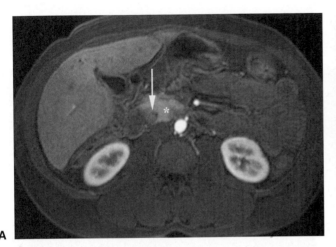
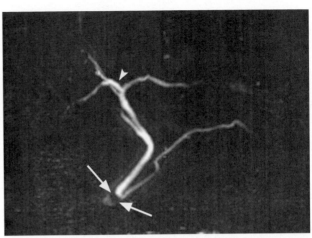

FIGURE 11-104 Pseudolesion caused by complex anatomy at junction of common bile duct (CBD), pancreatic duct, and ampulla. **A:** Axial fat-suppressed, enhanced T1-weighted image raises question of distal CBD tumor or stone (*arrow*) (*Pancreatic head = asterisk*). **B:** MRCP image shows a prominent ampulla (*arrows*), but nothing in the duct. Notice variant posterior right hepatic duct anatomy (*arrowhead*).

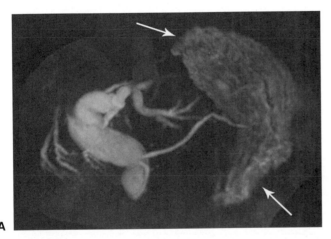
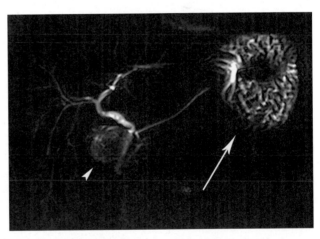

FIGURE 11-105 Fluid outlines bowel mucosa, creating the potential for confusion. **A** and **B:** MRCP images from two different patients show gastric rugae (*arrows*) and duodenal bulb (*arrowhead*). Negative oral contrast had been administered to reduce signal from gut, but interval mucosal secretion has occurred.

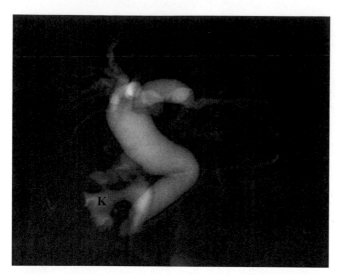

FIGURE 11-106 Asymptomatic bile duct dilatation after cholecystectomy. This phenomenon occurs in a significant minority of postcholecystectomy patients. Gallbladder was removed 20 years prior in this patient and serum liver function tests were within normal range (*Fluid in renal collecting system = K*).

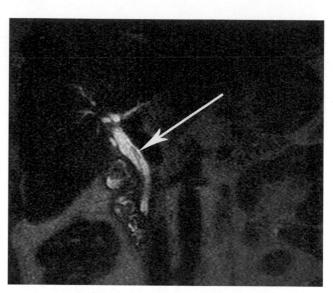

FIGURE 11-107 Biliary stents are easily missed on MRI. Thin-slice imaging is the most sensitive method of identifying a stent (*arrow*), which can otherwise be very subtle.

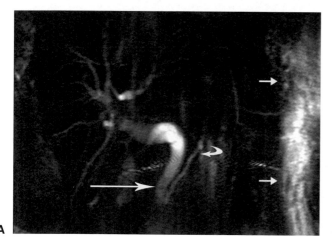

A

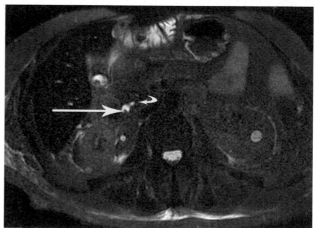

B

FIGURE 11-108 Small stone versus artifact. A: Subtle common bile duct (CBD) filling defect (*long arrow*) on projectional coronal MRCP image (*Pancreatic duct = curved arrow, Wraparound artifact from lateral abdominal wall edema = short arrows*). **B:** Correlation with axial plane confirms dependent stone (*arrow*) (*Pancreatic duct = curved arrow*).

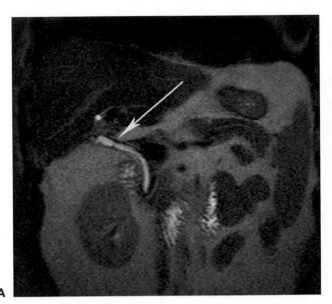
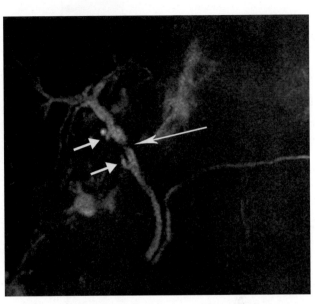

FIGURE 11-109 Typical appearance of duct-to-duct biliary anastomosis in liver transplant. **A:** Minimal narrowing (*arrow*) on thin-slice MRCP image, an unusually good result. **B:** Mild-to-moderate narrowing (*arrow*), a more typical appearance, and completely asymptomatic. Donor and recipient cystic duct remnants are visible (*short arrows*).

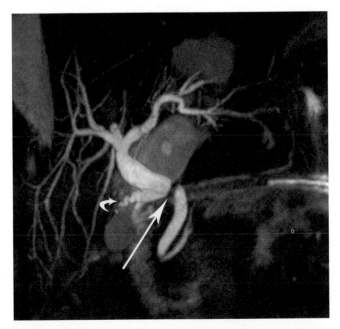

FIGURE 11-110 A pitfall in diagnosis of anastomotic stricture: donor bile ducts do not dilate as readily as native ducts. The transplant ducts in cases of high-grade stenosis (*arrow*) are unusually compliant, showing mild-to-moderate upstream dilatation (*Cystic duct remnant = curved arrow*).

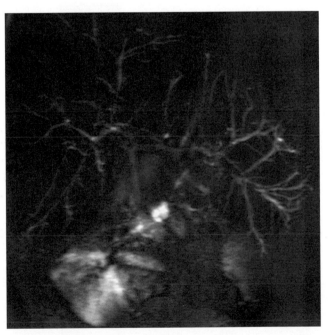

FIGURE 11-111 Ischemic duct alterations in transplant liver simulate primary sclerosing cholangitis. Conventional MRCP demonstrates extrahepatic duct effacement, along with central intrahepatic strictures.

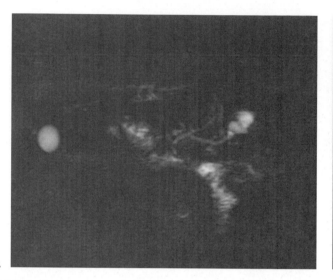

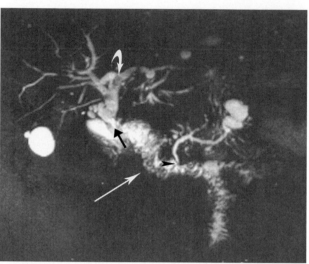

FIGURE 11-112 **Pneumobilia in surgically altered anatomy, a diagnostic challenge. A:** Conventional MRCP image in a patient who has undergone Whipple procedure. Extrahepatic duct is obscured by intraluminal air. **B:** Maximum intensity projection (MIP) reconstruction of a volumetric T2-weighted slab obtained later during examination, when air has redistributed. (*Roux limb = white arrow, Biliary-enteric anastomosis = black arrow, Pancreatic-jejunal reconstruction = arrowhead, Pneumobilia = curved arrow.*)

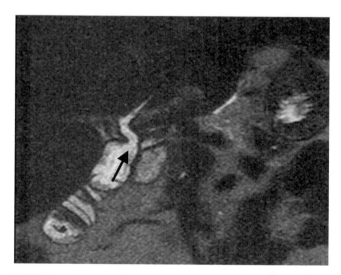

FIGURE 11-113 **Biliary-enteric anastomosis.** The biliary-enteric anastomosis (*arrow*) in another patient is well demonstrated on thin-slice coronal MRCP.

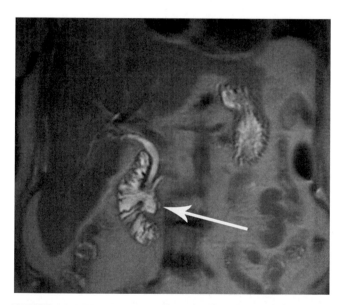

FIGURE 11-114 **Periampullary duodenal diverticulum can mimic a cystic mass.** Coronal thin-slice MRCP depicts medial outpouching from descending duodenum (*arrow*). Common bile duct (CBD) and pancreatic duct insert into the upper aspect of the diverticulum.

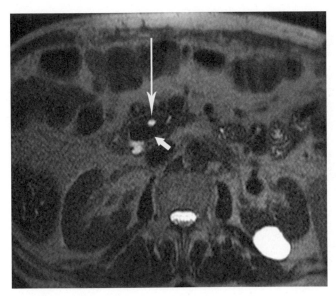

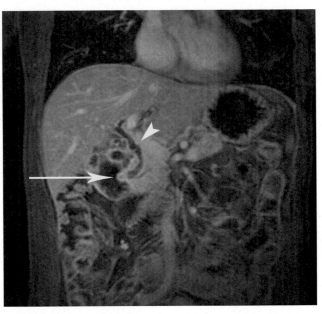

FIGURE 11-115 Air or negative contrast in a periampullary diverticulum can create diagnostic confusion. Axial T2-weighted image through head of pancreas shows intrapancreatic collection of negative oral contrast (*short arrow*) (*common bile duct in cross-section = arrow*).

FIGURE 11-116 Prominent, enhancing duodenal papilla following stone passage should not be mistaken for malignancy. Papilla (*arrow*) bulges into duodenal lumen (*Common bile duct = arrowhead*).

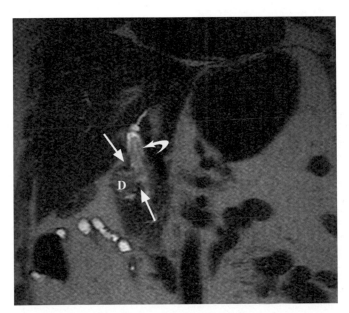

FIGURE 11-117 Food fills and obscures common bile duct. Isointense ingested material (*curved arrow*) from duodenum extends into the common bile duct (CBD) through the prominent choledochoduodenostomy (*arrows*) (*Duodenum = D*).

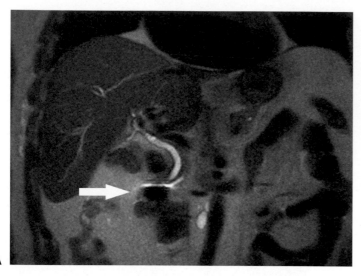
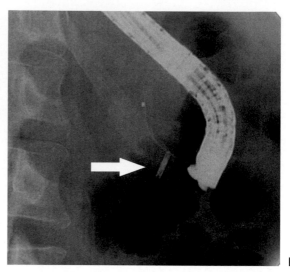

FIGURE 11-118 New MR safety issue, the endoscopic hemostasis clip. A: Coronal T2 image through the common duct shows a small focus of metal artifact (*arrow*) near the ampulla. **B:** ERCP image confirms the presence of a metal clip (*arrow*). All currently available versions are ferromagnetic but are purported to detach and pass out of the body within a day or two. However, this clip had been endoscopically placed more than 7 months before imaging.

Suggested Readings

Ayuso JR, Ayuso C, Bombuy E, et al. Preoperative evaluation of biliary anatomy in adult live liver donors with volumetric mangafodipir trisodium enhanced magnetic resonance cholangiography. *Liver Transpl.* 2004;10:1391–1397.

Chen WJ, Ying DJ, Liu ZJ, et al. Analysis of the arterial supply of the extrahepatic bile ducts and its clinical significance. *Clin Anat.* 1999; 12:245–249.

Colagrande S, Centi N, Galdiero R, et al. Transient hepatic intensity differences: Part 2, those not associated with focal lesions. *AJR Am J Roentgenol.* 2007;188:160–166.

Covey AM, Brody LA, Getrajdman GI, et al. Incidence, patterns, and clinical relevance of variant portal vein anatomy. *AJR Am J Roentgenol.* 2004;183:1055–1064.

Dasgupta D, Stringer MD. Cystic duct and Heister's "valves." *Clin Anat.* 2005;18:81–87.

Douard R, Chevallier JM, Delmas V, et al. Laparoscopic detection of aberrant left hepatic artery: A prospective study in 300 consecutive patients. *Surg Radiol Anat.* 2006;28; 13–17.

Gillard JH, Patel MC, Abrahams PH, et al. Riedel's lobe of the liver: Fact or fiction? *Clin Anat.* 1998;11:47–49.

Hamer OW, Aguirre DA, Casola G, et al. Fatty liver: Imaging patterns and pitfalls. *RadioGraphics.* 2006;26:1637–1653.

Hata F, Hirata K, Murakami G, et al. Identification of segments VI and VII of the liver based on the ramification patterns of the intrahepatic portal and hepatic veins. *Clin Anat.* 1999;12:229–244.

Hoeffel C, Azizi L, Lewin M, et al. Normal and pathologic features of the postoperative biliary tract at 3D MRCP and MRI. *RadioGraphics.* 2006;26:1603–1620.

Ishibashi Y, Murakami G, Honma T, et al. Morphometric study of the sphincter of Oddi (hepatopancreatic) and configuration of the submucosal portion of the sphincteric muscle mass. *Clin Anat.* 2000;13: 159–167.

Kitagawa S, Murakami G, Hata F. Configuration of the right portion of the caudate lobe with special reference to identification of its right margin. *Clin Anat.* 2000;13:321–340.

Lamah M, Karanjia ND, Dickson GH. Anatomical variations of the extrahepatic biliary tree: Review of the world literature. *Clin Anat.* 2001; 14:167–172.

Limamond P, Raman SS, Ghobrial RM, et al. The utility of MRCP in preoperative mapping of biliary anatomy in adult-to-adult living related liver transplant donors. *J Magn Reson Imaging.* 2004;19:209–215.

Limamond P, Zimmerman P, Raman SS, et al. Interpretation of CT and MRI after radiofrequency ablation of hepatic malignancies. *AJR Am J Roentgenol.* 2003;181:1625–1640.

Losanoff JE, Jones JW, Richman BW, et al. Hepaticocystic duct: A rare anomaly of the extrahepatic biliary system. *Clin Anat.* 2002;15:314–315.

Macchi V, Porzionato A, Parenti A, et al. Main accessory sulcus of the liver. *Clin Anat.* 2005;18:39–45.

Mehran R, Schneider R, Franchebois P. The minor hepatic veins: Anatomy and classification. *Clin Anat.* 2000;13:416–421.

Meyers WC, Peterseim DS, Pappas TN, et al. Low insertion of hepatic segmental duct VII-VIII is an important cause of major biliary injury or misdiagnosis. *Am J Surg.* 1996;171:187–191.

Newatia A, Khatri G, Friedman B, et al. Subtraction imaging: Applications for nonvascular abdominal MRI. *AJR Am J Roentgenol.* 2007; 188(4):1018–1025.

Remer EM, Motta-Ramirez GA, Henderson JM. Imaging findings in incidental intrahepatic portal venous shunts. *AJR Am J Roentgenol*. 2007;188:502.

Sheporaitis L, Freeny PC. Hepatic and portal surface veins: A new anatomic variant revealed during abdominal CT. *AJR Am J Roentgenol*. 1998;17:1559–1564.

Singh B, Ramsaroop L, Allopi L, et al. Duplicate gall bladder: An unusual case report. *Surg Radiol Anat*. 2006;28:654–657.

Uva P, Arvelakis A, Rodriguez-Laiz G. Common hepatic artery arising from the left gastric artery: A rare anatomic variation identified on a cadaveric liver donor. *Surg Radiol Anat*. 2007;29:93–95.

Westphalen ACA, Qayyum A, Yeh BM, et al. Liver fat: Effect of hepatic iron deposition on evaluation with opposed-phase MRI. *Radiology*. 2007;242:450–455.

Yu J, Turner MA, Fulcher AS. Congenital anomalies and normal variants of the pancreaticobiliary tract and the pancreas in adults: Part 1, biliary tract. *AJR Am J Roentgenol*. 2006;187:1536–1543.

Zhang J, Israel GM, Hecht EM, et al. Isotropic 3D T2-weighted MRCP with parallel imaging: Feasibility study. *AJR Am J Roentgenol*. 2006; 187:1564–1570.

Chapter 12

Gallbladder

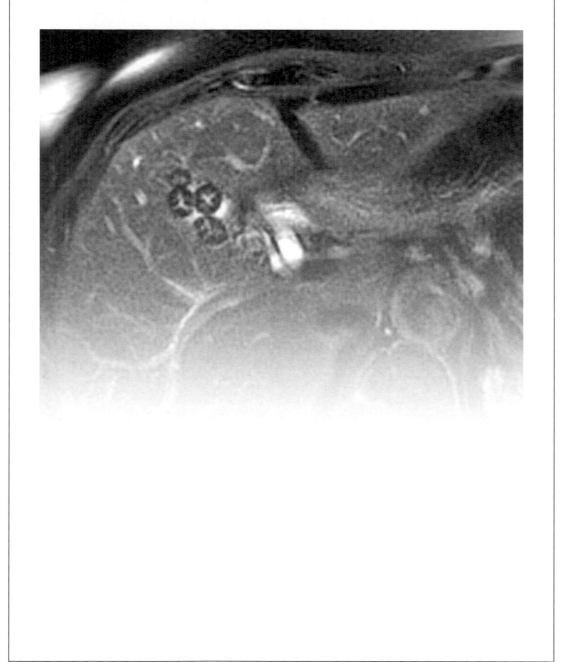

Mellena D. Bridges

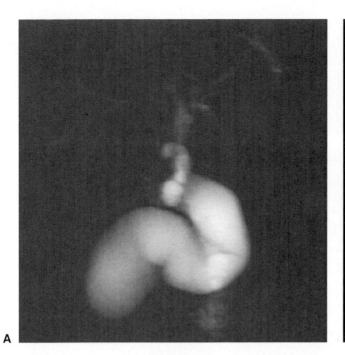
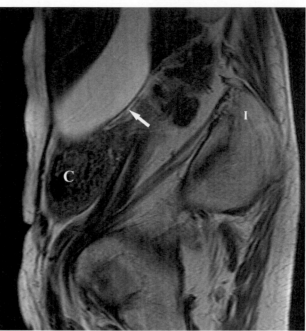

FIGURE 12-1 Unusual gallbladder shapes can result from developmental anomalies, acquired disease, or simply from the lie of adjacent organs. **A:** S-shaped gallbladder with a nicely demonstrated cystic duct. **B:** Sagittal T2-weighted pelvic image in a kyphotic woman shows a low-lying gallbladder (*short arrow*) draped over the cecum (*C*) (*Ilium = I*).

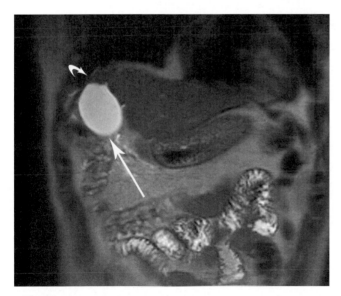

FIGURE 12-2 Fundus of gallbladder under diaphragm due to liver atrophy. In cirrhosis, the gallbladder can lie very high and/or very posteriorly, depending on the pattern of atrophy and hypertrophy (*Gallbladder = arrow, Right hemidiaphragm = curved arrow*).

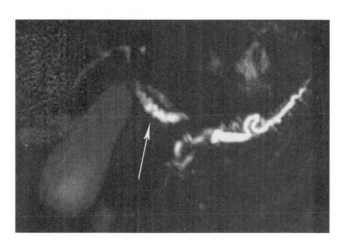

FIGURE 12-3 Very long cystic duct can be misinterpreted as a strictured or beaded common duct (*arrow*). Notice changes of chronic pancreatitis in the pancreatic duct.

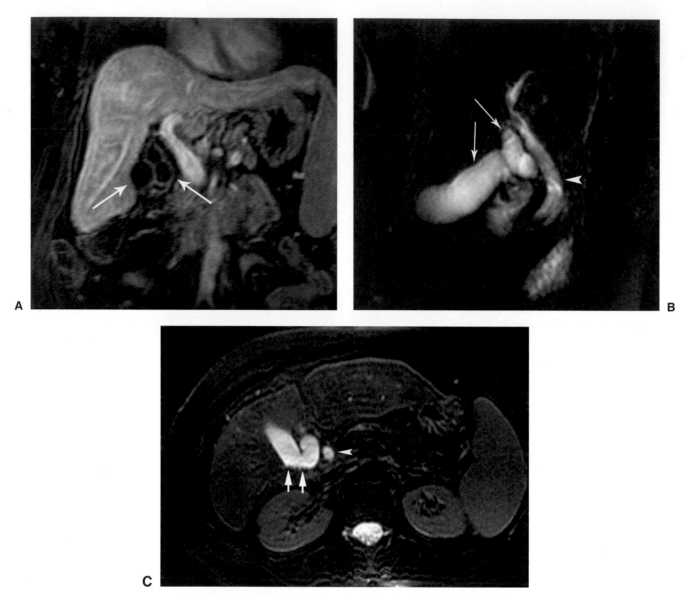

FIGURE 12-4 Hairpin turn of gallbladder neck simulates gallbladder multiplicity or cystic focus. **A:** Coronal enhanced T1-weighted image reveals an apparently multilocular cystic structure in the gallbladder fossa (*arrows*). **B:** Coronal thick-slab MRCP does not clarify (*Common hepatic duct = arrowhead*). **C:** Axial heavily T2-weighted image shows the hairpin turn in the gallbladder neck, along with tiny layering stones (*arrows*).

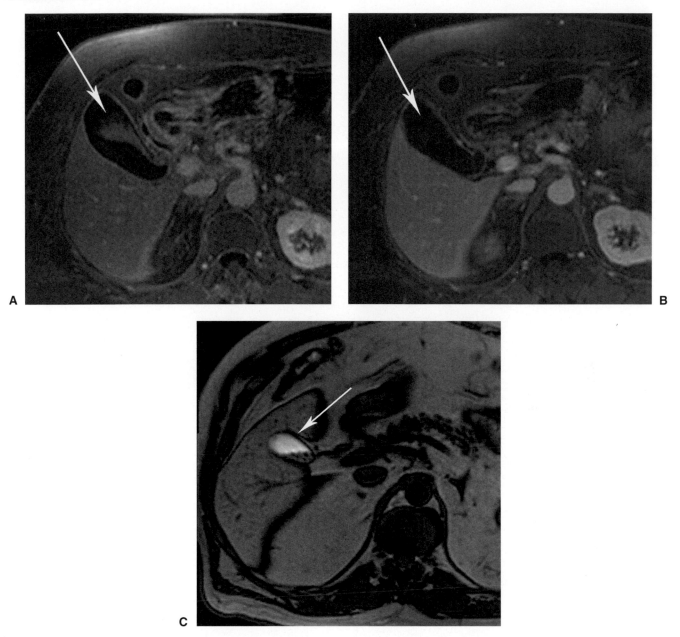

FIGURE 12-5 **Contrast excretion into gallbladder simulates enhancement. A:** A plume of contrast (*arrow*) is demonstrated in the gallbladder on fat-suppressed T1-weighted image obtained after a 15-minute delay. Two percent to 4% of this particular gadolinium formulation (gadobenate) is excreted into the bile. **B:** Image obtained less than 15 minutes earlier showed no contrast in the gallbladder (*arrow*). **C:** Opposed-phase T1-weighted image shows gallbladder contrast accumulation (*arrow*) in another patient who had received gadobenate the previous day.

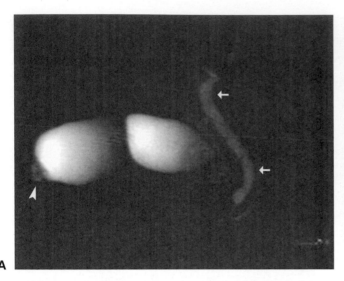

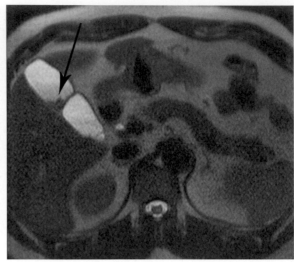

A   **B**

FIGURE 12-6 **Compartmentalization of the gallbladder. A:** Conventional thick slice MRCP shows two apparent chambers to the gallbladder (*Fundal adenomyoma = arrowhead, Common duct = short arrows*). **B:** Axial multislice sequence confirms separation and depicts layering stones in each compartment (*black arrow*). Appearance is most often due to annular adenomyomatosis.

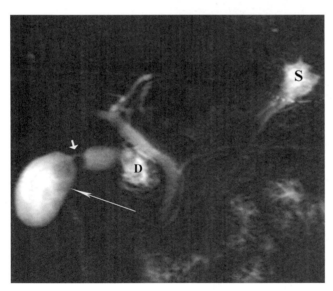

FIGURE 12-7 **Annular adenomyomatosis.** Thick-slab MRCP in another patient shows thread-like channel between compartments (*short arrow*) as well as stones in the distal chamber (*long arrow*) (*Stomach lumen = S, Duodenal bulb = D*).

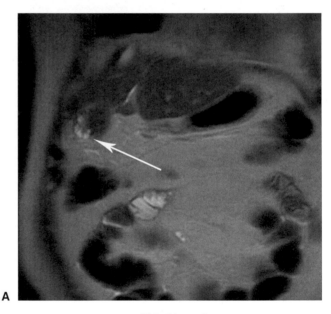

A

FIGURE 12-8 **Benign gallbladder adenomyoma, a potential pitfall. A:** Coronal T2-weighted image through anterior abdomen shows a cystic mass at the gallbladder fundus (*arrow*).

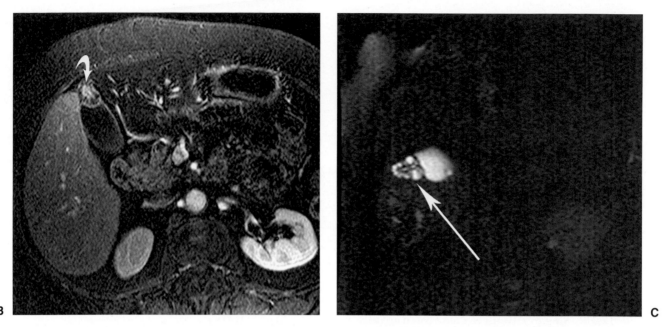

FIGURE 12-8 **Benign gallbladder adenomyoma, a potential pitfall.** (*continued*) **B:** Axial enhanced T1-weighted image shows a small mass with central enhancement (*curved arrow*). **C:** Sagittal fat-suppressed heavily T2-weighted image shows the typical fibrovascular core of the adenomyoma surrounded by small cysts (*arrow*). This has been described as a Christmas tree configuration.

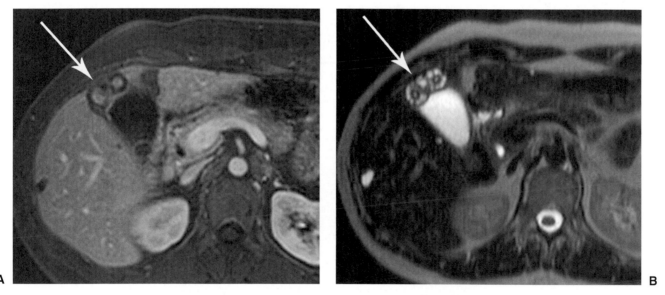

FIGURE 12-9 **Complex fundal adenomyoma. A:** Incidentally discovered, complex fundal mass (*arrow*) on axial enhanced T1-weighted image. **B:** T2-weighted image clearly shows clusters of mural cysts (*arrow*) organized around a pair of fibrovascular cores.

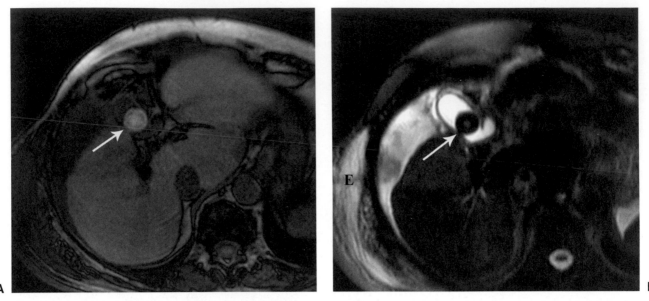

FIGURE 12-10 **Single gallstone has lamellated architecture and T1-hyperintensity.** Axial fat-suppressed unenhanced **(A)** T1- and **(B)** T2-weighted images depict a large, round gallstone with a target appearance (*arrows*). Biliary stones often show increased T1 signal, presumably due to cholesterol content, unless heavily calcified. Notice edema (*E*) in the body wall as well as cirrhotic hepatic morphology.

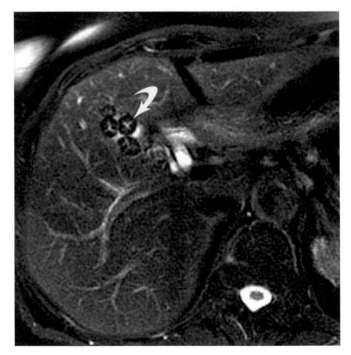

FIGURE 12-11 **MRI version of the gallstone Mercedes-Benz sign.** Radiating central fissures (*curved arrow*) in these T2-hypointense stones are visible because they have filled with hyperintense bile.

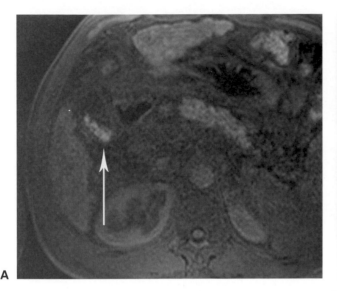

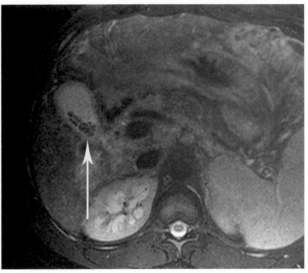

FIGURE 12-12 **T1-hyperintense gallstones. A:** Fat-suppressed unenhanced axial image reveals a cluster of hyperintense foci in the right upper quadrant (*arrow*). **B:** Fat-suppressed T2-weighted image shows these to be small hypointense gallstones (*arrow*), likely cholesterol stones.

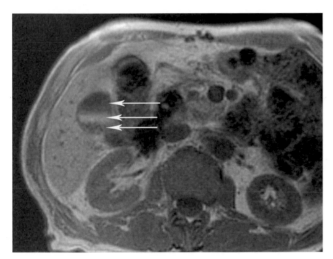

FIGURE 12-13 **Trilaminar appearance of the gallbladder** (*arrows*). Tiny dependent gallstones are topped by T1-hyperintense concentrated bile, which is in turn topped by a layer of more typically T1-hypointense bile.

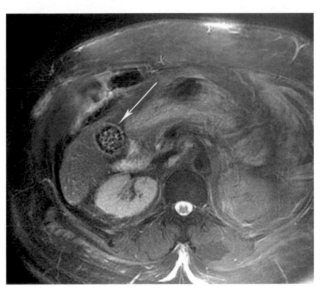

FIGURE 12-14 **Gallstones difficult to see in absence of surrounding bile.** T2-weighted axial image shows gallbladder packed with tiny hypointense stones (*arrow*).

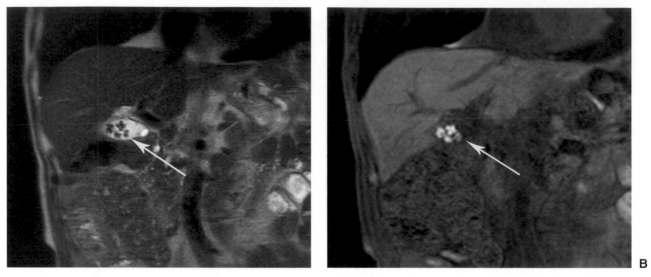

FIGURE 12-15   Cholesterol stones shaped like crosses or jacks. Coronal **(A)** T2-weighted and **(B)** precontrast T1-weighted images show stones that vary from the usual faceted or round configuration (*arrows*). Notice high T1 signal.

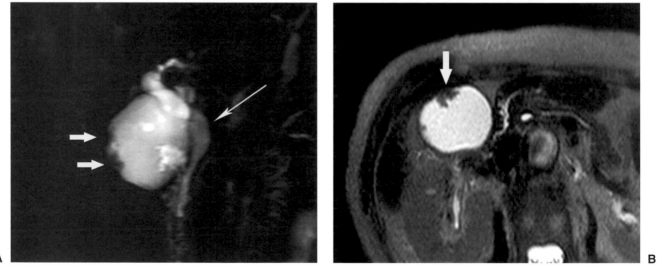

FIGURE 12-16   Floating sludge simulates polypoid gallbladder wall mass. A: Sagittal conventional MRCP image shows apparent irregularity and focal thickening of the anterior gallbladder wall (*short arrows*) (*Common bile duct = long arrow*). **B:** Axial thin-slice MRCP image shows nondependent tumefactive sludge (*arrow*). On occasion, stones and/or sludge will be lighter than bile.

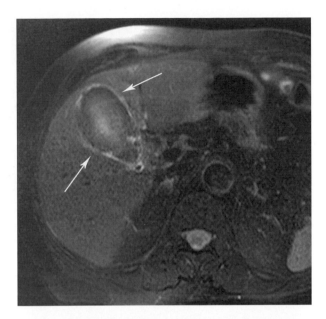

FIGURE 12-17 **Sludge-filled gallbladder simulates mass** on T2-weighted imaging. Normal high signal intensity of bile (*arrows*) is markedly reduced by inspissation.

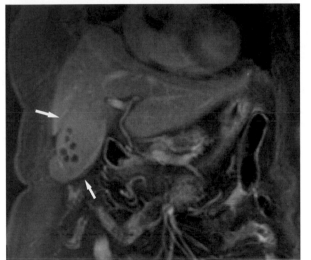

A

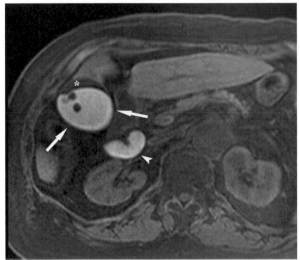

B

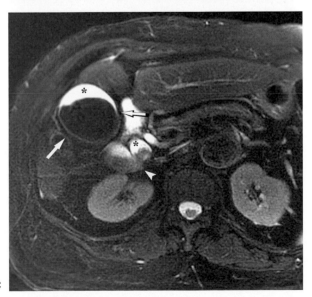

C

FIGURE 12-18 **Tumefactive gallbladder sludge with embedded stones. A:** Gallbladder (*arrows*) is hyperintense even to liver on this enhanced, fat-suppressed coronal T1-weighted image. **B:** Precontrast imaging shows that the hyperintensity was pre-existing, and not due to later enhancement. Notice hypointense calcified stones suspended in the sludge, along with more sludge in the distended gallbladder neck (*arrowhead*) (*Liquid bile = asterisk*). **C:** The sludge is quite hypointense on this fat-suppressed T2-weighted image, in contrast to the hyperintense bile collecting anteriorly (*asterisk*) (*Gallbladder neck = arrowhead*).

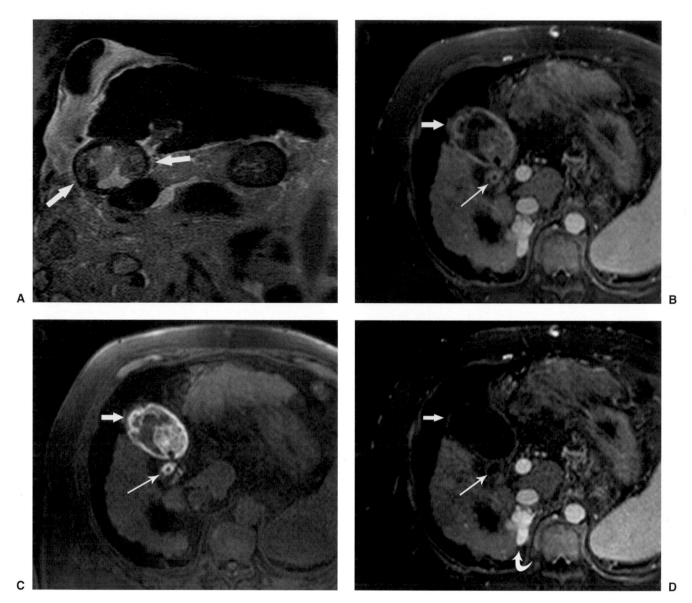

FIGURE 12-19   Porcelain gallbladder simulates malignancy. A: Distended gallbladder with poorly defined wall and apparent mural material (*arrows*) on coronal T2-weighted image. **B:** Axial postcontrast T1-weighted image suggests heterogeneous enhancement of the gallbladder (*short arrow*) and cystic duct (*long arrow*). **C:** However, marked hyperintensity is observed on precontrast imaging in the gallbladder (*short arrow*) and cystic duct (*long arrow*). **D:** Underlying enhancement is excluded by subtraction technique. Notice large portosystemic shunt (*curved arrow*) in this cirrhotic patient (*Gallbladder = short arrow, Cystic duct = long arrow*).

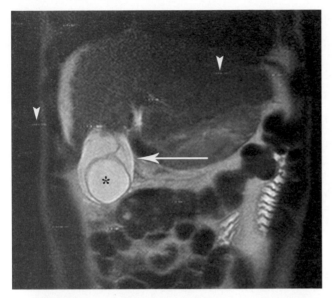

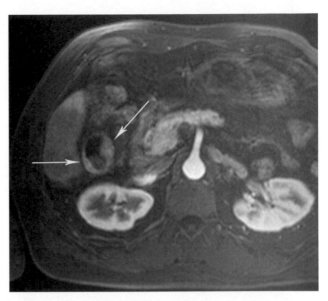

FIGURE 12-20 Gallbladder wall edema simulates chole-cystitis. Portal hypertension in this cirrhotic patient is evidenced by dramatic gallbladder wall edema (*arrow*). Notice lack of inflammatory changes in the pericholecystic fat, a clue to the true diagnosis (*Gallbladder lumen = asterisk, Artifact from RF leak = arrowheads*). RF, radiofrequency.

FIGURE 12-21 Lymphoma mimics gallbladder carcinoma in patient with primary sclerosing cholangitis. Enhanced T1-weighted axial image demonstrates incidentally discovered, smooth, enhancing thickening of the gallbladder wall (*arrows*).

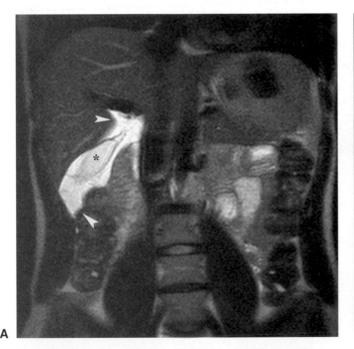

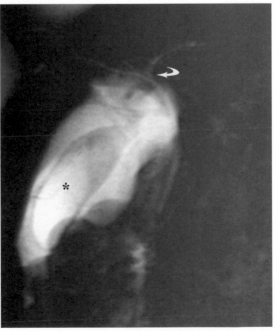

FIGURE 12-22 Lymphangioma mimics gallbladder wall edema. A: Coronal T2-weighted image shows a large, surgically proven lymphangioma (*arrowheads*) encasing the gallbladder (*asterisk*). **B:** Thick-slab MRCP image shows its relationship to the bile ducts and gallbladder lumen (*asterisk*) (*Biliary hilum = curved arrow*).

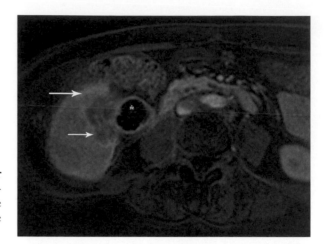

FIGURE 12-23 Gallbladder carcinoma mistaken for cholecystitis. Gallbladder malignancy (*arrows*) often invades the liver fairly early in development. In this case, the gallbladder lumen (*asterisk*) remains patent despite wide penetration of tumor into liver.

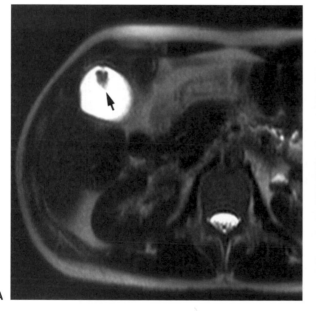

A

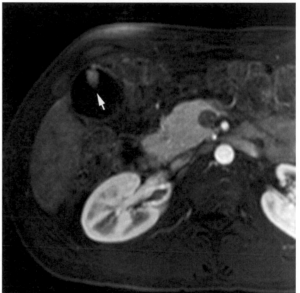

B

FIGURE 12-24 Adenoma simulates polypoid gallbladder malignancy in patient with primary sclerosing cholangitis (PSC). **A:** Filling defect (*arrow*) extends from the anterior gallbladder wall on axial T2-weighted image. **B:** Correlative T1-weighted image demonstrates brisk enhancement of the nodule (*arrow*), subsequently proven surgically to be an adenoma. **C:** MRCP depicts intrahepatic ductal changes of PSC.

C

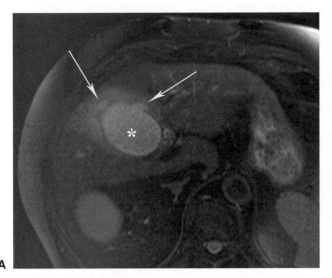

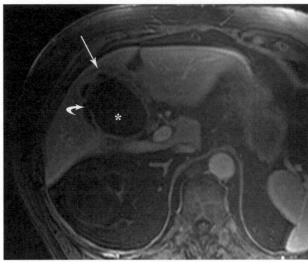

FIGURE 12-25 **Gangrenous cholecystitis mistaken for malignancy.** MRI performed to exclude liver metastases in asymptomatic elderly patient. **A:** Axial fat-suppressed T2-weighted image shows a distended gallbladder (*asterisk*) with outpouchings of fluid (*arrows*) and diffusely hyperintense adjacent liver tissue. **B:** Irregular thickening and focal necrosis of the gallbladder wall (*curved arrow*) is more clearly demonstrated on enhanced T1-weighted image at slightly different level (*Gallbladder lumen = asterisk*).

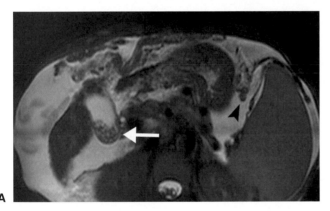

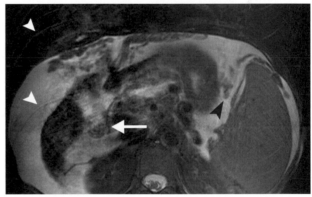

FIGURE 12-26 **Potential solutions for motion artifact are numerous** and include breathholding, respiratory and cardiac gating, antiperistaltics, and various saturation pulses like fat suppression. The **(A)** single-shot image uses a technique for acquiring single images separately and rapidly, and avoids much of the degradation from complex motion obvious in the **(B)** 4-minute turbo spin echo (TSE) T2 image, despite respiratory gating (*Motion artifact = arrowheads, Gallstones = arrows, Gastrosplenic ligament = black arrowhead*).

Suggested Readings

Boscak AR, Al-Hawary M, Ramsburgh SR. Best cases from the AFIP: Adenomyomatosis of the gallbladder. *Radiographics.* 2006;26(3):941–946.

Dasgupta D, Stringer MD. Cystic duct and Heister's "valves". *Clin Anat.* 2005;18:81–87.

Elsayes KM, Oliveira EP, Narra VR, et al. Magnetic resonance imaging of the gallbladder: Spectrum of abnormalities. *Acta Radiol.* 2007; 48(5):476–482.

Heller SL, Lee VS. MR imaging of the gallbladder and biliary system. *Magn Reson Imaging Clin N Am.* 2005;13(2):295–311.

van Breda Vriesman AC, Engelbrecht MR, Smithuis RH. Diffuse gallbladder wall thickening: Differential diagnosis. *AJR Am J Roentgenol.* 2007;188(2):495–501.

Yu J, Turner MA, Fulcher AS, et al. Congenital anomalies and normal variants of the pancreaticobiliary tract and the pancreas in adults: Part 1, biliary tract. *AJR Am J Roentgenol.* 2006;187:1536–1543.

Chapter 13

Pancreas

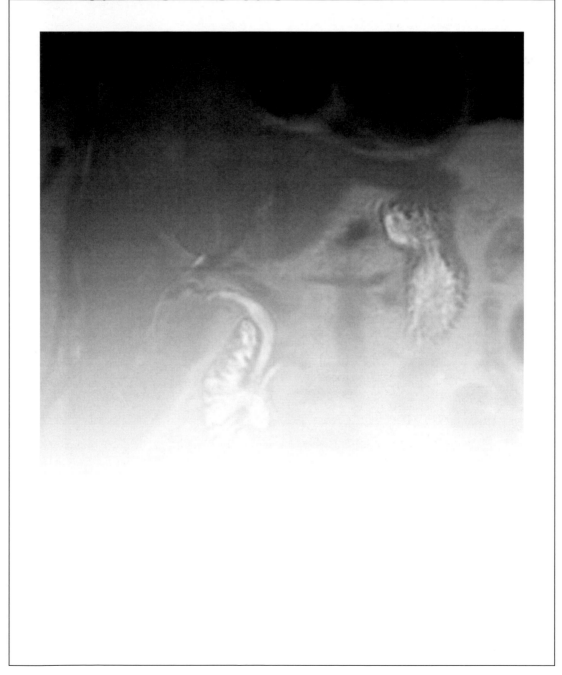

Mellena D. Bridges

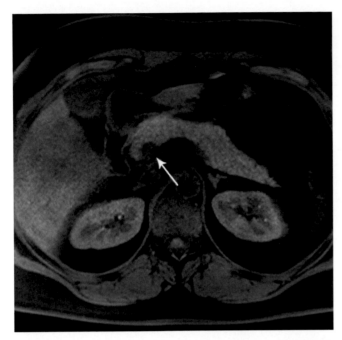

FIGURE 13-1 Normally hyperintense pancreatic signal in T1-weighted image. The pancreas demonstrates very high signal intensity on T1-weighted images, especially when fat is suppressed. The neck, body, and tail often lie in the same plane, with the neck arching over the portal confluence (*arrow*).

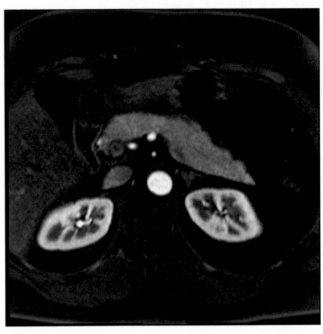

FIGURE 13-2 Normal brisk and uniform pancreatic enhancement. Note the uniform hyperintense signal throughout the pancreas on enhanced T1-weighted fat suppressed image.

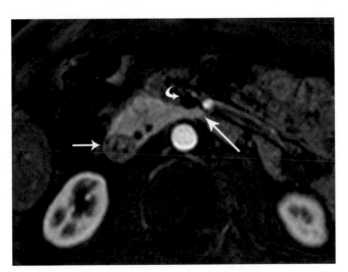

FIGURE 13-3 Normal pancreatic head enhances uniformly, and lies in close association to the duodenum (*short arrow*). The uncinate process (*long arrow*) is a tongue of tissue between the aorta and unenhanced superior mesenteric vein (*curved arrow*).

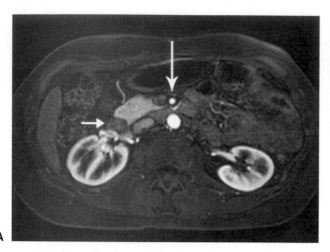
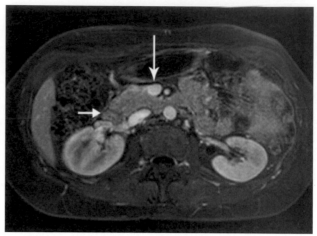

FIGURE 13-4   Normal dramatic change in relative signal intensity with phase of contrast. A: Arterial-dominant phase image through the pancreatic head clearly differentiates the pancreas from the duodenum (*short arrow*) (*Superior mesenteric artery = long arrow*). **B:** This difference is nearly absent by the portal dominant phase (*Duodenum = short arrow, Superior mesenteric vein = long arrow*).

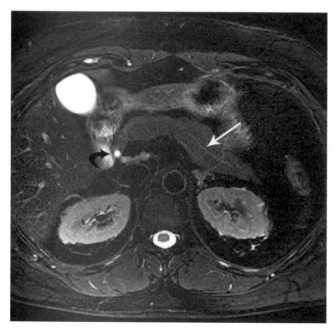

FIGURE 13-5   Normal pancreas on T2-weighted imaging. The pancreas is isointense to liver and hypointense to the kidneys and spleen (not shown), especially when fat signal is suppressed. The common bile duct (*curved arrow*) and slender pancreatic duct (*arrow*) can now be seen.

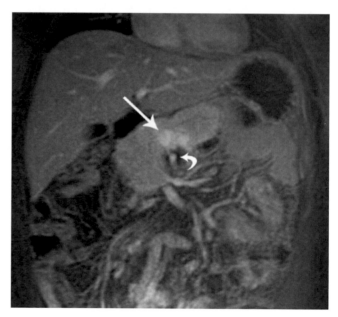

FIGURE 13-6   Coronal imaging of the pancreas. Coronal enhanced image shows the head, neck, and body in this pancreas enlarged by autoimmune pancreatitis. Notice the intimate association with the portal confluence (*arrow*) and superior mesenteric artery (*curved arrow*).

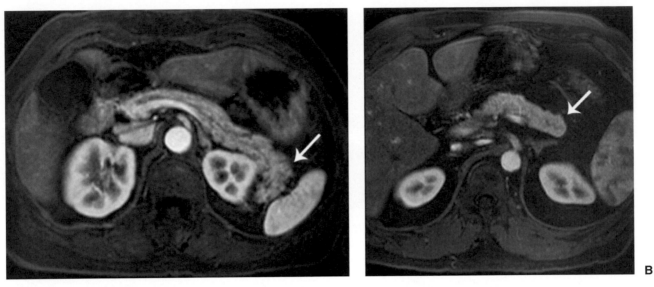

FIGURE 13-7 **Variations of the pancreatic tail.** The pancreatic tail (*arrow*) can be **(A)** long, **(B)** short, or absent. The term *dorsal agenesis* is used when the body is also absent.

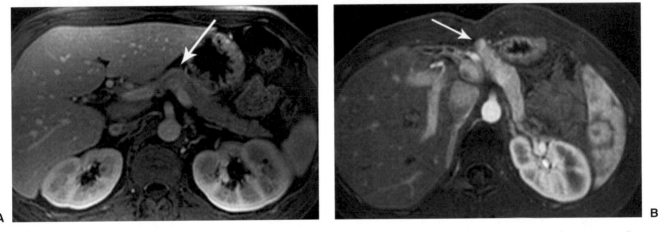

FIGURE 13-8 **Variations in pancreatic shape. A–B:** Bulges, peaks (*arrows*), and attenuated segments can be seen as adjacent organs move or are resected, especially in slender patients.

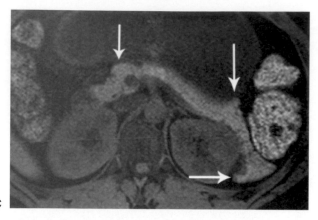

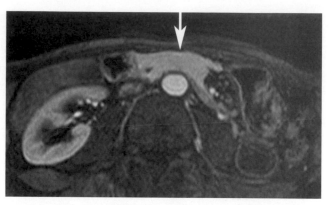

FIGURE 13-8 Variations in pancreatic shape. (*continued*) **C:** Bulges, peaks (*arrows*), and attenuated segments can be seen as adjacent organs move or are resected, especially in slender patients.

FIGURE 13-9 Variation in pancreatic location. The pancreatic head (*arrow*) can be displaced to the midline or even to the left of the aorta. Body habitus, scoliosis, abdominal masses, and size and lie of abdominal and retroperitoneal organs can affect the shape and position of the pancreas.

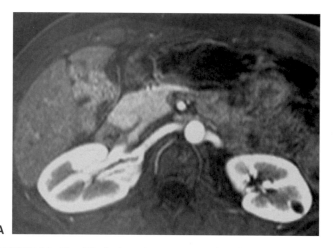

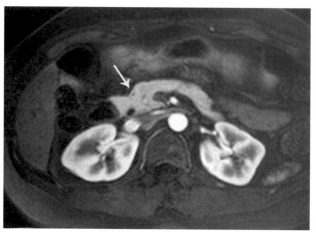

FIGURE 13-10 Variations in pancreatic head shape. A–B: Pancreatic head shape variations originate embryologically, when the head forms by fusing dorsal and ventral anlages. This development can be reflected as a cleft of variable depth, usually containing the gastroduodenal artery (*arrow*).

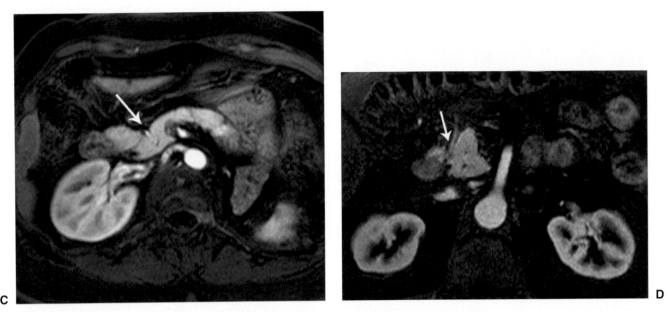

FIGURE 13-10 **Variations in pancreatic head shape.** (*continued*) **C–D:** Pancreatic head shape variations originate embryologically, when the head forms by fusing dorsal and ventral anlages. This development can be reflected as a cleft of variable depth, usually containing the gastroduodenal artery (*arrow*).

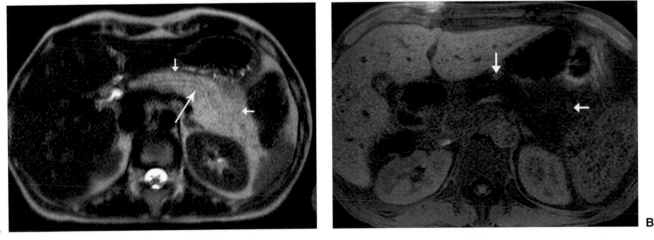

FIGURE 13-11 **Fatty pancreas. A:** Pancreatic volume is preserved (*short arrows*), but the parenchyma is nearly completely replaced by relatively high-signal tissue on this single-shot T2-weighted image (*Pancreatic duct = arrow*). **B:** The profound signal loss with chemical fat saturation proves that this tissue is predominantly fat (*arrows*).

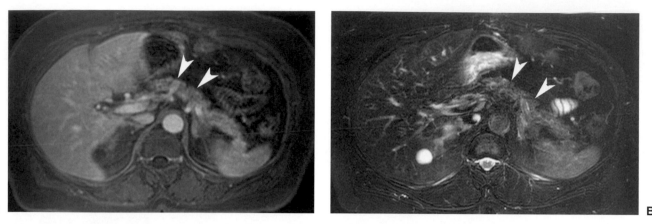

FIGURE 13-12 Pancreatic atrophy, presumably age-related. T2-weighted fat-suppressed **(A)** and T1-weighted enhanced **(B)** images demonstrate a diffusely atrophic pancreas (*arrowheads*) without duct abnormality in an asymptomatic, elderly patient.

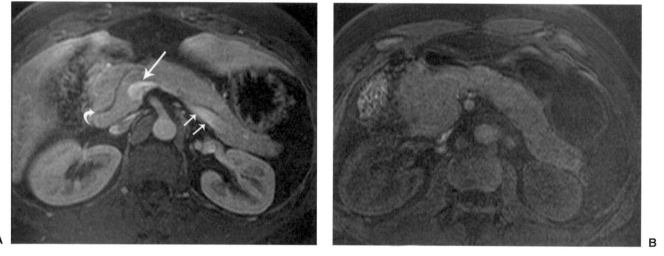

FIGURE 13-13 Enlarged pancreas due to autoimmune pancreatitis. A: Enhanced T1-weighted image demonstrates a fairly horizontal lie of the pancreas, including the head on this image (*Pancreatic duct = curved arrow, Portal confluence = long arrow, Splenic vein = short arrows*). **B:** Notice the abnormally reduced signal intensity of the entire pancreas on unenhanced T1-weighed image.

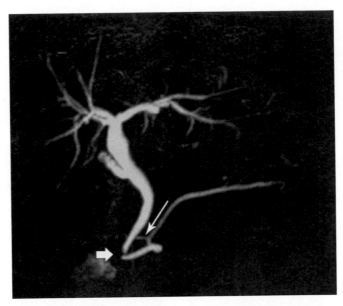

FIGURE 13-14 **Normal pancreaticobiliary ductal anatomy.** Projectional MRCP image shows the confluence of the bile duct and main pancreatic duct at the ampulla (*short arrow*). The minor duct of Santorini (*long arrow*) drains more cephalad through the minor duodenal papilla.

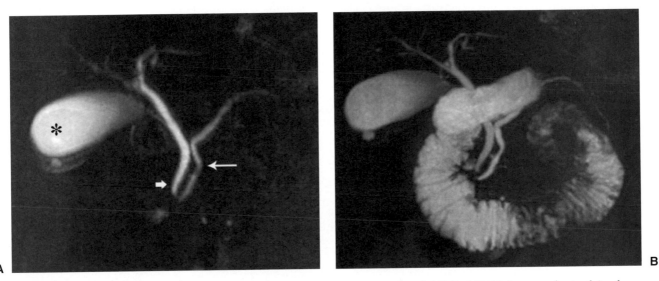

FIGURE 13-15 **Normal pancreatic exocrine function on secretin-stimulated MRI.** MRCP images obtained in the same patient before **(A)** and after **(B)** secretin administration show copious excretion of pancreatic fluid into the small bowel (*Pancreatic duct = long arrow, Distal common bile duct = short arrow, Gallbladder = asterisk*).

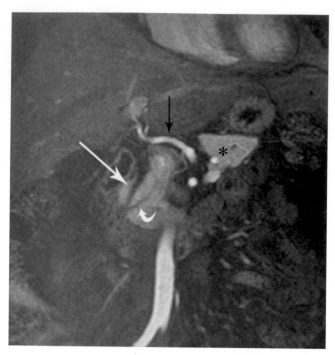

FIGURE 13-16 Normal confluence of the common bile duct and pancreatic duct in the pancreatic head. Coronal enhanced T1-weighted image shows the common bile duct (*white arrow*) and pancreatic duct (*curved arrow*) descending normally through the pancreatic head to merge at the duodenal ampulla (*Body of pancreas = asterisk, Hepatic artery = black arrow*).

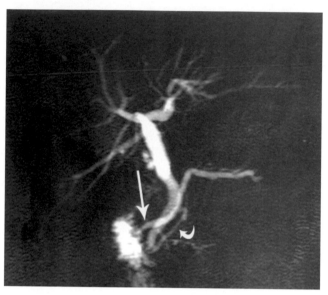

FIGURE 13-17 Preferential flow of pancreatic secretions through the minor papilla. Projectional MRCP image demonstrates a normal anatomic variant in which the ducts are joined (*curved arrow*), but most of the drainage of pancreatic secretions (*straight arrow*) occurs through the minor papilla.

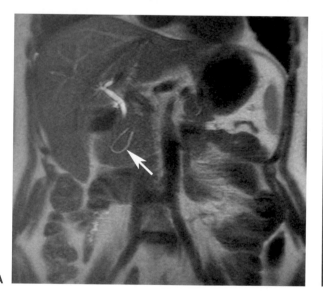

A

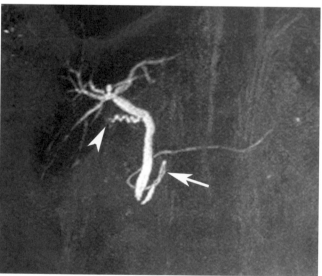

B

FIGURE 13-18 Normal tortuosity of the pancreatic duct. Apparent loop in the pancreatic duct (*arrow*) on **(A)** coronal MRI and **(B)** projectional MRCP image reflects the tortuous course it takes through the pancreatic head (approximately 3 cm in anteroposterior depth). Notice the cystic duct remnant (*arrowhead*) in this postcholecystectomy patient.

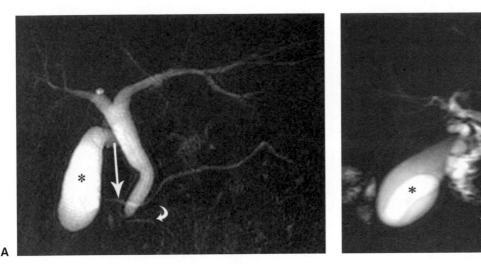

FIGURE 13-19 **Pancreas divisum. A** and **B:** Pancreas divisum is a common variant and controversial risk factor for pancreatitis. Projectional MRCP in two patients demonstrate failed developmental fusion between the dorsal and ventral ducts (*Main pancreatic duct = arrow, Separate ventral duct = curved arrow, CBD = short arrow, Gallbladder = asterisk*). Notice the fluid-coated gastric rugae (*arrowheads*) in the second patient **(B)**. CBD, common bile duct.

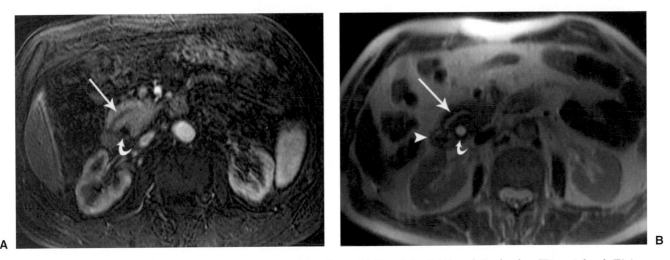

FIGURE 13-20 **Pancreas divisum on axial imaging.** Axial enhanced T1-weighted **(A)** and single-shot T2-weighted **(B)** images delineate the main pancreatic duct (*long arrow*) traveling horizontally through the upper pancreatic head to the minor papilla (*arrowhead*). Common bile duct (*curved arrow*) descends to the major papilla and is completely independent of the main pancreatic duct.

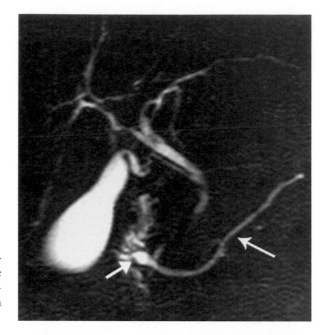

FIGURE 13-21   Santorinicele associated with pancreas divisum. Bulbous protrusion (*short arrow*) of the distal duct (*long arrow*) into the duodenum on projectional MRCP image has an appearance similar to a choledochocele or ureterocele.

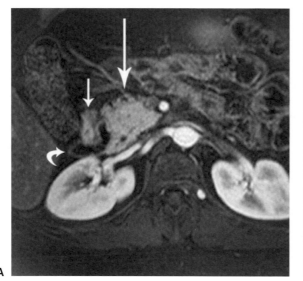

A

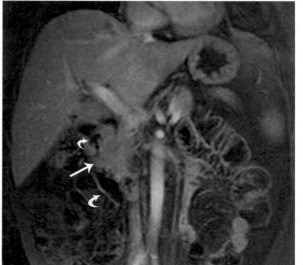

B

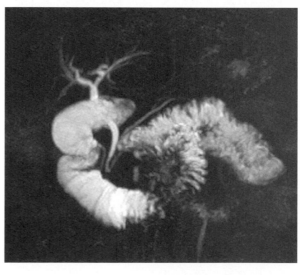

C

FIGURE 13-22   Annular pancreas. Enhanced axial **(A)** and coronal **(B)** images show a small band of pancreatic head tissue (*short arrow*) on its way around the second portion of the duodenum (*curved arrow*) (*Pancreatic head = long arrow*). **C:** Coronal maximum intensity projection (MIP) MRCP images show a circumferential impression on the descending duodenum (*arrow*) and the tiny duct that drains the annular portion (*curved arrow*).

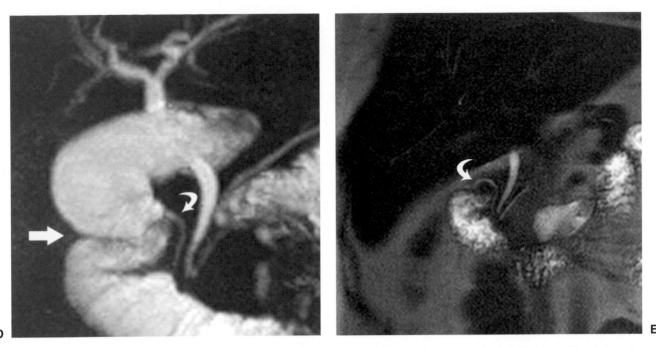

FIGURE 13-22 **Annular pancreas.** (*continued*) **D** and **E:** Coronal maximum intensity projection (MIP) MRCP images show a circumferential impression on the descending duodenum (*arrow*) and the tiny duct that drains the annular portion (*curved arrow*), better seen on the thin section image (**E**).

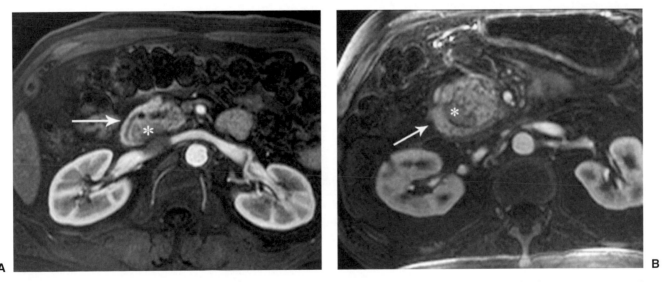

FIGURE 13-23 **Annular pancreas.** Enhancing pancreatic tissue (*arrows*) is circumferential around duodenum (*asterisk*) in three additional patients. **A:** Hypointense aberrant duct courses horizontally in this asymptomatic patient. **B:** This patient with an incidental annular pancreas (*arrow*) was scanned to evaluate for possible gallstone pancreatitis, which was confirmed.

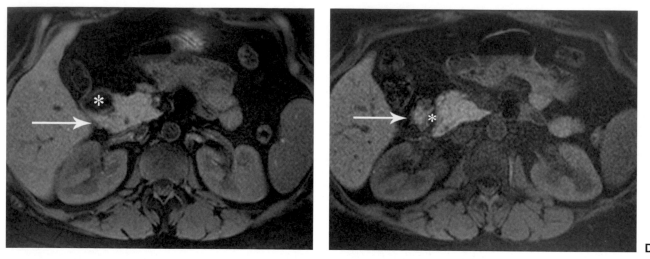

FIGURE 13-23 **Annular pancreas.** (*continued*) **C** and **D**: Sequential unenhanced T1-weighted images in a third patient show segments of a more obliquely oriented annulus (*arrows*). Notice the high intrinsic T1-weighted signal intensity of the pancreatic tissue (Duodenum = asterisk).

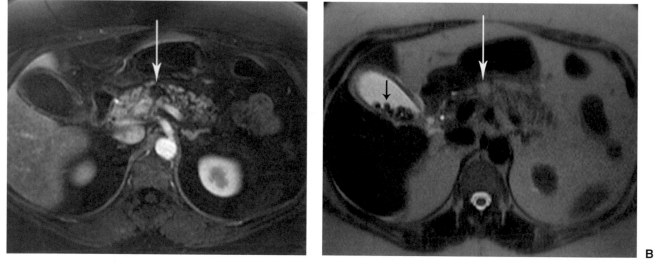

FIGURE 13-24 **Pancreatic lipoma.** This small pancreatic lipoma (*white arrow*) is isointense on **(A)** enhanced fat-suppressed T1-weighted and **(B)** T2-weighted images, and was mistaken for a hypoenhancing mass on CT. Notice the cholelithiasis (*black arrow*) and thickened gallbladder wall from chronic inflammation.

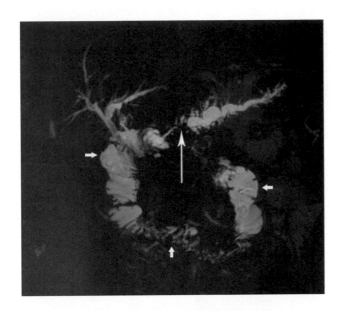

FIGURE 13-25 Prior Whipple procedure. Maximum intensity projection (MIP) image reconstructed from a 3-D MRCP acquisition following secretin stimulation. Notice the pancreaticojejunostomy and hepaticojejunostomy with fluid filling the afferent limb (*short arrows*). Tumor obstructs the pancreatic duct (*long arrow*) upstream from the pancreaticojejunal anastomosis.

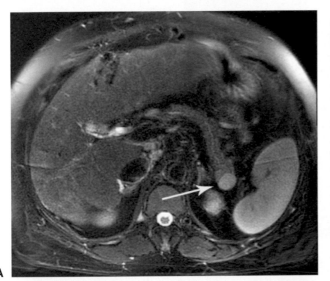

A

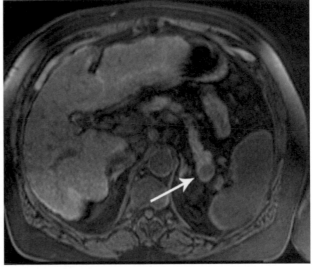

B

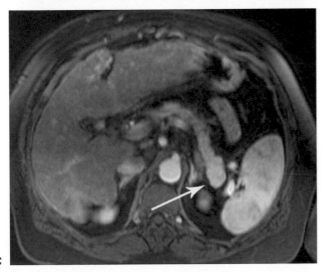

C

FIGURE 13-26 Splenule in the pancreatic tail simulates a hypervascular mass. T2-weighted fat-suppressed **(A)**, T1-weighted fat suppressed **(B)** and enhanced T1-weighted fat suppressed **(C)** images demonstrate a well-circumscribed nodule (*arrow*), which remains isointense to the spleen on all pulse sequences.

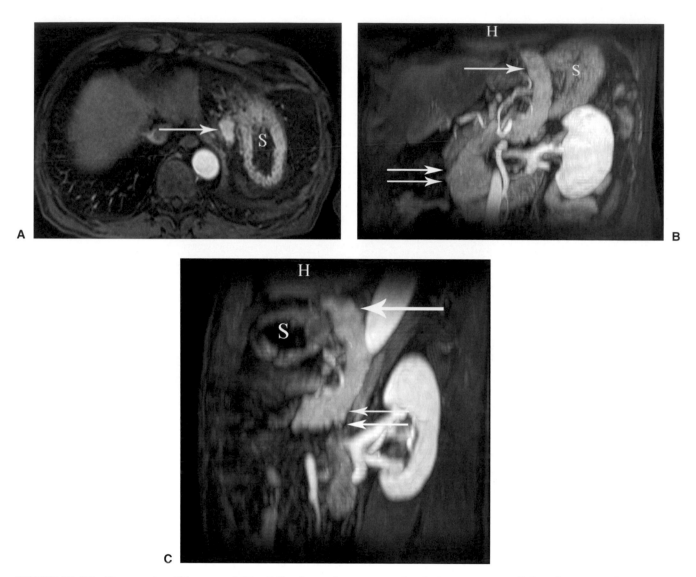

FIGURE 13-27 **Pancreatic tail hypermobility following splenectomy, simulating a mass medial to the gastric fundus.** Axial (**A**), coronal oblique (**B**), and sagittal (**C**) reconstructions show a vertically oriented body and tail (*single arrows*) reaching the diaphragm (*Pancreatic head = double arrows, Heart = H, Stomach = S*).

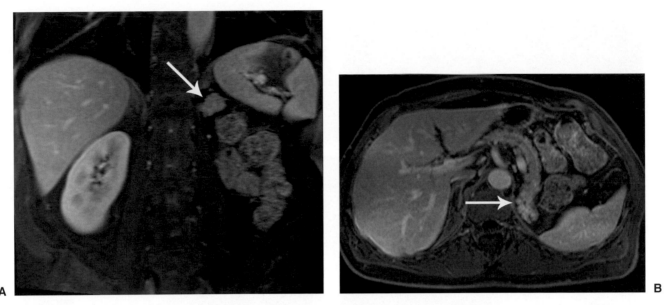

FIGURE 13-28 **Pancreatic tail simulates a left upper quadrant (LUQ) mass.** Coronal enhanced **(A)** and axial T2-weighted **(B)** images demonstrate a small portion of the pancreatic tail (*arrow*) that simulates a left adrenal nodule.

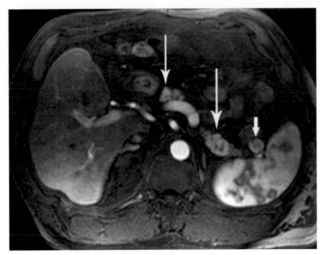

FIGURE 13-29 **Renal cell carcinoma metastases to the pancreas.** Small metastases (*long arrows*) to the pancreas simulate islet cell tumor. Renal cell carcinoma metastases strongly enhance, can be multiple and very small. Note the splenule (*short arrow*).

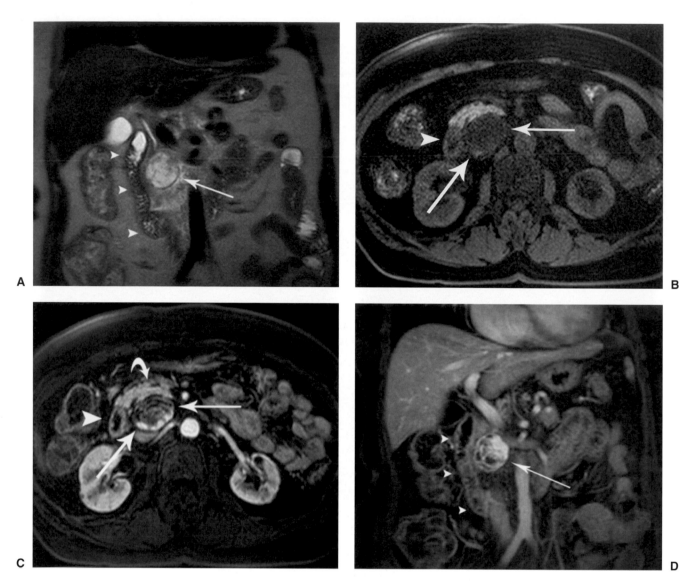

FIGURE 13-30 **Precaval hemangioma simulating a pancreatic mass. A:** Coronal T2-weighted, **(B)** T1-weighted, and **(C and D)** sequential enhanced images demonstrate a well-circumscribed, relatively T2-hyperintense mass (*arrow*) that displaces the normal pancreatic head anteriorly (*curved arrow*) and progressively enhances (*Duodenum = arrowheads*). **C:** Arterial phase shows characteristic discontinuous, nodular peripheral enhancement of the hemangioma.

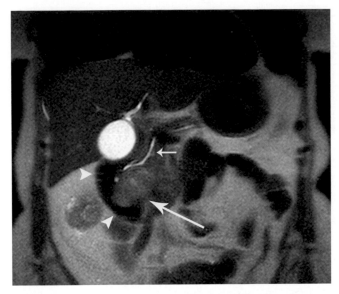

FIGURE 13-31 Duodenal gastrointestinal stromal tumor (GIST) simulating a pancreatic head mass. Peripancreatic masses can easily invaginate the relatively soft pancreas tissue and simulate a pancreas tumor. Duodenal lumen (*arrowheads*) hypointensity is due to negative oral contrast agent. Notice how the mass (*long arrow*) superiorly displaces the pancreatic duct (*short arrow*).

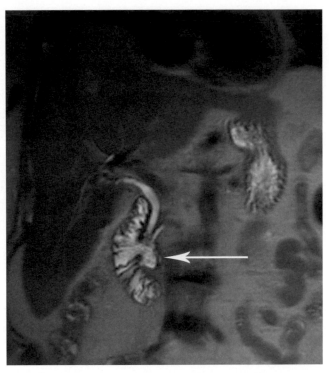

FIGURE 13-32 Periampullary duodenal diverticulum. Thin slice coronal MRCP image demonstrates a periampullary duodenal diverticulum (*arrow*), which can mimic a cystic pancreatic head lesion. Since duodenal diverticula contain various mixtures of air, fluid, and solid material, their appearance can be very confusing. CT may confirm the presence of air, solidifying the diagnosis.

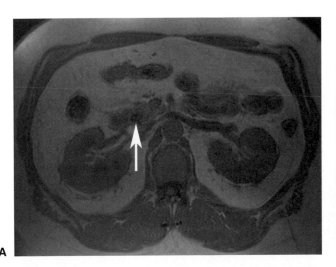

A

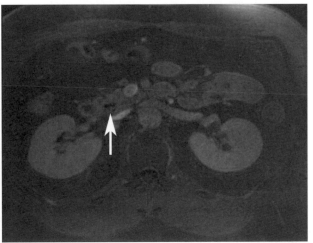

B

FIGURE 13-33 Duodenal diverticulum simulating a pancreatic head cystic lesion. Axial T1-weighted images before (**A**) and after (**B**) contrast demonstrate a small hypointense focus (*arrow*) within the pancreatic head, due to a small duodenal diverticulum. Peripheral enhancement of the diverticular mucosa can be confused with a pancreatic cystic lesion.

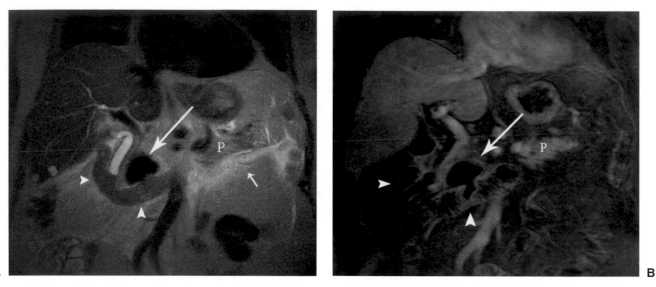

FIGURE 13-34 **Duodenal diverticulum. A:** Coronal T2-weighted images demonstrate a diverticulum (*long arrow*) arising from the duodenum (*arrowheads*) in a patient with incidental acute pancreatitis. Notice the peripancreatic edema (*short arrow*). **B:** Enhanced T1-weighted fat suppressed image clearly shows the discontinuous superior duodenal wall at the point of origin of the hypointense, air-filled diverticulum (*arrow*) (*Pancreas = P, Duodenum = arrowheads*).

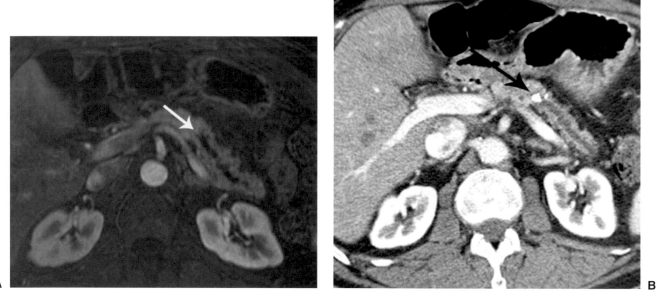

FIGURE 13-35 **Pancreatic ductal stone missed on MRI. A:** Enhanced T1-weighted axial image demonstrates ductal dilatation within the pancreatic tail without obvious obstructing lesion. **B:** Enhanced CT reveals a large pancreatic ductal stone (*arrow*) in an obvious case of calcific pancreatitis. Unless surrounded by fluid, calcium can be invisible on MRI.

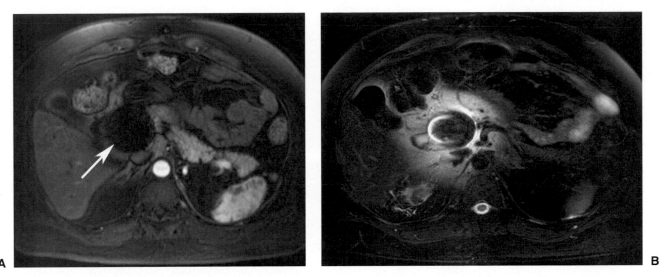

FIGURE 13-36 Metallic clip artifact obscures the pancreatic head. Axial T2-weighted **(A)** and enhanced T1-weighted fat-suppressed **(B)** images demonstrate varying degrees of susceptibility artifact (*arrow*) which obscure the pancreatic head. In general, artifact can be decreased by increasing the bandwidth, increasing the matrix, using FSE sequencing, and avoiding chemical fat suppression and gradient echo techniques. If gradient echo sequences are used, a low echo time (TE) improves image quality.

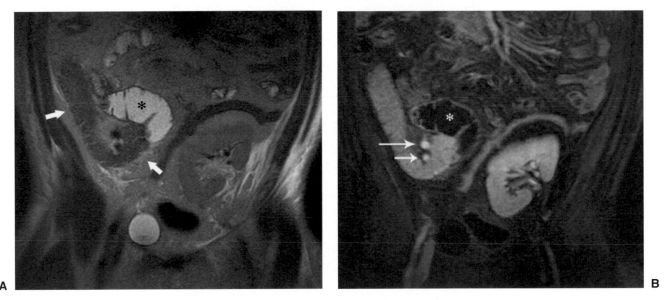

FIGURE 13-37 Pancreas transplant in the right lower quadrant. A: Coronal T2-weighted image shows an isointense gland (*arrows*) with its fluid-filled donor duodenal segment (*asterisk*). **B:** Enhanced T1-weighted image shows normal enhancement. The pancreatic head and neck are curled around donor superior mesenteric vein (SMV) and superior mesenteric artery (SMA) (*arrows*). Notice the left pelvic renal transplant.

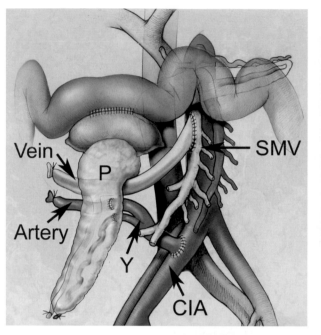

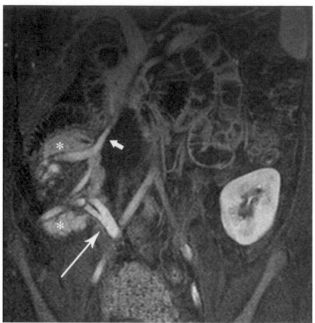

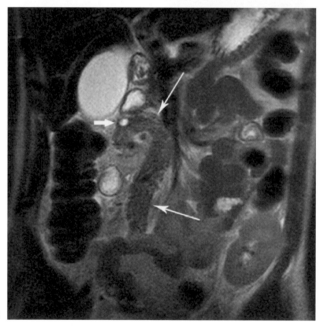

FIGURE 13-38 **Pancreas transplant with venous drainage into portal system.** **A:** Diagram of alternate surgical approach (*Pancreas transplant = P, Superior mesenteric vein = SMV, Common iliac artery = CIA, Donor iliac Y-graft = Y*). **B:** Coronal image demonstrates venous drainage of the pancreas transplant (*asterisk*) into the portal system through the SMV (*short arrow*) (*Donor iliac Y-graft = long arrow*). **C:** Image from another patient also shows the usual vertical orientation of the graft (*long arrows*), but in this arrangement with pancreatic head more cephalad (*Oversewn donor CBD in cross-section = short arrow*). CBD, common bile duct.

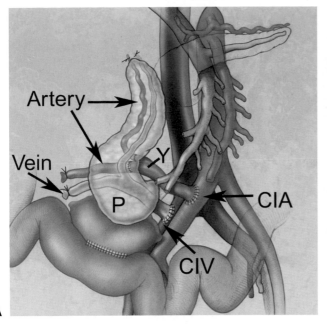 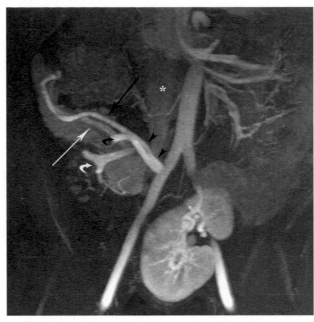

FIGURE 13-39 **Pancreas transplant with venous drainage to the iliac vein. A:** Diagram illustrates the venous drainage of the transplant inferiorly to the recipient iliac vein. Arterial supply is from the external iliac artery through a donor iliac Y graft (*Y*). (*Pancreas transplant = P, Common iliac vein = CIV, Common iliac artery = CIA*). **B:** Coronal MR demonstrates corresponding anatomy (*Donor splenic artery = black arrow, Donor splenic vein = white arrow, Donor SMA = curved arrow, Donor iliac Y graft = arrowheads, Inferior vena cava = asterisk*).

Suggested Readings

Akisik MF, Sandrasegaran K, Aisen AA, et al. Dynamic secretin-enhanced MR cholangiopancreatography. *Radiographics*. 2006;26(3):665–677.

Alempijevic T, Stimec B, Kovacevic N. Anatomical features of the minor duodenal papilla in pancreas divisum. *Surg Radiol Anat*. 2006;28:620–623.

Balci NC, Alkaade S, Akduman IE, Bilgin M, Murdock CP, Burton FR. Serial contrast-enhanced MRI of the pancreas: Correlation with secretin-stimulated endoscopic pancreatic function test. *Acad Radiol*. 2006;13(11):1367–1372.

Boraschi P, Donati F, Gigoni R, et al. Pancreatic transplants: Secretin-stimulated MR pancreatography. *Abdom Imaging*. 2007;32(2):207–214.

Hagspiel KD, Nandalur K, Burkholder B, et al. Contrast-enhanced MR angiography after pancreas transplantation: Normal appearance and vascular complications. *AJR Am J Roentgenol*. 2005;184(2):465–473.

Hagspiel KD, Nandalur K, Pruett TL, et al. Evaluation of vascular complications of pancreas transplantation with high spatial resolution contrast-enhanced MR angiography. *Radiology*. 2007;242:590–599.

Heverhagen JT, Wagner HJ, Ebel H, et al. Pancreatic transplants: Non-invasive evaluation with secretin-augmented MR pancreatography and MR perfusion measurements–preliminary results. *Radiology*. 2004;233(1):273–280.

Kim JK, Altun E, Elias J, Jr., et al. Focal pancreatic mass: Distinction of pancreatic cancer from chronic pancreatitis using gadolinium-enhanced 3D-gradient-echo MRI. *J Magn Reson Imaging*. 2007;26(2):313–322.

Kim HJ, Byun JH, Park SH, et al. Focal fatty replacement of the pancreas: Usefulness of chemical shift MRI. *AJR Am J Roentgenol*. 2007;188:429–432.

Kim MH, Lee SS, Kim CD, et al. Incomplete pancreas divisum: Is it merely a normal anatomic variant without clinical implications? *Endoscopy*. 2001;22:778–785.

Miller FH, Rini NJ, Keppke AL. MRI of adenocarcinoma of the pancreas. *AJR Am J Roentgenol*. 2006;187(4):W365–W374.

Nijs EL, Callahan MJ. Congenital and developmental pancreatic anomalies: Ultrasound, computed tomography, and magnetic resonance imaging features. *Semin Ultrasound CT MR*. 2007;28(5):395–401.

Tozbikian G, Bloomston M, Stevens R, et al. Accessory spleen presenting as a mass in the tail of the pancreas. *Ann Diagn Pathol*. 2007;11(4):277–281.

Singh B, Ramsaroop L, Allopi L, et al. Duplicate gallbladder: An unusual case report. *Surg Radiol Anat*. 2006;28:654–657.

L Van Hoe L, Gryspeerdt S, Vanbeckevoort D, et al. Normal Vaterian sphincter complex: Evaluation of morphology and contractility with dynamic single-shot MR cholangiopancreatography. *AJR Am J Roentgenol*. 1998;170:1497–1450.

Yu J, Turner MA, Fulcher AS, et al. Congenital anomalies and normal variants of the pancreaticobiliary tract and the pancreas in adults: Part 2, pancreatic duct and pancreas. *AJR Am J Roentgenol*. 2006;187:1544–1553.

Chapter 14

Kidneys and Adrenals

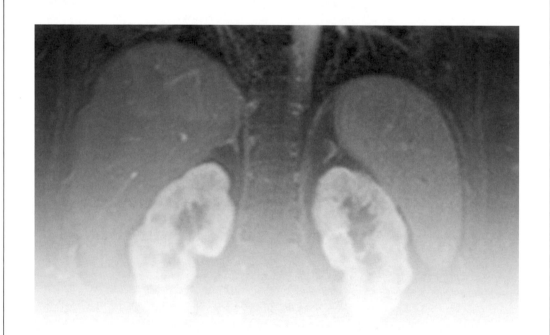

Kidneys

Ureters

Adrenals

Mellena D. Bridges and Joseph G. Cernigliaro

Kidneys

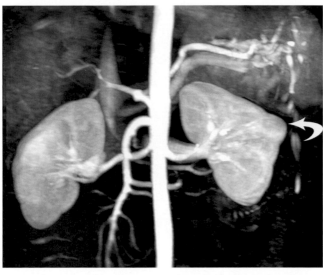

FIGURE 14-1 Dromedary hump, a pseudolesion of the left kidney. Maximum intensity projection (MIP) reconstruction of an abdominal MRA demonstrates a focal bulge in the lateral aspect of this kidney (*curved arrow*). This occurs over time in response to downward flattening pressure from the adjacent spleen.

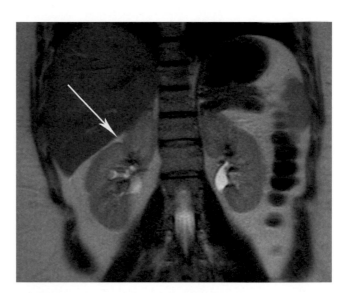

FIGURE 14-2 Focal fetal lobulation. Focal fetal lobulation (*arrow*) is a subtle variant. This is more obvious on sonography, when it is described as the hyperechogenic junctional line.

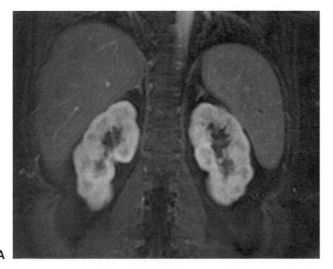

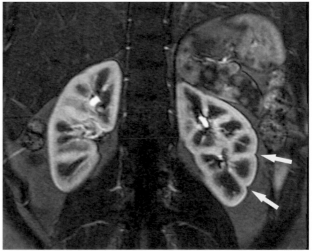

FIGURE 14-3 Bilateral fetal lobulation, a normal variant and potential mimic of renal mass or cortical scar. **A:** Coronal enhanced T1-weighted image in the nephrographic phase depicts an undulating surface contour bilaterally. **B:** Coronal image from another patient in early corticomedullary phase shows more lobulation on the left (*arrows*). Importantly, there is no underlying cortical thinning or calyceal abnormality.

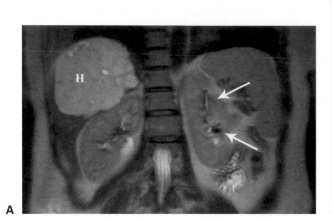
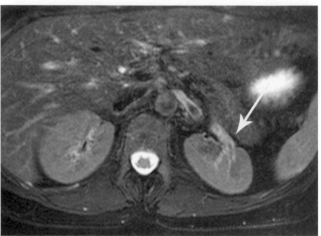

A   B

FIGURE 14-4 **Malrotated left kidney, a common variant. A:** Coronal and **(B)** axial fat-suppressed T2-weighted images depict the hilum of left kidney (*arrows*) oriented anterolaterally, rather than medially. The kidney is otherwise at its normal level (*Hepatic hemangioma = H*).

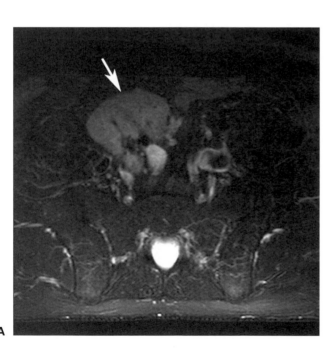
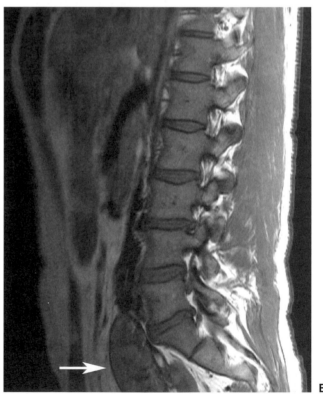

A   B

FIGURE 14-5 **Pelvic kidney,** incidentally discovered on routine lumbar spine MRI. **A:** Axial fat-suppressed T2-weighted and **(B)** sagittal T1-weighted images show a soft tissue focus anterior to the right common iliac vessels, consistent with a pelvic kidney (*arrows*), which failed to ascend out of the pelvis *in utero*.

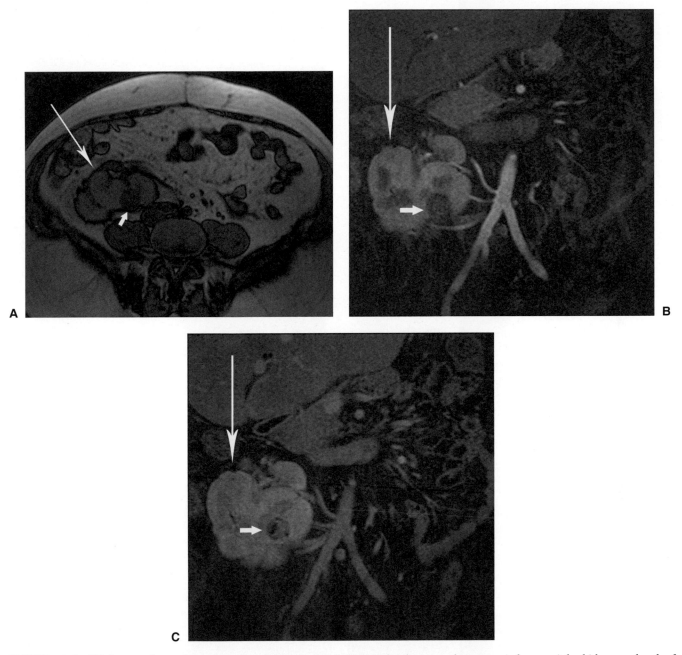

FIGURE 14-6 **Right renal ptosis and malrotation. A:** Axial T1-weighted image shows a misshapen right kidney at level of iliac crest (*arrow*). **B:** Coronal maximum intensity projection (MIP) reconstruction of arterial phase-enhanced data set shows multiple right renal arteries supplying the kidney (*long arrow*), arising from distal aorta and proximal common iliac artery. Note the concomitant renal cell carcinoma (*short arrow*). **C:** Right renal veins become visible on venous phase MIP (*Renal cell carcinoma = short arrow, Kidney = long arrow*).

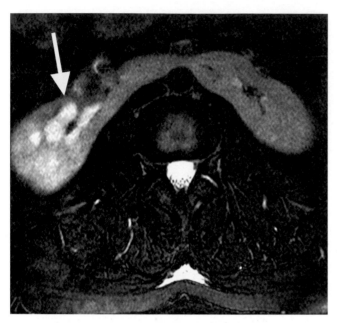

FIGURE 14-7 **Horseshoe kidney with mild dilatation of the right collecting system.** Fat-suppressed T2-weighted axial image from a lumbar spine examination shows a band of hyperintense tissue draped across the spine and great vessels. Fluid fills the right pelvocalyceal system (*arrow*). Anterior rotation of the pelves puts the horseshoe kidney at some risk for stasis and stones.

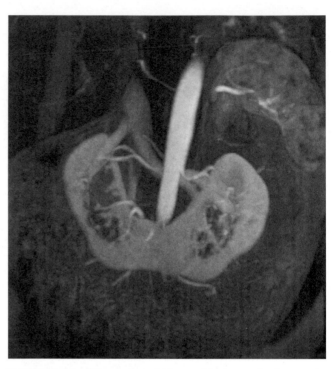

FIGURE 14-8 **Horseshoe kidney.** Notice multiple arteries and veins, typical in this variant. The inferior mesenteric artery originating from the aorta creates a block to further migration of the kidneys.

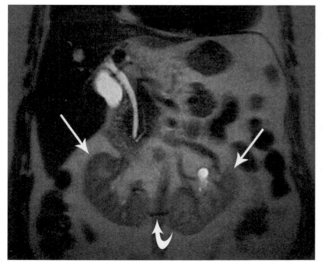

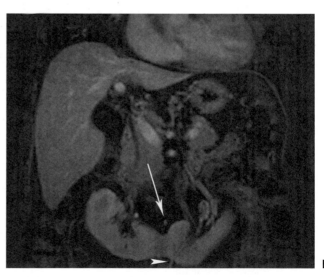

FIGURE 14-9 **Horseshoe kidney** requires low positioning of the imaging volume. **A:** Coronal T2-weighted image of a horseshoe kidney (*arrows*) shows medial tilt of each lower pole to fuse in the midline (*Bridging artery = curved arrow*). **B:** Ureter (*arrowhead*) courses anteriorly, and is nearly excluded from coronal enhanced T1-weighted acquisition. Inferior mesenteric artery (*arrow*) marks the upper border of the fusion.

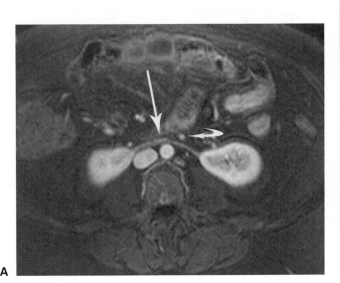
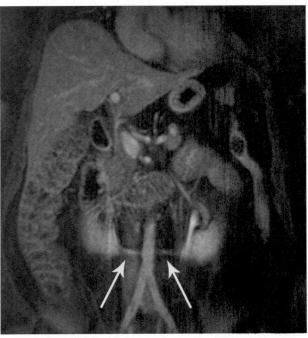

FIGURE 14-10 Fibrous band in this horseshoe kidney is the only tissue connection between right and left moieties. **A:** Axial and **(B)** coronal fat-suppressed, enhanced T1-weighted images depict the horizontal band between the lower poles (*arrows*), just above the aortic bifurcation, and just under the inferior mesenteric artery (IMA) origin (*curved arrow*).

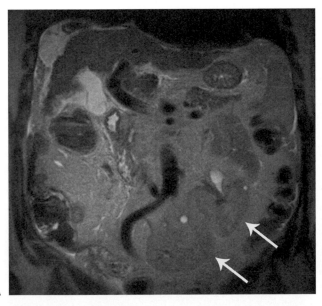
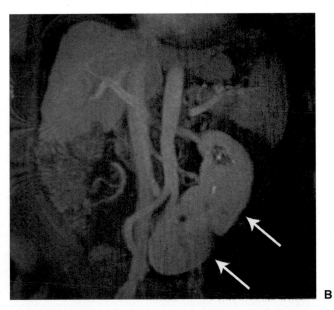

FIGURE 14-11 Crossed-fused ectopia. Both kidneys lie to the left of midline, fused at their poles. Coronal **(A)** T2 and **(B)** T1-weighted enhanced maximum intensity projection (MIP) shows the fused kidneys to the left of midline (*arrows*).

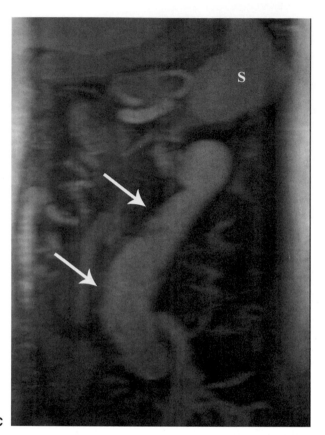

C

FIGURE 14-11 **Crossed-fused ectopia.** (*continued*) **C:** Sagittal MIP reconstruction shows the typical anterior rotation of the fused kidneys (*Spleen = S*).

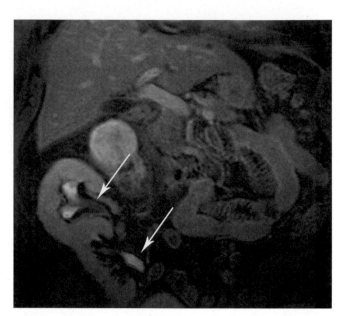

FIGURE 14-12 **Crossed-fused ectopia on the right.** The two separate collecting systems (*arrows*) are depicted on this excretory phase image from a coronal enhanced T1-weighted acquisition.

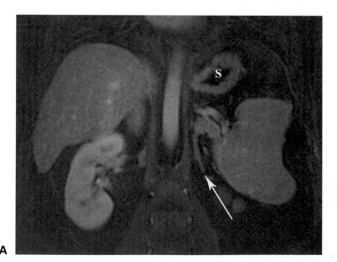

A

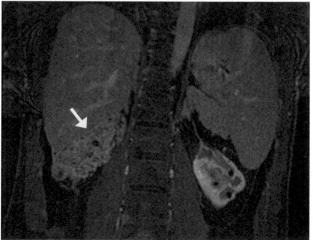

B

FIGURE 14-13 **Unilateral renal agenesis alters regional anatomy. A:** Absence of the left kidney results in pancake adrenal (*arrow*). Notice also alterations in position of stomach (*S*), pancreas and (without a splenorenal ligament) the spleen. **B:** Absence of the right kidney allows the hepatic flexure to become displaced inferior to the liver (*short arrow*). Contralateral kidney is small and scarred.

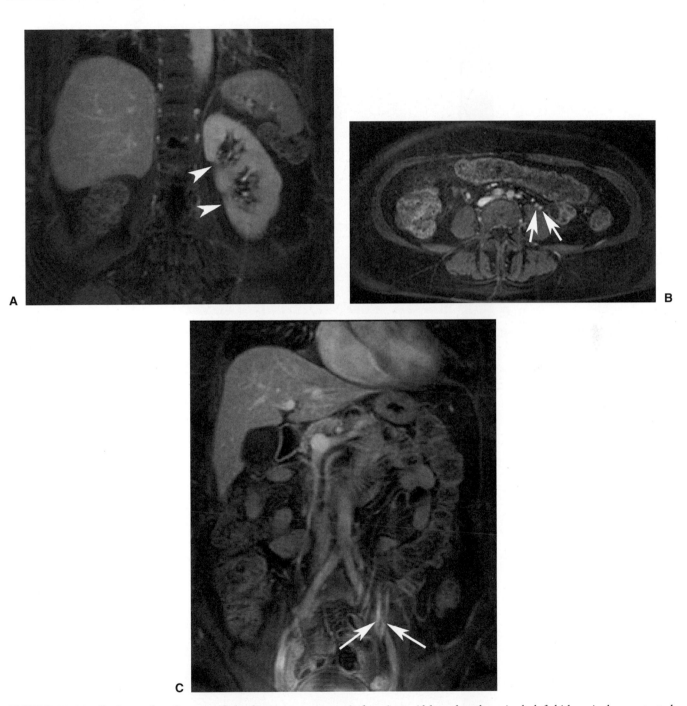

FIGURE 14-14 Left renal and ureteral duplication, a congenital variant. Although only a single left kidney is demonstrated, the renal pelvis is at least partially duplicated, and there are two draining ureters. **A:** Coronal enhanced image shows two left renal hila (*arrowheads*). **B:** Axial and **(C)** large field-of-view coronal enhanced images show duplication of unobstructed ureter (*arrows*) into the pelvis.

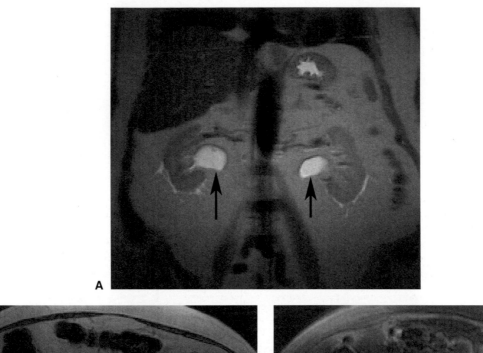

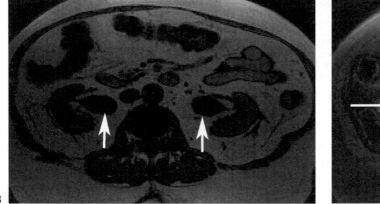

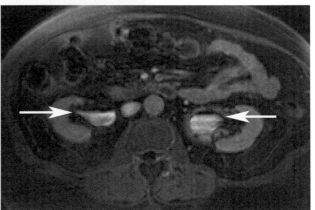

FIGURE 14-15 **Extrarenal pelves, a normal variant, can simulate uteropelvic junction (UPJ) obstruction. A:** Coronal T2-weighted and **(B)** axial T1-weighted images show fullness of both renal pelves (*arrows*), but without any calyceal dilatation. **C:** Notice pelvic fluid–fluid levels (*arrows*) on delayed enhanced T1-weighted image from dependent layering of contrast.

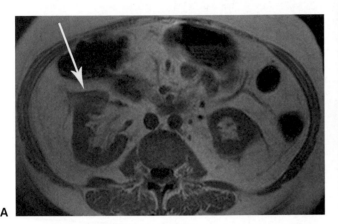

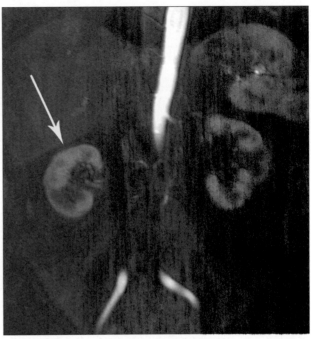

FIGURE 14-16 **Horizontal orientation simulates renal enlargement. A:** On axial imaging, the right kidney (*arrow*) looks larger than the left. **B:** In contrast, coronal source image from MRA suggests that the right kidney (*arrow*) is actually smaller. The explanation is that the renal axis is in the horizontal plane.

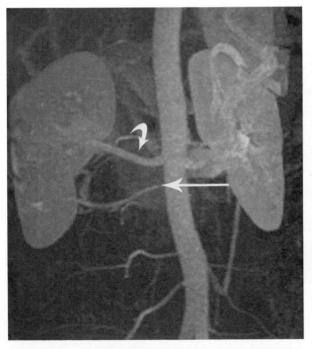

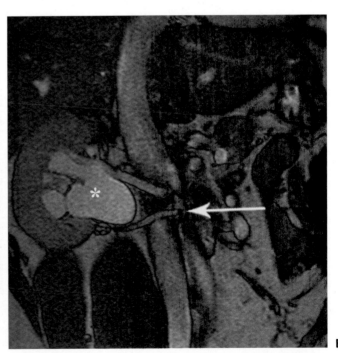

FIGURE 14-17 **Ureteropelvic junction (UPJ) obstruction due to crossing artery. A:** Coronal maximum intensity projection (MIP) image from renal MRA demonstrates two right renal arteries separated by several centimeters (*Upper artery = curved arrow, Lower artery = arrow*). **B:** Steady-state free precession (True FISP) coronal image reveals the hydronephrosis (*asterisk*) caused by the more inferior of the two arteries (*arrow*). FISP, fast imaging with steady state precession.

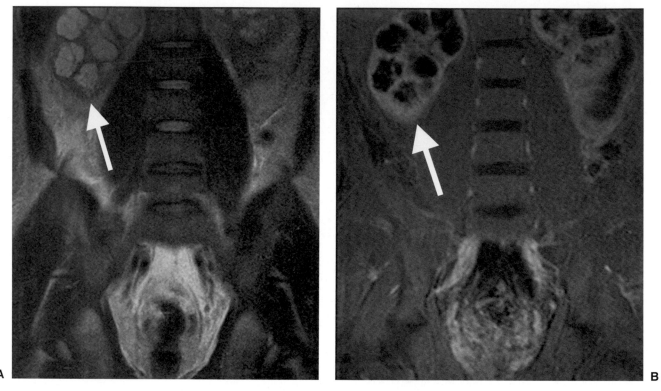

FIGURE 14-18 **Medullary cystic disease simulates hydronephrosis. A:** Coronal T2-weighted and **(B)** enhanced T1-weighted images obtained during a routine pelvic scan reveal abnormal kidneys at the top of the imaging volume (*arrows*). The clues to the diagnosis of medullary cystic disease are the lack of renal pelvis involvement and the complexity of the cysts.

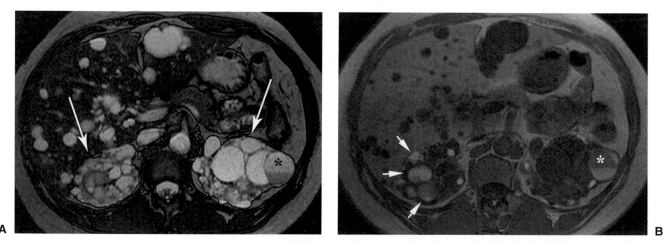

FIGURE 14-19 **The cysts of autosomal dominant polycystic disease** demonstrate a variety of signal intensities, often because of internal hemorrhage. The appearance on enhanced images can thus easily mimic a soft tissue mass. **A:** Axial True FISP image shows the kidneys to be replaced by innumerable cysts of varying signal intensities (*arrows*). **B:** A number of these cysts (*arrows*) are T1-hyperintense, consistent with internal hemorrhage. Differentiation between a hemorrhagic cyst and a true enhancing mass can be made by using subtraction techniques. FISP, fast imaging with steady state precession.

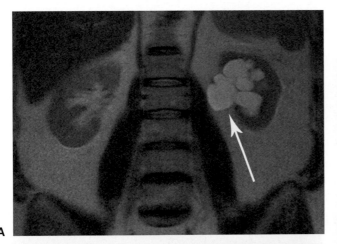

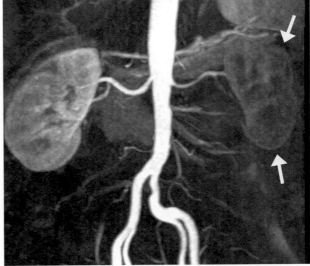

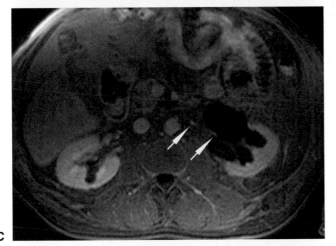

FIGURE 14-20 **Large parapelvic cysts simulate hydro-nephrosis. A:** Coronal T2-weighted image shows lobulated high signal intensity fluid filling the left pelvis and calyces (*arrow*). **B:** Enhancement of the left kidney lags on a coronal renal MRA (*short arrows*). **C:** Axial T1-weighted image obtained 5 minutes following contrast injection shows the normal-sized ureter (*arrows*) emerging from among the symptomatic cysts. Examination requested to locate a possible crossing vessel responsible for the presumed uteropelvic junction (UPJ) obstruction.

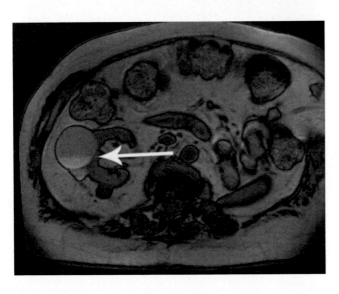

FIGURE 14-21 **Fluid–fluid level in hemorrhagic cyst.** A fluid–fluid level (*arrow*) is present, with the heavier blood products layered dependently on this axial T1-weighted image in a patient with multiple renal cysts.

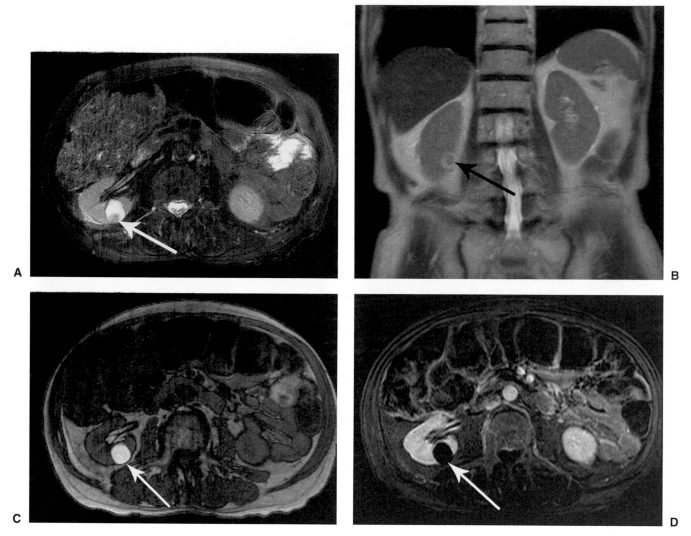

FIGURE 14-22 **Dependent clot simulates mural nodule. A:** Nodule (*arrow*) is identified in posterior aspect of right renal cyst on axial fat-suppressed T2-weighted image. **B:** Similar appearance on coronal T2-weighted image. **C:** Cyst (*arrow*) is very hyperintense on T1-weighted image, consistent with hemorrhage or proteinaceous fluid. Nodule is poorly seen. **D:** Postcontrast subtraction image confirms lack of viable soft tissue in the cyst (*arrow*).

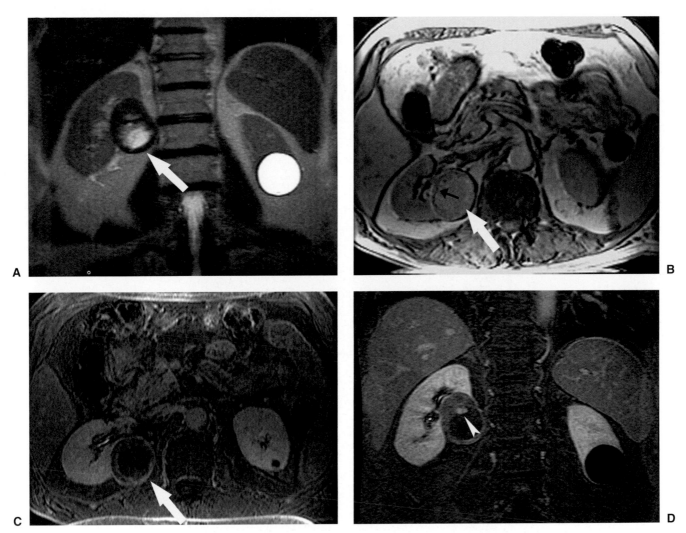

FIGURE 14-23 **Hemorrhagic malignancy simulates chronic hemorrhagic cyst. A:** Well-circumscribed partially cystic lesion in right kidney includes a thick peripheral component of extremely low T2 signal intensity (*arrow*). **B:** Axial T1-weighted image demonstrates high signal throughout the mass (*large arrow*), except for a thick isointense rind anteriorly (*small arrow*). **C:** Axial and **(D)** coronal subtracted enhanced images also show a thick rind of poorly enhancing tissue (*arrow*) and a single brightly enhancing nodule (*arrowhead*). At resection, this was a cystic malignancy with a thick, hemosiderin-laden rind and a single viable tumor nodule (*arrowhead*).

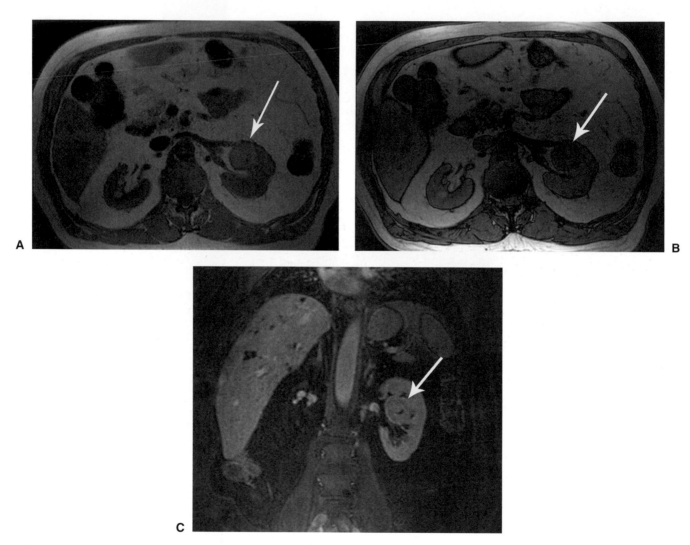

FIGURE 14-24 **Signal loss on opposed phase imaging is *not* sufficient to diagnose benignity.** Round renal mass (*arrows*) is hyperintense to kidney on **(A)** in-phase image, and hypointense on **(B)** opposed-phase imaging, consistent with intralesional lipid or glycogen. **C:** Mass (*arrow*) proves to be solid lesion on coronal enhanced image, and resected specimen was a clear cell renal cell carcinoma (RCC).

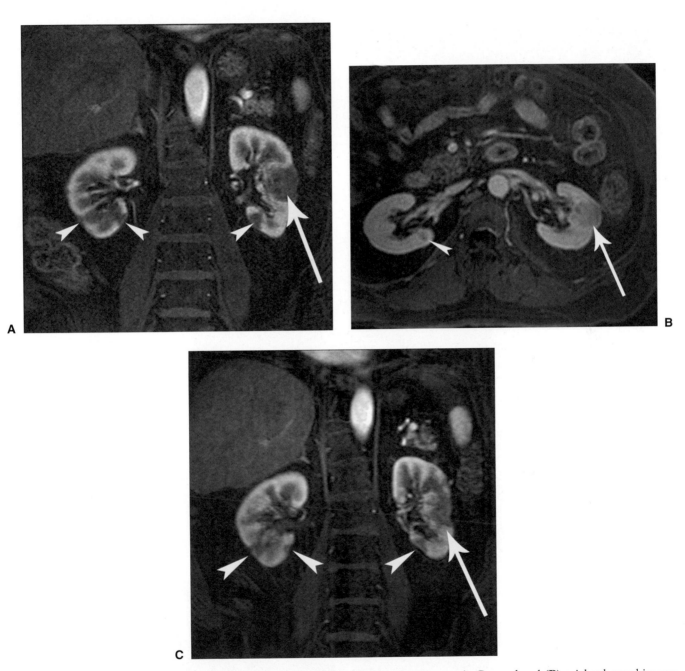

FIGURE 14-25 **Inflammatory pseudotumor mimics multifocal infiltrative tumor. A:** Coronal and **(B)** axial enhanced images show a sizable area of diminished enhancement and slight mass effect in the left kidney (*long arrow*). Additional smaller foci are present bilaterally (*arrowheads*). **C:** Posttreatment scan shows lesion shrinkage, as well as associated capsular retraction.

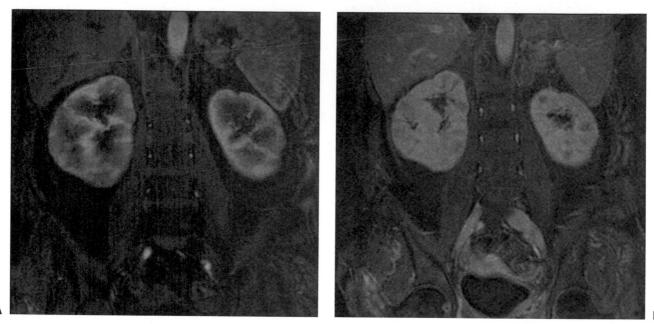

FIGURE 14-26 **Interstitial nephritis mimics pyelonephritis. A** and **B:** Not all patchy or striated nephrograms are caused by bacterial pyelonephritis. Coronal enhanced T1-weighted images captured during two phases of contrast enhancement in this patient with interstitial nephritis.

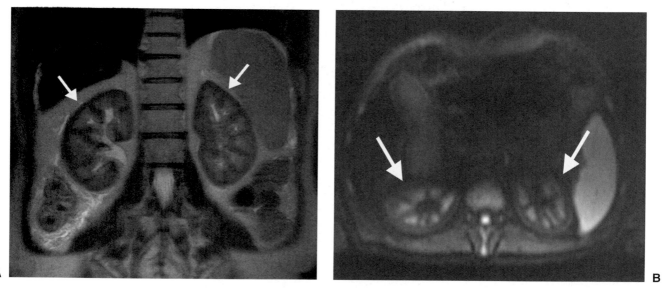

FIGURE 14-27 **Abnormal corticomedullary differentiation** in this patient with nocturnal paroxysmal hemoglobinuria. **A:** Coronal T2-weighted image shows loss of cortical signal in both kidneys (*arrows*). **B:** Contrast (*arrows*) is even more striking on iron-sensitive axial echoplanar diffusion-weighted image (b = 500).

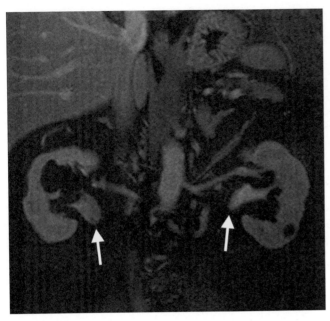

FIGURE 14-28 **Excreted renal pelvis contrast mimics enhancing masses** in collecting system. A 2-mL timing bolus injection given earlier is responsible for this appearance (*arrows*) on nephrographic phase T2-weighted image.

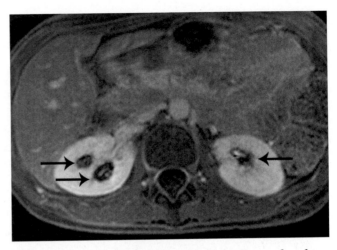

FIGURE 14-29 **Hypointense, "blooming" renal calyces** (*arrows*) **on enhanced image.** At high enough concentrations of gadolinium, for example in concentrated urine, T2* effects become strong enough to overwhelm T1-shortening effects. The result is profound hypointensity.

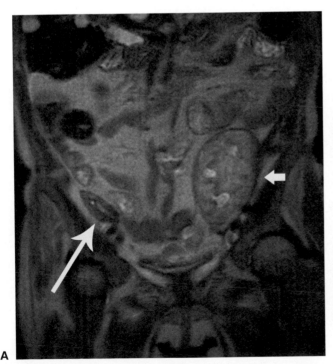

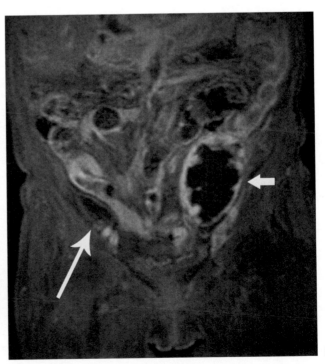

A

B

FIGURE 14-30 **Failed renal transplant simulates pelvic mass. A:** Coronal single-shot T2-weighted image shows a small, fusiform soft tissue mass (*long arrow*) in the anterior right lower quadrant. More recent transplant in the left lower quadrant (*short arrow*) shows no clear corticomedullary organization. **B:** Coronal enhanced image reveals very faint cortical enhancement in the nonfunctioning right lower quadrant (RLQ) graft (*long arrow*) and central infarction in the newer graft (*short arrow*).

▣ Ureters

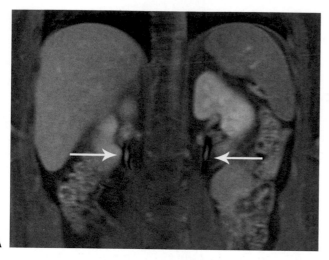
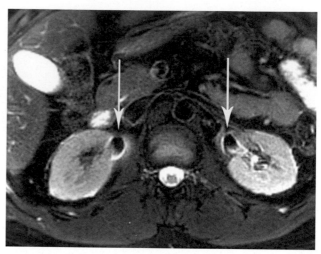

FIGURE 14-31 **Signal loss in ureteral walls due to concentrated gadolinium. A:** Linear hypointensities follow the walls of both proximal ureters on coronal enhanced T1-weighted image (*arrows*). **B:** Even on a spin echo image, signal loss can be appreciated in renal pelvis.

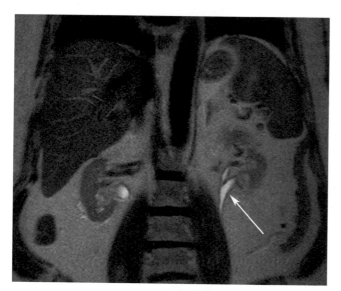

FIGURE 14-32 **Bifid renal pelvis, a normal variant.** The left renal pelvis (*arrow*) fuses itself into a single chamber just above the ureteropelvic junction (UPJ) on this coronal single shot T2-weighted image.

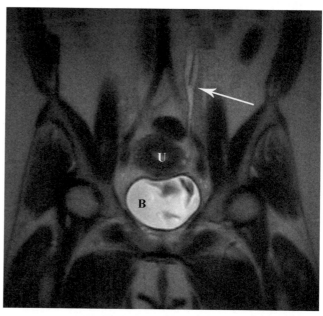

FIGURE 14-33 **Partial duplication of ureter, a common variant.** Coronal T2-weighted image demonstrates fusion of the bifid ureter (*arrow*) just as it enters the pelvis (*Fluid-filled bladder = B, Uterus = U*).

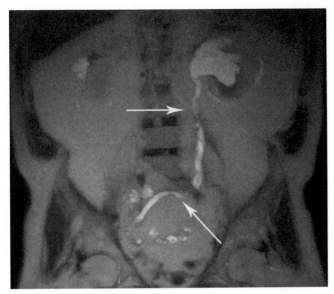

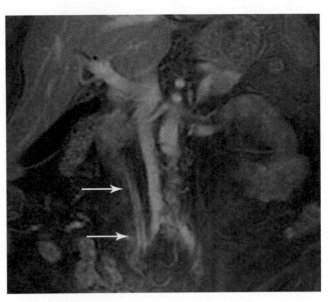

FIGURE 14-34 **Ureter crosses the midline** *en route* **to the right lower quadrant (RLQ) ileal conduit.** Thin maximum intensity projection (MIP) reconstruction of a T2-weighted coronal sequence shows hydroureteronephrosis (*arrows*) caused by a stricture at the anastomosis (*arrows*) with the RLQ ileal conduit (not depicted).

FIGURE 14-35 **Diffuse, intense enhancement of ureter wall in presence of ureteral stent,** a potential mimic of malignancy or infection. Notice parallel enhancing lines along the course of the ureter on coronal enhanced T1-weighted image (*arrows*). Stent itself is poorly discernible on MRI.

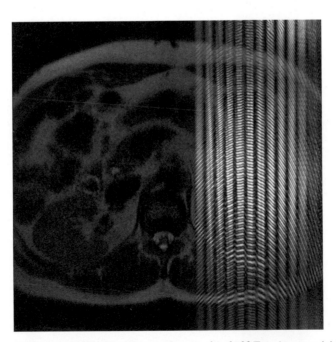

FIGURE 14-36 **Radiofrequency (RF) interference.** The artifact in this half-Fourier acquisition single-shot turbo spin-echo (HASTE) sequence is caused by RF cross talk from an adjacent scanner. The artifact bands are parallel to the phase-encoding direction, and each band occurs at a different frequency (in the left to right frequency-encoding direction) which corresponds to the transmitted RF excitation frequency during slice-selection in the adjacent scanner.

■ Adrenals

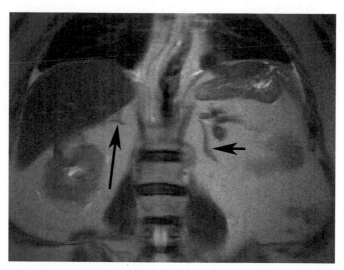

FIGURE 14-37   In absence of left kidney, the left adrenal is flattened. Coronal T2-weighted image depicts both adrenals. The right adrenal (*long arrow*) has been molded by the presence of the subjacent kidney. The left adrenal is long and slab-like (*short arrow*).

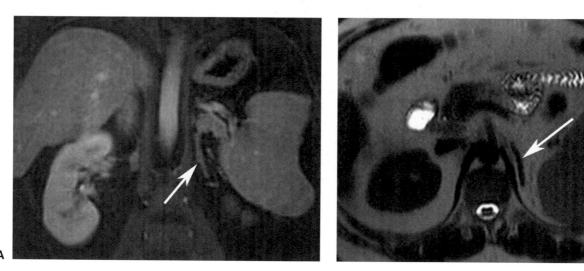

FIGURE 14-38   Pancake adrenal in left renal agenesis. A: Coronal enhanced T1-weighted and **(B)** axial T2-weighted images. Without a companion kidney to mold it into the usual Y- or T-configuration, this adrenal (*arrows*) developed into a flat slab of tissue. Males can also lack the ipsilateral seminal vesicles.

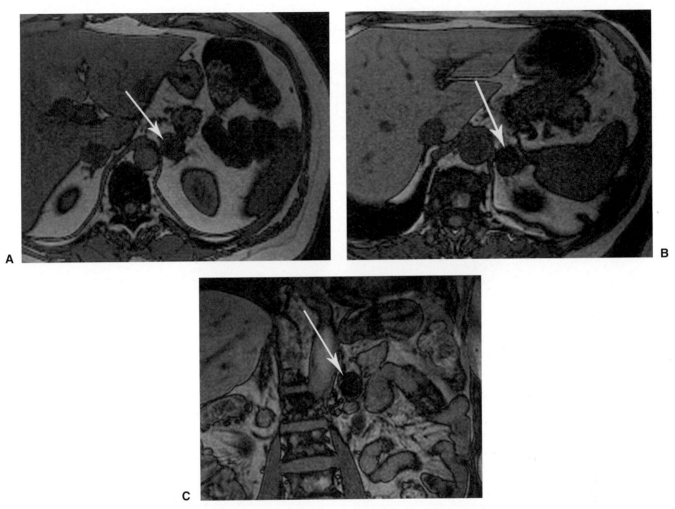

FIGURE 14-39 **Uniform signal drop on opposed-phase image is not a requirement for adenoma diagnosis. A–C:** T1-weighted opposed-phase gradient echo images in three different patients display benign adenomas (*arrows*). Intracellular lipid can be homogeneously or heterogeneously distributed.

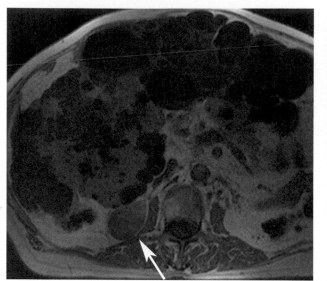
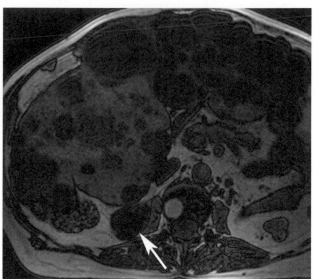

FIGURE 14-40 In- and opposed-phase sequences are much less useful in isolation than when acquired together. Taken together, these matching **(A)** in-phase and **(B)** opposed-phase images through the right adrenal together confirm a large adenoma (*arrows*). However, in-phase imaging alone is nonspecific. Further, on opposed-phase imaging, the differential diagnosis would include a cyst (especially in the presence of polycystic liver disease, as here), iron-containing nodule or old hematoma.

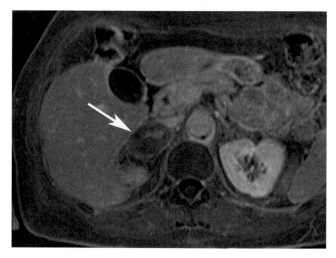
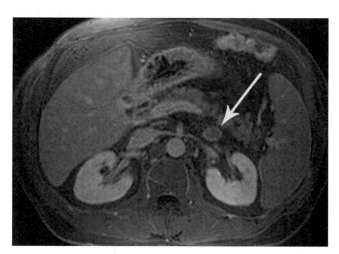

FIGURE 14-41 As with CT, contrast washout is a MR feature of adenoma. Axial enhanced image shows a moderately large, solid adrenal adenoma (*arrow*) that has become quite hypointense after a 15-minute delay.

FIGURE 14-42 Washout criteria should be used with caution in the setting of hypervascular tumors like hepatocellular carcinoma. Adrenal metastases from these sorts of primaries can also show washout after a 15-minute delay, as had this hepatocellular carcinoma (HCC) metastasis (*arrow*).

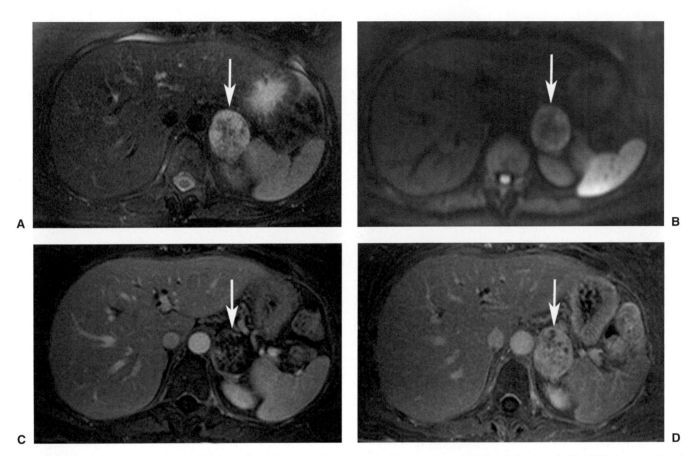

FIGURE 14-43 Large, atypical adenoma simulates malignancy. A: Fat-suppressed T2-weighted and **(B)** diffusion-weighted images delineate a well-circumscribed, heterogeneously hyperintense adrenal mass (*arrows*). **C:** Portal and **(D)** delayed phase T1-weighted images show very gradual enhancement of the lesion (*arrows*). Neither T2-hyperintensity nor delayed enhancement is characteristic of adenoma, although the lesion was a surgically proven partially necrotic adenoma.

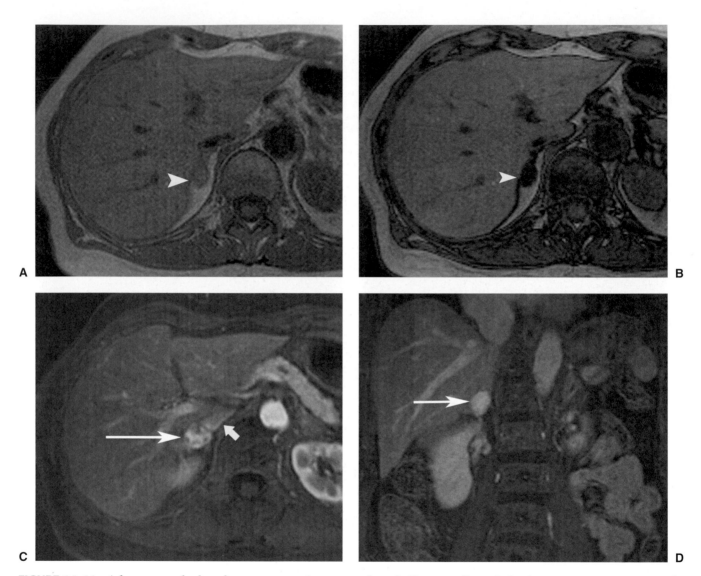

FIGURE 14-44 Adenoma and pheochromocytoma in same adrenal. Since small cortical adenomas are so common, the coexistence of two lesions is not rare. Tiny adenoma (*arrowhead*) in the lateral right adrenal limb on **(A)** in-phase image appropriately loses signal on **(B)** opposed-phase axial image. **C:** Axial and **(D)** coronal T1-weighted enhanced images reveal intensely enhancing anterior adrenal lesion (*arrow*), a proven pheochromocytoma (*IVC = short arrow*). IVC, inferior vena cava.

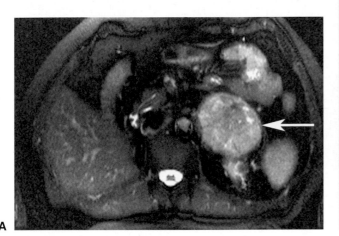

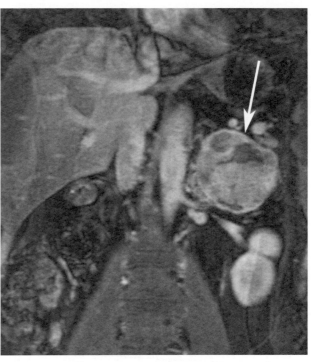

FIGURE 14-45 **Solitary metastasis to left adrenal from remote contralateral renal cell carcinoma. A:** Lacking a central area of necrosis, this heterogeneously T2-hyperintense metastasis (*arrow*) could be mistaken for a primary adrenal tumor, such as pheochromocytoma. **B:** Coronal T1-weighted enhanced image shows a heterogeneously hypervascular tumor.

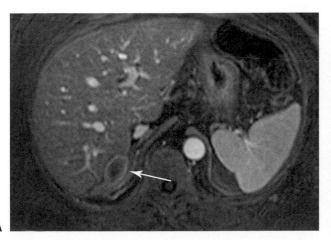

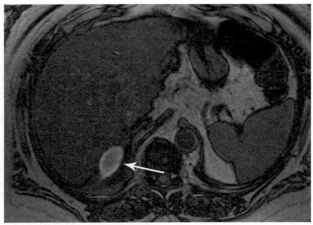

FIGURE 14-46 **Adrenal hematoma simulates ring-enhancing lesion. A:** Axial fat-suppressed enhanced T1-weighted image demonstrates oval, apparently enhancing lesion (*arrow*) posteromedial to the liver. **B:** Unenhanced T1-weighted image reveals an underlying lesion hyperintensity that increases peripherally, consistent with hematoma (*arrow*).

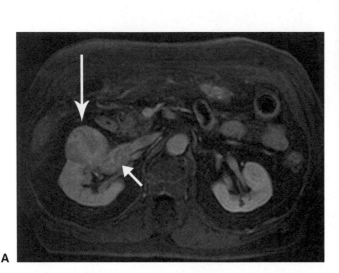

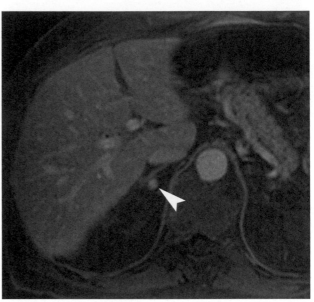

FIGURE 14-47 **Tiny adrenal hemangioma simulates metastasis from renal cell carcinoma.** **A:** Solid, vascular mass (*long arrow*) in the right kidney (renal cell carcinoma) with venous extension (*short arrow*). **B:** Punctate, hyperenhancing nodule in the medial limb right adrenal (*arrowhead*) later proved at radical nephrectomy to be an adrenal hemangioma.

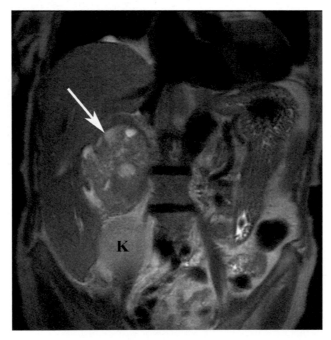

FIGURE 14-48 **Para-adrenal lesion simulates adrenal lesion** through mass-effect on the normal gland. Large, heterogeneously T2-hyperintense mass (*arrow*) in the right suprarenal space effaced the normal right adrenal gland. Retroperitoneal adenopathy was the tissue diagnosis (*Right kidney = K*).

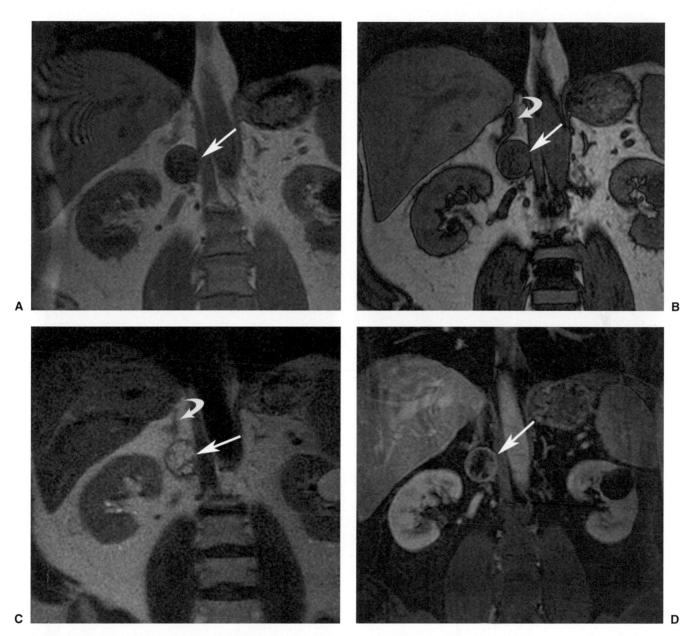

FIGURE 14-49 **Coronal imaging can differentiate between periadrenal and adrenal lesions. A:** In- and **(B)** opposed-phase images nicely differentiate a round, non–lipid-containing right retroperitoneal mass (*arrow*) from the right adrenal (*curved arrow*) above. **C:** High T2 signal and **(D)** peripheral enhancement pattern would be atypical for adenoma. Lesion proved to be an extraadrenal schwannoma.

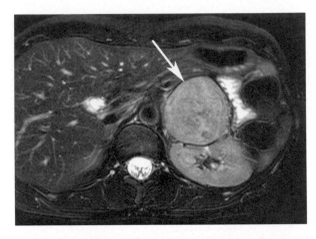

FIGURE 14-50 Left adrenal pheochromocytoma mistaken for pancreatic tail mass. Because of its position anterior to the kidney, adrenal pathology (*arrow*) can be difficult to distinguish from pancreas or stomach. Sagittal imaging is often very helpful.

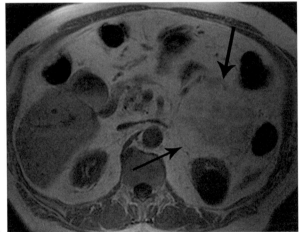

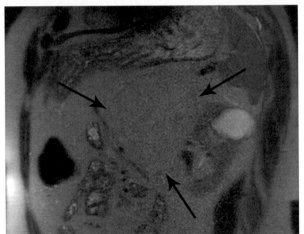

A

B

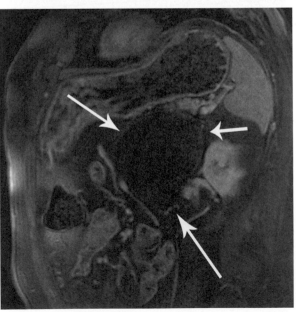

FIGURE 14-51 Large left adrenal myelolipoma mimics well-differentiated retroperitoneal liposarcoma. Multiplanar imaging can be very helpful for localizing the adrenal and relationship to a perirenal mass. **A:** Axial T2-weighted image shows a large myelolipoma (*arrows*) which is anterior to the left kidney and nearly isointense to mesenteric fat. Sagittal **(B)** T2 and **(C)** fat-suppressed enhanced images through the mass show a thin capsule and confirm that it is largely adipose tissue.

C

Suggested Readings

Kidneys

Bamac B, Colak T. Bilateral accessory renal arteries with retroaortic left renal vein: Report of an elderly cadaver case. *Clin Anat*. 2006;19: 714–715.

Gunenc C, Denk CC. Combined unusual anatomical variations of the superior mesenteric and right renal arteries. *Clin Anat*. 2006;19:716–717.

Herborn CU, Watkins DM, Runge VM, et al. Renal arteries: Comparison of steady-state free precession MR angiography and contrast-enhanced MR angiography. *Radiology*. 2006;239:263–268.

Knutson T, Hawas B. Horseshoe kidney with a circumcaval ureter. *Scand J Urol Nephrol*. 2004;38(4):348–350.

Loukas M, Aparicio S, Beck A, et al. Rare case of right accessory renal artery originating as a common trunk with the inferior mesenteric artery: A case report. *Clin Anat*. 2005;18:530–535.

Macchi V, Parenti A, DeCaro R. Pivotal role of the sub-supracardinal anastomosis in the development and course of the left renal vein. *Clin Anat*. 2004;16:358–361.

Michaely HJ, Kramer H, Attenberger U, et al. Renal magnetic resonance angiography at 3 T: Technical feasibility and clinical perspectives. *Top Magn Reson Imaging*. 2007;18(2):117–125.

Nikken JJ, Krestin GP. MRI of the kidney-state of the art. *Eur Radiol*. 2007;17(11):2780–2793.

Pilcher JM, Padhani AR. Problem in diagnostic imaging: Behind the left renal vein. *Clin Anat*. 1997;10:349–352.

Rossi UG, Romano M, Ferro C. Seven renal arteries. *Clin Anat*. 2006; 19:632–633.

Satyapal KS, Haffejee AA, Naidoo ML, et al. Rare additional renal artery in live-related transplantation. *Clin Anat*. 2006;19:363–364.

Shakeri AB, Tubbs RS, Shoja MM, et al. Bipolar supernumerary renal artery. *Surg Radiol Anat*. 2007;29:89–92.

Shaw MBK, Cutress M, Papavassilious V, et al. Duplicated inferior vena cava and crossed renal actopia with abdominal aortic aneurysm: Preoperative anatomic studies facilitate surgery. *Clin Anat*. 2004;16:355–357.

Singh G, Ng YK, Bay BH. Bilateral accessory renal arteries associated with some anomalies of the ovarian arteries: A case study. *Clin Anat*. 1998;11:417–420.

Wolfram-Gabel R, Kahn J-L, Rapp E. Is the renal space closed? *Clin Anat*. 2000;13:168–176.

Adrenals

Glazer GM, Woolsey EJ, Borrello J, et al. Adrenal tissue characterization using MRI. *Radiology*. 1986;158:73.

Israel GM, Korobkin M, Wang C, et al. Comparison of unenhanced CT and chemical shift MRI in evaluating lipid-rich adrenal adenomas. *Am J Roentgenol*. 2004;183:215–219.

Namimoto T, Yamashita Y, Mitsuzaki K, et al. Adrenal masses: Quantification of fat content with double-echo chemical shift in-phase and opposed-phase FLASH MR images for differentiation of adrenal adenomas. *Radiology*. 2001;218:642.

Savci G, Yazici Z, Sahin N, et al. Value of chemical shift subtraction MRI in characterization of adrenal masses. *Am J Roentgenol*. 2006; 186:130–135.

Chapter 15

Spleen

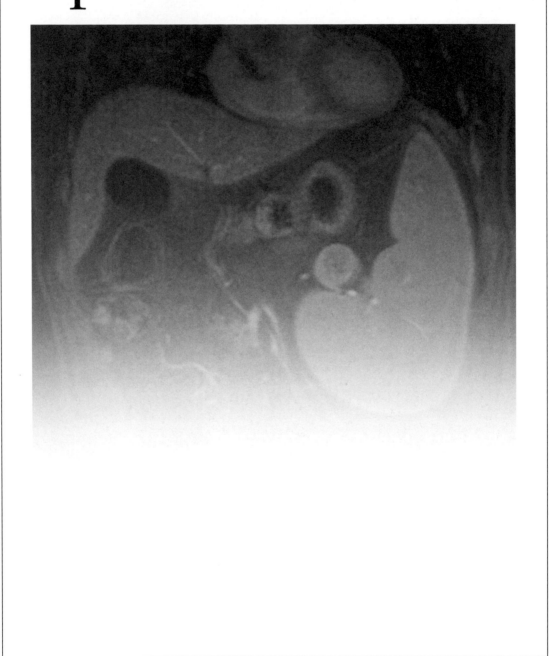

Mellena D. Bridges

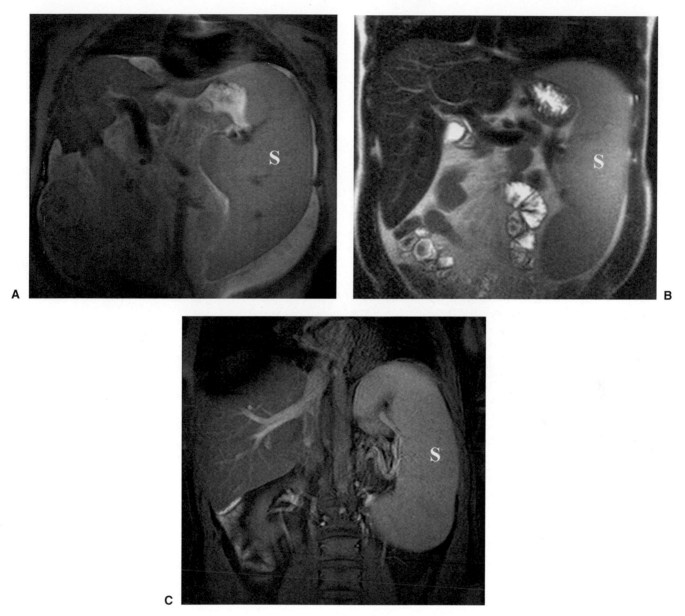

FIGURE 15-1 Enlargement of the spleen is nonspecific, with causes ranging from portal hypertension to malignancy to infiltrative disease. **A:** Coronal T2-weighted image in a patient with cirrhosis and portal hypertension (*Spleen* = S). **B:** Gaucher's disease of the spleen (S). **C:** Lymphoma of the spleen (S) in a balanced steady-state free precession image.

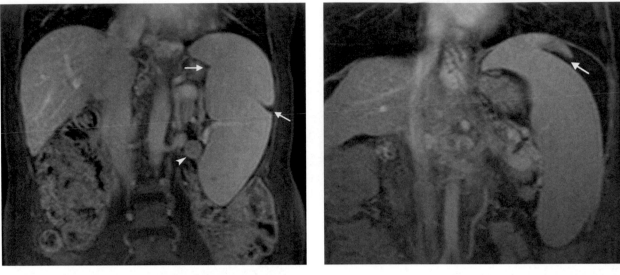

FIGURE 15-2 **Splenic cleft, common normal variant. A** and **B:** Coronal fat-suppressed, enhanced T1-weighted images in two different patients show deep peripheral splenic clefts (*arrows*) (*Splenule = arrowhead*).

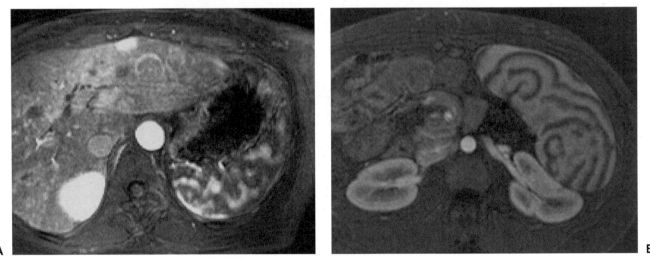

FIGURE 15-3 **Early enhancement pattern after contrast administration is quite variable.** By the portal phase, however, most spleens will appear homogeneous again. **A** and **B:** Arterial dominant phase through the spleen in four different patients (*Spleen = arrow*).

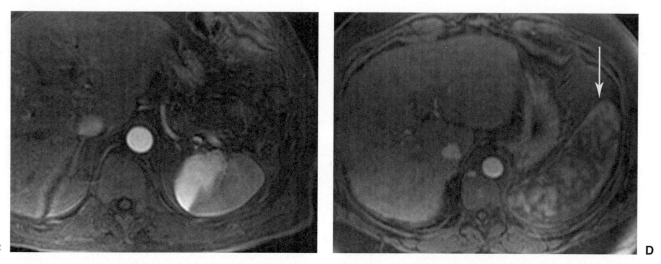

C   D

FIGURE 15-3   Early enhancement pattern after contrast administration is quite variable. (*continued*) By the portal phase, however, most spleens will appear homogeneous again. **C** and **D:** Arterial dominant phase through the spleen in several different patients (*Spleen = arrow*).

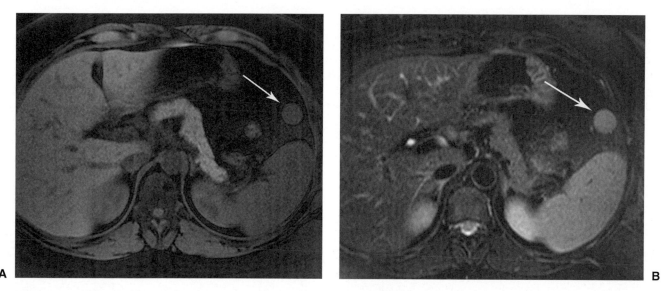

A   B

FIGURE 15-4   Splenule (accessory spleen), normal variant. Recognition depends on the isointensity of the splenule to the spleen on all imaging sequences. Fat-suppressed **(A)** T1- and **(B)** T2-weighted images show a round nodule that is isointense to spleen (*arrows*).

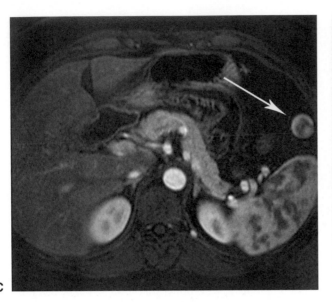

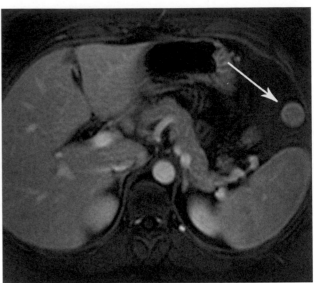

C

D

FIGURE 15-4 **Splenule (accessory spleen), normal variant.** (*continued*) Splenule (*arrows*) matches enhancement pattern of spleen on (**C**) arterial and (**D**) portal phase enhanced T1-weighted images.

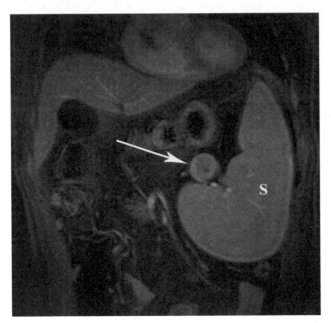

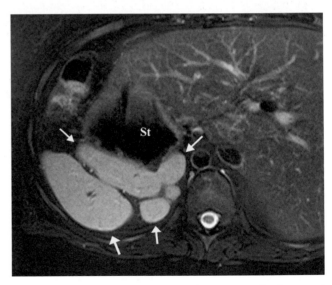

FIGURE 15-5 **Splenules enlarge along with the spleen.** Coronal fat-suppressed enhanced T1-weighted image depicts splenic enlargement and a hypertrophied companion splenule (*arrow*) (*Spleen = S*).

FIGURE 15-6 **Polysplenia.** Polysplenia or multiple splenic nodules (*arrows*), is commonly associated with situs abnormalities (as here) and with other congenital anomalies (*Spleen = arrows, Stomach = St*).

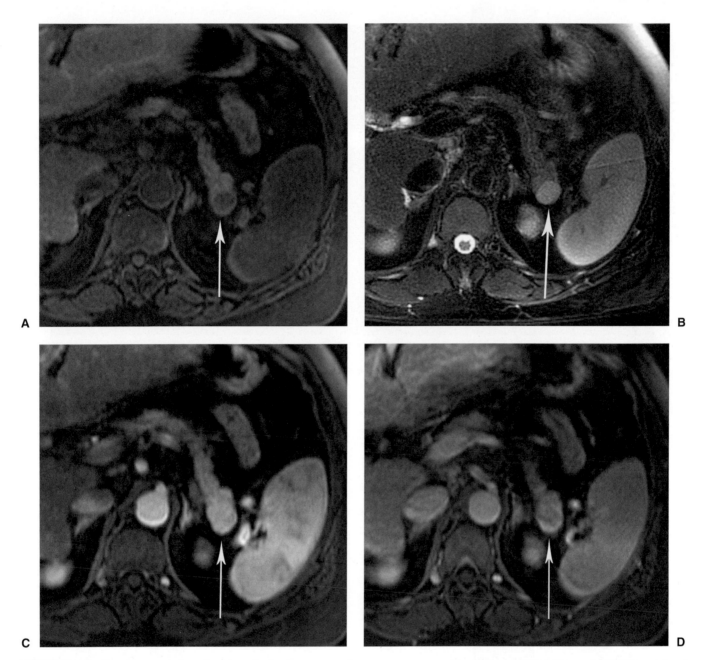

FIGURE 15-7   Intrapancreatic splenule mimics hypervascular pancreas mass. Fat-suppressed **(A)** T1- and **(B)** T2-weighted images show round lesion (*arrow*) in pancreatic tail with signal intensity identical to spleen. **C:** Late arterial and **(D)** delayed phase images show an enhancement pattern of the splenule (*arrows*) that closely parallels the spleen.

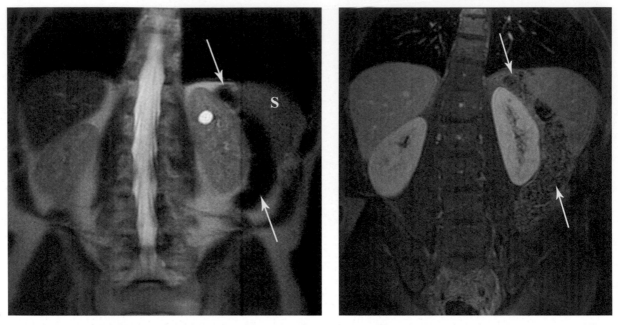

FIGURE 15-8 Excessively mobile spleen. With looseness or defects in the splenic mesentery, colon can migrate up to the diaphragm between kidney and spleen, or even behind the spleen. **A** and **B:** Air-filled hepatic flexure (*arrows*) is sandwiched between spleen (*S*) and kidney on coronal and contrast-enhanced T1-weighted imaging. Extreme versions are termed *wandering spleen*.

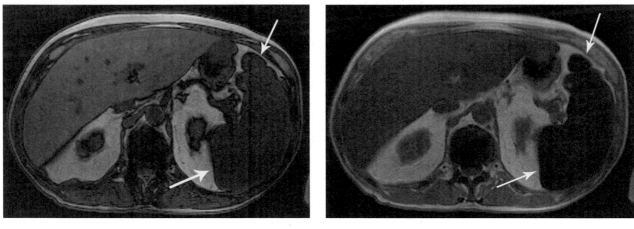

FIGURE 15-9 Parenchymal iron deposition poorly demonstrated at very low echo time (TE). The gradient echo T1-weighted techniques currently applied to the abdomen can suppress susceptibility artifact because of their very short echo times. **A:** Opposed-phase image obtained at a relatively low TE of 2.3 milliseconds shows splenic enlargement and only mildly reduced signal intensity (*arrow*). **B:** In-phase image with TE 4.8 demonstrates dramatic splenic signal loss (*arrows*) in a patient with hemosiderosis.

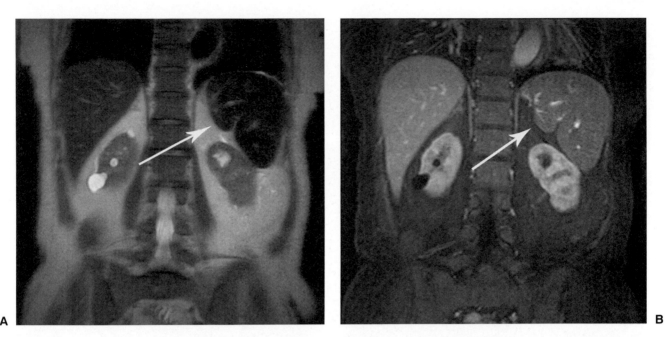

FIGURE 15-10 Further iron deposition reduces signal on spin echo and enhanced sequences as well. The spleen (*arrows*) is markedly hypointense on **(A)** single-shot TSE T2 image and slightly hypointense on **(B)** enhanced T1-weighted fat-suppressed image.

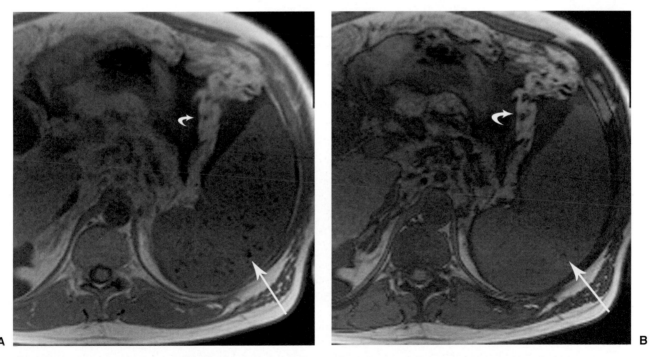

FIGURE 15-11 Gamna-Gandy bodies pockmark spleen on in-phase image. A: Small foci of hemorrhage (*arrow*) due to splenic congestion show profound signal loss on in-phase T1-weighted image because of susceptibility artifact. **B:** Finding (*arrow*) is less conspicuous on opposed phase image obtained at lower echo time (TE) setting (*Gastrosplenic ligament = curved arrow*).

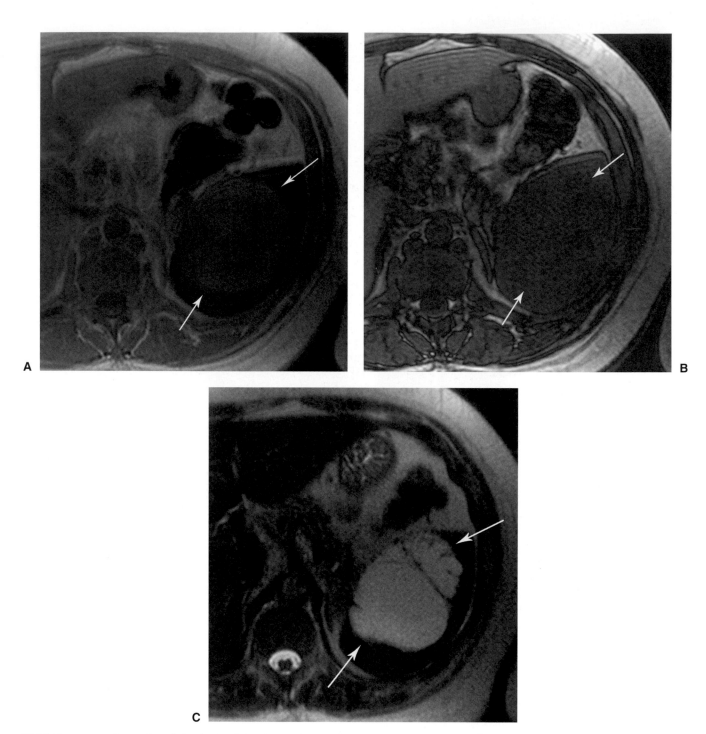

FIGURE 15-12 **Example of the lack of fixed signal intensities in MRI: large lymphangioma in a siderotic spleen. A:** On in-phase image gradient echo T1-weighted image, exaggeration of intensity differences between the cyst (*arrows*) and the background spleen is due to the lipid component of the cyst contents and parenchymal signal suppression (because of susceptibility artifact). **B:** The spleen is isointense to the cyst on opposed-phase T1-weighted image, as the spleen increases in signal (less T2* effect) and the cyst signal decreases. **C:** T2-weighted image shows the multilocularity of the lymphangioma (*arrows*).

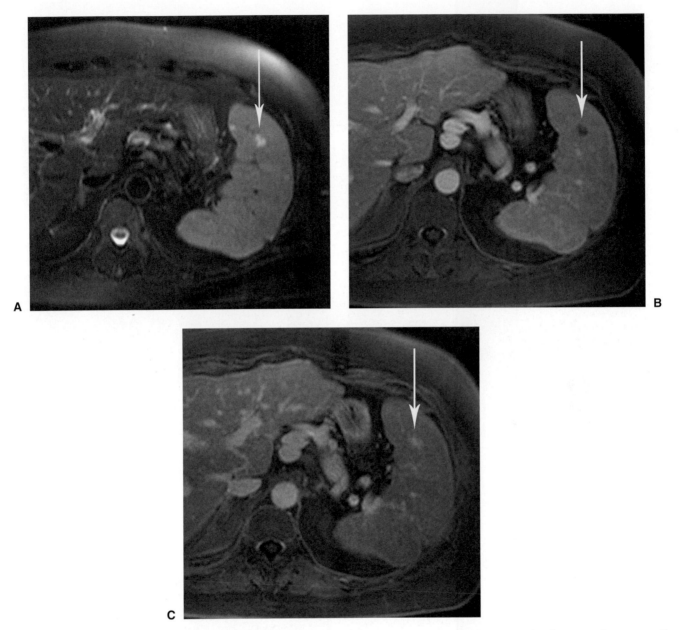

FIGURE 15-13 Hemangioma, a common benign splenic lesion. A: Fat-suppressed T2-weighted image shows a well-circumscribed, hyperintense lesion (*arrow*). **B:** Arterial and **(C)** delayed phase T1-weighted images demonstrate gradual complete fill-in of the hemangioma (*arrow*), when signal intensity becomes equivalent to blood vessels.

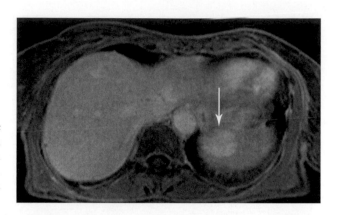

FIGURE 15-14 **True delayed imaging can be diagnostic of splenic hemangioma.** T1-weighted image obtained in same patient 15 minutes following contrast administration now shows uniform, well-defined hyperenhancement (*arrow*), contributing to confident diagnosis of splenic hemangioma in an otherwise nonspecific lesion.

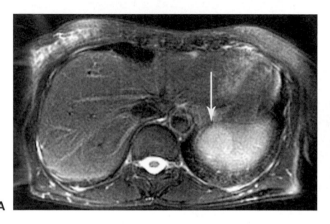

A

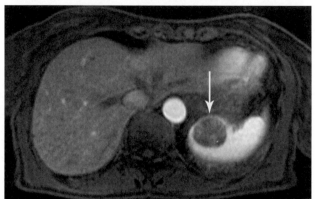

B

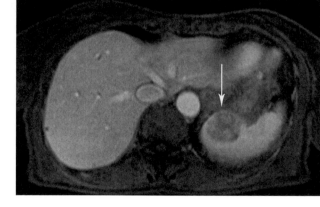

C

FIGURE 15-15 **Discontinuous nodular or puddling enhancement pattern rarely seen in hemangiomas of the spleen.** This is in contrast to the liver. **A:** Large, round lesion (*arrow*) is hyperintense on axial T2-weighted image. **B:** Arterial and (**C**) portal phase T1-weighted images show gradual, ill-defined internal enhancement of the hemangioma (*arrows*).

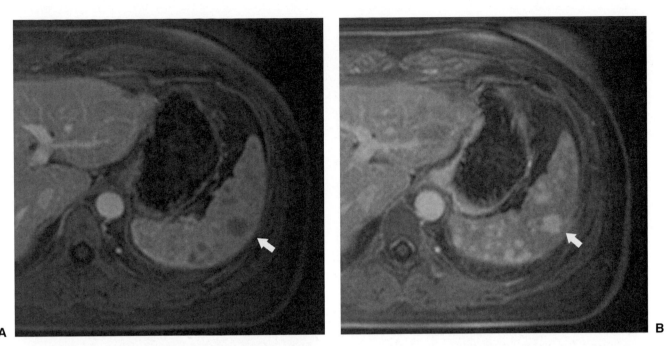

FIGURE 15-16 **Hemangiomatosis simulates splenic metastases** in patient with melanoma. **A:** Multiple indeterminate lesions (*arrow*) are demonstrated on enhanced fat-suppressed T1-weighted image. **(B)** Typical uniform, well-defined hyperenhancement (*arrow*) is seen after a delay, confirming multiple hemangiomas.

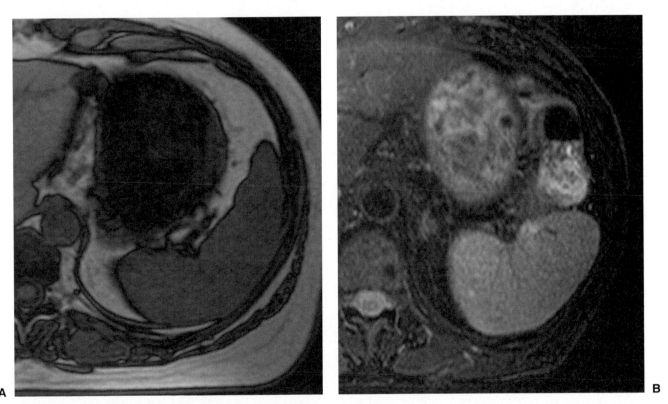

FIGURE 15-17 **Conspicuity of hemangiomas compromised by lack of contrast with spleen parenchyma. A** and **B:** Multiple small hemangiomas in two different patients are fairly subtle on T1-weighted and T2-weighted images, respectively.

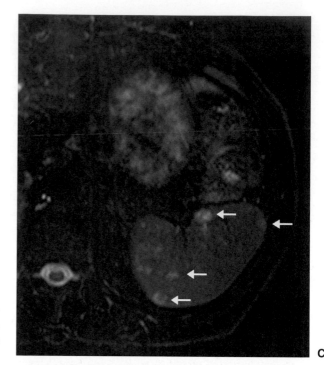

FIGURE 15-17 Conspicuity of hemangiomas compromised by lack of contrast with spleen parenchyma. (*continued*) **C:** Conspicuity of the lesions (*arrows*) can be improved by heavier T2-weighting.

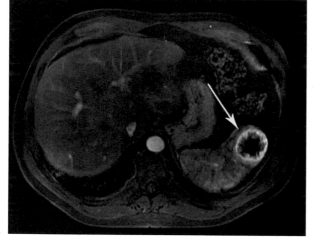

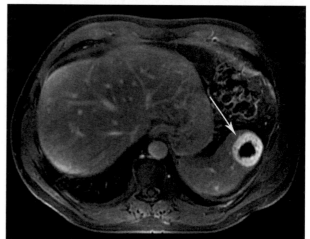

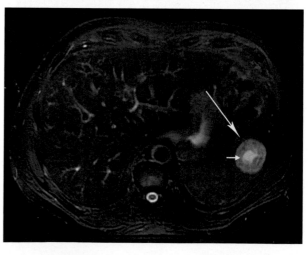

FIGURE 15-18 Hemangioma mimics ring-enhancing splenic metastasis. **A:** Ring-enhancing lesion (*arrow*) is demonstrated on arterial dominant, fat-suppressed axial image. **B:** The lesion is better defined following a delay. There is a hyperintense periphery, but the center has not filled in with contrast. **C:** The surgically proven centrally hyalinized hemangioma is centrally hypointense (*short arrow*) on correlative T2-weighted image.

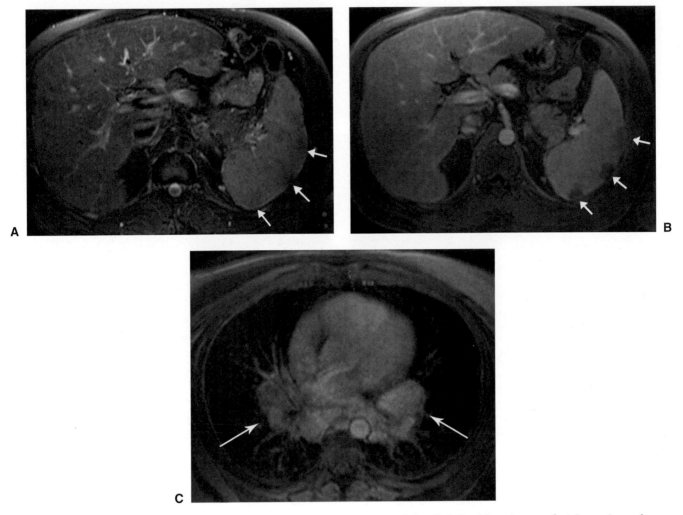

FIGURE 15-19 **Sarcoid granulomas simulate splenic malignancy. A:** Subtle, ill-defined hypointense foci (*arrows*) are demonstrated along lateral margin of spleen. **B:** Following contrast administration, T1-weighted image shows the poorly enhancing lesions (*arrows*) to better advantage. **C:** Massive enhancing hilar adenopathy (*arrows*) is consistent with sarcoidosis.

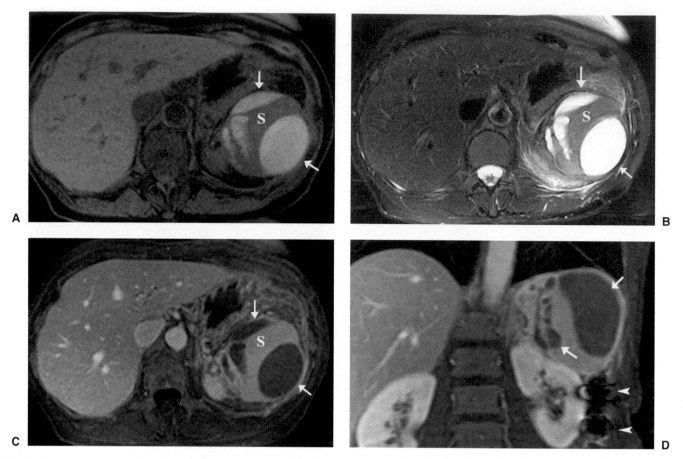

FIGURE 15-20 **Pancreatic-splenic fistula with pseudocysts mistaken for subcapsular splenic hematomas.** Axial **(A)** T1- and **(B)** T2-weighted images depict several hyperintense collections (*arrows*) in the spleen (*S*). T1-hyperintensity indicates proteinaceous or hemorrhagic fluid. No enhancement on **(C)** axial or **(D)** coronal postcontrast T1-weighted image (*Air artifact from bowel = arrowheads, Spleen = S*).

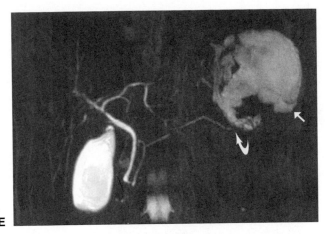

E

FIGURE 15-20 **Pancreatic-splenic fistula with pseudocysts mistaken for subcapsular splenic hematomas.** (*continued*) **E:** Maximum intensity projection (MIP) reconstruction of a 3-D TSE T2 acquisition shows disrupted duct in pancreatic tail (*curved arrow*) with fluid rising to the spleen.

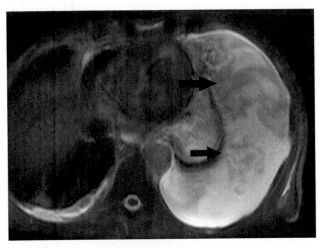

FIGURE 15-21 **Motion artifact in ascites simulates spleen.** Motion in ascites (*arrows*) creates complex patterns of signal loss on T2-weighted single-shot image that simulates the spleen on this single image.

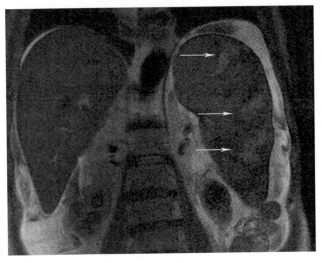

A

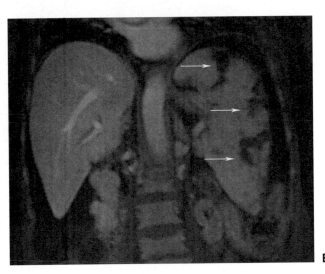

B

FIGURE 15-22 **Splenic infarcts mimic mass lesions. A:** Coronal T2-weighted image demonstrates splenomegaly with three indistinct wedge-shaped hyperintense regions peripherally (*arrows*). **B:** These areas (*arrows*) fail to enhance following contrast administration, consistent with necrosis.

Suggested Readings

Betal D, Hughes ML, Whitehouse GH, et al. Postprandial decrease in splenic volume demonstrated by magnetic resonance imaging and stereology. *Clin Anat.* 2000;13:404–409.

Kim SH, Lee JM, Lee JY, et al. Contrast-enhanced sonography of intrapancreatic accessory spleen in six patients. *AJR Am J Roentgenol.* 2007;188:422–428.

Pandey SK, Bhattacharya S, Mishra RN, et al. Anatomical variations of the splenic artery and its clinical implications. *Clin Anat.* 2004;17:497–502.

Sahni AD, Jit BI, Gupta CNM, et al. Branches of the splenic artery and splenic arterial segments. *Clin Anat.* 2003;16:371–377.

Chapter 16

Vasculature

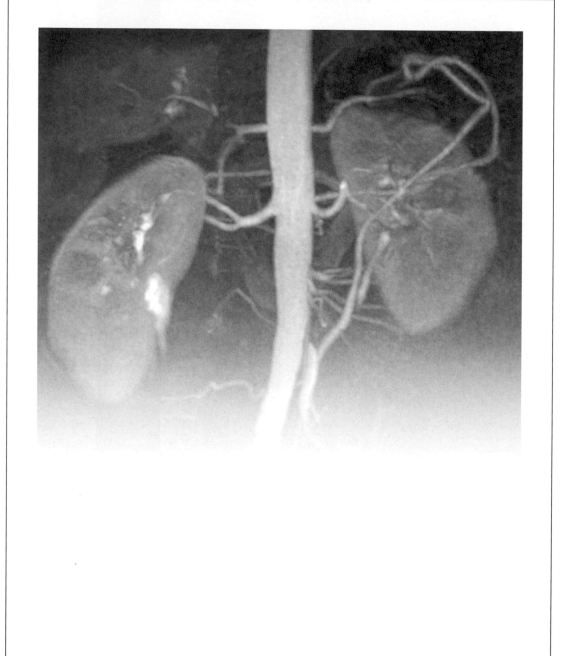

Mellena D. Bridges, J. Mark McKinney, and Eric M. Walser

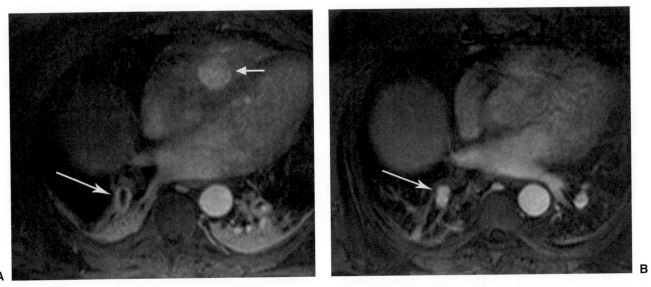

FIGURE 16-1 **Pulmonary embolus incidentally discovered during abdominal MRI. A:** Axial T1-weighted image through the liver dome obtained following contrast injection shows a filling defect in the posteromedial segmental pulmonary artery (*arrow*) (*Aortic pulsation artifact = short arrow*). **B:** Examination 4 months later demonstrates interval resolution of the clot.

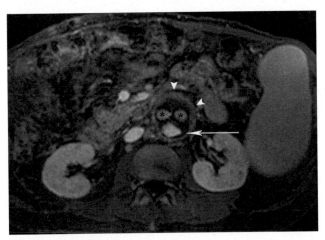

FIGURE 16-2 **Type II endoleak from an aortic stent-graft simulates a third vessel or graft limb in abdominal aortic aneurysm sac.** Axial enhanced T-weighted image shows the aneurysm sac (*arrowheads*) enclosing the pair of graft limbs (*asterisk*) as well as an endoleak (*arrow*), evidenced by an oval collection of contrast posteriorly. Notice the serrated margin of the graft limbs.

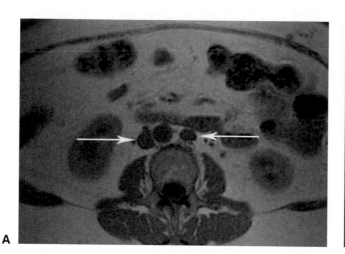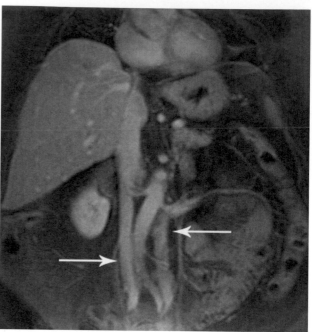

FIGURE 16-3 **Duplicated inferior vena cava (IVC), a normal variant.** Axial unenhanced **(A)** and coronal enhanced, fat-suppressed **(B)** T1-weighted images demonstrate two large vessels on either side of the infrarenal aorta (*arrows*). Left-sided IVC joins the left renal vein, and then merges with the right-sided IVC to create a single suprarenal IVC. This variant is due to persistence of both the left and right supracardinal veins and occurs in 2% of individuals.

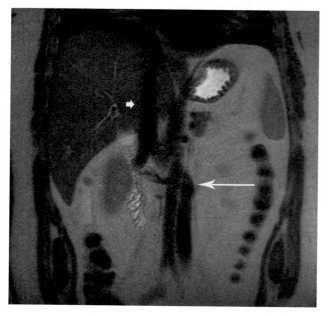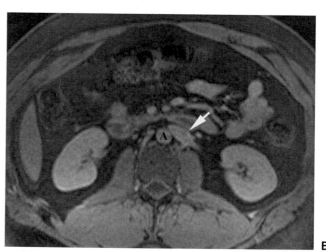

FIGURE 16-4 **Left inferior vena cava (IVC), a variant anatomy. A:** On coronal T2-weighted image, the IVC appears as a large vessel (*arrow*) to the left of the infrarenal aorta that merges with the left renal vein, then crosses the midline to assume its normal suprarenal position (*thick arrow*). **B:** Axial fat-suppressed T1-weighted gradient echo image shows the IVC–left renal vein confluence beginning to cross from left to right (*short arrow*) (*Aorta = A*). This variant is due to persistence of the lower left supracardinal vein and occurs in 0.5% of individuals.

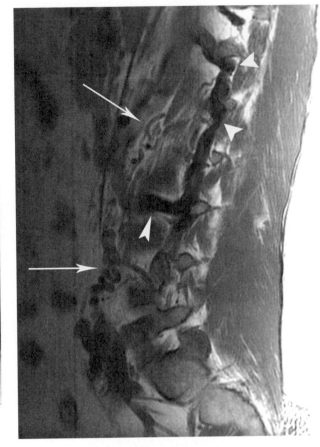

FIGURE 16-5 **Congenital partial absence of the infrarenal inferior vena cava (IVC). A:** Axial T1-weighted image from a lumbar spine MRI demonstrates only a few small vessels in the expected position of the IVC (*arrow*) (*Aorta = A*). **B:** Sagittal T1-weighted image shows these vessels as well as very large paravertebral collateral veins (*arrowheads*).

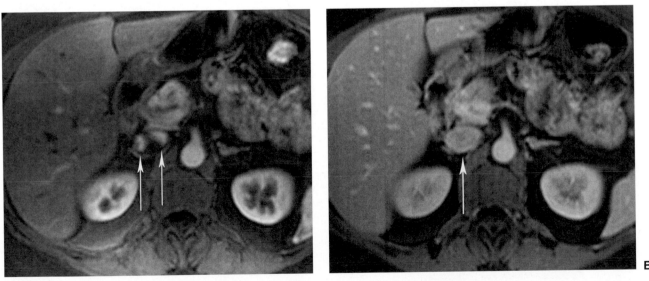

FIGURE 16-6 **Laminar flow in inferior vena cava (IVC) simulates thrombus. A:** Rapid contrast transit through the kidneys results in two columns of contrast (*arrows*) appearing in the suprarenal IVC on this axial arterial phase T1-weighted image. The impression of an intervening filling defect is created. **B:** Similar image obtained in a later phase shows contrast filling the entire IVC lumen (*arrow*).

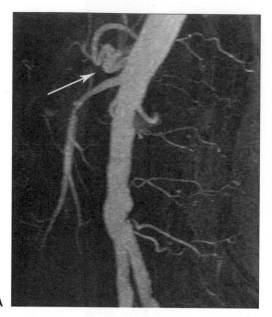

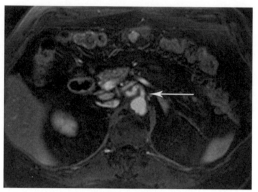

A **B**

FIGURE 16-7 **Tortuous celiac trunk simulates aneurysm. A:** Maximum intensity projection (MIP) image from a sagittal MRA demonstrates tortuosity of the celiac trunk (*arrow*), interpreted as an aneurysm on prior CT. **B:** Axial enhanced T1-weighted image shows hairpin turn of the vessel (*arrow*).

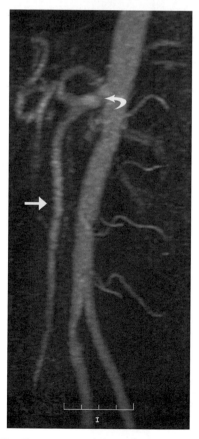

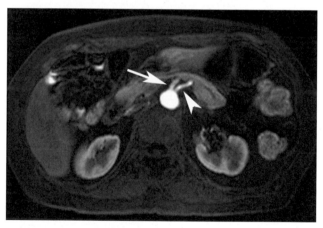

FIGURE 16-9 **Side-by-side origins of hepatic and splenic arteries.** Axial enhanced image shows separate origins of the hepatic (*arrow*) and splenic (*arrowhead*) arteries from the aorta, without a celiac trunk.

FIGURE 16-8 **Common origin of superior mesenteric artery (SMA) and celiac trunk, a normal variant.** Sagittal maximum intensity projection (MIP) image from an MRA shows a single trunk (*curved arrow*) from which the celiac vessels and the SMA (*arrow*) emerge. This occurs in less than 1% of the population.

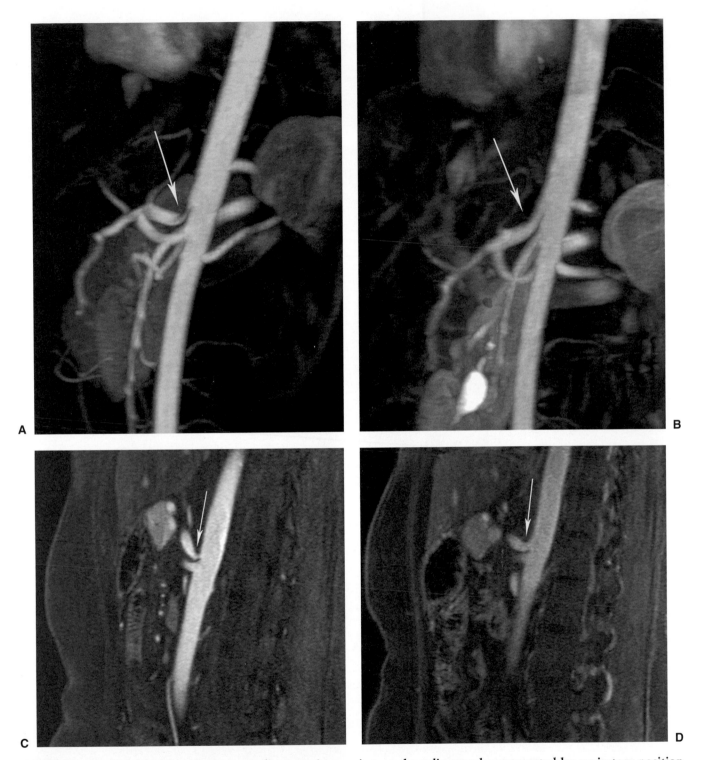

FIGURE 16-10 **Severity of median arcuate ligament impression on the celiac trunk exaggerated by expiratory position.** **A:** Maximum intensity projection (MIP) image of a sagittal MRA data set obtained in expiration suggests significant narrowing of the proximal celiac (*arrow*). **B:** Impression resolves on inspiration. Paired **(C)** expiratory and **(D)** inspiratory images from another patient demonstrate the same phenomenon (*Celiac artery = arrow*).

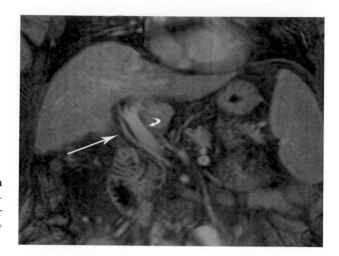

FIGURE 16-11   Replaced right hepatic artery, a common normal variant. Coronal contrast enhanced T1-weighted image depicts course of the right hepatic artery (*arrow*) inferior to the portal vein (*curved arrow*). These variants become very important if a pancreatic head resection is planned.

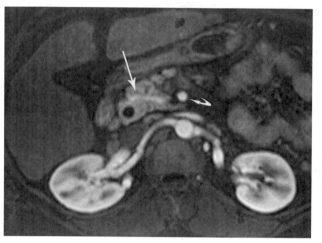

A

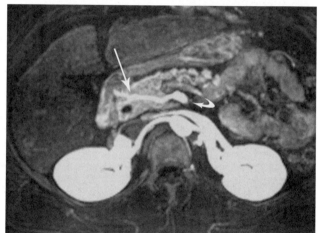

B

FIGURE 16-12   Replaced proper hepatic artery, a normal variant. A: Axial enhanced T1-weighted image shows a sizable artery (*arrow*) coursing horizontally through the pancreatic head at the level of the superior mesenteric artery (SMA) (*curved arrow*). **B:** Axial and **(C)** coronal maximum intensity projection (MIP) images confirm origin and course of the hepatic artery (*arrow*). This normal variant occurs in 15% to 20% of the population (*SMA = curved arrow, Pancreas = P*).

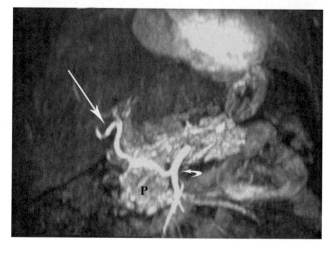

C

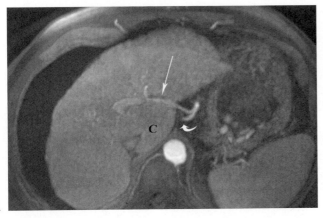

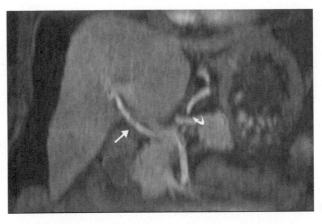

FIGURE 16-13 **Replaced left hepatic artery (LHA) and right hepatic artery (RHA). A:** Axial subvolume maximum intensity projection (MIP) shows origin of the left hepatic artery from the left gastric (*curved arrow*). Notice how the LHA courses through the fissure for the ligamentum venosum (*arrow*) (*Caudate lobe = C*). **B:** Coronal reconstruction shows course of replaced RHA (*arrow*). The left gastric artery (*curved arrow*) courses vertically and is larger than usual.

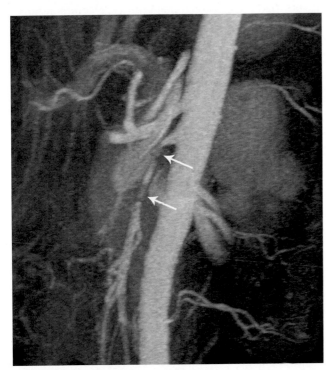

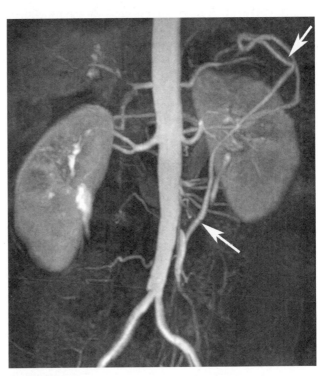

FIGURE 16-14 **Artifact from superior mesenteric artery (SMA) stent simulates segmental occlusions.** Maximum intensity projection reconstruction of MRA data set shows interruptions of the contrast column (*arrows*) within the SMA, suggesting stenoses/occlusions. However, this was artifactual and due to the presence of a stent.

FIGURE 16-15 **Arc of Riolan.** Coronal MRA demonstrates an arc of Riolan (*arrows*), which directly connects the superior and inferior mesenteric arteries through the middle and left colic arteries at the splenic flexure.

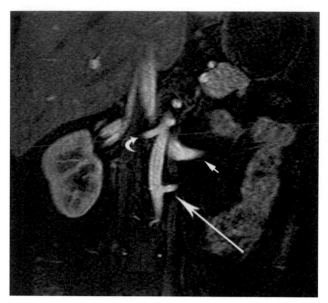

FIGURE 16-16 **Low origin of the left renal artery, a normal variant.** Source image from a coronal MRA shows left renal artery (*long arrow*) arising from the aorta several centimeters below its usual origin just distal to the superior mesenteric artery (SMA). In approximately 75% of the population, the renal arteries arise elsewhere from the aorta, anywhere from the T12 to L2 vertebral levels (*Right renal artery = curved arrow, Left renal vein = short arrow*).

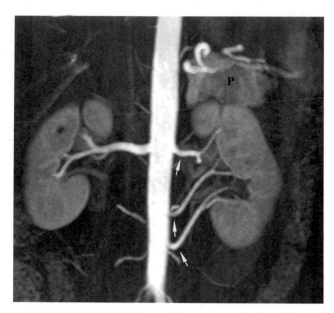

FIGURE 16-17 **Multiple renal arteries, a common normal variant.** Maximum intensity projection (MIP) reconstruction from a coronal MRA data set demonstrates three left renal arteries (*arrows*) and one on the right. Multiple renal arteries occur in approximately 30% of the population. Notice how including the anterior portion of the data set in the MIP results in the appearance of pancreatic tissue (*P*) perched on the left renal upper pole.

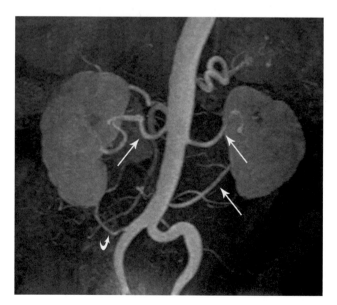

FIGURE 16-18 **Multiple bilateral renal arteries.** Maximum intensity projection (MIP) image from a coronal MRA data set demonstrates multiple renal arteries (*arrows*), including one arising from the right common iliac artery (*curved arrow*) to supply the right renal lower pole. Multiple renal arteries are unilateral in approximately 30% of the population and bilateral in approximately 10% of the population.

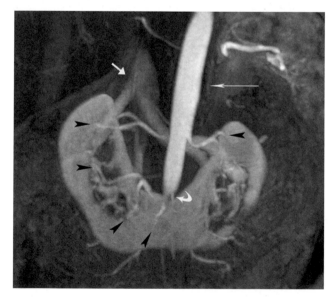

FIGURE 16-19 **Horseshoe kidney typically has multiple arteries and veins.** Maximum intensity projection (MIP) image from a coronal MRA shows multiple arteries (*arrowheads*) arising bilaterally from multiple levels of the aorta (*long arrow*). Inferior mesenteric artery (*curved arrow*) is always just above the fusion (*IVC = short arrow*).

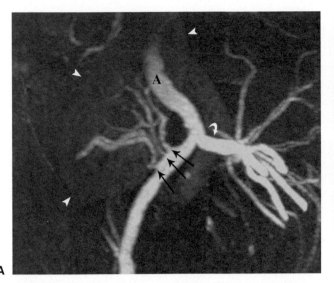

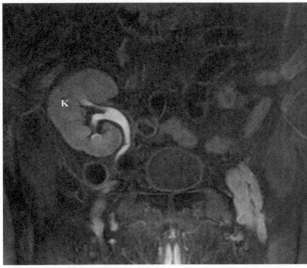

FIGURE 16-20 **Multiple arteries in kidney transplant. A:** Maximum intensity projection reconstruction of a coronal pelvic MRA demonstrates all three donor kidney arteries (*black arrows*) anastomosed to the external iliac artery (*Internal iliac artery = curved arrow, Common iliac artery = A, Kidney = arrowheads*). **B:** Coronal T1-weighted image in later phase of contrast shows enhancing graft kidney (*K*) and opacified donor ureter.

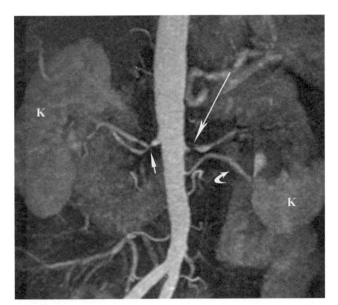

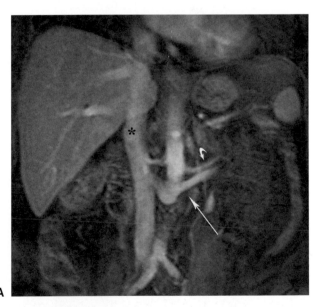

FIGURE 16-21 **Lower pole of left kidney simulates a mass** because it is the only normal part of this kidney. The rest of the kidney is atrophic due to high-grade stenosis of the uppermost renal artery (*long arrow*). The left lower renal artery (*curved arrow*) is normal in caliber. Right renal artery is moderately narrowed just before its early bifurcation (*short arrow*) (*Kidneys = K*).

FIGURE 16-22 **Retroaortic left renal vein (LRV), a common normal variant. A:** Coronal enhanced T1-weighted image demonstrates the typical curved course and low position of a retroaortic LRV (*arrow*). Retroaortic LRV occurs in approximately 3% of individuals (*Left renal artery = curved arrow, IVC = asterisk*).

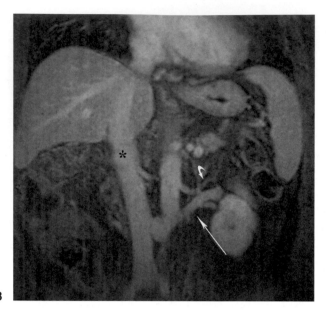

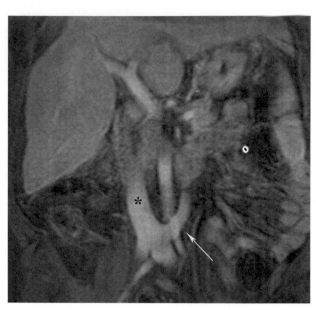

B

C

FIGURE 16-22 Retroaortic left renal vein (LRV), a common normal variant. (*continued*) **B:** Another retroaortic LRV (*arrow*), with lower caval insertion (*Left renal artery = curved arrow, IVC = asterisk*). **C:** A third retroaortic LRV (*arrow*) joins the IVC just above the iliac confluence (*IVC = asterisk*). IVC, inferior vena cava.

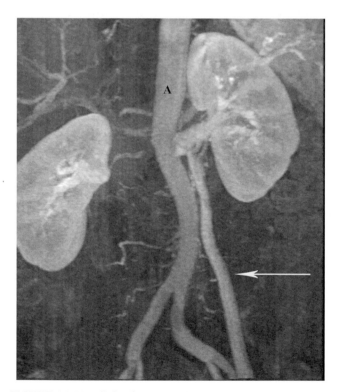

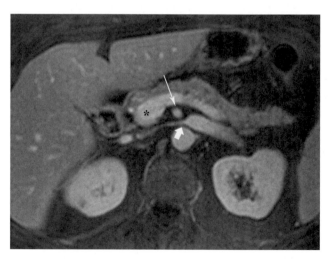

FIGURE 16-24 Nutcracker phenomenon of the left renal vein. The left renal vein (*thick arrow*) is narrowed as it crosses between the descending superior mesenteric artery (SMA) (*long arrow*) and aorta (*Portal confluence = asterisk*).

FIGURE 16-23 Subvolume maximum intensity projection (MIP) improves visualization of individual vessels. Use of only a part of 3-D data set subtracts overlying vessels and defines an incompetent left gonadal vein (*arrow*), which was the cause of massive pelvic varices (*Aorta = A*).

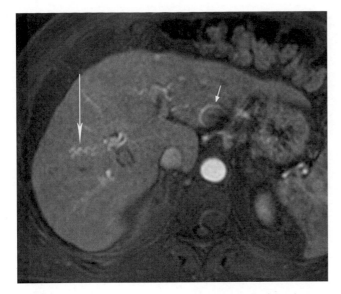

FIGURE 16-25 **Spiral hepatic arteries in cirrhosis.** As arteries hypertrophy, they sometimes also take a tortuous course (*long arrow*) (*Aortic pulsation artifact = short arrow*).

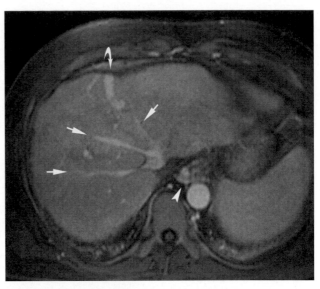

FIGURE 16-26 **Hepatic vein attenuation, common in cirrhosis.** Axial contrast-enhanced T1-weighted image demonstrates narrowed hepatic veins (*arrows*) with a large paraumbilical collateral (*curved arrow*) and small paraesophageal varices (*arrowhead*), due to portal hypertension. Notice how parenchymal atrophy has reduced the space between veins.

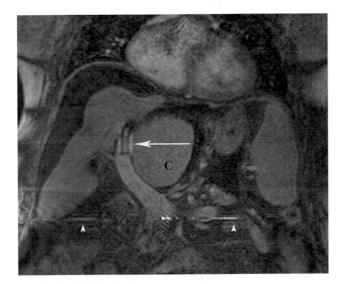

FIGURE 16-27 **Covered transjugular intrahepatic portosystemic shunt (TIPS).** Coronal contrast-enhanced T1-weighted image through the portal vein shows the opacified blood in the proximal end of a patent shunt (*arrow*). Notice radiofrequency (RF) artifact (*arrowheads*) and peripheral loss of fat suppression in this 360-pound patient (*Caudate lobe = C*).

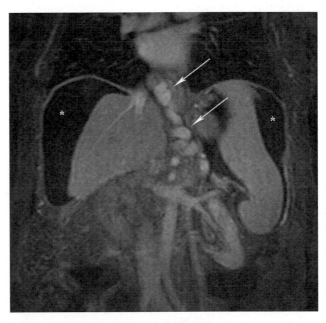

FIGURE 16-28 **Esophageal varices, one of a number of possible collateral pathways in portal hypertension.** Enlarged tortuous vessel (*arrows*) flows to the gastroesophageal junction from the left gastric vein in a patient with cirrhosis (*Ascites = asterisk*).

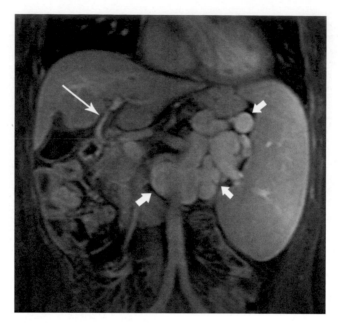

FIGURE 16-29 **Spontaneous splenorenal shunt in portal hypertension.** Shunting from splenic vein to left renal vein is very common in portal hypertension and usually associated with a confusing cluster of intervening enlarged, tortuous vessels (*short arrows*) (*Attenuated main portal vein = long arrow*).

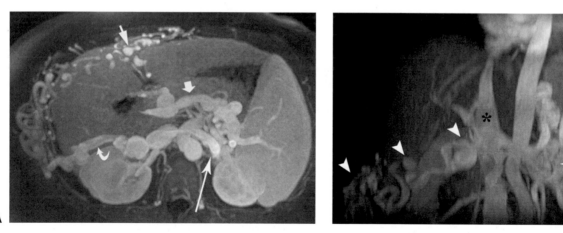

FIGURE 16-30 **Bilateral portal-renal shunts, additional vascular pathways in portal hypertension. A:** Maximum intensity projection (MIP) reconstruction of an axial 3-D enhanced T1-weighted data set shows pathway from a paraumbilical collateral (*short arrow*) to the right renal vein (*curved arrow*) and a pathway from the splenic vein (*thick arrow*) to the left renal vein (*long arrow*). **B:** Coronal maximum intensity projection (MIP) redemonstrates the paraumbilical collateral (*arrowheads*) and the splenorenal shunt (*arrow*) (*IVC = asterisk, Spleen = S*). IVC, inferior vena cava.

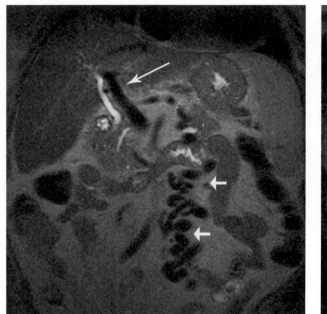

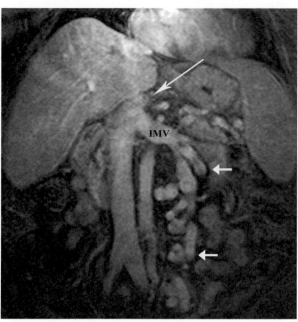

FIGURE 16-31 Inferior mesenteric vein (IMV) collaterals, another alternative drainage pathway in portal hypertension. **A:** Coronal T2-weighted image show the portal vein (*long arrow*) and a tangle of flow-void collaterals (*short arrows*) in the left abdomen. **B:** Coronal enhanced T1-weighted image shows the collateral (*short arrows*) leading into the *IMV* (*Portal vein = long arrow*).

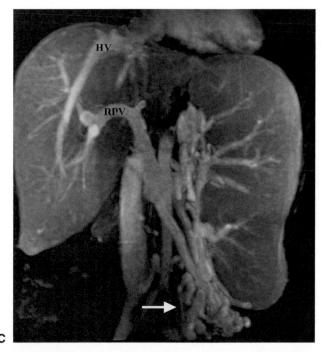

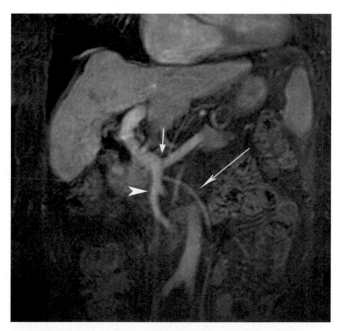

FIGURE 16-31 Inferior mesenteric vein (IMV) collaterals, another alternative drainage pathway in portal hypertension. **C:** Maximum intensity projection (MIP) image from MRA/magnetic resonance venogram (MRV) shows bunching of large collaterals (*Right portal vein = RPV, Right hepatic vein = HV*).

FIGURE 16-32 Inferior mesenteric vein drains into superior mesenteric vein, a normal variant. Coronal T2-weighted image shows the inferior mesenteric vein (*long arrow*) draining into the superior mesenteric vein (*arrowhead*) Portal confluence = *short arrow*).

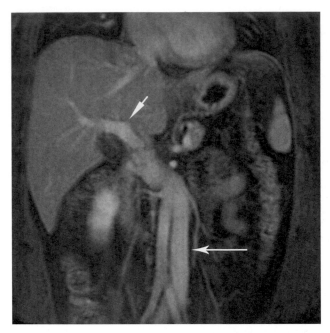

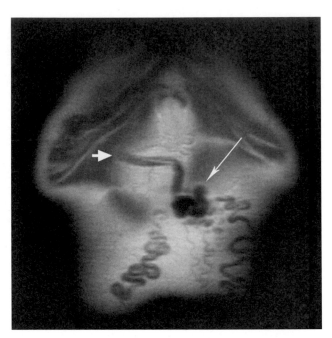

FIGURE 16-33 **Apparent portal continuation of the left inferior vena cava (IVC), a pitfall of coronal imaging.** Volume averaging results in apparent continuity of left IVC (*arrow*) and portal vein (*short arrow*). The IVC actually courses with the left renal vein to its normal suprarenal caval position.

FIGURE 16-34 **Anterior abdominal wall collaterals are signal voids** on T2-weighted image. Coronal single-shot T2-weighted image through the anterior abdominal wall shows tubular low signal in the paraumbilical collateral (*short arrow*), caput medusae (*long arrow*), and tortuous subcutaneous varices.

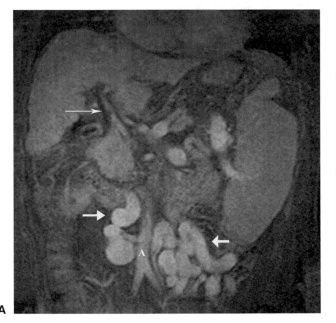

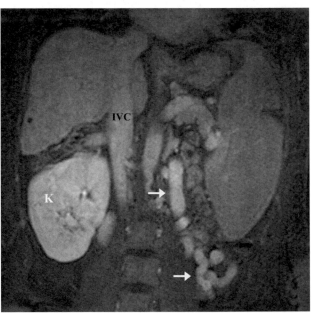

FIGURE 16-35 **Crossed-fused ectopic kidney provides portal drainage. A:** Coronal T1-weighted image demonstrates a tangle of huge vessels (*short arrows*) in the lower left abdomen (*Portal vein = long arrow, Aorta = A*). **B:** More posterior coronal image shows descending side of collateral network (*arrows*) and the ectopic moiety of a crossed fused ectopic kidney (*K*). Portal flow courses into the ectopic renal vein and then inferior vena cava (IVC).

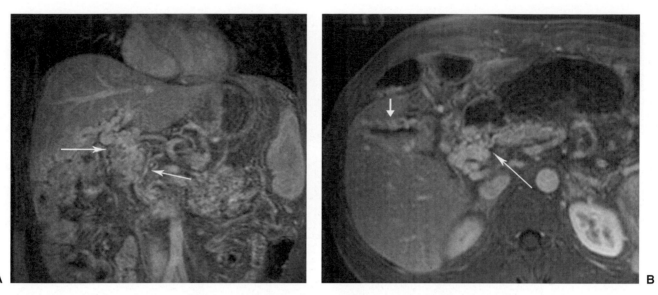

FIGURE 16-36 **Cavernous transformation of the portal vein simulates a vascular mass. A:** Coronal enhanced T1-weighted image demonstrates a complex network of small vessels (*arrows*), difficult to resolve due to motion artifact. **B:** Axial image also shows gallbladder varices (*short arrow*) in addition to the cavernous transformation (*long arrow*).

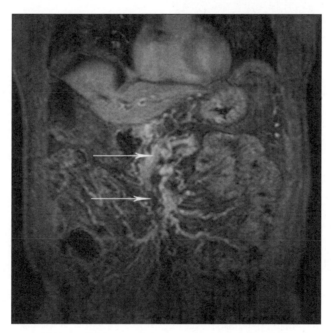

FIGURE 16-37 **Chronic thrombosis of the entire portal system.** Coronal enhanced fat-suppressed T1-weighted image demonstrates a network of tortuous vessels in the small bowel mesentery (*arrows*), due to "cavernous transformation" of the entire portal circulation.

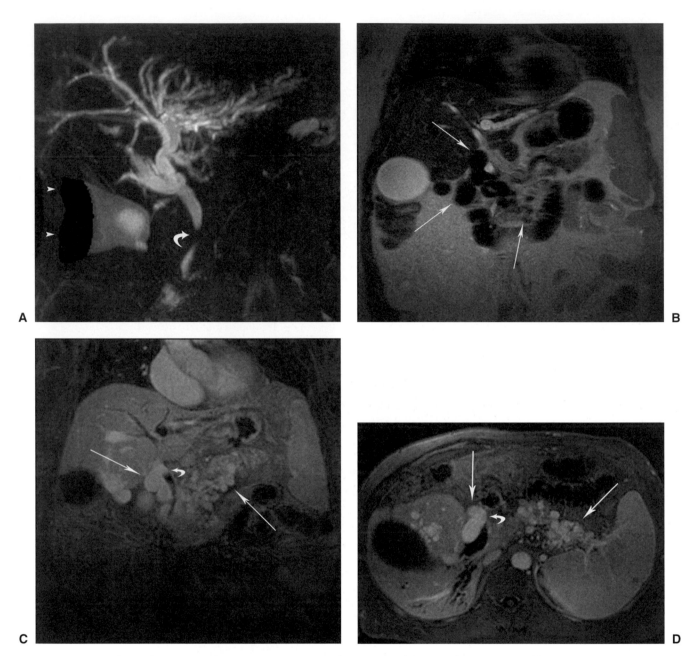

FIGURE 16-38 Biliary obstruction due to cavernous transformation of the portal system (portal biliopathy). **A:** MRCP image shows the tapered common bile duct (CBD) stricture (*curved arrow*) and dilated upstream biliary tree (*Reconstruction artifact = arrowheads*). **B:** Coronal T2-weighted image demonstrates a tangle of large signal voids (*arrows*) within the pancreatic head that compress the CBD. **C:** Coronal and **(D)** axial enhanced T1-weighted images confirm these as vessels (*long arrows*) (*Narrowed CBD = curved arrow*).

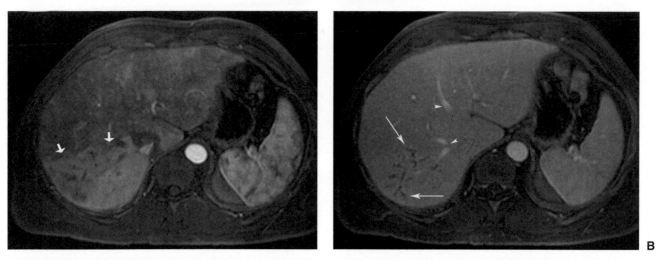

FIGURE 16-39 Occlusion of portal veins in hepatic segment VII simulates bile duct dilatation and beading. **A:** Axial enhanced T1-weighted image shows rapid early enhancement (*arrows*) in segment VII of the liver. Since the hepatic artery has to provide much of the inflow to this segment, this is a clue to the real explanation of findings. **B:** In a later phase, liver enhancement has normalized, but small, occluded branching portal veins (*arrows*) are revealed (*Normal hepatic veins = arrowheads*).

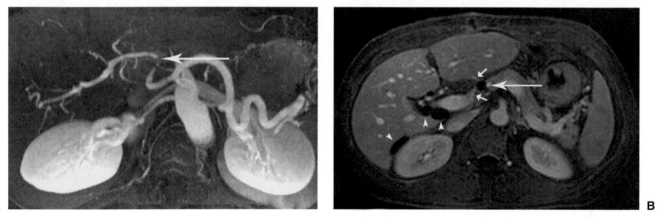

FIGURE 16-40 Artifact from surgical clip simulates hepatic artery anastomotic occlusion. A: Maximum intensity projection (MIP) image from an axial MRA data set shows apparent hepatic artery interruption (*arrow*) at the anastomosis in a transplant patient. **B:** Axial enhanced T1-weighted image shows susceptibility artifact from clip (*arrow*) adjacent to the hepatic artery (*short arrows*) (*Other clips = arrowheads*).

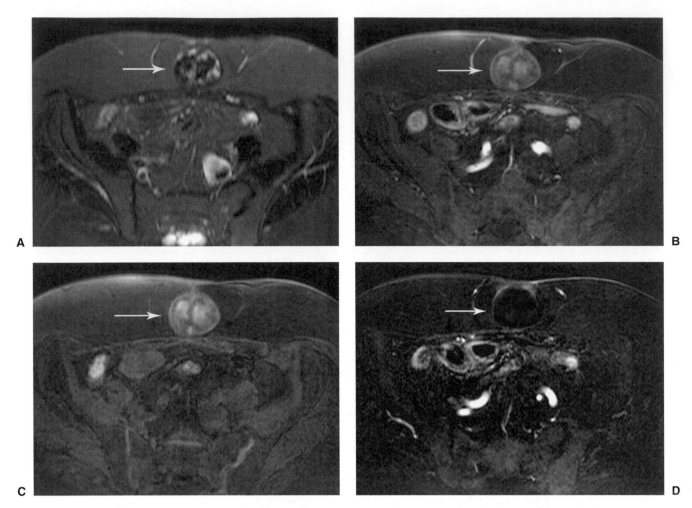

FIGURE 16-41 **Thrombosed abdominal wall venous collateral simulates mass in liver transplant patient. A:** Axial T2-weighted fat-suppressed image through upper pelvis shows a round, heterogeneous mass (*arrow*) in the anterior midline. **B:** Axial contrast-enhanced image suggests internal enhancement (*arrow*). **C:** However, precontrast image shows preexisting hyperintensity (*arrow*). **D:** Subtraction image confirms complete lack of enhancement (*arrow*) in this collateral that thrombosed following transplant.

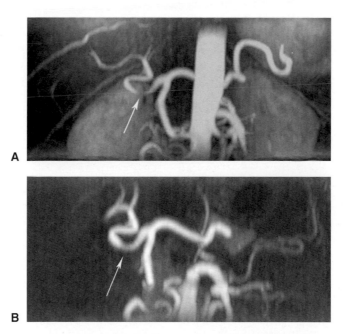

FIGURE 16-42 Maximum intensity projection (MIP) reconstruction overestimates hepatic arterial anastomotic narrowing. **A:** MIP of an axial MRA suggests high-grade stricture of the anastomosis (*arrow*) in this transplant patient. **B:** Subvolume MIP shows widely patent anastomosis (*arrow*).

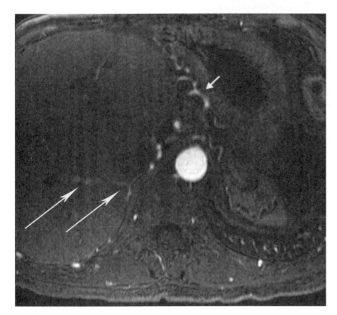

FIGURE 16-43 Collateral filling of graft artery in hepatic arterial occlusion. Back-filling of segmental right hepatic artery from a subcapsular vessel (*arrows*) in a donor liver. Although ostensibly impossible, a liver graft occasionally finds collateral supply from vessels other than the hepatic artery (*Enlarged gastric arteries = short arrow*).

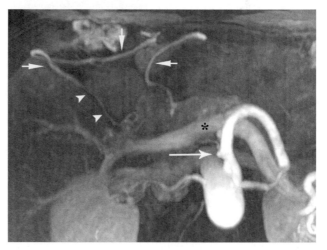

FIGURE 16-44 Another case of hepatic artery occlusion with collateral filling. Oblique axial maximum intensity projection (MIP) image from a subvolume hepatic arterial MRA demonstrates complete occlusion (*long arrow*) at the hepatic artery origin from the celiac trunk. Collateral (*short arrows*), likely from the native gastroduodenal, retrograde fills the intrahepatic artery (*arrowheads*) (*Portal vein = asterisk*).

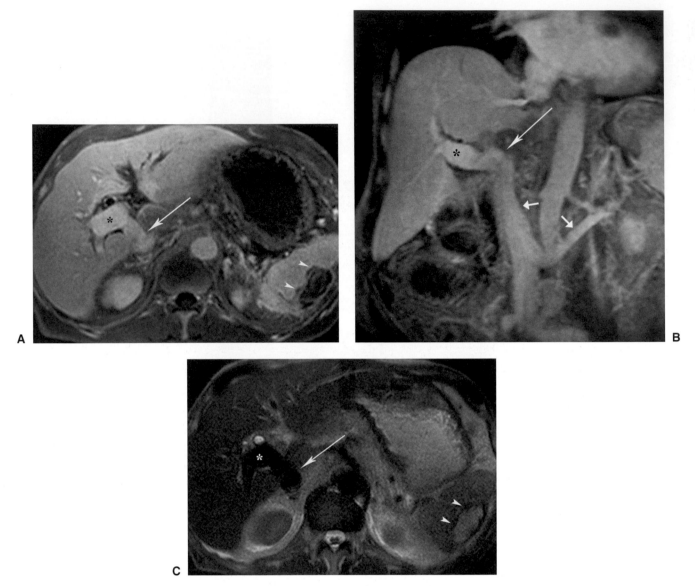

FIGURE 16-45   Surgically created portocaval shunt. A: Axial enhanced T1-weighted image shows shunt (*arrow*) as large vessel spanning the right portal vein (*asterisk*) and infrahepatic vena cava. **B:** Coronal image shows the inferior vena cava (IVC) and retroaortic left renal vein (*short arrows*) (*Shunt = long arrow, right portal vein = asterisk*). **C:** Axial T2-weighted image shows shunt (*long arrow*) as signal void coursing posteromedially from the liver hilum (*Right portal vein = asterisk, Splenic infarct = arrowheads*).

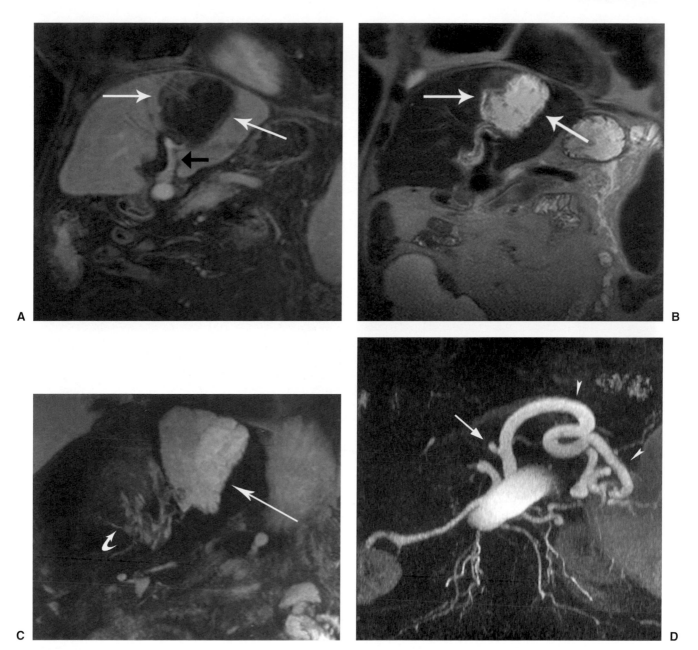

FIGURE 16-46 Ischemic necrosis simulates hypovascular tumor in transplant liver. A: Coronal enhanced T1-weighted image shows large liver mass with variable signal intensity (*white arrows*) (*Left portal vein = black arrow*). Coronal **(B)** T2-weighted and **(C)** MRCP images delineate the necrosis cavity (*long arrows*) in addition to a number of abnormal intrahepatic bile ducts (*curved arrow*). **D:** Oblique coronal maximum intensity projection (MIP) MRA shows abrupt occlusion of the hepatic artery (*arrow*) just after its origin from the celiac trunk (*Splenic artery = arrowheads*).

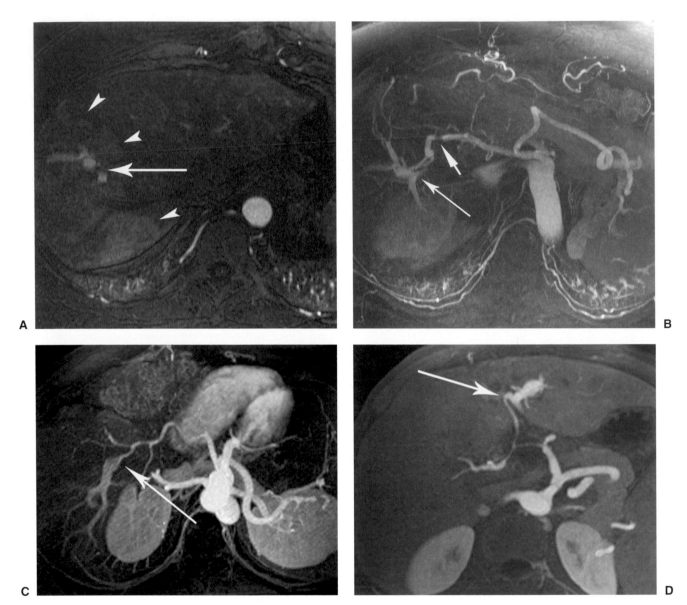

FIGURE 16-47 Arterioportal fistula, a common complication of percutaneous liver biopsy. A: Regional early arterial enhancement (*arrowheads*) is seen in association with the fistula (*arrow*). **B:** Maximum intensity projection (MIP) reconstruction shows narrowed anastomosis (*short arrow*) and fistula (*long arrow*). **C:** Rapid filling of fistula (*arrow*) from the artery in another transplant patient. **D:** Another biopsy-related fistula (*arrow*) in the left lobe.

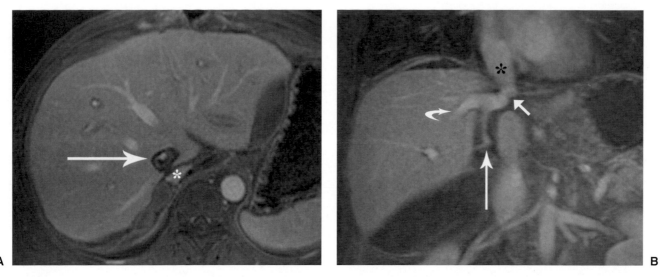

FIGURE 16-48 **Target appearance of donor inferior vena cava (IVC) in liver transplant with piggy-back reconstruction.** **A:** Axial contrast-enhanced T1-weighted image shows donor IVC (*arrow*) below the level of the hepatic vein insertions. Target appearance results from thrombus around the patent channel of an accessory hepatic vein. Native IVC (*asterisk*) is normal. **B:** Coronal subvolume maximum intensity projection (MIP) image delineates the vascular flow pattern in this piggyback reconstruction (*Accessory donor hepatic vein = long arrow, IVC-IVC anastomosis = short arrow, Donor hepatic vein = curved arrow, Suprahepatic IVC = asterisk*).

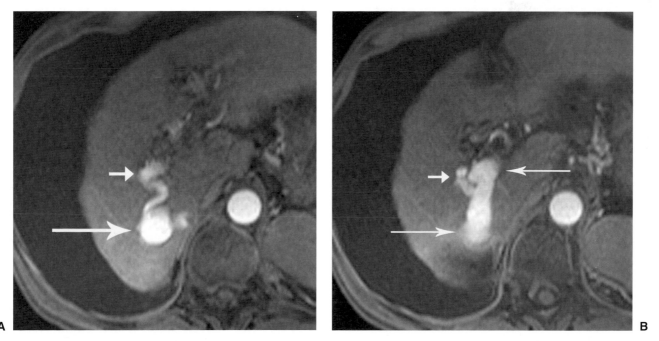

FIGURE 16-49 **Massive postbiopsy hepatoportal fistula in cirrhotic patient simulates congenital vascular malformation.** **A:** Massive round collection of contrast (*long arrow*) connects with tortuous vessel (*short arrow*) moving toward the hilum. **B:** Lower slice shows dilated portal vein (*long arrows*) and enlarged feeding hepatic vein (*short arrow*).

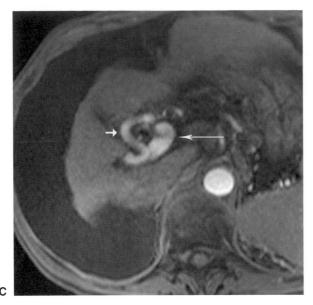

FIGURE 16-49 Massive postbiopsy hepatoportal fistula in cirrhotic patient simulates congenital vascular malformation. (*continued*) **C:** Image through the hilum confirms that the larger of the vessels is the right portal vein (*long arrow*) and the smaller is the right hepatic artery (*short arrow*)

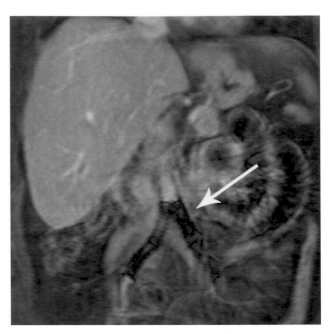

FIGURE 16-50 Artifact from "kissing" iliac stents. Coronal enhanced T1-weighted gradient echo image shows tubular signal voids from the pair of iliac stents (*arrow*).

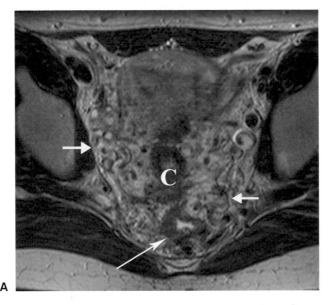

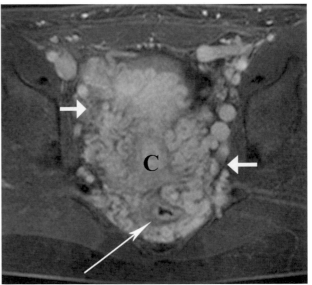

FIGURE 16-51 Massive varices simulate a vascular pelvic mass. Axial (**A**) T2-weighted and (**B**) enhanced T1-weighted images show massive, bilateral varices (*short arrows*) filling the pelvis (*Cervix = C, Rectum = long arrow*).

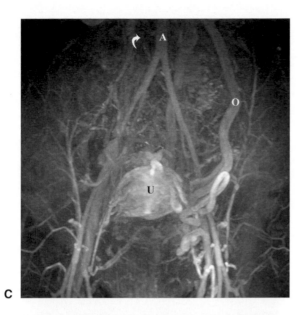

C

FIGURE 16-51 Massive varices simulate a vascular pelvic mass. (*continued*) **C:** Maximum intensity projection from a MR venogram reveals the etiology, which is an occluded IVC (*curved arrow*) (*Uterus = U, Dilated left ovarian vein = O, Aorta = A*). IVC, inferior vena cava.

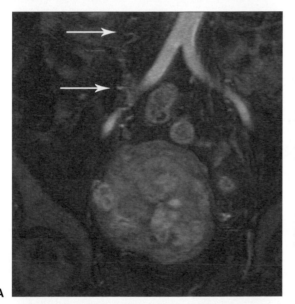

A

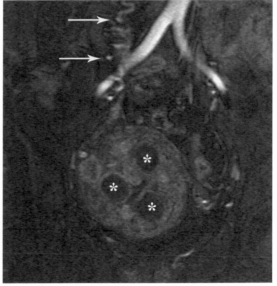

B

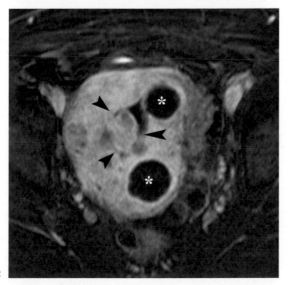

C

FIGURE 16-52 Ovarian artery visible because of high flow to fibroid uterus. A: Spiral course of the right ovarian artery (*arrows*) toward enlarged uterus is shown on subvolume magnetic resonance projection (MIP) from a pelvic MRA. **B:** Following uterine artery embolization, a few of the fibroids (*asterisk*) have been devascularized, but the ovarian artery (*arrow*) is even more prominent. **C:** Subtraction image confirms necrosis in some fibroids (*asterisk*), but not the intracavitary submucosal tumor (*arrowheads*) or other lesions in the right uterus.

Suggested Readings

Ashton E, Ellis K, McDonald SW. Course of the short gastric veins and their suitability for pancreatic islet transplantation. *Clin Anat*. 2004; 17:651–657.

Barberini F, Ripani M, Heyn R, et al. A singular pancreatico-colic artery: Anatomical report and clinical implications. *Surg Radiol Anat*. 2006;28:328–331.

Deepthinath R, Nayak BS, Mehta RB, et al. Multiple variations in the paired arteries of the abdominal aorta. *Clin Anat*. 2006;19:566–568.

El-Sherif AM, Dixon AK. Interesting inferior vena cava. *Clin Anat*. 1999;12:427–429.

Epstein J, Arora A, Ellis H. Surface anatomy of the inferior epigastric artery in relation to laparoscopic injury. *Clin Anat*. 2004;17:400–408.

Gunenc C, Denk CC. Combined unusual anatomical variations of the superior mesenteric and right renal arteries. *Clin Anat*. 2006;19:716–717.

Kadir S. The kidneys. In: Kadir S, ed. *Atlas of normal and variant angiographic anatomy*. Philadelphia: WB Saunders; 1991:387–428.

Kadir S, Lundell C, Saeed M. Celiac, superior, and inferior mesenteric arteries. In: Kadir S, ed. *Atlas of normal and variant angiographic anatomy*. Philadelphia: WB Saunders; 1991:297–364.

Kim HJ, Ko YT, Lim JW, et al. Radiologic anatomy of the superior mesenteric vein and branching patterns of the first jejunal trunk: Evaluation using multi-detector row CT venography. *Surg Radiol Anat*. 2007;29:67–75.

Loukas M, Jordan R. An unusual arterial connection between the celiac trunk and the gastroduodenal artery. *Clin Anat*. 2006; 712–713.

Lundell C, Kadir S. The portal venous system and hepatic veins. In: Kadir S, ed. *Atlas of normal and variant angiographic anatomy*. Philadelphia: WB Saunders; 1991:365–385.

Nael K, Ruehm SG, Michaely HJ, et al. Multistation whole-body high-spatial resolution MR angiography using a 32-channel MR system. *AJR Am J Roentgenol*. 2007;188:529–539.

Ohkubo M. Aberrant left gastric vein directly draining into the liver. *Clin Anat*. 2000;13:134–137.

Osawa T, Feng X-Y, Sasaki N, et al. Rare care of the inferior mesenteric artery and the common hepatic artery arising from the superior mesenteric artery. *Clin Anat*. 2004;17:518–521.

Pan X, Saida Y, Kurosaki Y, et al. Fatty mass in the inferior vena cava at CT: Lipoma or normal variant? *Radiat Med*. 1995;13:251–253.

Perry JN, Williams MP, Dubbins PA, et al. Lipomata of the inferior vena cava: A normal variant? *Clinic Radiol*. 1994;49:341–342.

Potthast S, Bongartz GM, Huegli R, et al. Intraarterial contrast-enhanced MR aortography with and without parallel acquisition technique in patients with peripheral arterial occlusive disease. *AJR Am J Roentgenol*. 2007;188:823–829.

Saeed M, Murshid KR, Rufai AA, et al. Coexistence of multiple anomalies in the celiac mesenteric arterial system. *Clin Anat*. 2003;16:30–36.

Shaw MBK, Cutress M, Papavassilious V, et al. Duplicated inferior vena cava and crossed renal actopia with abdominal aortic aneurysm: Pre-operative anatomic studies facilitate surgery. *Clin Anat*. 2004;16:355–357.

Singh G, NG YK, Bay BH. Bilateral accessory renal arteries associated with some anomalies of the ovarian arteries: A case study. *Clin Anat*. 1998;11:417–420.

Yahel J, Arensburg B. The topographic relationships of the unpaired visceral branches of the aorta. *Clin Anat*. 1998;11:304–309.

Chapter 17

Lumbar Spine

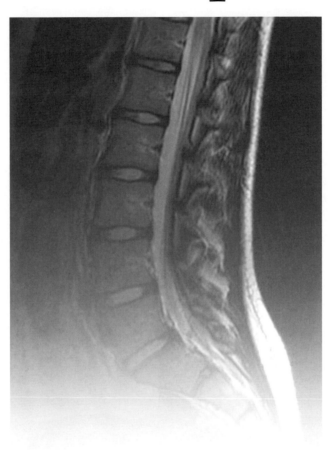

Laura W. Bancroft and Debbie J. Merinbaum

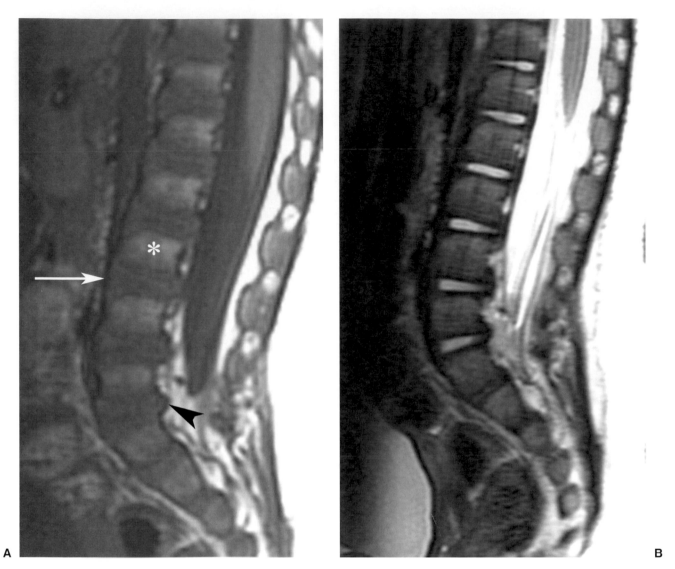

FIGURE 17-1   Infant lumbar spine. Sagittal **(A)** T1- and **(B)** T2-weighted images in a 7-month-old child. Signal intensities on the **(A)** T1-weighted image make the intervertebral discs (*arrow*) appear almost as tall as the vertebral bodies (*asterisk*) and appear to protrude posteriorly (*arrowhead*).

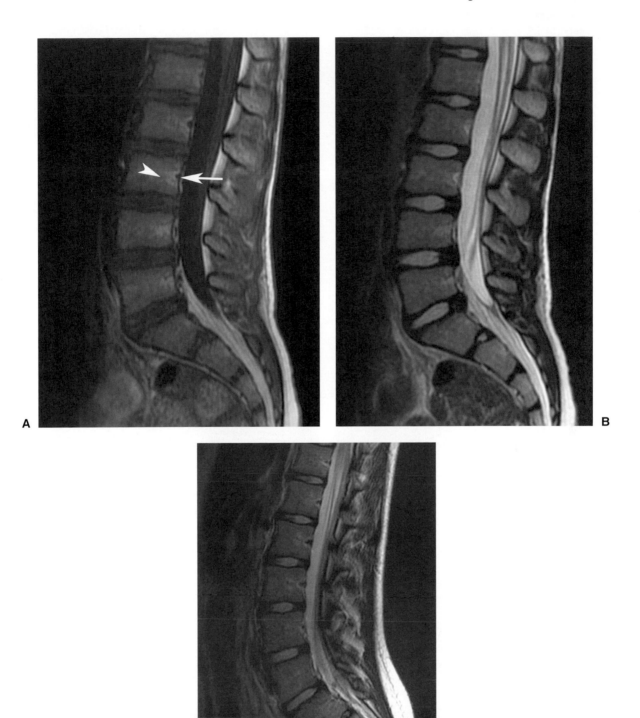

FIGURE 17-2 **Pediatric spine.** Sagittal **(A)** T1- and **(B)** T2-weighed images in a 10-year-old child show development of the vertebrae and discs, which now have a more adult-like proportion. Notice the yellow marrow (*arrowhead*) that has developed around the basivertebral veins (*arrow*). **C:** Further marrow changes in the mid-vertebral body are apparent in this 15-year-old child.

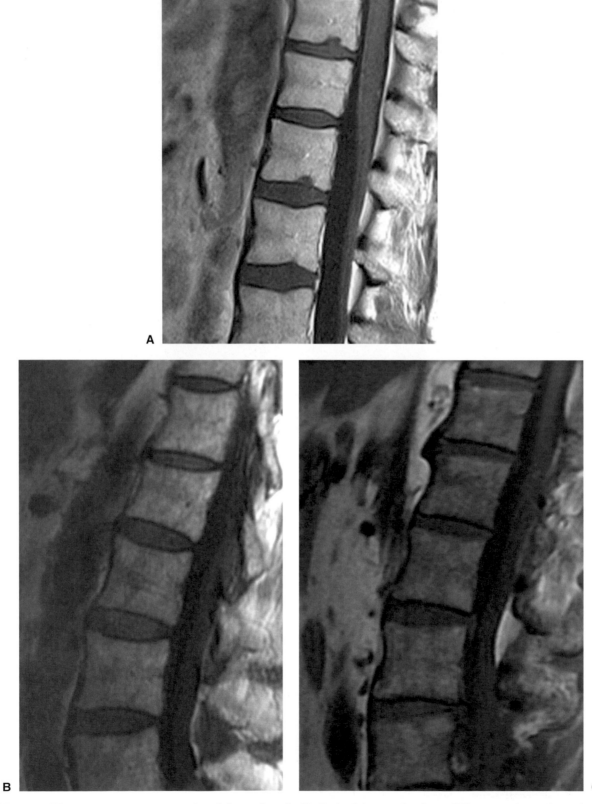

FIGURE 17-3 Heterogeneous marrow signal intensity. A–C: Sagittal images in three different patients show the normal variation of yellow and red marrow that can be present within the adult spine.

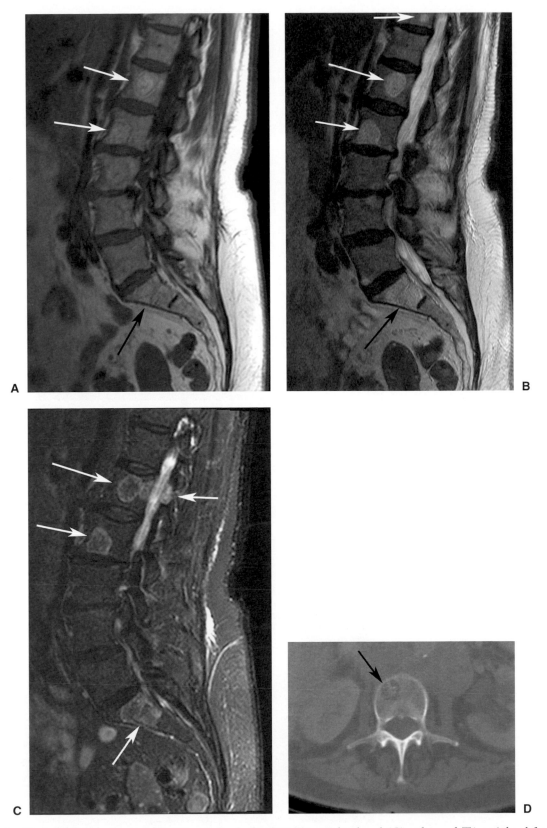

FIGURE 17-4 **Hemangiomas.** Sagittal **(A)** T1-weighted, **(B)** FSE T2-weighted and **(C)** enhanced T1-weighted fat-suppressed images show multiple vertebral foci (*arrows*), which are primarily of fatty intensity and show peripheral enhancement. **D:** Correlating CT shows the classic appearance of a hemangioma (*arrow*). The coarsened trabeculae are seen in cross-section and there is a background of fat.

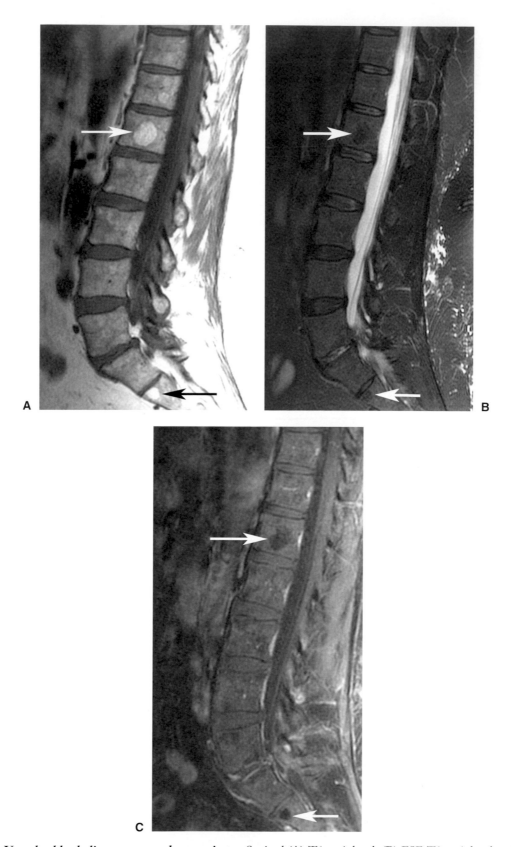

FIGURE 17-5   Vertebral body lipoma versus hemangioma. Sagittal **(A)** T1-weighted, **(B)** FSE T2-weighted and **(C)** enhanced T1-weighted fat suppressed images show a fatty focus (*arrows*) in the L1 vertebral body, which does not appreciably enhance. Finding is benign and is either an intraosseous lipoma or hemangioma.

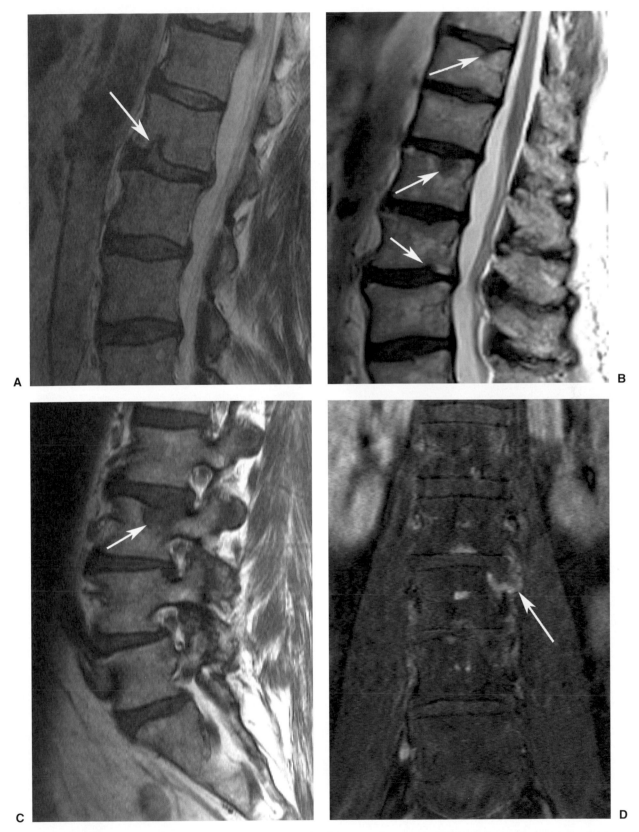

FIGURE 17-6 **Schmorl's nodes. A** and **B:** Sagittal T2-weighted images show typical Schmorl's nodes (*arrows*), which are foci of herniated disc material. **C:** Sagittal T1-weighted image shows a Schmorl's node (*arrow*) involving the superior endplate of L3. **D:** Coronal T1-weighted enhanced fat-suppressed image shows a displaced vessel (*arrow*) inferior to the herniated disc material, which is somewhat unusual.

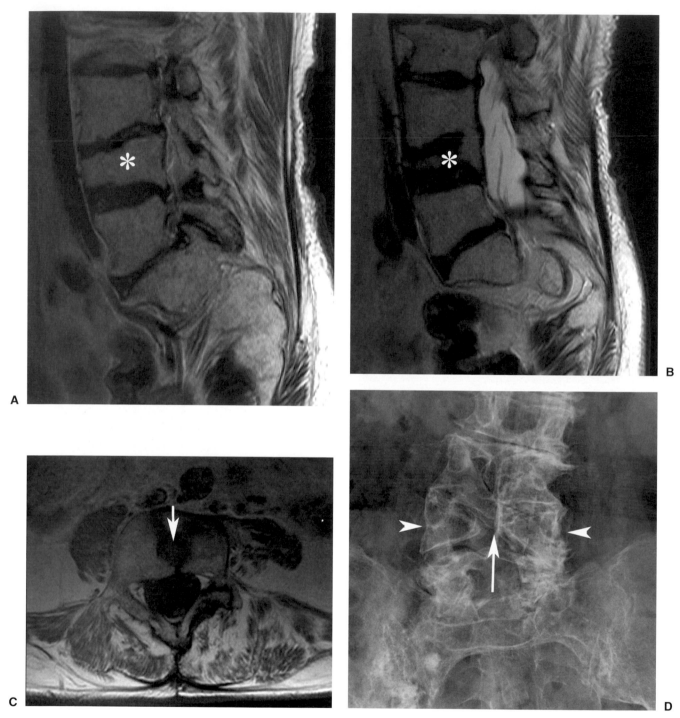

FIGURE 17-7   Butterfly vertebra. Sagittal images through the **(A)** lateral and **(B)** central spine show the bilaterally wedge-shaped vertebral body (*asterisk*), with greatest deformity centrally. **C:** Axial T1-weighted image shows a central defect (*arrow*) corresponding to the cleft within the variant butterfly vertebra. **D:** Corresponding radiograph shows the central cleft (*arrow*) and laterally wedge-shaped vertebra (*arrowheads*).

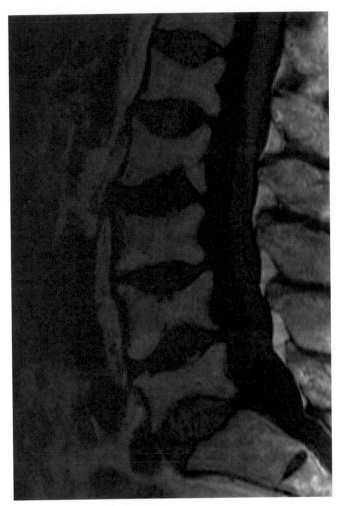

FIGURE 17-8 Fishmouth vertebrae due to osteopenic compression fractures. Sagittal T1-weighted image shows fishmouth configuration of all vertebral bodies due to osteopenic compression fractures. The diffusely abnormal vertebral configuration should not be confused with a dysplastic process.

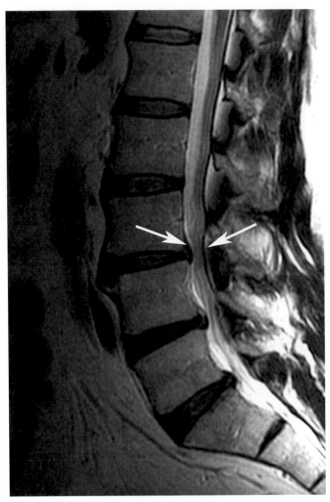

FIGURE 17-9 Congenitally narrowed central canal. Congenitally short pedicles can narrow the anterior to posterior dimension of the central canal and result in premature canal stenosis (*arrows*) when degenerative disc disease occurs.

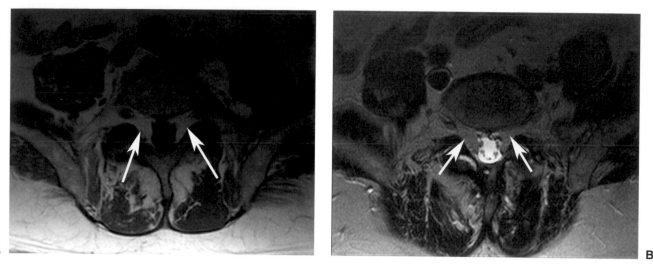

FIGURE 17-10   Epidural lipomatosis. Axial **(A)** T1- and **(B)** FSE T2-weighted images show prominent epidural fat (*arrows*), of no clinical significance.

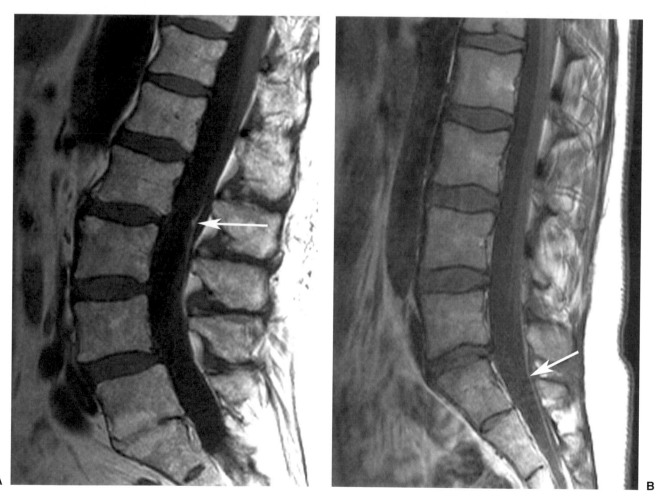

FIGURE 17-11   Fatty filum terminalis. A and **B:** Sagittal T1-weighted images in different patients show fat (*arrows*) within the filum terminalis.

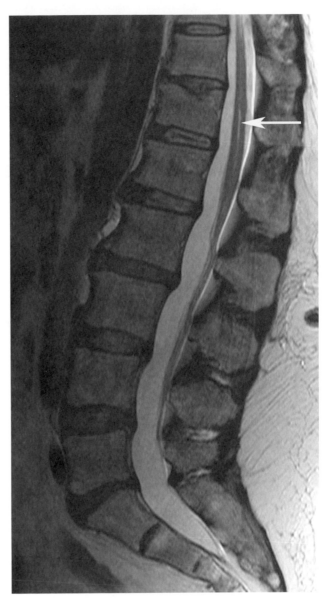

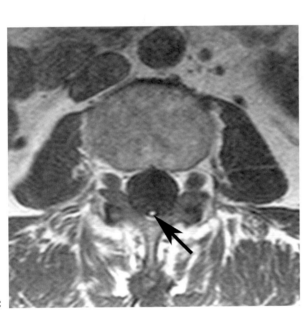

FIGURE 17-11 Fatty filum terminalis. (*continued*) **C:** Axial image shows the posterior position of the fat (*arrow*) within the canal.

FIGURE 17-12 Prominent central canal. The central canal of the cord (*arrow*) can be visualized in the normal patient.

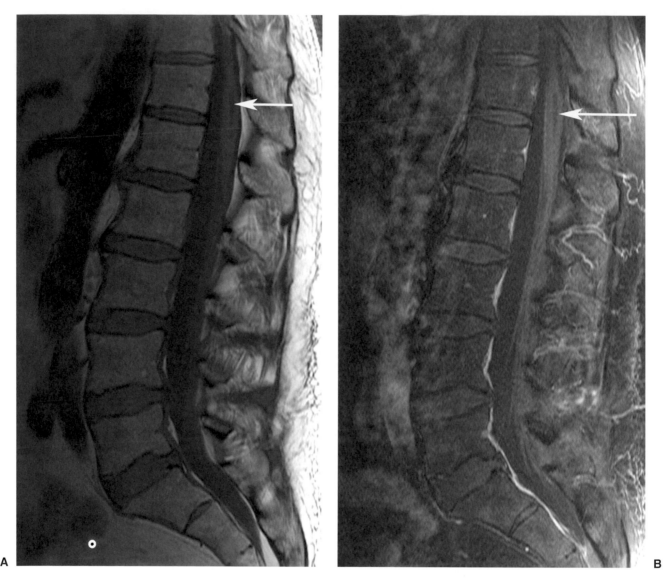

FIGURE 17-13 **Terminal ventricle.** Sagittal T1-weighted images **(A)** before and **(B)** after contrast administration shows a focally dilated distal central canal (*arrows*) that extends below the tip of the conus medullaris into the filum terminale, termed the *terminal ventricle*.

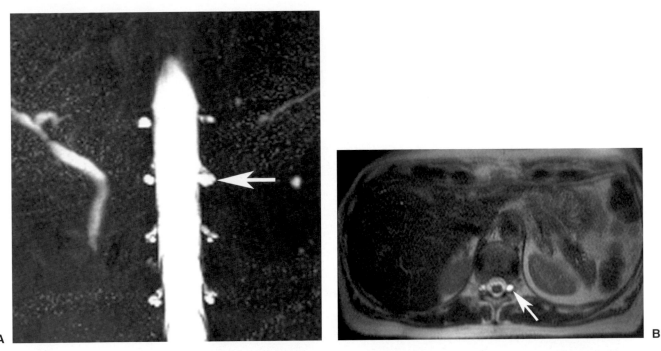

FIGURE 17-14 **Asymmetric nerve sheaths. A:** Coronal maximum intensity projection (MIP) projection of a heavily fluid-sensitive image has a MR myelographic effect. Note the mild asymmetric enlargement of a left upper lumbar nerve sheath (*arrow*) compared with the other levels. **B:** Axial T2-weighted image in the same patient demonstrates the enlarged nerve sheath (*arrow*).

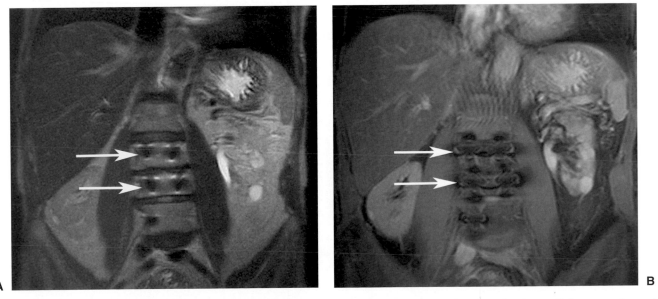

FIGURE 17-15 **Susceptibility artifact created by lumbar pedicle screws. A:** The artifact from lumbar pedicle screws (*arrows*) appears quite focal on the spin-echo coronal image. **B:** On a gradient echo–based image at the same anatomic level, the focal artifacts (*arrows*) fuse into a much larger area of distortion and signal loss.

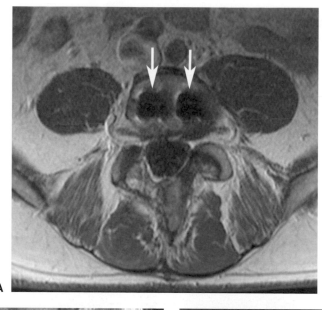

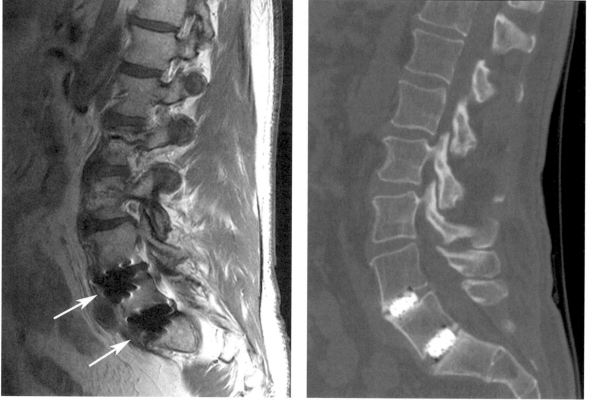

FIGURE 17-16 Lumbar intervertebral disc cages artifact. A: Axial and **(B** and **C)** sagittal T1-weighted images show artifact from intervertebral disc cages (*arrows*) that have been placed to achieve more normal disc heights and stabilization.

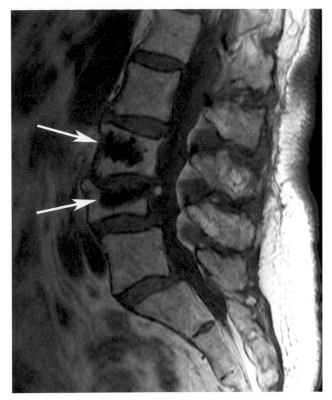

FIGURE 17-17 Vertebroplasty. Sagittal T1-weighted image shows L3 and L4 signal voids (*arrows*) from vertebroplasty cement within nonacute compression fractures. Notice the normal fatty signal within the adjacent vertebrae.

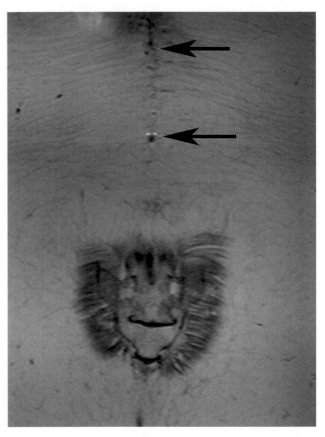

FIGURE 17-18 Skin incision artifact. Coronal image shows minimal artifact (*arrows*) in the skin and subcutaneous tissues after lumbar surgery.

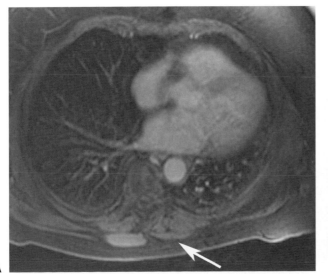

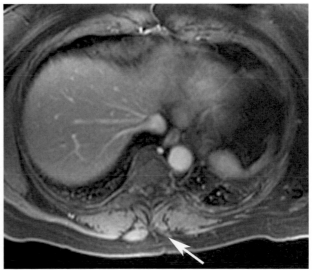

A

B

FIGURE 17-19 Partial absence of the trapezius. A and **B:** Axial images show absence of the inferior portion of the left trapezius (*arrows*), which is a normal variant. A supernumerary right sided trapezius muscle was originally considered.

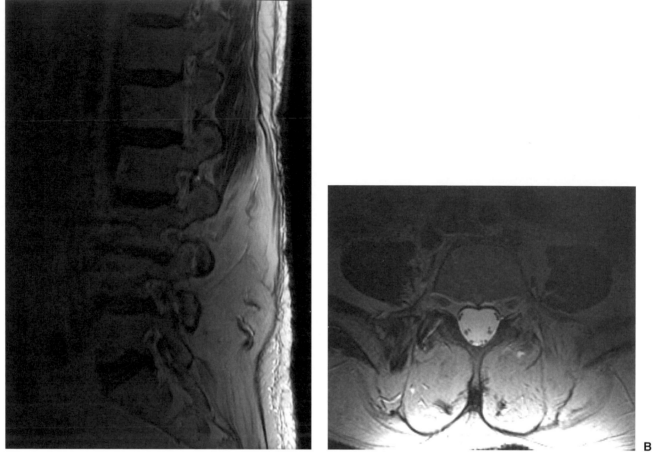

FIGURE 17-20 Paraspinal muscle atrophy. A: Sagittal and **(B)** axial images depict marked atrophy of the lower paraspinal musculature in this patient with long-standing back pain and disuse. Findings should not be misinterpreted as a fatty mass.

Suggested Readings

Lumbar Spine

Bergman RA, Thompson SA, Afifi AK, et al., ed. *Compendium of human anatomic variation*. Baltimore: Urban & Schwarzenberg; 1988.

Chandraraj S, Briggs CA, Opeskin K. Disc herniations in young and end-plate vascularity. *Clin Anat*. 1998;11:171–176.

Christodoulou AG, Apostolou T, Ploumis A, et al. Pedicle dimensions of the thoracic and lumbar vertebrae in the Greek population. *Clin Anat*. 2005;18:404–408.

Griffith JF, Yeung DWK, Antonio GE, et al. Vertebral marrow fat content and diffusion and perfusion indexes in women with varying bone density: MR evaluation. *Radiology*. 2006;241:831–839.

Hauger O, Cotten A, Chateil JF, et al. Giant cystic Schmorl's nodes: Imaging findings in six patients. *AJR Am J Roentgenol*. 2001;176(4):969–972.

Hughes RJ, Saiffusin A. Numbering of lumbosacral transitional vertebrae on MRI: Role of the iliolumbar ligaments. *AJR Am J Roentgenol*. 2006;187:W59–W66.

Kershner DE, Binhammer RT. Lumbar intrathecal ligaments. *Clin Anat*. 2002;15:82–87.

Krueger EC, Perry JO, Wu Y, et al. Changes in T2 relaxation times associated with maturation of the human intervertebral disk. *AJNR Am J Neuroradiol*. 2007;28:1237–1241.

Loughenbury PR, Wadhwani S, Soames RW. The posterior longitudinal ligament and peridural (epidural) membrane. *Clin Anat*. 2006;19:487–492.

MacDonald A, Chatrath P, Spector T, et al. Level of termination of the spinal cord and the dural sac: A magnetic resonance study. *Clin Anat*. 1999;12:149–152.

Medina LS, Al-Orfali M, Zurakowski D, et al. Occult lumbosacral dysraphism in children and young adults: Diagnostic performance of fast screening and conventional MR imaging. *Radiology*. 1999;211:767–771.

Montazei JL, Divine M, Lepage E, et al. Normal spinal bone marrow in adults: Dynamic gadolinium-enhanced MR imaging. *Radiology*. 2003;229:703–709.

Newell RLM. The spinal epidural space. *Clin Anat*. 1999;12:375–379.

Parke WW, Settles HE, Bunger PC, et al. Lumbosacral anterolateral spinal arteries and brief review of "accessory" longitudinal arteries of the spinal cord. *Clin Anat*. 1999;12:171–178.

Petit-Lacour MC, Lasjaunias P, Iffenecker C, et al. Visibility of the central canal on MRI. *Neuroradiology*. 2000;42:756–761.

Pfirrmann CWA, Resnick D. Schmorl nodes of the thoracic and lumbar spine: Radiographic-pathologic study of prevalence, characterization, and correlation with degenerative changes of 1,650 spinal levels in 100 cadavers. *Radiology*. 2001;219:368.

Roberts N, Hogg D, Whitehouse GH, et al. Quantitative analysis of diurnal variation in volume and water content of lumbar intervertebral discs. *Clin Anat*. 1998;11:1–8.

Sonel B, Yalçin P, Ozturk EA, et al. Butterfly vertebra: A case report. *Clin Imaging*. 2001;25(3):206–208.

Wu HTH, Morrison WB, Schweitzer ME. Edematous Schmorl's nodes on thoracolumbar MR imaging: Characteristics patterns and changes over time. *Skeletal Radiol*. 2006;35:212–219.

Miscellaneous

Blachar A, Mahmud T, Arastu M, et al. Distribution of fluid within the peritoneal cavity: A cadaveric study. *Clin Anat*. 2005;18:443–445.

Uppot RN, Sahani DV, Hahn PF, et al. Impact of obesity on medical imaging and image-guided intervention. *AJR Am J Roentgenol*. 2007;188:433–440.

Section V

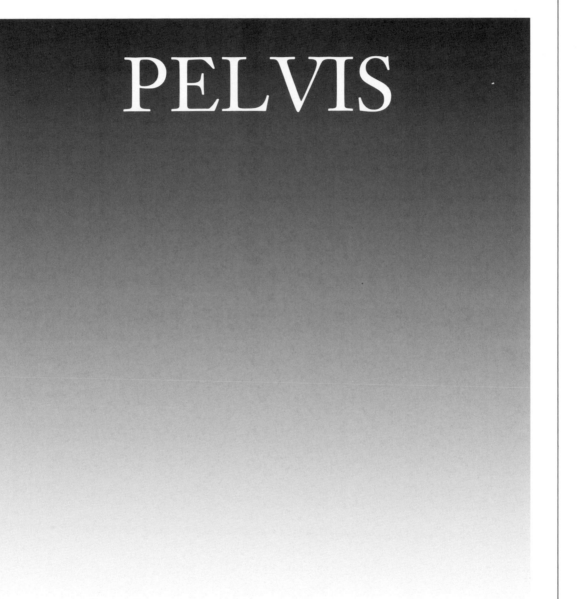

PELVIS

Chapter 18

Female

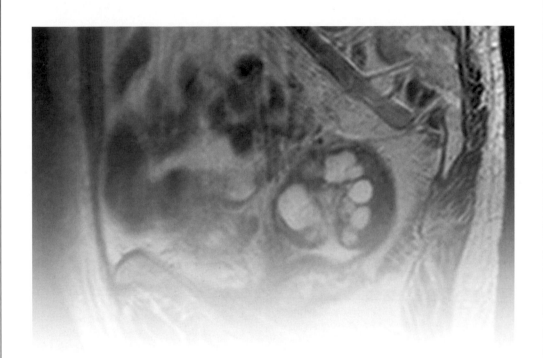

Uterus and Cervix
Ovaries and Adnexa
Vagina and Perineum

Mellena D. Bridges

■ Uterus and Cervix

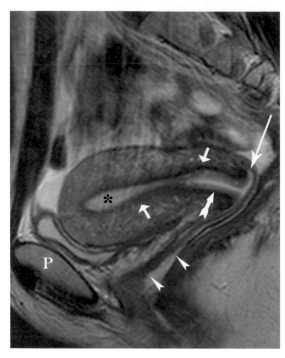

FIGURE 18-1 Normal anteverted uterus on sagittal T2-weighted image. Degree of anteversion will depend on bladder distension. Annotated image shows relatively hyperintense endometrium (*asterisk*) and cervical mucosa (*tailed arrow*). Short arrows show the hypointense inner myometrium, or junctional zone, in continuity with the hypointense fibrous stroma of the cervix (*Posterior vaginal fornix = long arrow, Vagina = arrowheads, Pubic bone = P*).

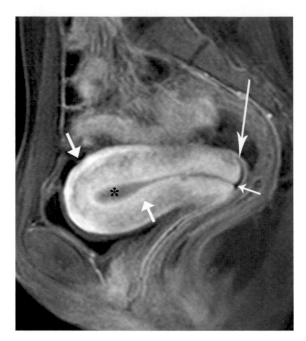

FIGURE 18-2 Normal anteverted uterus on fat-suppressed enhanced T1-weighted image. Notice intense enhancement of the uterine muscle when compared with the endometrium (*asterisk*). Short arrows show the junctional zone and serosal surface of the myometrium (*Posterior vaginal fornix = long arrow, External cervical os = small arrow*).

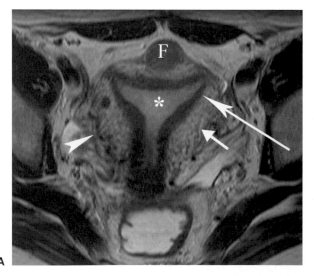

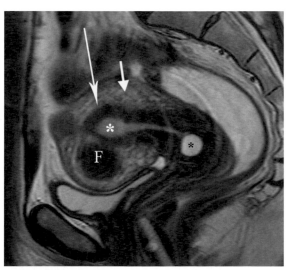

FIGURE 18-3 Anteverted uterus in another woman of child-bearing age. Endometrium (*asterisk*) has typical goblet shape in the axial plane (**A**) and frequently appears thicker toward the fundus in the sagittal plane (**B**). Zonal anatomy well demonstrated on these T2-weighted images, with hypointense junctional zone (*arrow*) and isointense outer myometrium (*short arrow*) (*Arcuate vessels in the outer third = arrowheads, Large nabothian cyst = black asterisk*).

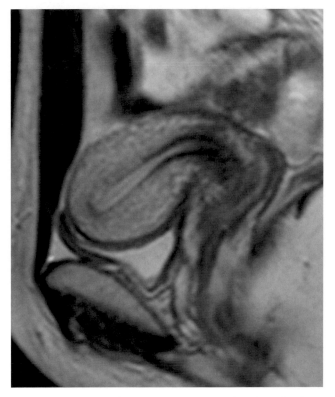

FIGURE 18-4 **Anteflexed uterus** is angulated at the lower uterine segment.

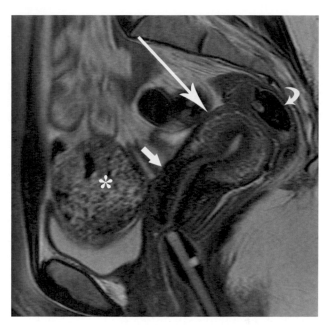

FIGURE 18-5 **Retroverted uterus**, a very common normal variant. Sagittal T2-weighted image shows the "tipped" uterus, with fundus near the rectum (*curved arrow*). Muscle in outer uterus (*arrow*) is arranged more loosely, resulting in higher signal intensity (*Cervix = short arrow, Stool in cecum = asterisk*).

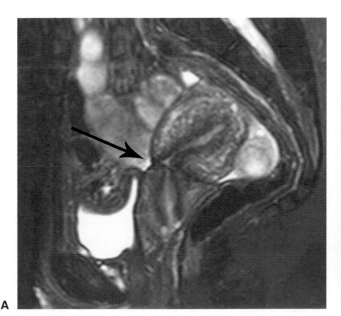

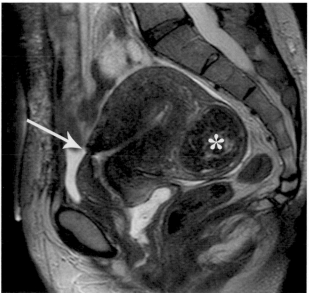

FIGURE 18-6 **Retroflexed uterus** shows angulation at the lower uterine segment, with the fundus directed posteriorly. **A:** Sagittal fat-suppressed T2-weighted image also demonstrates caesarean-section defect (*arrow*). **B:** Non–fat-suppressed image in another patient shows a hypointense fibroid posteriorly (*asterisk*) as well as a caesarean-section defect.

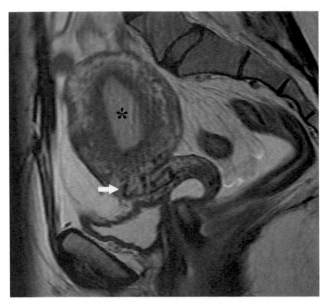

FIGURE 18-7 Anteverted, retroflexed uterus. Midline T2-weighted sagittal slice depicts the endometrium (*asterisk*) and then cuts more obliquely through the off-midline lower uterine segment (*Flow voids of arcuate vessels = arrow*).

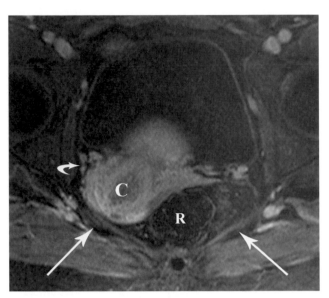

FIGURE 18-8 Uterine and cervical mobility, a potential pitfall. In one of many possible uterine orientations, the cervicovaginal junction lies next to the rectum and against the sacrospinous ligament (*Cervix = C, Rectum = R, Sacrospinous ligaments = arrows, Parametrial vessels = curved arrow*).

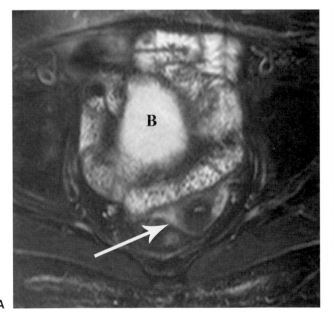

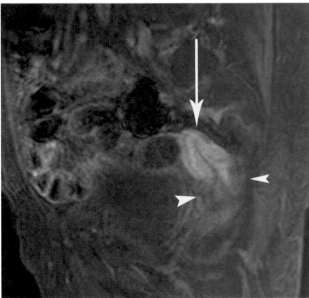

FIGURE 18-9 Uterine mobility results in presacral pseudomass. A and **B:** Uterus (*arrows*) of elderly woman is retroverted and displaced posteriorly by pelvic floor relaxation. **A:** Vestige of lower uterine segment zonal anatomy preserved on axial T2-weighted fat-suppressed (FS) image. **B:** Off-midline sagittal enhanced T1-weighted image shows strong uterine and poor cervical enhancement (*arrowheads*) in this small, fibrotic organ (*Bladder = B*).

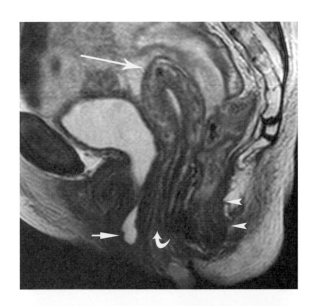

FIGURE 18-10 Uterine prolapse, Stage II. Unexpected position of pelvic organs can create pitfalls, and is a common problem among women with pelvic floor defects or relaxation. Mid-sagittal T2-weighted image demonstrates uterine fundus (*arrow*) posterior to the bladder. The exocervix (*curved arrow*) is located within the lower vagina (*Cystocele = short arrow, Hypointense anal sphincter = arrowheads*).

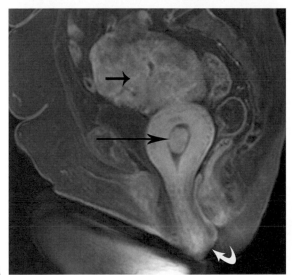

A

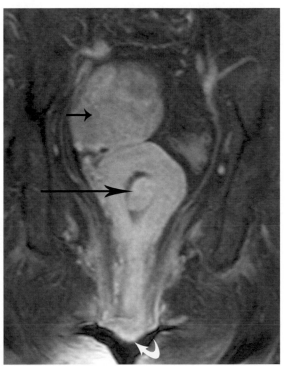

B

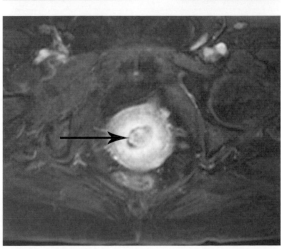

C

FIGURE 18-11 Uterine prolapse, Stage III. A, B, and **C:** Sagittal, coronal, and axial images from enhanced T1-weighted acquisition shows cervix beyond the introitus (*curved arrow*) in this symptomatic woman (*Submucosal fibroid = arrow, Brenner tumor right ovary = short arrow*).

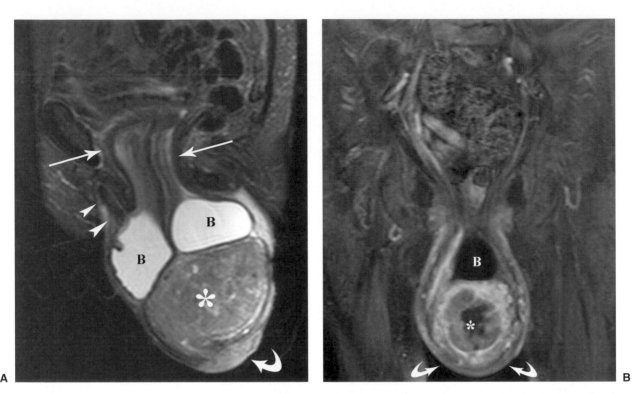

FIGURE 18-12 Uterine prolapse, Stage IV, or procidentia. A: Sagittal T2-weighted image and **(B)** coronal enhanced T1-weighted image, both with fat suppression, show intussuscepted uterus in this patient with irreducible prolapse and endometrial carcinoma (*asterisk*) (*Effaced cervix = curved arrow, Doubled vaginal wall = arrow, Trapped bladder = B, Urethra rotated 180 degrees from normal = arrowhead*).

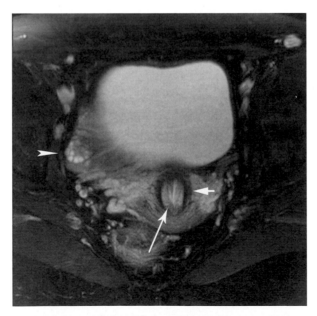

FIGURE 18-13   Normal zonal anatomy of the cervix is well demonstrated in an axial T2-weighted fat-suppressed image. Notice clear distinction between hyperintense mucosa (*arrow*) and hypointense fibromuscular stroma (*short arrow*), which is of variable thickness, depending on age (*Ovary = arrowhead*).

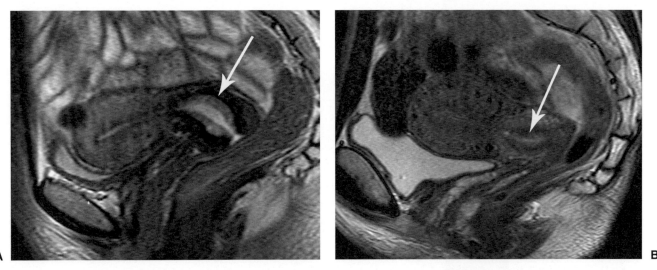

FIGURE 18-14   Normal variants in appearance of cervical mucosa and fibromuscular stroma. A and B: Depending on age and hormonal status, cervical mucosa (*arrows*) is variable in thickness and luminal secretions. The fibromuscular stroma of the cervical wall can vary from a markedly prominent and hypointense appearance, to ill defined and relatively thin, to atrophic and hypointense.

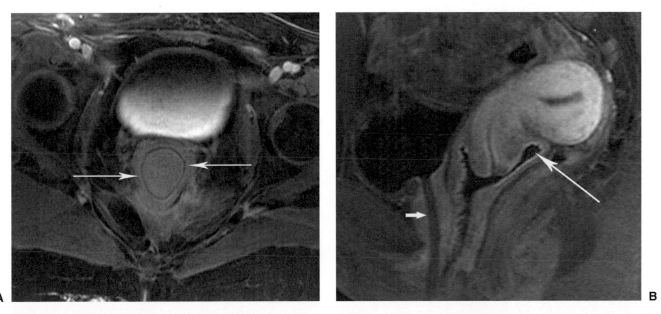

FIGURE 18-15   Cervix simulates a vaginal mass. A: Axial contrast-enhanced image demonstrates the exocervix surrounded by the vaginal fornices (*arrows*). **B:** Coronal plane confirms the position of the cervix (*Urethral catheter = short arrow*).

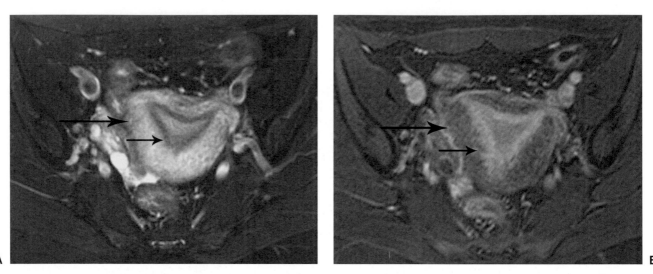

FIGURE 18-16 **Hormonal effects on uterus at mid-cycle. A:** Axial T2-weighted and **(B)** axial contrast-enhanced T1-weighted images, both with fat suppression, depict normal well-hydrated myometrium (*arrow*) along with distinct, enhancing junctional zone (*short arrow*).

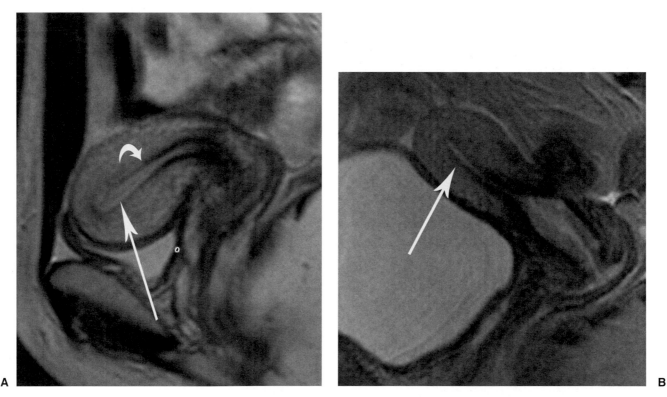

FIGURE 18-17 **Oral contraceptive effects on uterus** include thin endometrium and poorly demonstrated uterine zonal anatomy. **A** and **B:** Sagittal T2-weighted images show narrow endometrial stripe (*arrow*) and loss of hypointense junctional zone (*curved arrow*).

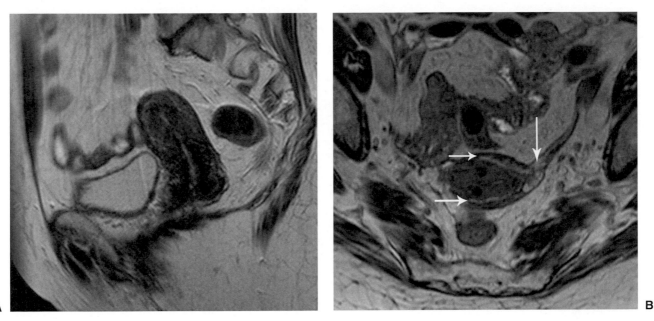

FIGURE 18-18 **Age-related changes in the uterus** include atrophy and thinning of the endometrium. **A:** Sagittal T2-weighted image shows small, low signal intensity organ. **B:** Axial T2-weighted image through the atrophic fundus of another patient with typical, relatively prominent uterine vessels. These enter through the broad ligament to traverse the outer myometrium as arcuate vessels (*arrows*).

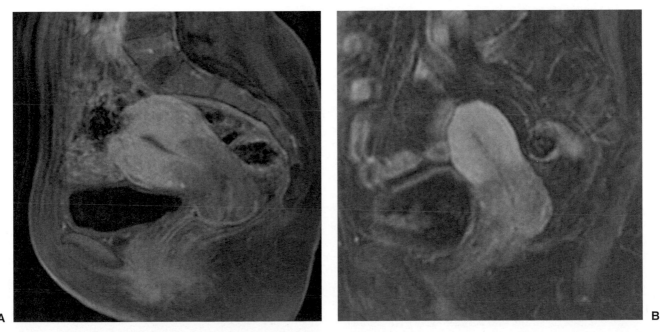

FIGURE 18-19 **Abrupt change in enhancement at the lower uterine segment, a common variant appearance, simulates an infiltrating cervical mass.** This pattern clearly differentiates corpus from cervix. Enhanced sagittal T1-weighted images in, respectively, a 22-year-old **(A)**, a 48-year-old **(B)**. Notice progressive decrease in size of the corpus relative to the cervix as the patients age.

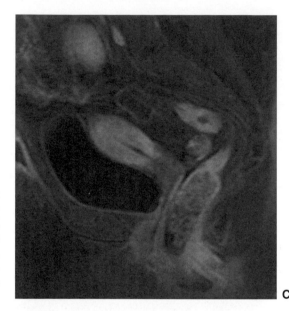

C

FIGURE 18-19 Abrupt change in enhancement at the lower uterine segment, a common variant appearance, simulates an infiltrating cervical mass. (*continued*) This pattern clearly differentiates corpus from cervix. Enhanced sagittal T1-weighted images in a 75-year-old (**C**). Notice progressive decrease in size of the corpus relative to the cervix as the patients age.

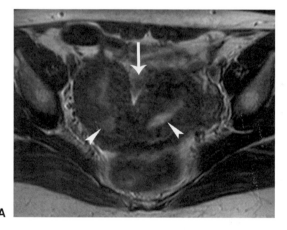

A

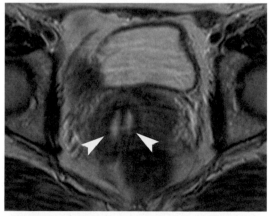

B

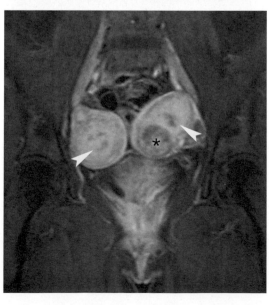

C

FIGURE 18-20 Bicornuate uterus, another Müllerian anomaly. **A:** Axial T2-weighted image demonstrates a definite fundal cleft (*arrow*), required for distinction between bicornuate and septate uterus. Paired endometrial cavities are well seen (*arrowheads*). **B:** Axial image obtained more inferiorly shows paired endocervical canals (*arrowheads*), defining this as bicornuate bicollis. **C:** Coronal enhanced T1-weighted image shows the two separate horns in this fibroid (*asterisk*) uterus.

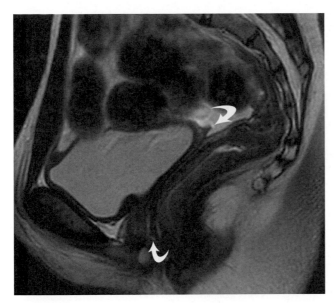

FIGURE 18-21 **Uterine and cervical agenesis** in a 15-year-old girl with primary amenorrhea. Early failure in Müllerian duct development results in varying combinations of uterine, cervical and upper vaginal agenesis/hypoplasia. Sagittal T2-weighted image shows abrupt termination of the hypoplastic vagina (*curved arrow*). Neither cervix nor uterus are discernible.

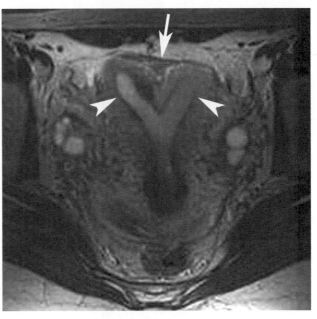

FIGURE 18-22 **Subseptate uterus.** In this case, the septum involves only the fundus, but the cornua are slightly more splayed (*arrowheads*).

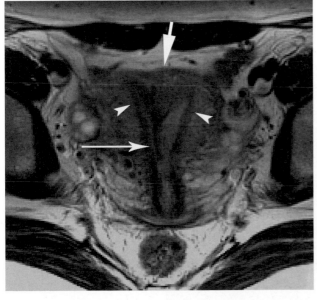

A

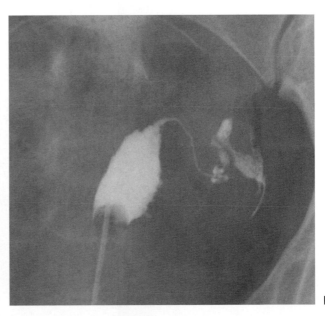

B

FIGURE 18-23 **Septate uterus. A:** Absence of a significant fundal cleft (*short arrow*) is diagnostic of septate uterus. In this example, the lower septum is thin and fibrous (*arrow*) and the cornua are barely splayed (*arrowheads*). **B:** Correlative hysterosalpingogram was interpreted as a unicornuate uterus, due to failure to fill to the right of the septum.

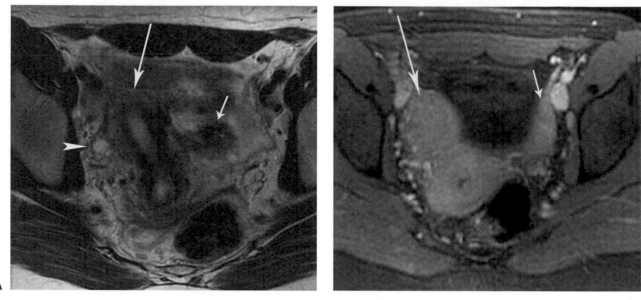

FIGURE 18-24 **Unicornuate uterus with rudimentary horn.** **A:** Axial T2-weighted image reveals well-developed right horn (*arrow*) with hyperintense endometrium and a normal right ovary (*arrowhead*). The small, abnormal left horn is a potential pseudomass and occurs in more than half the cases of unicornuate uterus. **B:** Axial enhanced image at a slightly different level also shows the two horns, both of which enhance avidly.

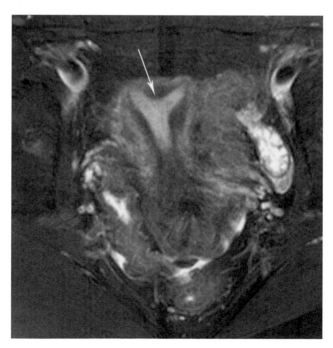

FIGURE 18-25 **Arcuate uterus, a common variant.** Axial fat-suppressed T2-weighted image shows an indentation (*arrow*) in the fundal endometrium, but a normal serosal fundal surface.

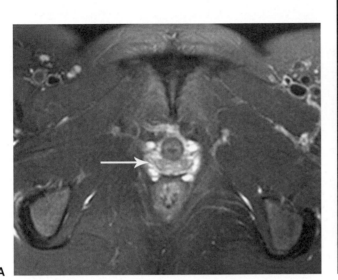

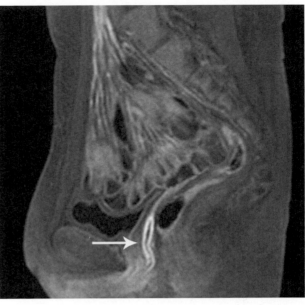

FIGURE 18-26   Testicular feminization in a young woman with primary amenorrhea. A: Axial fat-suppressed image shows ill-defined vaginal tissue (*arrow*) between urethra and anorectum. **B:** Mucosa of rudimentary distal vagina (*arrow*) enhances strongly in this sagittal T1-weighted fat-suppressed image. As would be expected, ovaries, uterus, cervix, and upper vagina are absent.

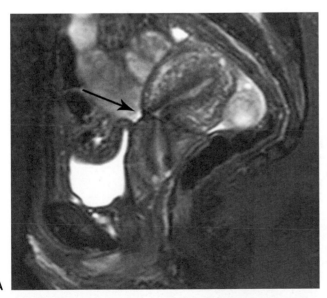

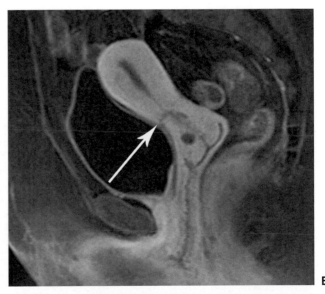

FIGURE 18-27   Caesarean-section defect in the lower uterine segment. A: Sagittal T2-weighted and **(B)** enhanced T1-weighted images demonstrate typical appearances of the low transverse incision scar (*arrows*). Notice the focal tissue thinning, reduced signal intensity, and reduced enhancement.

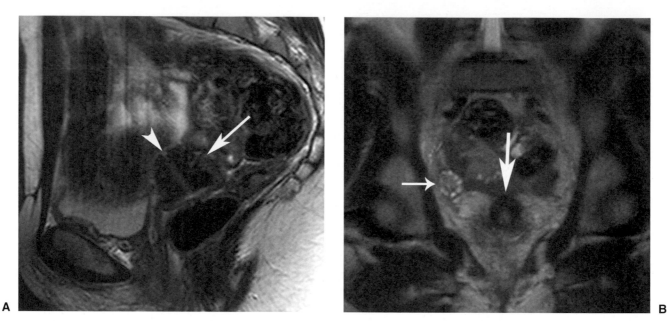

FIGURE 18-28 **Appearance after supracervical hysterectomy** can simulate a pelvic mass, especially in populations where complete hysterectomy is more the norm. **A** and **B:** Sagittal and coronal T2-weighted image demonstrates abrupt truncation of the cervical remnant (*Right ovary = small arrow, Cervical canal = arrowhead*).

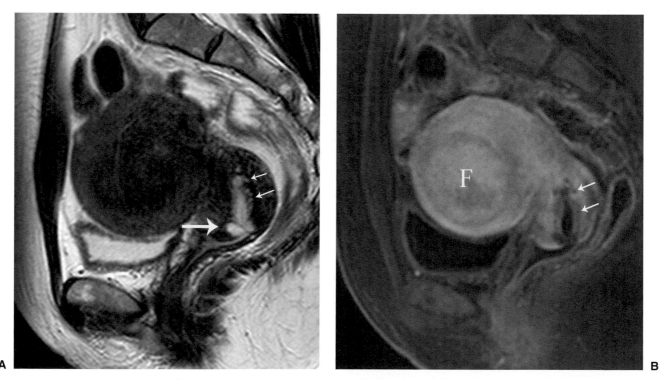

FIGURE 18-29 **Nabothian cysts of the cervix can be single or multiple,** and can simulate neoplasia. **A:** Sagittal T2-weighted image demonstrates a cervical canal lined with tiny cysts (*small arrows*) from the external to the internal os. Note the larger cyst (*arrow*) near the anterior margin external os. **B:** Sagittal enhanced T1-weighted image with fat suppression (*Uterine fibroid = F*).

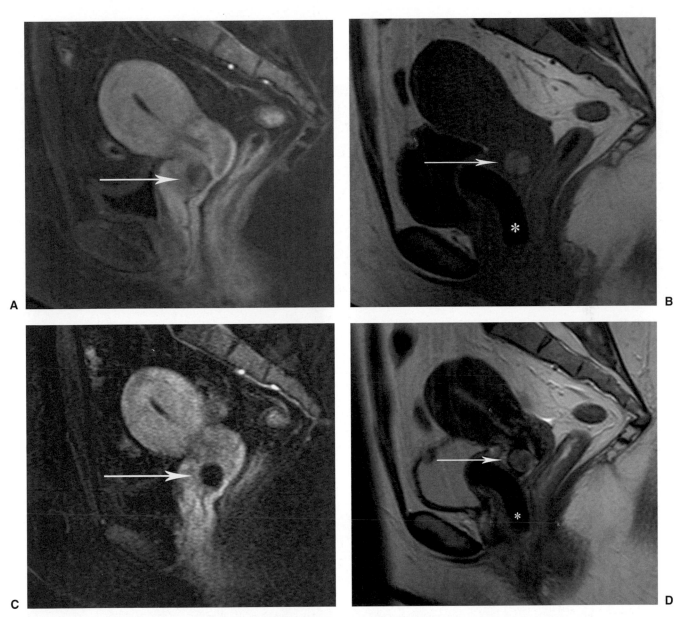

FIGURE 18-30 **Complicated Nabothian cyst simulates cervical mass. A:** Midline sagittal enhanced T1-weighted image with fat suppression suggests a hypoenhancing mass in the lower anterior cervix (*arrow*). **B:** Unenhanced T1-weighted image reveals high-signal material in the lesion, consistent with blood products/proteinaceous material. **C:** Subtraction image confirms lack of enhancement, consistent with a complicated cyst. **D:** Notice the vaginal tampon (*asterisk*) on this T2-weighted image (and in image B), which was removed before the enhanced sequences.

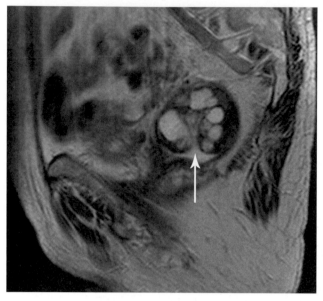

FIGURE 18-31 **Large cervical nabothian cysts** in a supra-cervical hysterectomy remnant. Finding had been interpreted as an ovarian mass on prior CT (*External os = arrow*).

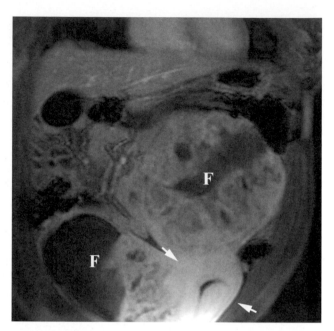

FIGURE 18-32 **Large exophytic leiomyoma simulates an abdominal mass.** Coronal enhanced image of the abdomen and upper pelvis demonstrates two partially degenerated fibroids (*F*) arising from a uterus (*arrows*) which is displaced out of the pelvis by other fibroids.

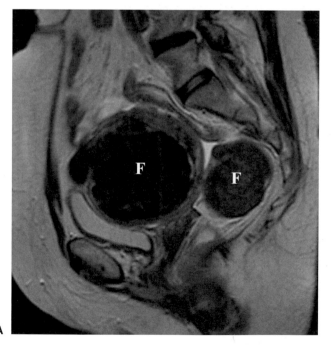

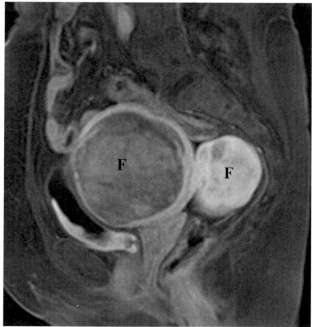

FIGURE 18-33 **Wide spectrum of fibroid imaging appearances can complicate diagnosis. A:** T2-weighted sagittal image shows a profoundly hypointense myometrial mass as well as a more posterior, more mildly hypointense exophytic mass. Both are fibroids (*F*). **B:** T1 appearance of same lesions following contrast administration shows one enhancing only moderately, but the other very intensely (*Fibroids = F*).

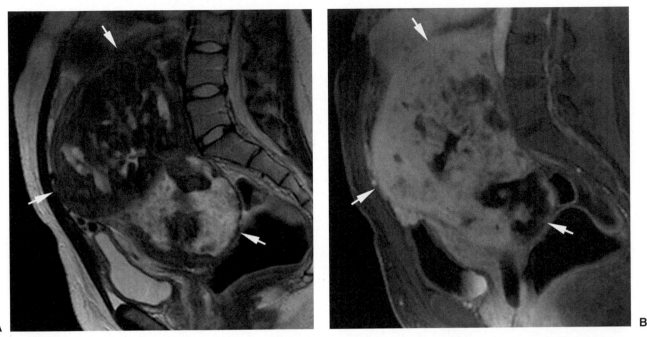

FIGURE 18-34 **Large, partially degenerated fibroid simulates sarcoma or extrauterine mass. A** and **B:** Sagittal T2-weighted and enhanced images reveal a strikingly heterogenous pelvic mass (*arrows*). Very low T2 signal intensity preserved in viable areas, as is strong enhancement, consistent with degenerated leiomyoma.

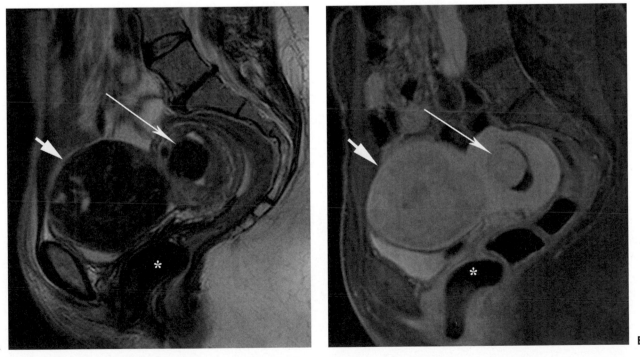

FIGURE 18-35 **Exophytic subserosal and submucosal leiomyomas mimic extrauterine and endometrial masses. A** and **B:** T2-weighted and enhanced sagittal images demonstrate large, T2-hypointense, avidly enhancing exophytic (*short arrow*) and intracavitary (*long arrow*) fibroids. Multiplanar imaging is essential for establishing origin of these lesions (*Tampon in vagina =* *asterisk*).

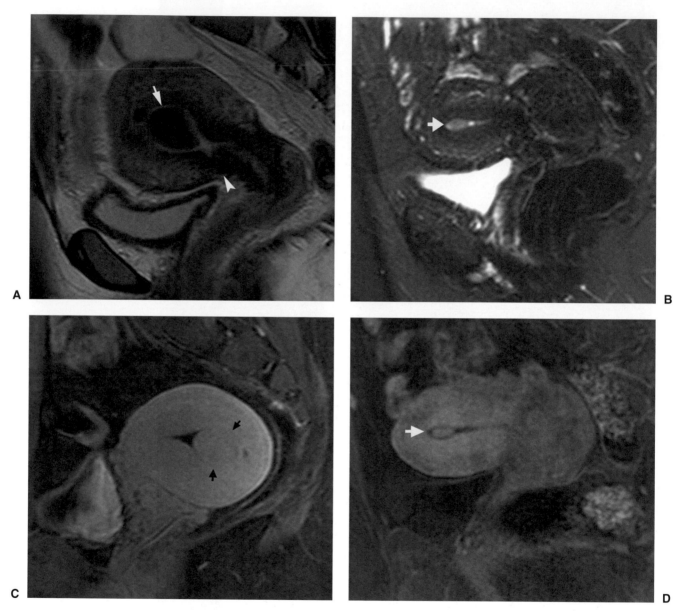

FIGURE 18-36 **Submucosal leiomyoma can be mistaken for endometrial polyp.** Sagittal T2-weighted images demonstrate two well-defined intracavitary masses (*arrows*). The leiomyoma in (**A**) has much lower signal intensity than the polyp in (**B**) (*caesarian-section scar = arrowhead*). Similarly, sagittal enhanced images show more intense enhancement in the fibroid (**C**) than in the polyp (**D**).

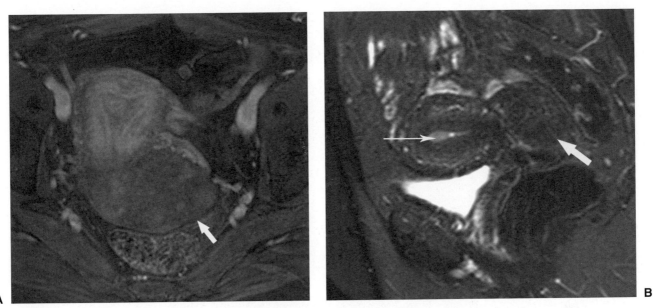

FIGURE 18-37   Cervical fibroid simulates an infiltrating mass. A: Axial T1-weighted enhanced image shows cervical enlargement and heterogeneity (*short arrow*). **B:** Sagittal T2-weighted image reveals mass to be quite hypointense, consistent with leiomyoma (*Endometrial polyp = long arrow*).

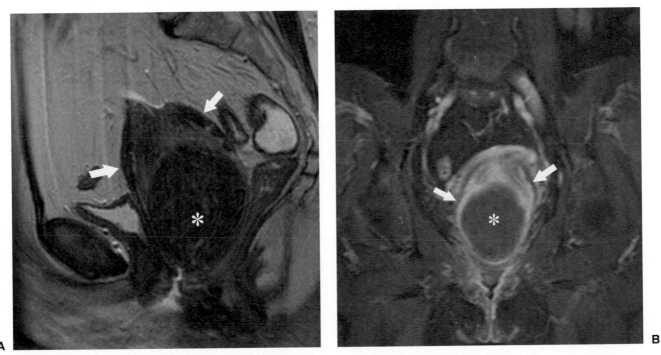

FIGURE 18-38   Intussuscepting submucosal fibroid simulates a cervical mass. A: Sagittal T2-weighted image demonstrates a large lesion (*asterisk*) filling and distending the cervix (*small arrows*). **B:** Coronal enhanced T1-weighted image and later subtractions prove the fibroid to be necrotic.

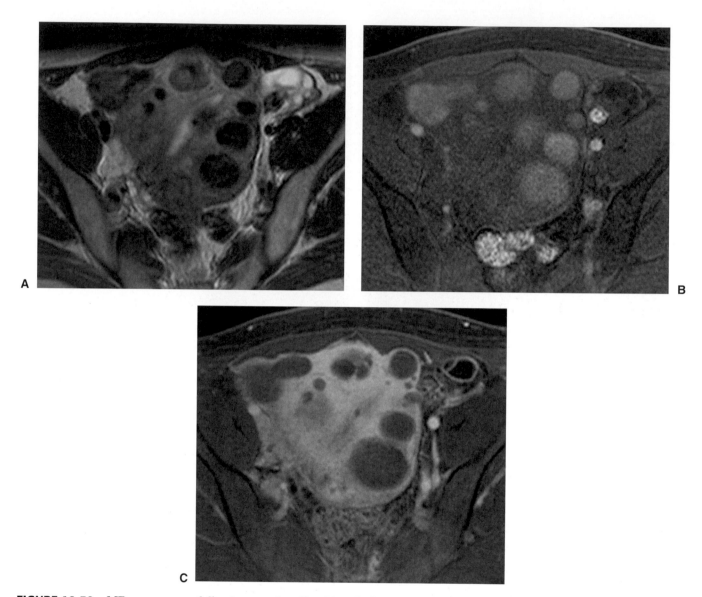

FIGURE 18-39 MR appearance following uterine fibroid embolization. **A:** Axial T2-weighted image demonstrates multiple typically hypointense fibroids. **B:** However, these are hyperintense with fat-suppressed T1-weighting, consistent with hemorrhagic necrosis. **C:** Necrosis confirmed by lack of enhancement following contrast administration. Pregnancy- or hormone-induced necrosis has the same appearance.

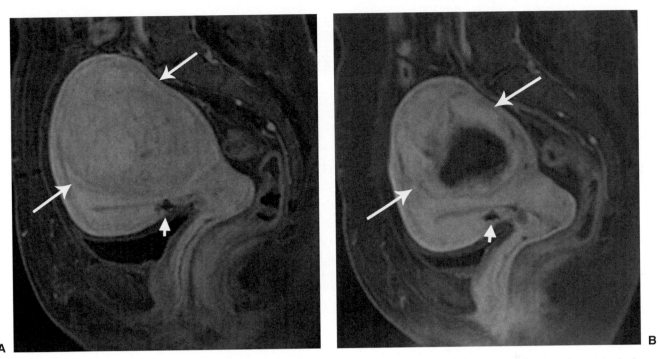

FIGURE 18-40 **Partial response to uterine fibroid embolization. A:** Preprocedure sagittal-enhanced image shows single, large, intensely enhancing leimyoma (*arrows*). **B:** Nine months later, the fibroid is smaller, but with sizable regions of viable tissue. These can regrow (*caesarian-section defect = small arrow*).

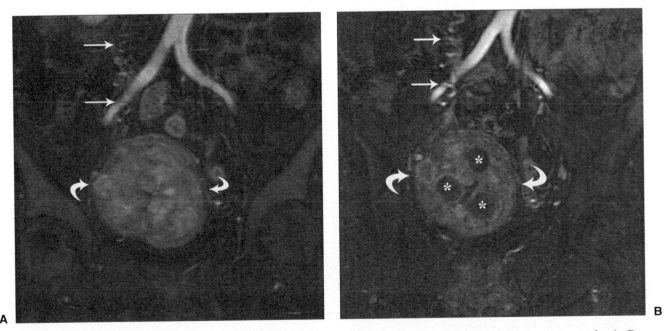

FIGURE 18-41 **Partial fibroid response to uterine artery embolization** due to prominent ovarian artery supply. **A:** Preembolization and **(B)** postembolization coronal T1-weighted images obtained in the arterial phase show an enlarged right ovarian artery (*arrows*). Following treatment, only small portions of the confluent fibroids are necrotic (*asterisk*).

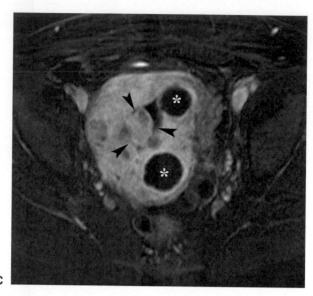

FIGURE 18-41 Partial fibroid response to uterine artery embolization due to prominent ovarian artery supply. (*continued*) **C:** Subtraction image confirms necrosis in some fibroids (*asterisk*), but not the intracavitary submucosal tumor (*arrowheads*) or other lesions in the right uterus.

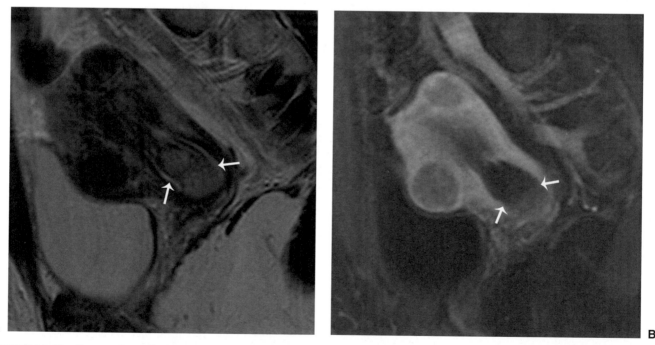

FIGURE 18-42 Incomplete abortion simulates cervical mass. A: T2-isointense material (*arrows*) fills and distends the cervical canal. **B:** Sagittal enhanced image demonstrates poor enhancement, consistent with necrotic products of conception and/or clot (*arrows*). Notice that the low-signal intensity inner cervical wall is preserved, if stretched.

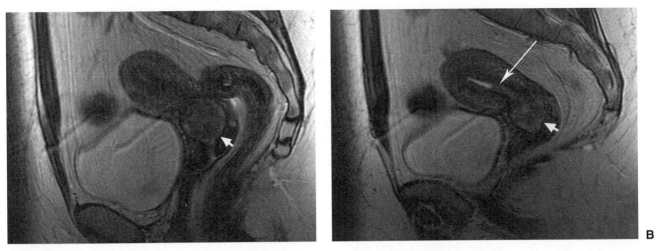

FIGURE 18-43 Endometrial polyp simulates a cervical mass. A: Isointense, mass (*short arrow*) distends the central cervix in this sagittal T2-weighted image. **B:** The next slice shows the telltale stalk (*long arrow*) of the pedunculated polyp (*short arrow*), which has prolapsed into the cervical canal.

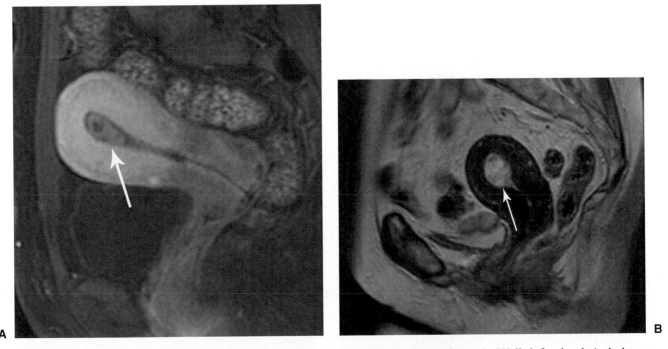

FIGURE 18-44 Endometrial polyp or hyperplasia can simulate endometrial neoplasia. A: Well-defined, relatively hypoenhancing, intracavitary polyp (*arrow*). Patient was receiving hormone replacement therapy. **B:** High T2-signal intensity hyperplastic material distends the endometrial cavity, with sparing of the hypointense inner myometrium. Patient was receiving tamoxifen therapy. Note that endometrial biopsy is often required to distinguish between hyperplasia and stage 1A endometrial carcinoma.

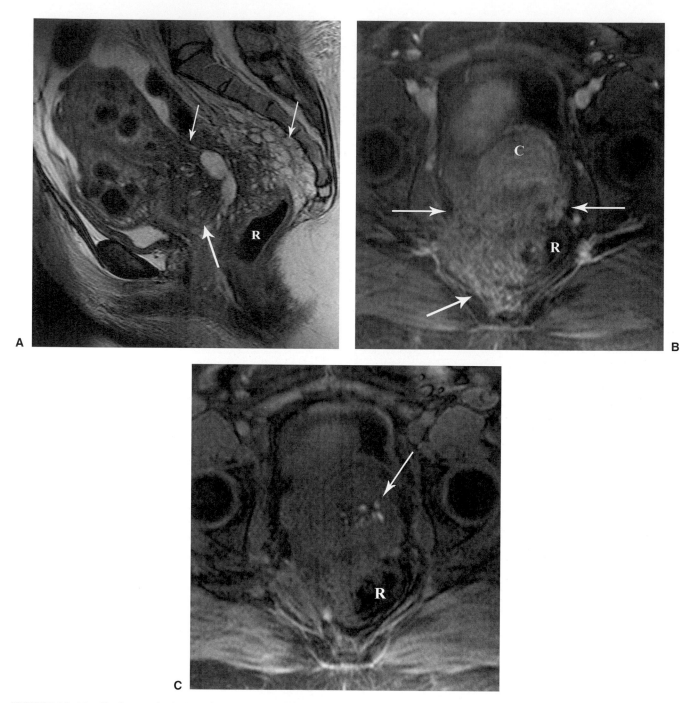

FIGURE 18-45 Endometriosis invades cervix and simulates infiltrating tumor. **A:** Sagittal T2-weighted image shows enlarged fibroid uterus with a bulky, heterogeneous posterior cervix. **B:** Infiltrating mass involves cervix, rectum and parametria. **C:** Unenhanced fat-suppressed T1-weighted image reveals a collection of hyperintense, hemorrhagic foci in the bulky tissue, a good clue to the diagnosis (*Invasive endometriosis = arrows, Rectum = R, Cervix = C*).

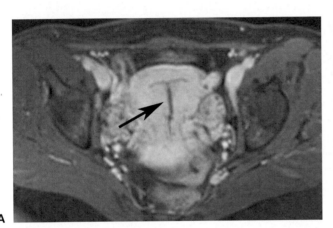

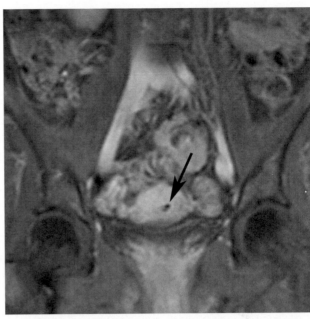

FIGURE 18-46 **Intrauterine device (IUD) fills the endometrial cavity.** **A** and **B**: Axial and coronal enhanced T1-weighted images reveal a clearly-defined, T-shaped signal void (*arrow*), too clearly defined and too poorly enhancing to be endometrium.

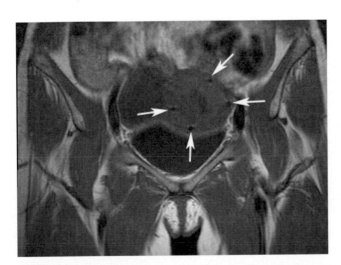

FIGURE 18-47 **Punctate myometrial signal voids are evidence of this patient's prior multiple myomectomies.** Tiny flecks of metal or other surgical hardware create foci of susceptibility (*arrows*).

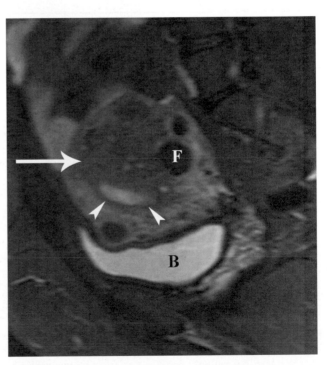

FIGURE 18-48 **Focal adenomyosis.** T2-weighted fat suppressed technique reveals a low signal intensity, poorly marginated uterine mass (*arrow*) indistinguishable from the junctional zone. Unlike a fibroid, it is poorly marginated, and contains tiny cystic foci (*arrowheads*) representing the ectopic basal endometrial tissue (*Fibroid = F, Bladder = B*).

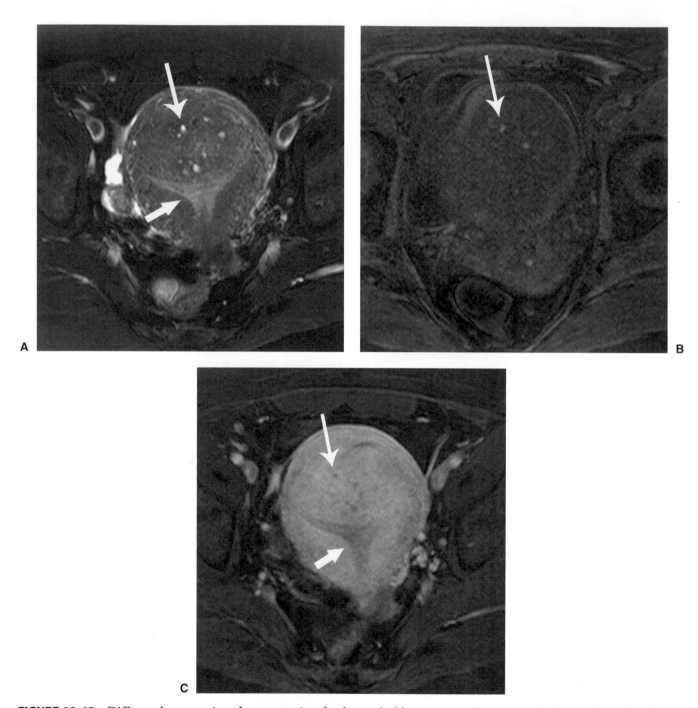

FIGURE 18-49 Diffuse adenomyosis enlarges uterine fundus and obliterates zonal anatomy. A: Axial T2-weighted image with fat suppression confirms low T2 signal intensity with scattered cystic foci (*arrow*) (*Endometrium = short arrow*). **B:** These tiny foci are relatively hyperintense on the correlative unenhanced T1-weighted image, consistent with hemorrhagic contents. **C:** Following contrast administration, the lesion enhances intensely, but is poorly delineated from surrounding myometrium.

Ovaries and Adnexa

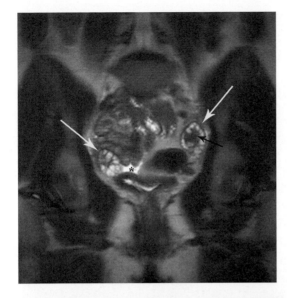

FIGURE 18-50 **Normal ovaries** (*white arrows*) on a coronal single-shot T2-weighted image. Confident identification of the ovary is facilitated by the multiple, primarily peripheral fluid-containing follicles surrounding a more central stroma (*black arrow*) (*Free fluid = asterisk*).

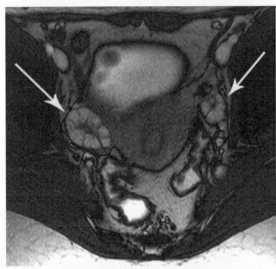

A

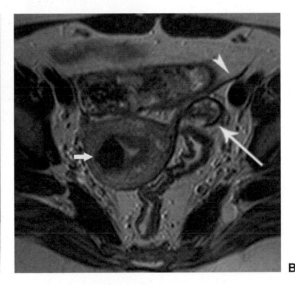

B

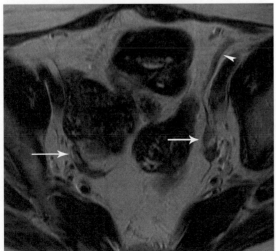

C

FIGURE 18-51 **Age-related changes in normal ovaries. A:** Axial fluid-sensitive steady-state free precession image in a 20-year-old shows normally prominent ovaries (*arrows*) with multiple peripheral follicles. **B:** Axial T2-weighted image in a perimenopausal woman shows decrease in ovarian (*long arrow*) and follicular size (*Submucosal fibroid = short arrow, Round ligament = arrowhead*). **C:** Axial T2-weighted image in an elderly woman demonstrates small, fusiform ovaries (*arrows*) without discernible follicles (*Round ligament = arrowheads*).

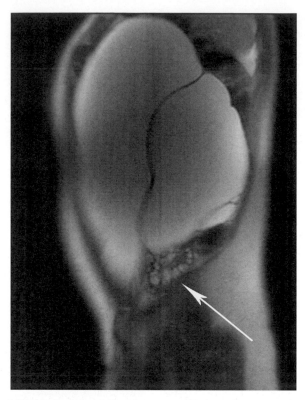

FIGURE 18-52 **T2-hyperintense follicles** facilitate identification of the ovary (*arrow*) at the inferior margin of a large serous cystadenoma.

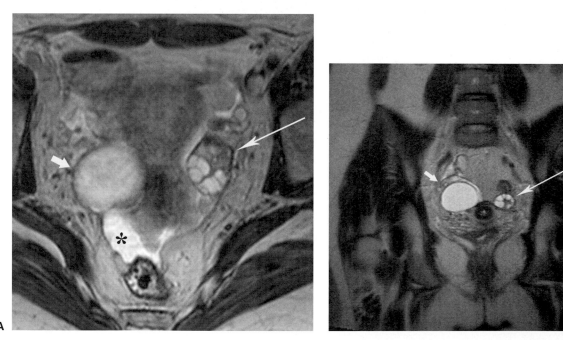

FIGURE 18-53 **Functional ovarian cyst. A:** Axial T2-weighted image in a premenopausal woman shows a normal left ovary (*long arrow*) and a volume-averaged functional right ovarian cyst (*short arrow*) (*Physiologic free fluid = asterisk*). **B:** Coronal projection more clearly depicts the right ovary draped over the high signal intensity cyst (*short arrow*) (*Left Ovary = long arrow*).

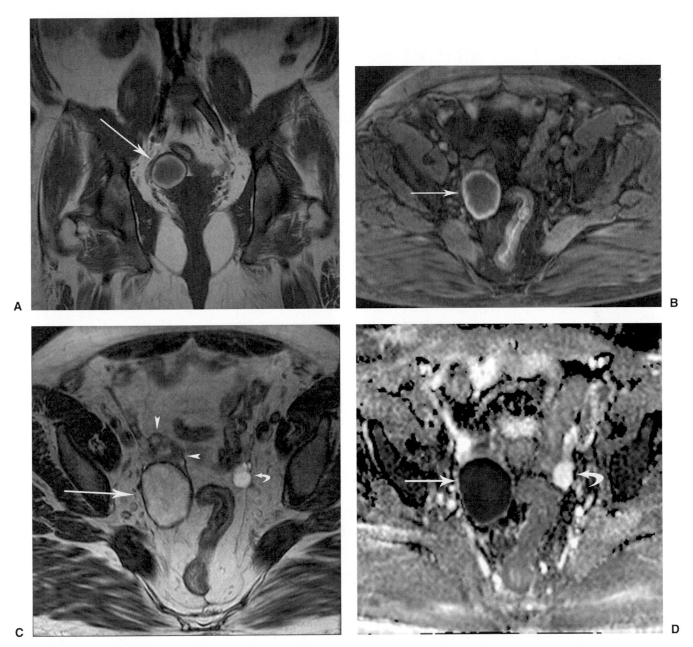

FIGURE 18-54 Hemorrhagic functional ovarian cyst. A: Coronal T1-weighted image shows a round mass with hyperintense rim (*arrow*). **B:** Axial fat-suppressed T1-weighted image confirms absence of fat and presence of intracystic hemorrhage, with characteristic hyperintense rim (*arrow*) and internal fading margin. **C:** Axial T2-weighted image demonstrates mild hypointensity and heterogeneity of the cyst (*long arrow*) within the right ovary (*arrowheads*), compared with simple cyst in left ovary (*curved arrow*) (*Ovarian tissue = arrowheads*). **D:** Diffusion-weighted apparent diffusion coefficient (ADC) map shows profound diffusion restriction in the cyst (*arrow*).

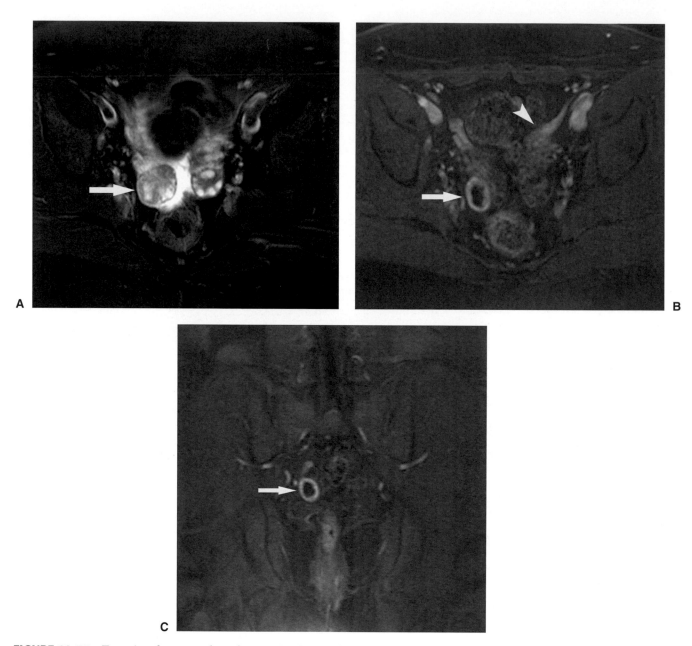

FIGURE 18-55 Functional corpus luteal cyst. A: Corpus luteal cyst (*arrow*) simulates an ill-defined intraovarian mass on T2-weighted axial imaging. **B:** Axial and **(C)** coronal T1-weighted, fat-suppressed, contrast-enhanced images show characteristic intense enhancement of the thick, often crenellated wall of the corpus luteum (*arrows*).

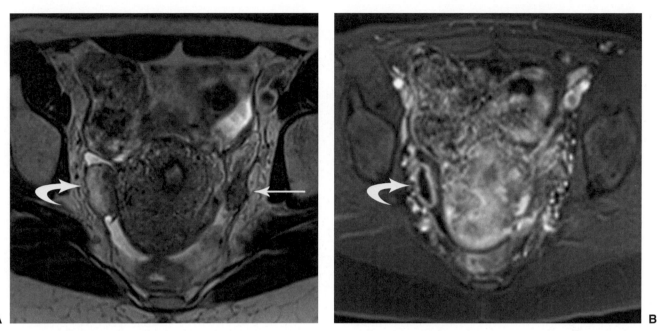

FIGURE 18-56 **Corpus luteal cyst enlarges right ovary. A:** Axial T2-weighted image shows enlargement and inhomogeneity of the right ovary (*curved arrow*) (*Left ovary = long arrow*). **B:** Correlative enhanced T1-weighted image clearly shows the underlying corpus luteum (*curved arrow*), with its thick, enhancing wall.

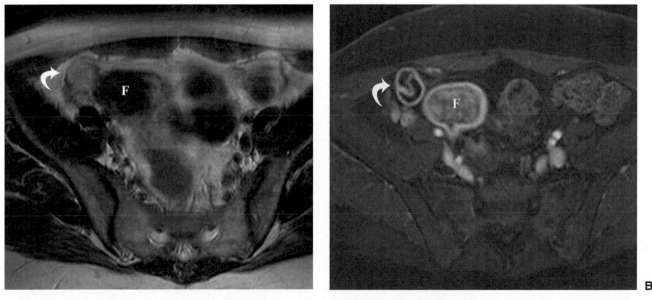

FIGURE 18-57 **Corpus luteal cyst simulates pelvic mass** in anteriorly positioned right ovary. **A:** T2-weighted image shows rounded, vaguely hyperintense lesion (*curved arrow*) anterior to the right psoas muscle (*Fibroid = F*). **B:** Correlative enhanced image shows mural enhancement typical of a corpus luteum (*curved arrow*), but with an apparently double wall.

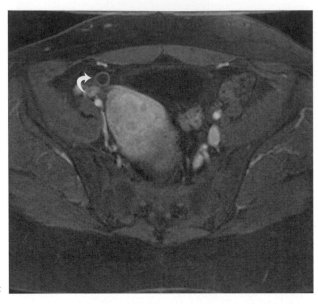

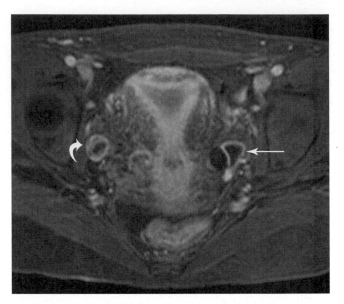

C

FIGURE 18-57 **Corpus luteal cyst simulates pelvic mass** in anteriorly positioned right ovary. (*continued*) **C:** Enhanced image obtained one month later shows typical resolution behavior of the cyst (*curved arrow*).

FIGURE 18-58 **Bilateral corpus luteal cysts.** Enhanced axial T1-weighted image demonstrates a thick-walled corpus luteum in the right ovary (*curved arrow*) and a thin-walled, presumably older corpus luteum in the left ovary (*long arrow*). Notice edematous myometrium and thickened endometrium, consistent with the luteal (secretory phase) of the menstrual cycle.

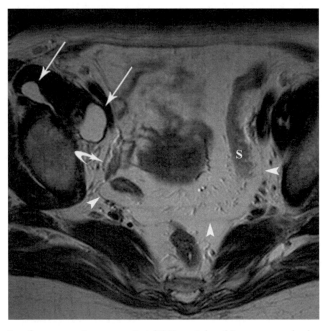

FIGURE 18-59 **Paralabral cyst simulates ovarian cyst.** Axial T2-weighted image reveals the intact right ovary (*curved arrow*) in close proximity to the medial component of a bilobed paralabral cyst (*arrows*) (*Sigmoid colon = S, Sigmoid mesocolon = arrowheads*).

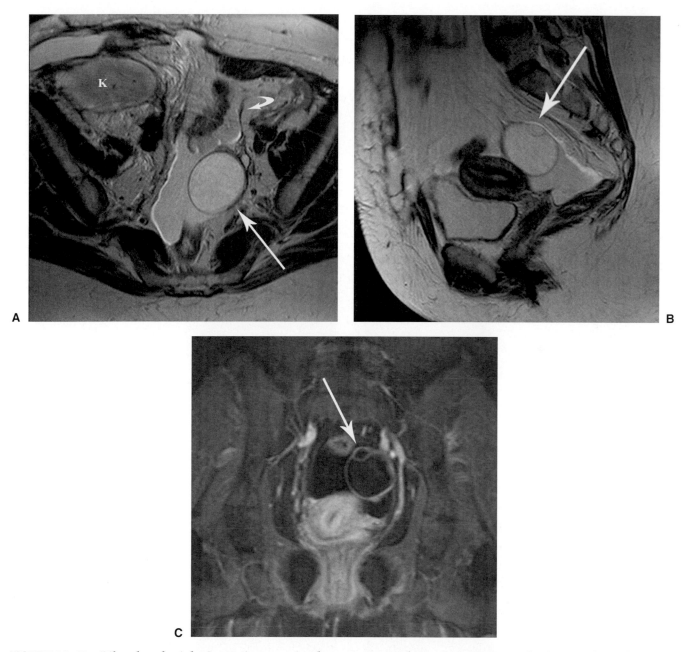

FIGURE 18-60 **Bilocular physiologic ovarian cyst simulates cystic neoplasm. A:** Axial T2-weighted image shows the typical thin-walled appearance of a physiologic ovarian cyst (*arrow*). Notice round ligament (*curved arrow*) leading to the ovary and the recent renal transplant (*K*). **B:** Sagittal T2-weighted and **(C)** coronal-enhanced images reveal a smaller cyst (*arrow*) at the upper margin of the larger cyst. On follow-up imaging, both had resolved.

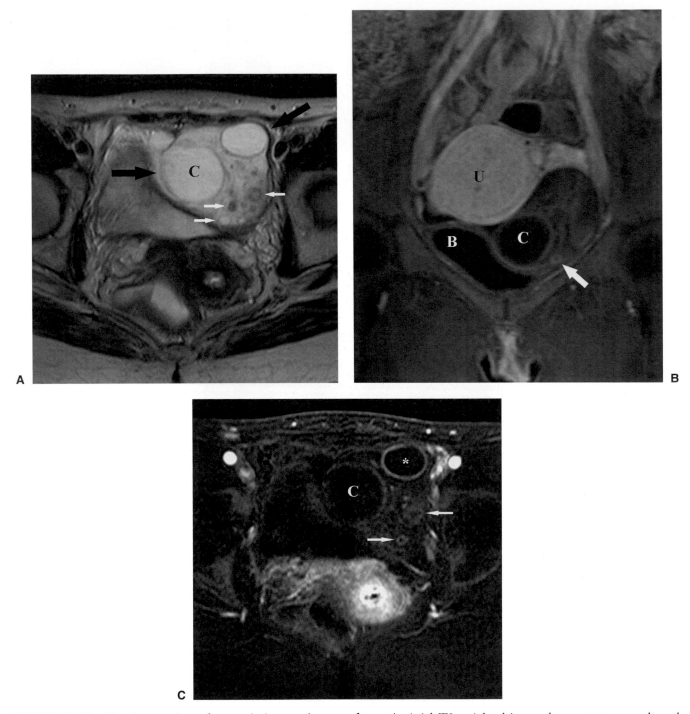

FIGURE 18-61 **Massive ovarian edema mimics ovarian neoplasm. A:** Axial T2-weighted image demonstrates an enlarged, edematous left ovary (*black arrows*). Internal follicles (*white arrows*) and physiologic cyst (*C*) are key to diagnosis. **B:** Typical appearance on enhanced coronal T1-weighted image includes reduced, but not absent, enhancement (*Follicle = arrow, Cyst = C, Uterus = U, Bladder = B*). **C:** Axial postcontrast subtracted image shows follicles (*arrows*) to better advantage (*Corpus luteal cyst = asterisk*).

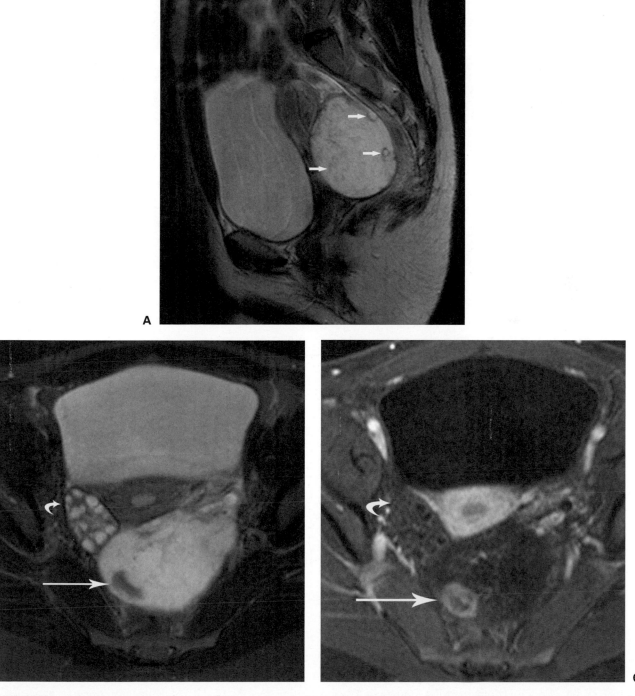

FIGURE 18-62 Massive ovarian edema reflects ovarian torsion without infarction. **A:** Sagittal T2-weighted image in another patient shows multiple small follicles (*arrows*) in edematous ovarian stroma. **B:** Axial fat-suppressed T2-weighted image reveals normal right ovary (*curved arrow*) and a corpus luteum (*long arrow*) in the torsed left ovary. **C:** Axial enhanced T1-weighted image with fat suppression shows the enlarged ovary (*arrow*) crossing the midline into the posterior right pelvis (*Right ovary = curved arrow*). Ovary regained normal appearance with trial of oral contraception.

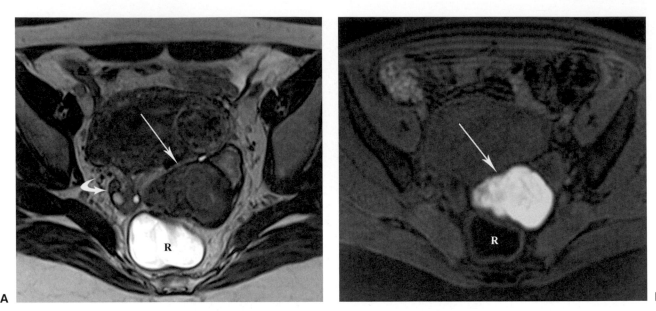

FIGURE 18-63 Endometrioma simulates solid ovarian mass. A: T2-weighted image demonstrates a large, hypointense left ovarian mass (*arrow*). Hypointensity is due to "T2-shading" (*Right ovary = curved arrow, Rectum = R*). **B:** Lesion is uniformly high signal intensity on correlative fat-suppressed unenhanced T1-weighted image, consistent with endometrioma (*Rectum = R*).

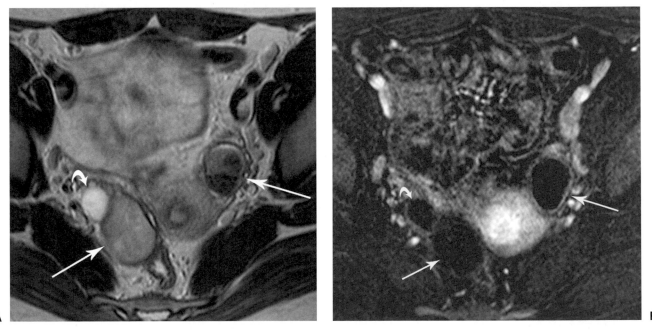

FIGURE 18-64 Endometriomas exhibit a range of T2 signal intensities. A: Axial T2-weighted image demonstrates markedly different appearances in bilateral endometriomas (*arrows*), which are both hypointense to the simple cyst (*curved arrow*). **B:** Correlative subtraction image confirms complete lack of enhancement in all three cysts (*arrows*).

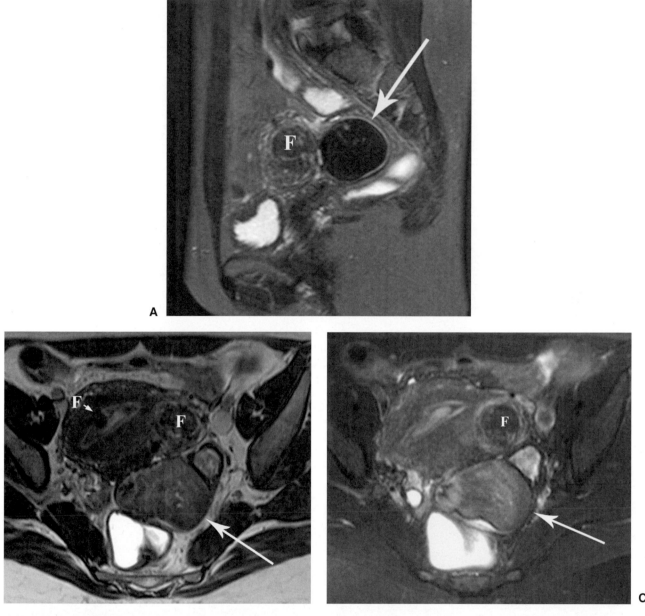

FIGURE 18-65 **Endometrioma often loses signal intensity on short tau inversion recovery (STIR) imaging,** potentially mimicking a fat-containing lesion. **A:** Sagittal STIR image depicts a *cul-de-sac* endometrioma (*arrow*) with markedly hypointense contents due to the T1-shortening effects of methemoglobin and concentrated protein (*Uterine fibroid = F*). On T2-weighted imaging performed **(B)** without and **(C)** with fat suppression, significant "shading" is seen, with no evidence of fat content.

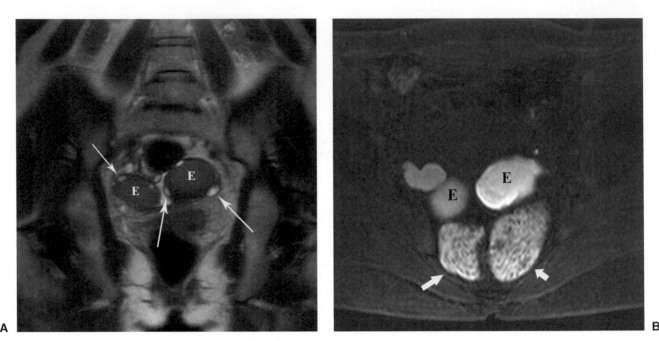

FIGURE 18-66 **"T2-shading" of endometriomas refers to T2 signal reduction, not a window shade appearance. A:** Coronal T2-weighted image shows relatively hypointense material within the endometriomas (*E*) displacing hyperintense follicles (*arrows*) into the periphery of the ovaries. **B:** Endometriomas (*E*) on axial T1-weighted fat suppressed image appear markedly hyperintense, as does fecal material in the rectum (*arrows*).

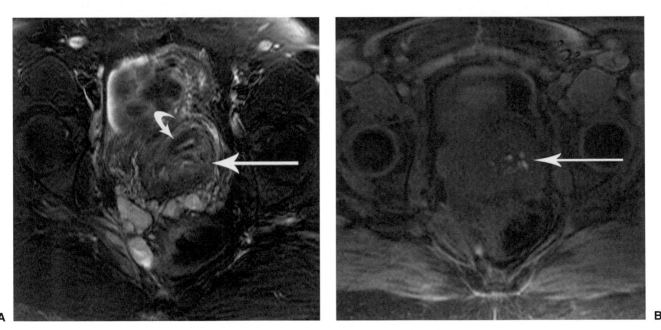

FIGURE 18-67 **Invasive endometriosis simulates cervical mass. A:** Axial fat-suppressed T2-weighted image shows ill-defined mass effect (*arrow*) in the posterior cervix (*Cervical canal = curved arrow*). **B:** Axial fat-suppressed T1-weighted image reveals punctate hemorrhagic foci (*arrow*), consistent with endometriosis.

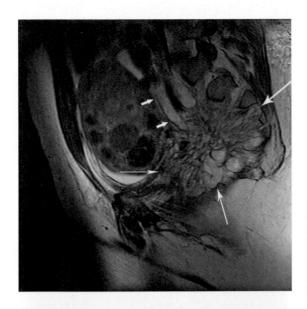

FIGURE 18-68 **Invasive endometriosis simulates multicystic presacral mass.** Sagittal T2-weighted image shows bizarre appearance of invasive endometriosis (*long arrows*). Fibrotic or invasive endometriosis may not demonstrate foci of characteristic high T1-signal intensity (*Obstructed ureter = short arrows*).

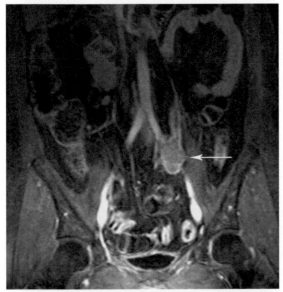

A

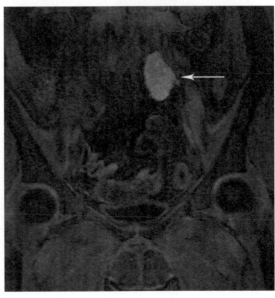

B

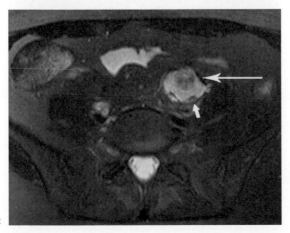

C

FIGURE 18-69 **Endometriosis mimics tumor obstructing ureter.** **A:** Coronal enhanced T1-weighted image demonstrates left ureteral mass (*arrow*). **B:** T1-weighted image obtained prior to contrast administration shows preexisting high T1 signal, consistent with endometriosis implant (*arrow*). **C:** Axial fat-suppressed T2-weighted image shows ureter (*short arrow*) nearly engulfed by heterogeneously hyperintense endometriosis (*long arrow*).

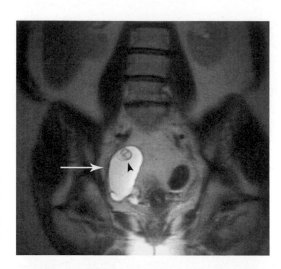

FIGURE 18-70 Peritoneal inclusion cyst simulates cystic neoplasm. Recognition of the right ovary (*arrowhead*) inside the large adnexal cyst (*arrow*) on this coronal T2-weighted image is key to diagnosis of peritoneal inclusion cyst in this elderly woman.

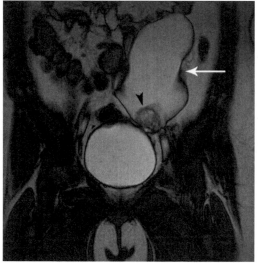

A

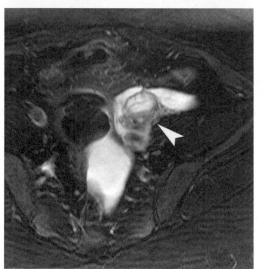

B

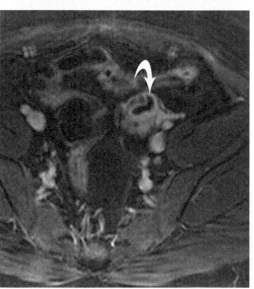

C

FIGURE 18-71 Peritoneal inclusion cyst in premenopausal woman. A: Coronal fluid-sensitive image shows typical lobulated cyst appearance (*arrow*), but a nonspecific appearance of the nodule inferiorly (*arrowhead*). **B:** Axial T2-weighted image again fails to define the nodule (*arrowhead*). **C:** Enhanced axial T1-weighted image shows typical enhancement pattern of a corpus luteum (*curved arrow*), confirming that the nodule is the left ovary.

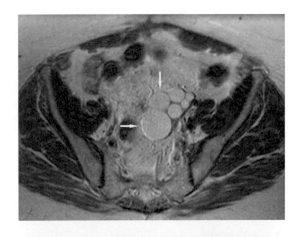

FIGURE 18-72 Imaging in less than optimal plane complicates diagnosis of hydrosalpinx. On axial T2-weighted sequence, hydrosalpinx (*arrows*) appears as multicystic mass.

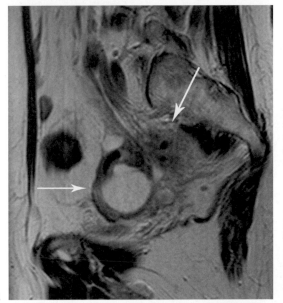

A

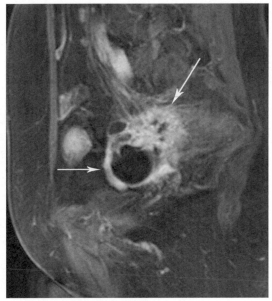

B

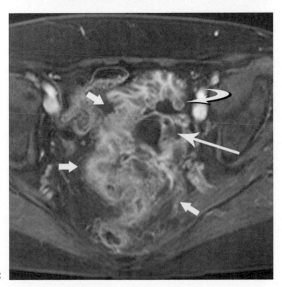

C

FIGURE 18-73 Sigmoid diverticulitis mimics ovarian tumor through effect on left ovary. Sagittal (**A**) T2-weighted and (**B**) enhanced fat-suppressed T1-weighted images depict an enlarged, poorly marginated left ovary (*arrows*), worrisome for ovarian neoplasm. **C:** Axial enhanced image reveals marked thickening and hyperemia of the sigmoid colon (*short arrows*) with inflammation extending to the ovary (*long arrow*), consistent with diverticulitis (*Normal mucosal enhancement = arrowhead, Intact diverticulum = curved arrow*).

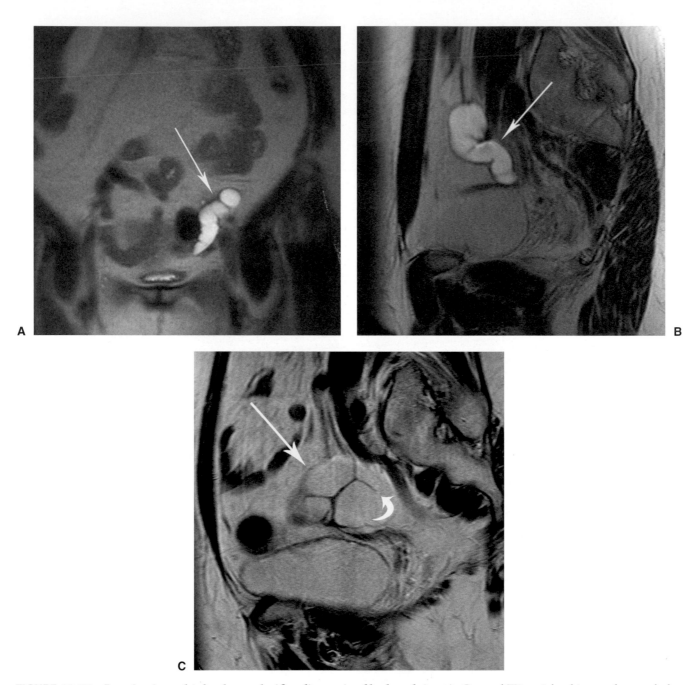

FIGURE 18-74 **Imaging in multiple planes clarifies diagnosis of hydrosalpinx. A:** Coronal T2-weighted image shows tubular, cystic structure rising out of the left pelvis (*arrow*). **B:** Similar appearance of hydrosalpinx (*arrow*) on sagittal T2-weighted image in another patient. **C:** As a hydrosalpinx grows, it folds further on itself, introducing uncertainty about its identity. Mucosal folds project into, but not across (*curved arrow*), the lumen of the folded tube.

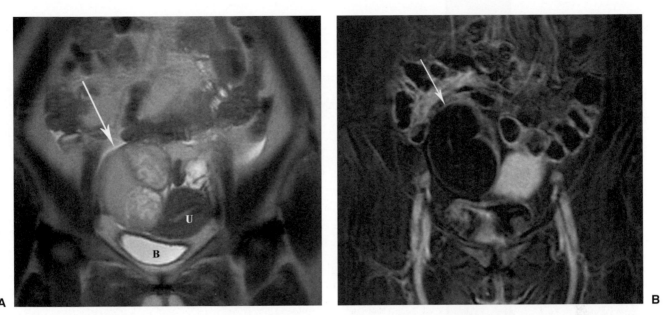

FIGURE 18-75 **Complicated fluid within hemosalpinx introduces uncertainty about its identity**, and raises questions about possible solidity. **A:** Coronal T2-weighted image demonstrates a large, lobulated right adnexal mass, with signal intensity lower than simple water (*arrow*) (*Uterus = U, Bladder = B*). **B:** Contrast administration, especially when used with subtraction, can settle the question. Coronal subtraction image shows complete lack of any enhancement in this endometriosis-related hemosalpinx (*arrow*).

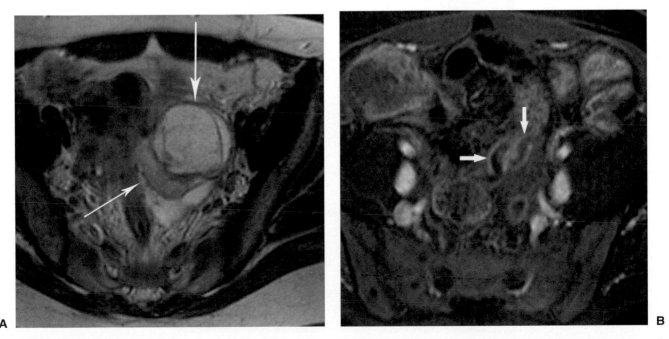

FIGURE 18-76 **Tubo-ovarian abscess enlarges left ovary and obscures its features. A:** The range of signal intensities with the left adnexal mass (*arrows*) on T2-weighted image is nonspecific, although the fine internal heterogeneity can be seen with pus. **B:** Axial enhanced image at a different level cuts through two segments of inflamed Fallopian tube (*arrows*).

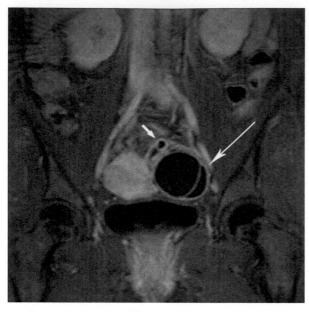

C

FIGURE 18-76 Tubo-ovarian abscess enlarges left ovary and obscures its features. (*continued*) **C:** Enhanced image shows these to be the dilated, thick-walled tube (*short arrow*) and nonenhancing tubo-ovarian abscess (*arrow*).

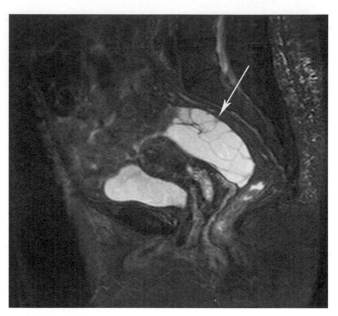

FIGURE 18-77 Ovarian cystadenoma can mimic a hydrosalpinx, especially when the thin septations are not appreciated. These are well demonstrated on a sagittal fat-suppressed T2-weighted image (*arrow*).

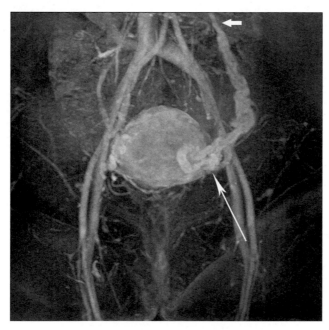

FIGURE 18-78 Common pelvic varices can obscure the ovary or function as a pseudomass (*long arrow*). Notice similarity to appearance of male varicocele as well as its origin from the incompetent ovarian vein (*short arrow*).

Vagina and Perineum

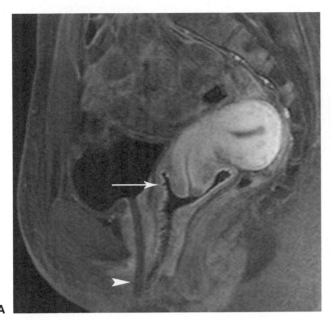

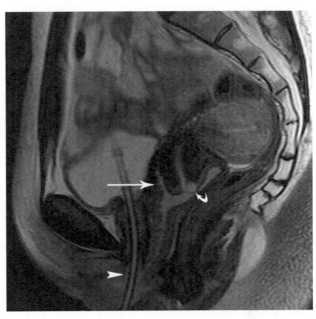

FIGURE 18-79 Normal vagina wall. A and **B:** Midline sagittal enhanced T1- **(A)** and T2-weighted **(B)** images show the normal, extensively rugated vaginal wall (*arrows*). The vagina has a feathery appearance, especially when the lumen is distended with fluid, as in this case (*Urethral catheter = arrowhead, Nabothian cyst = curved arrow*).

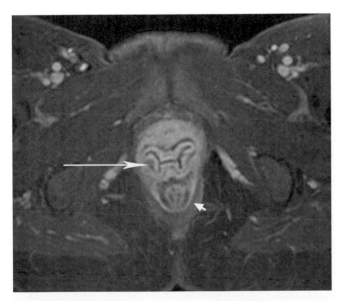

FIGURE 18-80 Mucosa of the premenopausal vagina enhances intensely (*arrow*), especially early after injection. Notice differential enhancement of the different elements of the anal sphincter (*short arrow*).

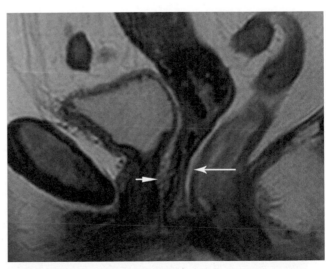

FIGURE 18-81 Normal postmenopausal vagina. Sagittal T2-weighted image demonstrates vaginal narrowing, shortening, and loss of folds. Rectovaginal (*long arrow*) and urethrovaginal (*short arrow*) septae become more clearly delineated.

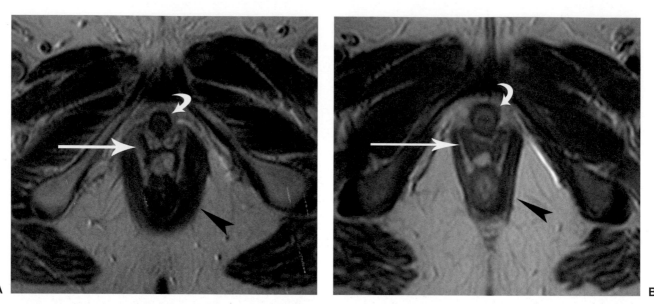

FIGURE 18-82 **Normal H-shape or butterfly shape of the vagina on axial imaging. A** and **B:** The "H" shape reflects the presence of good paravaginal support. Postmenopausal thinning of vaginal mucosa in **(B)** results in thinner limbs of the "H." (*Vagina = arrow, Puborectalis component of the levator muscle complex = arrowhead, Urethra = curved arrow*).

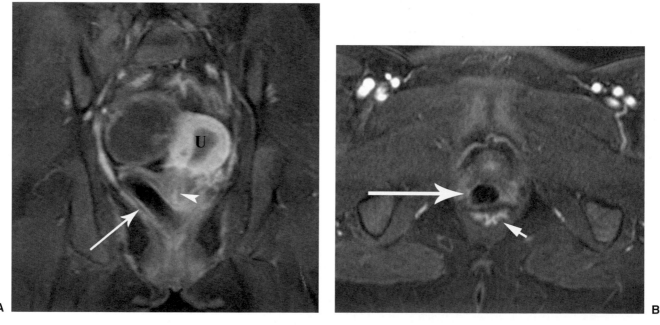

FIGURE 18-83 **Vaginal tampon. A:** Tampon (*arrow*) appears as a signal void cylinder on this coronal fat-suppressed enhanced T1-weighted image, where the end of the tampon is in the right lateral fornix (*Uterus = U, Enhancing cervical mucosa = arrowhead*). **B:** On an axial image obtained early in enhancement, the tampon is seen between urethra anteriorly and rectum posteriorly (*Enhancing rectal mucosa = short arrow*).

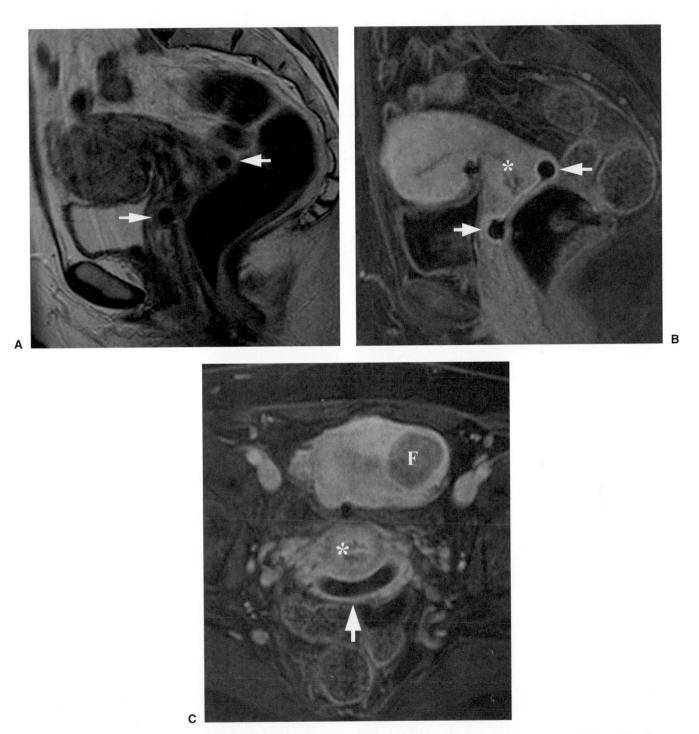

FIGURE 18-84 **Vaginal estrogen ring. A:** Round signal voids (*arrows*) in the vaginal fornices on this sagittal T2-weighted image represent a ring designed for slow release of estrogen. Correlative enhanced sagittal **(B)** and axial **(C)** images show the nonenhancing material circling the cervix (*Cervix = asterisk, Fibroid = F*).

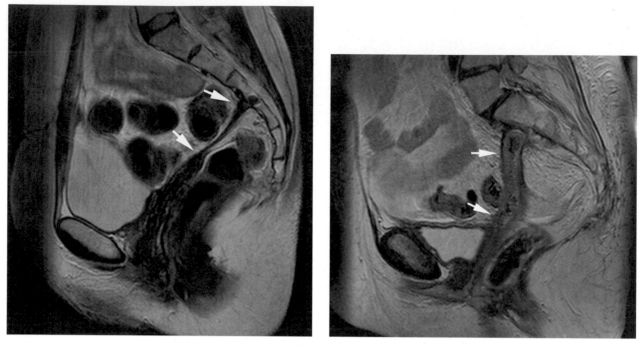

FIGURE 18-85 **Sacral colpopexy grafts for pelvic floor laxity. A** and **B:** Graft material (*short arrows*) suspends the posthysterec-
tomy vaginal vault from the sacrum. Appearance varies depending on material (tissue vs. manufactured meshes) and age of the graft.
Point of attachment varies from the first through the third sacral elements.

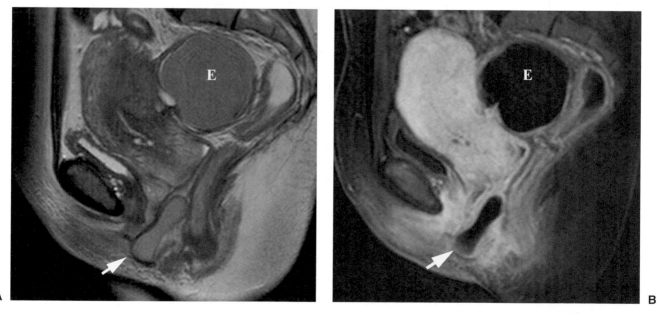

FIGURE 18-86 **Müllerian or inclusion cysts of the vagina** can occur anywhere in the vaginal wall. **A:** Sagittal T2-weighted
image demonstrates a large, prolapsing posterior vaginal wall mass (*arrow*) with signal intensity similar to the large *cul-de-sac*
endometrioma **(E). B:** Subtraction image proves the cystic nature of both lesions.

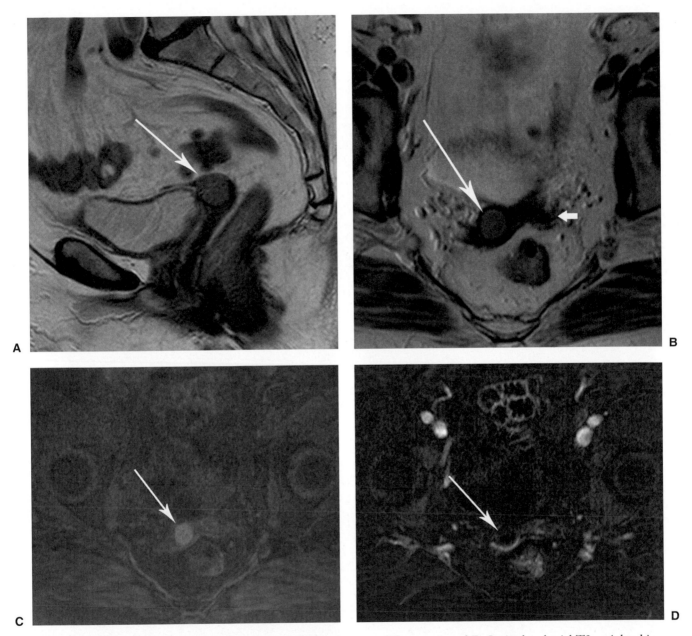

FIGURE 18-87 **Hemorrhagic cyst of the vaginal cuff simulates a solid mass. A** and **B:** Sagittal and axial T2-weighted images reveal a round, intermediate signal intensity mass (*long arrow*) in the vaginal cuff (*short arrow*). **C:** Fat-suppressed, precontrast T1-weighted image obtained before contrast injection shows the high signal intensity typical of hemorrhagic or proteinaceous fluid. **D:** Subtraction image proves complete lack of vascularity.

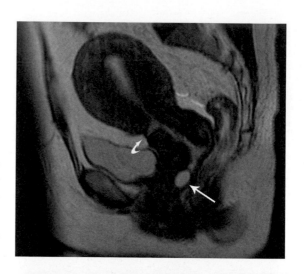

FIGURE 18-88 Incidentally discovered Gartner's duct cyst (*arrow*) in the expected position—anterolateral upper vaginal wall. These can be variable signal intensities depending on contents. Subtraction imaging will prove the lack of solid elements. Notice the caesarian-section scar in the lower uterine segment (*curved arrow*).

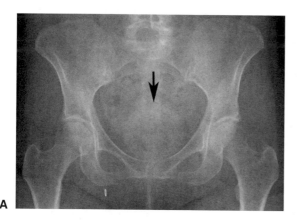

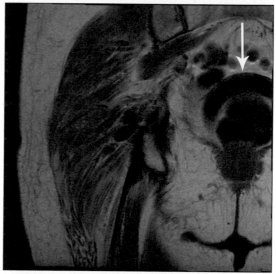

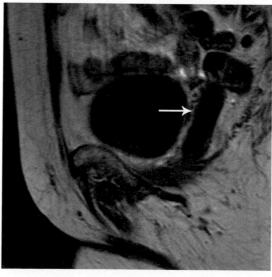

FIGURE 18-89 Vaginal pessary. A: Pelvic radiograph shows circular density (*arrow*) in the deep midline pelvis. B: Coronal T1-weighted image through the right hip reveals an arc of signal void (*arrow*). C: Sagittal T2-weighted image localizes the right side of the pessary (*arrow*) in the expected position of the vagina.

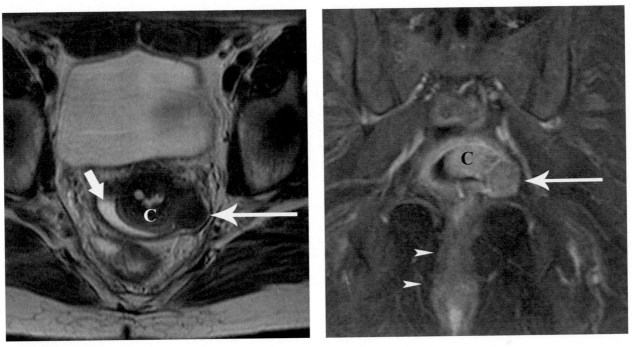

FIGURE 18-90 Small vaginal wall leiomyoma. A: The leiomyoma in the left lateral fornix (*arrow*) is uniformly low signal intensity on this axial T2-weighted image. Notice small amount of fluid in the contralateral fornix (*short arrow*). **B:** Following contrast injection, this coronal T1-weighted fat-suppressed image shows strong enhancement in the fibroid, similar to a typical uterine fibroid (*Cervix = C, Anal muscle = arrowheads*).

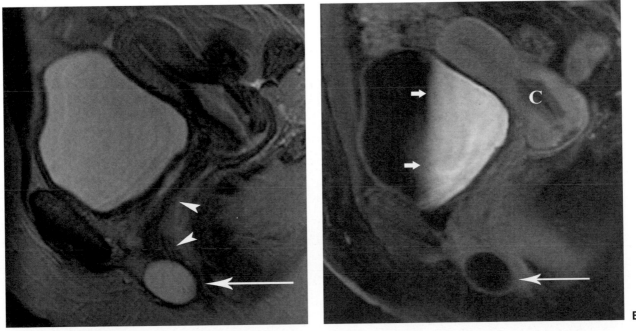

FIGURE 18-91 Bartholin's gland cyst of the vulva. A: Sagittal T2-weighted image demonstrates an oval, relatively high signal intensity cyst (*long arrow*) at the vaginal introitus (*Vagina = arrowheads*). **B:** Proteinaceous cyst contents are often high signal intensity on T1-weighted images, in which cases subtraction imaging will prove the cystic nature of the lesion (*long arrow*) (*Layering contrast in the bladder = short arrows, Cervix = C*).

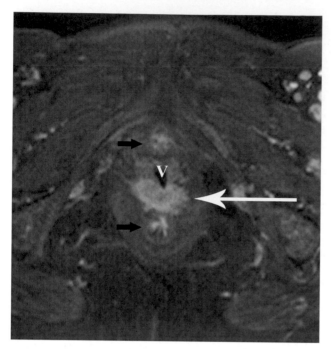

FIGURE 18-92 **Vulvar carcinoma in a woman thought to have vulvar infection.** The enhancing vulvar malignancy (*long arrow*) is depicted on an axial contrast-enhanced fat-suppressed T1-weighted image obtained immediately after injection. Notice bright mucosal enhancement of urethra and anus (*short arrows*) (*Vaginal lumen = V*).

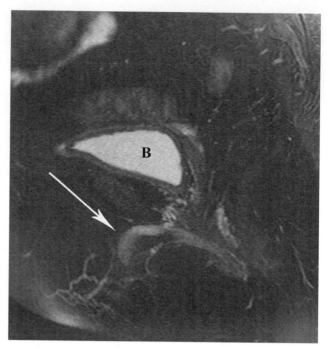

FIGURE 18-93 **Prominent clitoris.** The clitoris (*arrow*) is well seen on this sagittal fat-suppressed T2-weighted image as relatively high in signal intensity, immediately under the symphysis pubis. The clitoris will appear more prominent with age, as adjacent tissues atrophy and recede (*Bladder = B*).

Suggested Readings

Bergman RA, Thompson SA, Afifi AK, et al., ed. *Compendium of human anatomic variation*. Baltimore: Urban & Schwarzenberg; 1988.

Bridges MD, Petrou SP, Lightner DJ. Urethral bulking agents: Imaging review. *AJR Am J Roentgenol*. 2005;185:257–264.

El Jack AK, Siegelman ES. "Pseudoseptum" of the uterine cervix on MRI. *J Magn Reson Imaging*. 2007;26(4):963–965.

El-Sayed RF, Morsy MM, el-Mashed SM, et al. Anatomy of the urethral supporting ligaments defined by dissection, histology, and MRI of female cadavers and MRI of healthy nulliparous women. *AJR Am J Roentgenol*. 2007;189(5):1145–1157.

Elsayes KM, Mukundan G, Narra VR, et al. Endovaginal magnetic resonance imaging of the female urethra. *J Comput Assist Tomogr*. 2006; 30(1):1–6.

Elsayes KM, Narra VR, Dillman JR, et al. Vaginal masses: Magnetic resonance imaging features with pathologic correlation. *Acta Radiol*. 2007;48(8):921–933.

Hauth EA, Jaeger HJ, Libera H, et al. MR imaging of the uterus and cervix in healthy women: Determination of normal values. *Eur Radiol*. 2007;17(3):734–742.

Holloway BJ, López C, Balogun M. Technical report: A simple and reliable way to recognize the transient myometrial contraction–a common pitfall in MRI of the pelvis. *Clin Radiol*. 2007;62(6):596–599.

Huertas CP, Brown MA, Semelka RC. MR imaging evaluation of the adnexa. *Magn Reson Imaging Clin N Am*. 2006;14(4):471–487.

Imaoka I, Wada A, Matsuo M, et al. MR imaging of disorders associated with female infertility: Use in diagnosis, treatment, and management. *RadioGraphics*. 2003;23(6):1401–1421.

Jain KA. Imaging of peritoneal inclusion cysts. *AJR Am J Roentgenol*. 2000;174(6):1559–1563.

Kataoka M, Kido A, Koyama T, et al. MRI of the female pelvis at 3T compared to 1.5T: evaluation on high-resolution T2-weighted and HASTE images. *J Magn Reson Imaging*. 2007;25(3):527–534.

Katsumori T, Kasahara T, Kin Y, et al. Infarction of uterine fibroids after embolization: Relationship between postprocedural enhanced MRI findings and long-term clinical outcomes. *Cardiovasc Intervent Radiol*. 2007;[Epub ahead of print]. 2008;31(1):66–72.

Katsumori T, Kasahara T, Kin Y, et al. Magnetic resonance angiography of uterine artery: Changes with embolization using gelatin sponge particles alone for fibroids. *Cardiovasc Intervent Radiol*. 2007;30(3):398–404.

Kido A, Togashi K, Kataoka ML, et al. Intrauterine devices and uterine peristalsis: Evaluation with MRI. *Magn Reson Imaging*. 2007; [Epub ahead of print]. 2008;26(1):54–58.

Kin Y, Katsumori T, Kasahara T, et al. Hemodynamics of ovarian veins: MR angiography in women with uterine leiomyomata. *Eur J Radiol*. 2007;63(3):408–413.

Koyama T, Togashi K. Functional MR imaging of the female pelvis. *J Magn Reson Imaging*. 2007;25(6):1101–1112.

Lee JW, Fynes MM. Female urethral diverticula. *Best Pract Res Clin Obstet Gynaecol*. 2005;19(6):875–893.

Leyendecker JR, Gorengaut V, Brown JJ. MR imaging of maternal diseases of the abdomen and pelvis during pregnancy and the immediate postpartum period. *Radiographics*. 2004;24(5):1301–1316.

Llauger J, Palmer J, Pérez C, et al. The normal and pathologic ischiorectal fossa at CT and MR imaging. *Radiographics*. 1998;18(1):61–82.

Martin DR, Salman K, Wilmot CC, et al. MR imaging evaluation of the pelvic floor for the assessment of vaginal prolapse and urinary incontinence. *Magn Reson Imaging Clin N Am*. 2006;14(4):523–535.

Mauroy B, Demondion X, Bizet B, et al. The female inferior hypogastric (=pelvic) plexus: Anatomical and radiological description of the plexus and its differences—Applications to pelvic surgery. *Surg Radiol Anat*. 2007;29:55–66.

Mueller GC, Hussain HK, Smith YR, et al. Müllerian duct anomalies: Comparison of MRI diagnosis and clinical diagnosis. *AJR Am J Roentgenol*. 2007;189(6):1294–1302.

Nascimento AB, Mitchell DG, Holland G. Ovarian veins: Magnetic resonance imaging findings in an asymptomatic population. *J Magn Reson Imaging*. 2002;15(5):551–556.

O'Connell HE, DeLancey JO. Clitoral anatomy in nulliparous, healthy, premenopausal volunteers using unenhanced magnetic resonance imaging. *J Urol*. 2005;173(6):2060–2063.

Outwater EK, Siegelman ES, Chiowanich P, et al. Dilated fallopian tubes: MR imaging characteristics. *Radiology*. 1998;208(2):463–469.

Oztoprak I, Eqilmez H, Oztoprak B, et al. Complicated giant polycystic ovary mimicking tumor: MR imaging findings. *Pediatr Radiol*. 2007; 37(2):233–236.

Rizk DE, Czechowski J, Ekelund L. Magnetic resonance imaging of uterine version in a multiethnic, nulliparous, healthy female population. *J Reprod Med*. 2005;50(2):81–83.

Siegelman ES, Banner MP, Ramchandani P, et al. Multicoil MR imaging of symptomatic female urethral and periurethral disease. *Radiographics*. 1997;17(2):349–365.

Singh K, Reid WM, Berger LA. Assessment and grading of pelvic organ prolapse by use of dynamic magnetic resonance imaging. *Am J Obstet Gynecol*. 2001;185(1):71–77.

Suh DD, Yang CC, Cao Y, et al. Magnetic resonance imaging anatomy of the female genitalia in premenopausal and postmenopausal women. *J Urol*. 2003;170(1):138–144.

Takeuchi M, Matsuzaki K, Uehara H, et al. Pathologies of the uterine endometrial cavity: Usual and unusual manifestations and pitfalls on magnetic resonance imaging. *Eur Radiol*. 2005;15(11):2244–2255.

Tanaka YO, Saida TS, Minami R, et al. MR findings of ovarian tumors with hormonal activity, with emphasis on tumors other than sex cord-stromal tumors. *Eur J Radiol*. 2007;62(3):317–327.

Chapter 19

Male

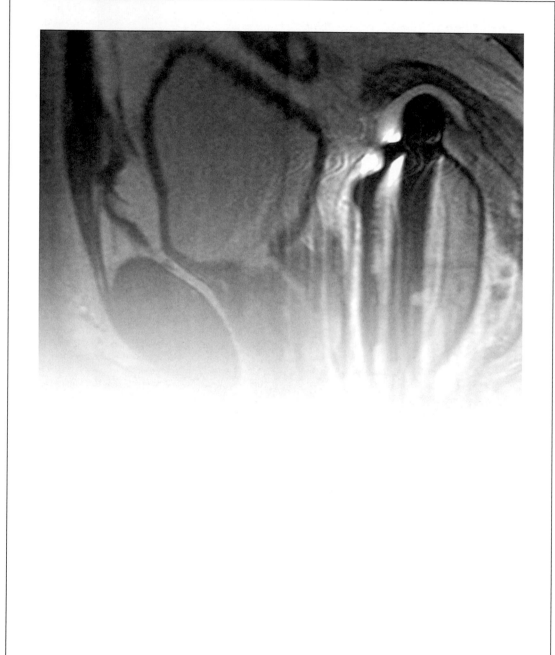

Mellena D. Bridges

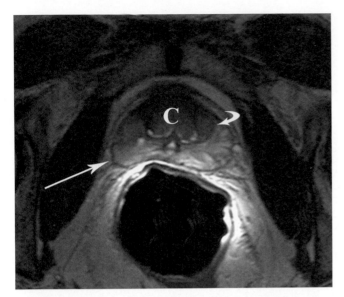

FIGURE 19-1 Zonal anatomy of the prostate demonstrated by axial T2-weighted imaging. High-resolution image through the prostate apex obtained using a combination of endorectal and surface array coils. Normal peripheral zone (*arrow*) is horseshoe-shaped, with a thin, well-defined hypointense capsule (*Central gland = C, Hypointense tumor nodule = curved arrow*).

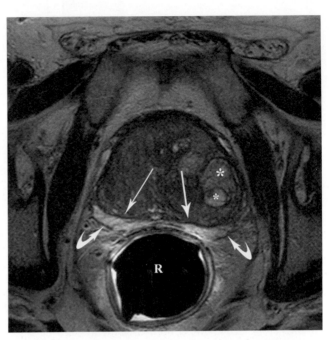

FIGURE 19-2 Benign prostatic hypertrophy (BPH) is a disease of the central gland. Axial T2-weighted image through the mid-gland shows typical heterogeneity and nodularity (*asterisk*), with compression of the hyperintense peripheral zone (*curved arrows*) (*Posterior margin of central gland = arrows, Rectum = R*).

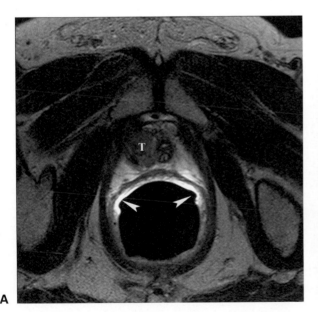

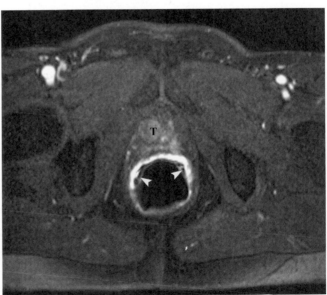

FIGURE 19-3 Near-field artifact from the directional endorectal coil. A: Axial T2-weighted image and **(B)** enhanced T1-weighted image with fat suppression demonstrate near-field artifact from the endorectal coil (*arrowheads*). Intense signal near the endoluminal coil is difficult to normalize (*Tumor = T*).

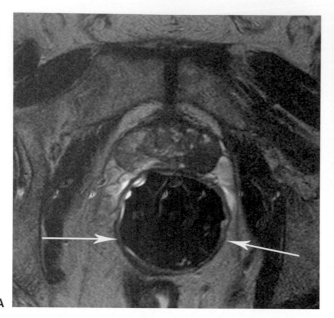

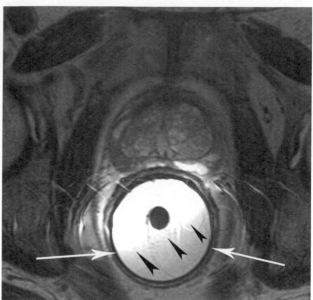

FIGURE 19-4   Inflatable balloon around an endorectal prostate coil. Axial T2-weighted images demonstrate inflatable balloon (*arrows*) filled with **(A)** signal-void air and **(B)** moderately hyperintense dilute barium mixture. Notice hyperintensity of fluid anteriorly (*arrowheads*) due to the directionality of the coil, which is also twisted in the rectum.

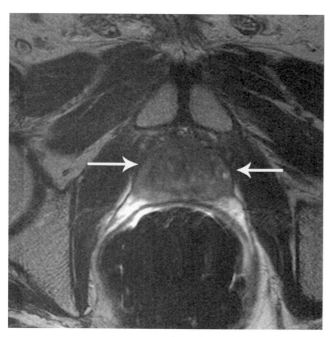

FIGURE 19-5   Radiation therapy results in loss of zonal anatomy on axial T2-weighted image. Notice diffuse loss of signal intensity, especially in peripheral zone (*arrows*).

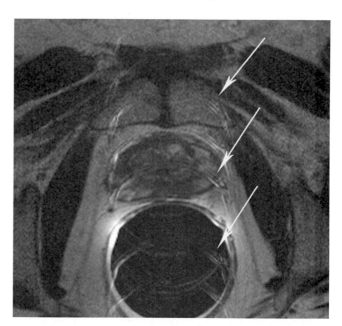

FIGURE 19-6   Ghosting artifact. Ghosting artifact (*arrows*) occurs from interface of the endorectal coil and rectal wall. Although most axial body MRI uses an anteroposterior phase-encoding direction, motion in this direction on prostate imaging can seriously compromise diagnostic quality.

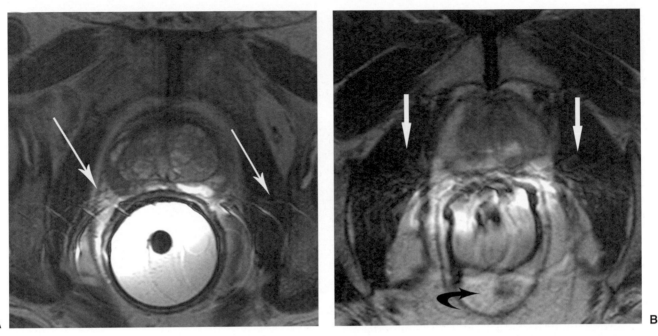

FIGURE 19-7   Ghosting artifact. Ghosting artifact (*arrows*) in the right-left direction usually compromises visualization only in the posterior peripheral zone **(A)**, but it can also reduce the quality of a broad swathe of the image. **(B)** Motion is exacerbated by the loose fit of this rectal balloon.

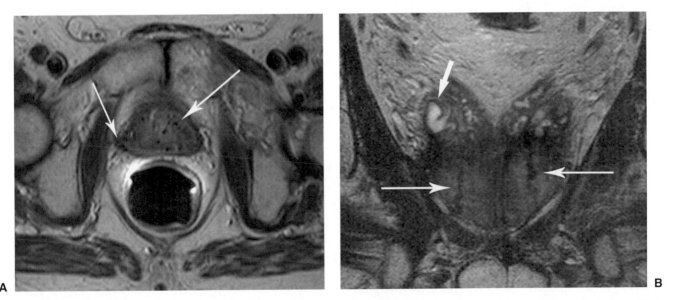

FIGURE 19-8   Brachytherapy seeds appear as tiny signal voids. Axial **(A)** and coronal **(B)** T2-weighted images show multiple well-defined hypointense foci (*arrows*), with the paths of the introducer needles better demonstrated in the coronal plane (*Right seminal vesicle = short arrow*).

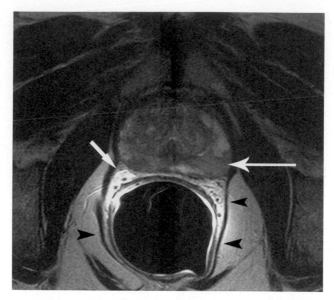

FIGURE 19-9 **Areas of low T2 signal intensity in the peripheral zone** (*long arrow*) are quite common, but nonspecific. Causes include prostatitis, trauma, biopsy-related hemorrhage, and malignancy (*Neurovascular bundle = short arrow, Levator ani muscle = black arrowheads*).

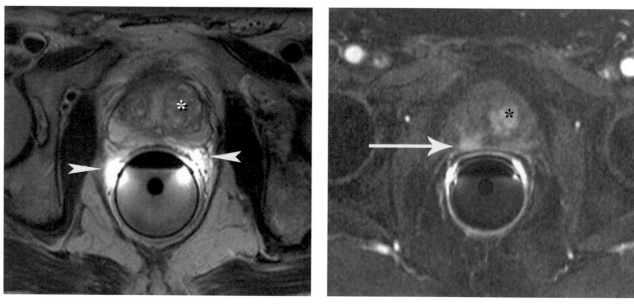

FIGURE 19-10 **T2-weighted image fails to localize prostate cancer. A:** A convincing focus of hypointensity is not demonstrated on this T2-weighted image (*Hypertrophic nodule in the central gland = asterisk, Near-field artifact from directional coil = arrowheads*). **B:** T1-weighted image obtained immediately following contrast administration reveals rapid, avid enhancement of the biopsy-proven carcinoma (*arrow*) (*Hypertrophic nodule in the central gland = asterisk*).

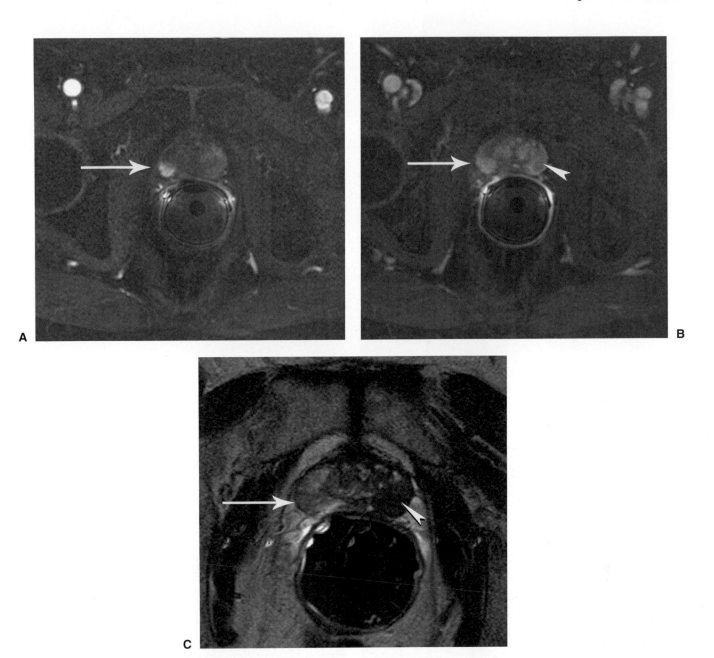

FIGURE 19-11 Postbiopsy hemorrhage simulates early enhancing tumor. A: T1-hyperintense focus of hemorrhage (*arrow*) appears to enhance during this very early phase following contrast injection. **B:** Several seconds later, its signal intensity has not increased, but the contralateral corner (*arrowhead*) now enhances strongly. **C:** T2-weighted image shows mild signal loss in the area of hemorrhage (*arrow*), and more profound hypointensity in the tumor (*arrowhead*).

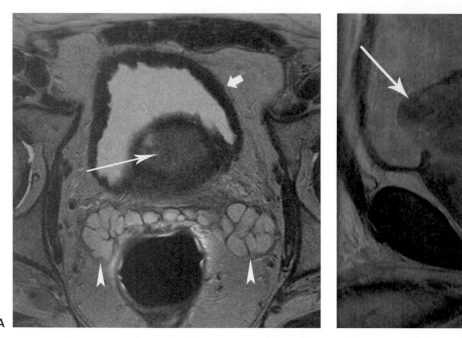

FIGURE 19-12   Benign prostate hypertrophy bulges into bladder base. Axial **(A)** and **(B)** sagittal T2-weighted images show prostate tissue (*long arrow*) occupying much of the trigone area. Notice associated bladder wall hypertrophy (*short arrow*) (*Seminal vesicles = arrowheads*).

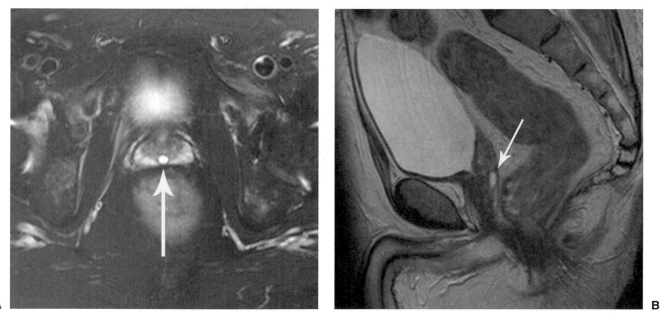

FIGURE 19-13   Utricle cyst of the prostate. A: Axial fat-suppressed T2-weighted image demonstrates small, midline cyst (*arrow*) in the posterior prostate. **B:** Sagittal midline T2-weighted image reveals the typical teardrop shape of a utricle cyst (*arrow*).

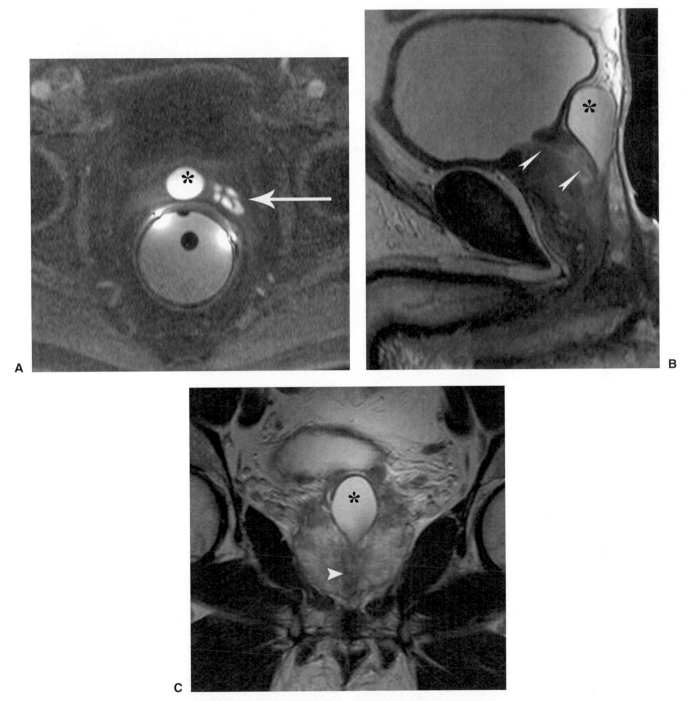

FIGURE 19-14 **High T1 signal intensity in larger midline cyst due to biopsy-related hemorrhage. A:** Axial T1-weighted image obtained without contrast shows hyperintense midline cyst (*asterisk*) and left seminal vesicles (*arrow*), both structures complicated by biopsy-related hemorrhage. Sagittal **(B)** and coronal **(C)** T2-weighted images demonstrate a hyperintense teardrop-shaped cyst rising well out of the prostate (*arrowheads*), suggesting Müllerian duct cyst.

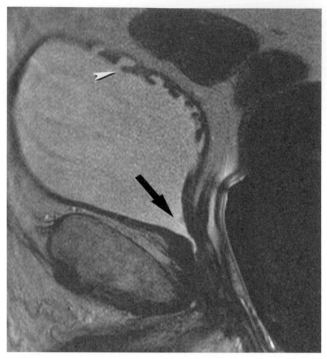

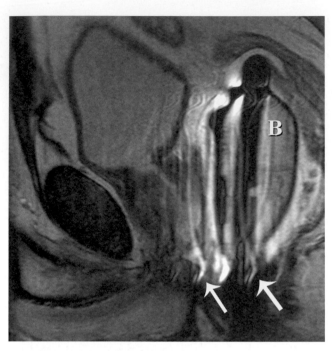

FIGURE 19-15 Transurethral resection of the prostate (TURP) defect. Midline sagittal T2-weighted image shows a funnel-shaped defect (*arrow*) at the bladder base due to transurethral resection of the prostate for symptomatic prostatomegaly. Notice trabeculation of bladder wall from long-term outlet obstruction (*arrowhead*).

FIGURE 19-16 Motion artifact obscures prostate. Ghosting of high near-field signal in the phase encoding direction (*arrows*) on sagittal T2-weighted image is from rectal peristalsis (*Rectal coil balloon = B*).

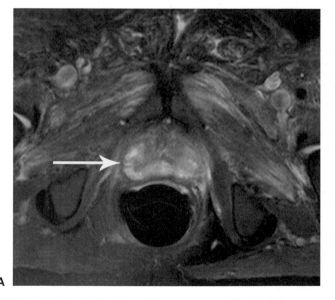

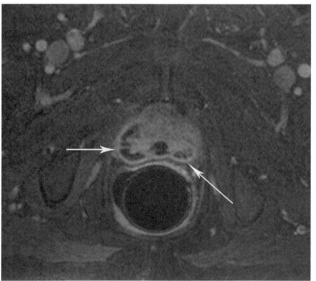

FIGURE 19-17 Infection of the prostate (A). Axial fat-suppressed T2-weighted image shows vague increased peripheral signal (*arrow*) with infiltration/edema of adjacent tissues. **B:** Enhanced T1-weighted images demonstrate ill-defined, nonenhancing areas (*arrows*), due to *Pseudomonas* infection.

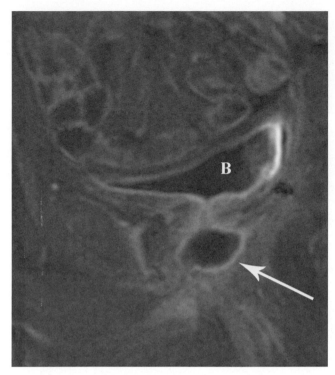

FIGURE 19-18   Radiation-induced prostate necrosis. Sagittal enhanced T1-weighted image in another patient shows complete absence of enhancement in a large portion of the prostate (*arrow*) (*Bladder = B*).

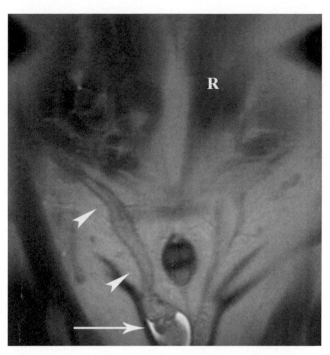

FIGURE 19-19   Normal course of the right spermatic cord (*arrowheads*) as it exits the inguinal canal and descends to the scrotal sac (*arrow*) (*Rectus abdominis = R*).

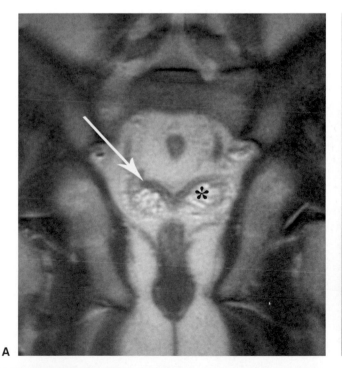

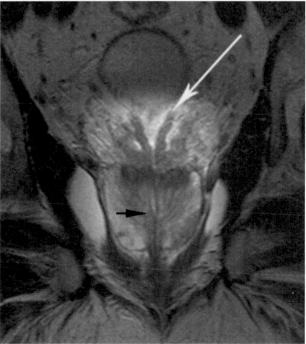

FIGURE 19-20   Low signal intensity of vas deferens does not indicate tumor infiltration. **A** and **B:** Coronal T2-weighted images show vas deferens in midline and above the higher signal intensity seminal vesicles (*Vas deferens = long arrow, Seminal vesicles = asterisk, Urethra = short arrow*).

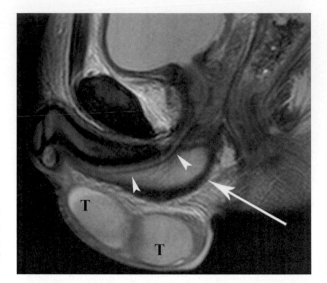

FIGURE 19-21 Normal scrotum and penis. Sagittal T2-weighted image demonstrates a pair of hyperintense testes *(T)* situated normally in the scrotum. Hyperintense penile bulb *(arrow)* sheathed in hypointense tunica *(Penile urethra = arrowheads)*.

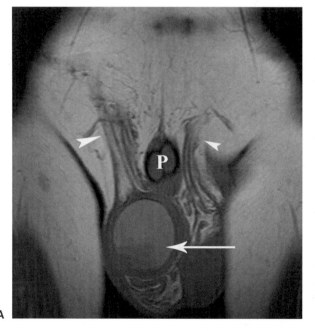

A

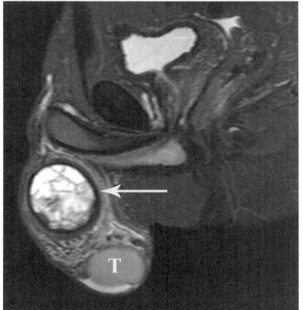

B

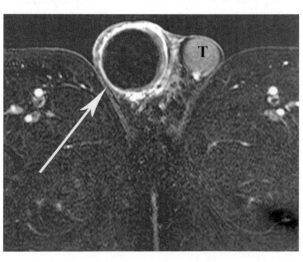

C

FIGURE 19-22 Hematoma in the right spermatic cord simulates tumor. A: Well-circumscribed, relatively hyperintense lesion *(arrow)* in the right hemiscrotum on coronal T1-weighted image. **B:** Sagittal T2-weighted image with fat suppression demonstrates high signal intensity with apparent internal septations. **C:** Axial postcontrast subtraction image reveals complete absence of enhancement *(Penis = P, Testis = T, Spermatic cords = arrowheads)*.

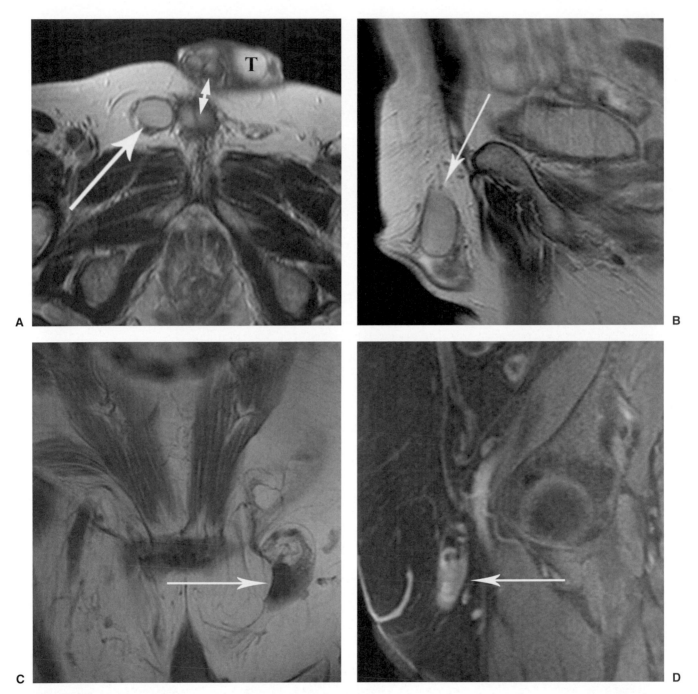

FIGURE 19-23 Varying degrees of atrophy in undescended testes. Axial **(A)** and sagittal **(B)** T2-weighted images reveal a small, but still relatively hyperintense, testis (*arrow*) in the right inguinal canal (*Left testis = T, Penis = double arrow*). Coronal T2 weighted **(C)** and sagittal enhanced T1-weighted **(D)** images demonstrate a tiny, atrophic, T2-hypointense testis (*arrow*) in the left groin of another patient.

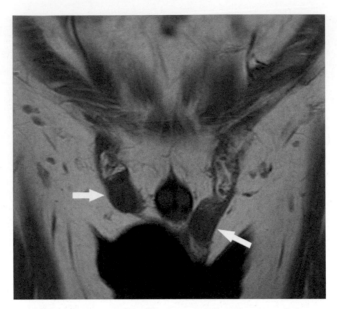

FIGURE 19-24 Hypoplastic scrotum with bilateral undescended testes. Coronal T2-weighted image demonstrates a small, hypointense testis (*arrows*) in each groin, well above the expected location of the scrotum.

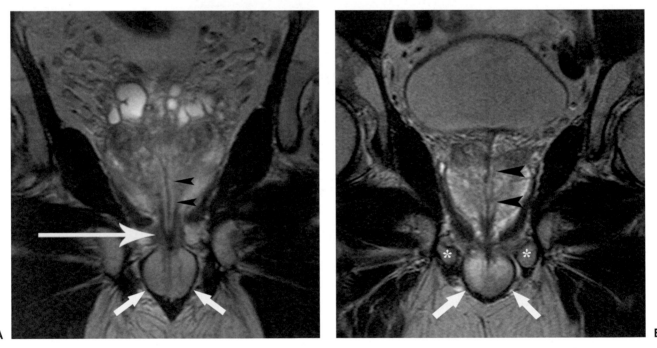

FIGURE 19-25 Normal bulbar penis. A: Coronal T2-weighted image through the prostatic (*arrowheads*) and membranous (*arrow*) urethra shows descent of the urethra into the penile bulb, the origin of the corpus spongiosum (*short arrows*). **B:** More anterior coronal image shows the bulb again, as well as the origins of the erectile cavernosal bodies along the inferior pubic rami (*asterisk*).

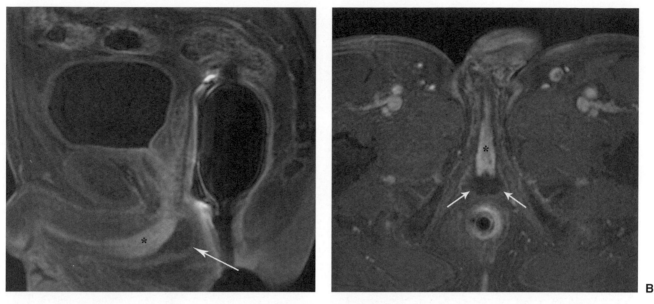

FIGURE 19-26 **Poor enhancement in the posterior penile bulb, a normal variant.** Sagittal **(A)** and axial **(B)** enhanced T1-weighted images demonstrate well-defined, persistent region of reduced enhancement, likely due to the differing blood supplies in the posterior bulb (*arrows*) and the rest of the bulbar penis (*asterisk*).

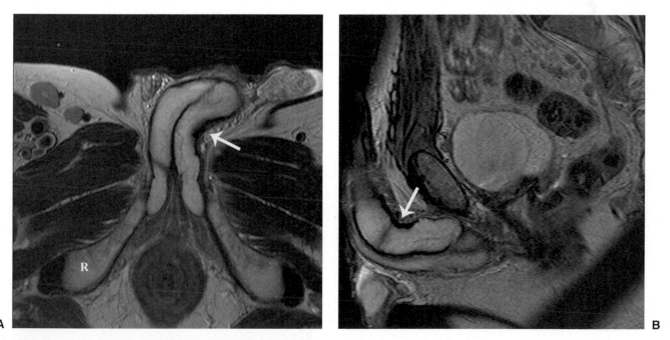

FIGURE 19-27 **Angulation of the penis** on imaging can be positional or fixed, as here, at the site of a Peyronie's plaque. Axial **(A)** and sagittal **(B)** T2-weighted images show hypointense thickening of the tunica albuginea and left corpus cavernosum (*arrow*) (*Inferior pubic ramus = R*).

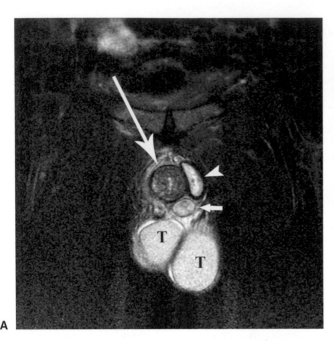

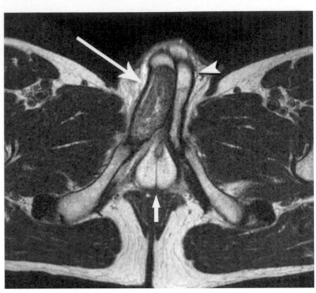

A   B

FIGURE 19-28 **Penile hematoma simulates tumor of the right cavernosal body.** Coronal fat-suppressed T2-weighted image **(A)** through the symphysis pubis and correlative axial T2-weighted image **(B)** show enlarged, hypointense left corpus cavernosum (*arrow*) and normal left cavernosal body (*arrowhead*). T1-weighted imaging performed with and without contrast will clarify these situations (*Corpus spongiosum = thick arrow, Testes = T*).

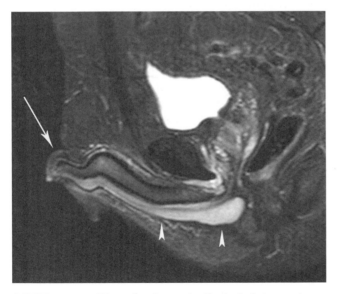

FIGURE 19-29 **Hypoplastic penis.** Sagittal short tau inversion recovery (STIR) image reveals a shortened distal penis (*arrow*), with decreased component volumes. Notice higher signal intensity of the corpus spongiosum (*arrowheads*).

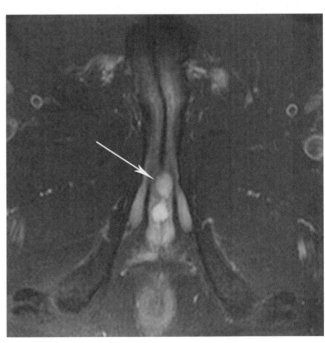

FIGURE 19-30 **Periurethral diverticulum.** Axial T2-weighted fat-suppressed image demonstrates bilobar high signal intensity diverticulum (*arrow*) in close association with the bulbar urethra.

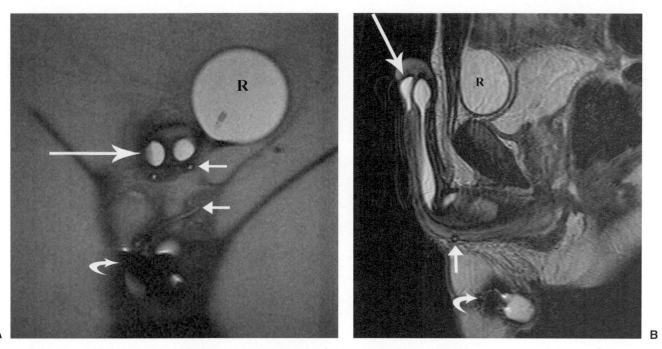

A   B

FIGURE 19-31   Inflatable penile prosthesis. Coronal **(A)** and sagittal **(B)** T2-weighted images demonstrate fluid-filled reservoir (*R*), cavernosal components (*arrow*) and connecting tubing (*short arrow*) (*Susceptibility artifact from scrotal pump = curved arrow*).

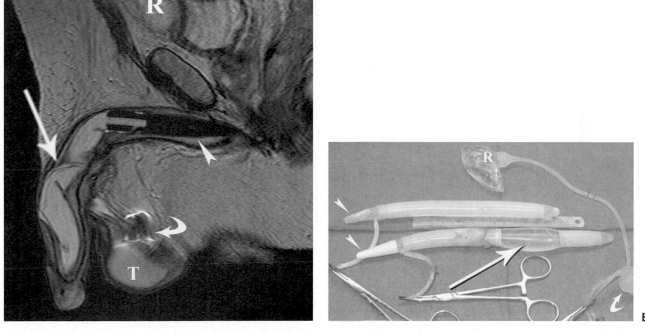

A   B

FIGURE 19-32   Aneurysm of corporal component. A: Sagittal T2-weighted image demonstrates enlarged, twisted segment of one component (*arrow*) (*Posterior extender = arrowhead, Testis = T, Pump = curved arrow, R = reservoir*). **B:** Correlative photograph of explanted components (*Posterior extender = arrowheads, Pump = curved arrow, R = reservoir*).

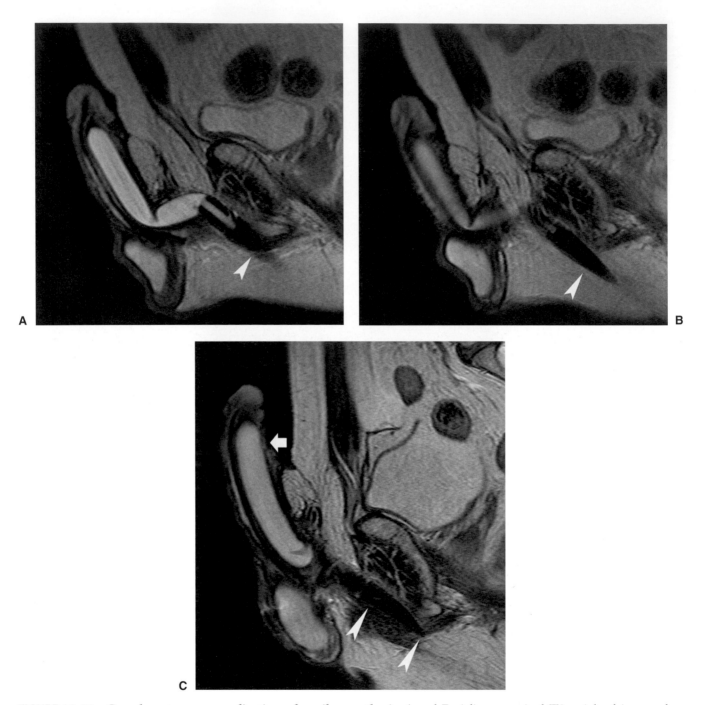

FIGURE 19-33 Crural rupture, a complication of penile prosthesis. A and **B:** Adjacent sagittal T2-weighted images show extender rupture through penile crus into buttock (*arrowheads*). **C:** Following repair, prosthesis is able to achieve complete inflation (*short arrow*).

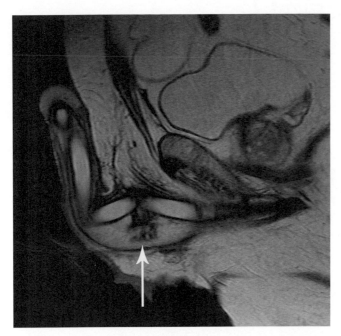

FIGURE 19-34   Cavernosal rupture, a complication of penile prosthesis. Component rupture through cavernosal body (*arrow*) is demonstrated on sagittal T2-weighted image.

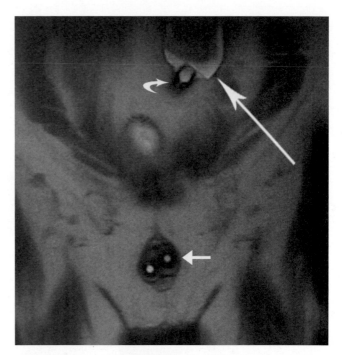

FIGURE 19-35   Penile prosthesis reservoir leak. Coronal T2-weighted image shows very little fluid in the reservoir (*arrow*), although the prosthesis itself is deflated (*Posterior extenders = short arrow, connecting tubing = curved arrow*).

Suggested Readings

Bergman RA, Thompson SA, Afifi AK, et al., ed. *Compendium of human anatomic variation*. Baltimore: Urban & Schwarzenberg; 1988.

Bhaskar PV, Basin V, Kumar S. Abnormal branch of the testicular artery. *Clin Anat*. 2006;19:569–570.

Deng J, Hall-Craggs MA, Craggs MD, et al. Three-dimensional MRI of the male urethrae with implanted artificial sphincters: Initial results. *Br J Radiol*. 2006;79(942):455–463.

Ikonen S, Kivisaari L, Vehmas T, et al. Optimal timing of post-biopsy MRI of the prostate. *Acta Radiol*. 2001;42(1):70–73.

Kaji Y, Kuroda K, Maeda T, et al. Anatomical and metabolic assessment of prostate using a 3-Tesla MR scanner with a custom-made external transceive coil: Healthy volunteer study. *J Magn Reson Imaging*. 2007; 25(3):517–526.

Kim B, Kawashima A, LeRoy AJ. Imaging of the male urethra. *Semin Ultrasound CT MR*. 2007;28(4):258–273.

Lapointe SP, Wei DC, Hricak H, et al. Magnetic resonance imaging in the evaluation of congenital anomalies of the external genitalia. *Urology*. 2001;58(3):452–456.

McDermott VG, Meakem TJ III, Stolpen AH, et al. Prostatic and periprostatic cysts: findings on MRI. *AJR Am J Roentgenol*. 1995; 164(1):123–127.

Noworolski SM, Henry RG, Vigneron DB, et al. Dynamic contrast-enhanced MRI in normal and abnormal prostate tissues as defined by biopsy, MRI, and 3D MRSI. *Magn Reson Med*. 2005;53(2):249–255.

Oh-oka H, Fujisawa M, Kin K, et al. Usefulness of MR-seminography using Gd-DTPA in intermediate magnetic field MRI equipment. *Magn Reson Imaging*. 2003;21(5):497–502.

Ozdemir MB, Celik HH, Aldur MM. Altered course of the right testicular artery. *Clin Anat*. 2004;17:67–69.

Tubbs RS, Salter EG, Oakes WJ. Unusual drainage of the testicular veins. *Clin Anat*. 2005;18:536–539.

Wachowicz K, Thomas SD, Fallone BG. Characterization of the susceptibility artifact around a prostate brachytherapy seed in MRI. *Med Phys*. 2006;33(12):4459–4467.

Wachsberg RH, Sebastiano LL, Sullivan BC, et al. Posterior urethral diverticulum presenting as a midline prostatic cyst: Sonographic and MRI appearance. *Abdom Imaging*. 1995;20:70–71.

Chapter 20

Unisex

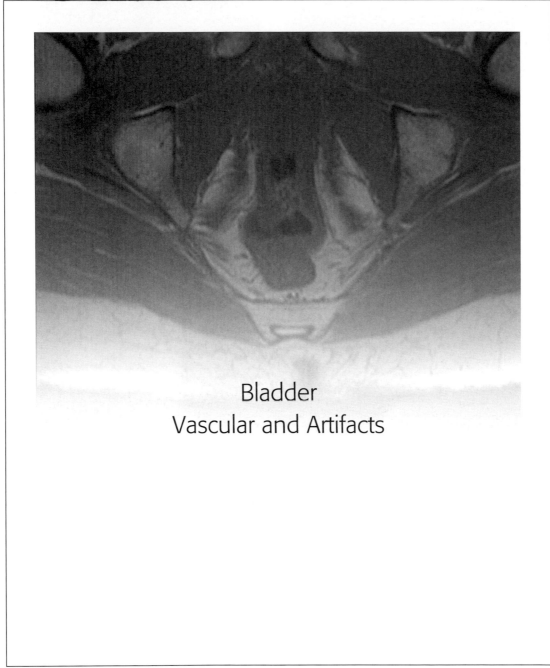

Bladder

Vascular and Artifacts

Mellena D. Bridges and Robert A. Pooley

▣ Bladder

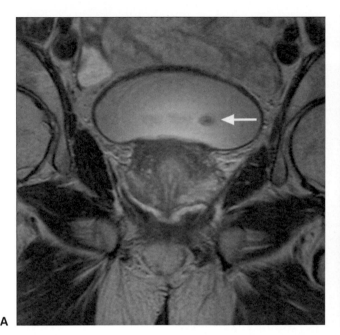

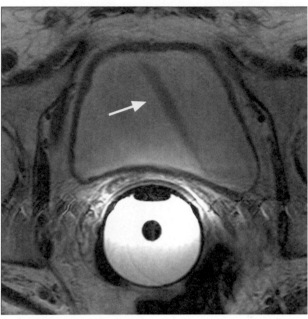

FIGURE 20-1   Ureteral jet by MR. A: Punctate focus of dephasing perpendicular to the coronal plane of this high-resolution T2-weighted image (*arrow*). **B:** Axial plane depicts the jet taking its normal trajectory (*arrow*) obliquely toward the midline.

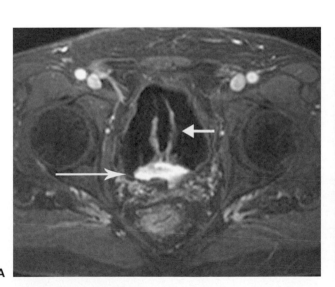

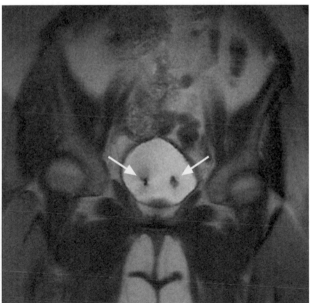

FIGURE 20-2   Bilateral ureteral jets. A: Axial enhanced T1-weighted image not only reveals the enhanced jets (*short arrow*) but also the dependent accumulation of dense contrast posteriorly (*long arrow*). **B:** Flow (*arrows*) appears punctate on coronal T2-weighted image.

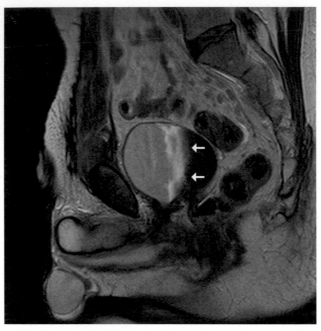

FIGURE 20-3 Fluid–fluid level of excreted gadolinium. When excreted, gadolinium is sufficiently concentrated for T2* effects to come into play. The result is the striking hypointensity of the most dependent portion of the gadolinium-concentrated urine will be profoundly hypointense (*arrows*).

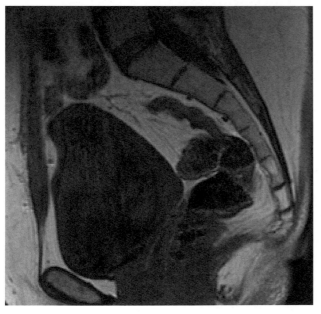

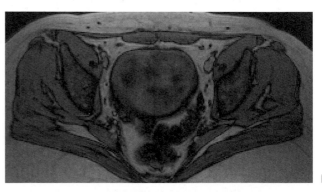

FIGURE 20-4 Urine artifact in bladder. A: Sagittal and **(B)** axial T1-weighted images show heterogeneous signal intensity of the urine within the bladder, due to motion artifact.

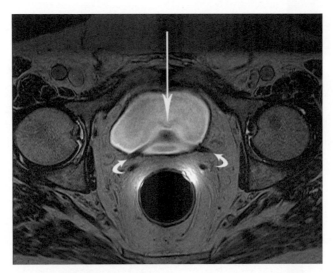

FIGURE 20-5 **Bladder trigone.** Central prostate hypertrophy has lifted the trigone (*arrow*) into the plane of the ureteral orifices (*curved arrows*).

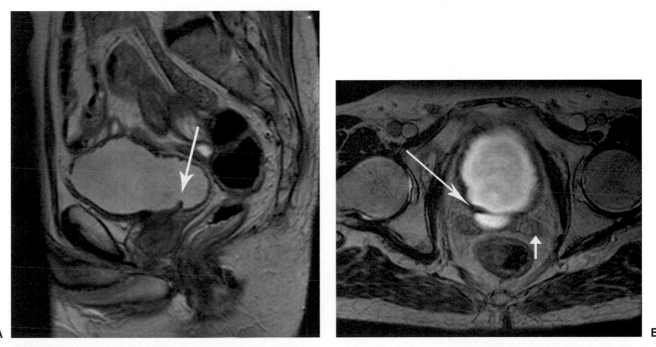

A   B

FIGURE 20-6 **Interureteric ridge prominent in trabeculated bladder. A:** Sagittal and **(B)** axial T2-weighted images show a prominent interureteric ridge (*long arrow*) and trabeculated bladder (*Seminal vesicle = short arrow*). Cystocele formation in women tends to occur just above the ridge.

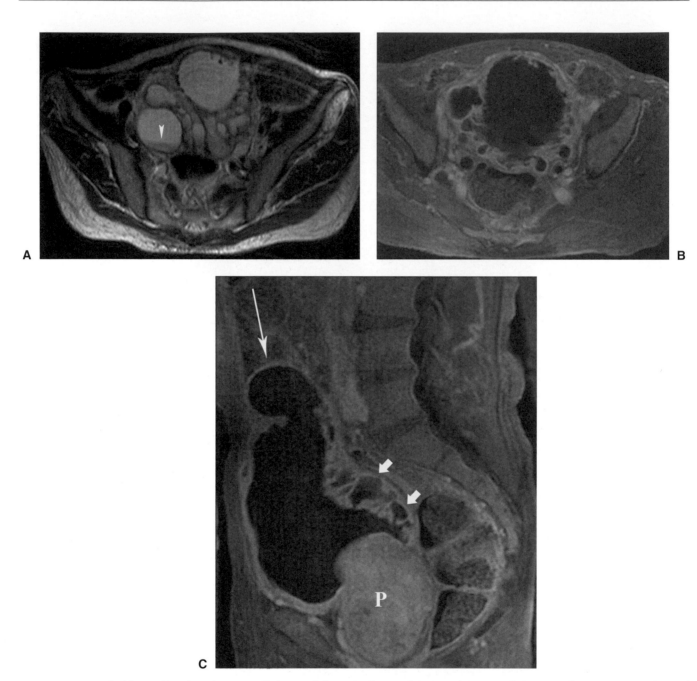

FIGURE 20-7   Bladder wall trabeculation, cellules, and diverticula simulate neoplasm. Axial **(A)** T2 and **(B)** contrast-enhanced T1-weighted images depict a complex, multicystic mass (*Fluid–fluid level = arrowhead*). **C:** An enhanced sagittal acquisition reveals the mass to be the bladder, its appearance altered by chronic outlet obstruction from the very large prostate (*P*) (*Diverticulum = long arrow, Cellules = short arrows*).

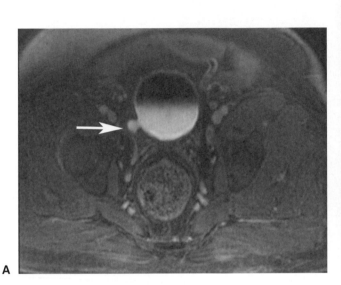
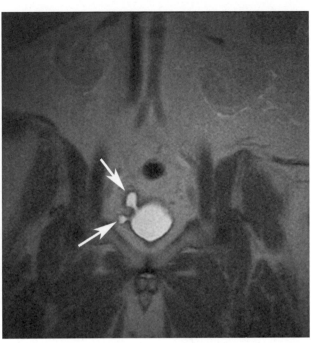

FIGURE 20-8   Bladder diverticula. A: Excreted contrast in the bladder communicates with a small right-sided bladder diverticulum (*arrow*), confirming its diagnosis. **B:** Coronal image shows two diverticula (*arrows*).

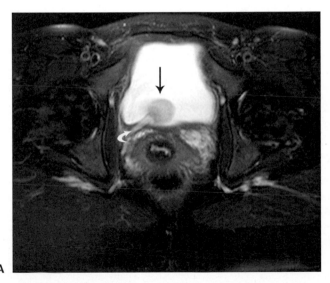
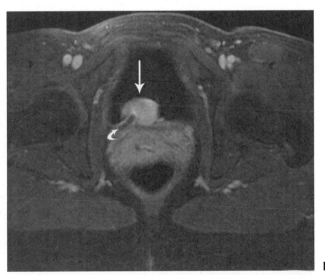

FIGURE 20-9   Chronically inflamed ureterocele mimics malignancy. A: A ureterocele (*arrow*) is capped by a large smooth nodule on axial fat-suppressed T2-weighted image. **B:** Mass (*arrow*) enhances avidly on axial fat-suppressed T1-weighted sequence (*Right ureter = curved arrow*).

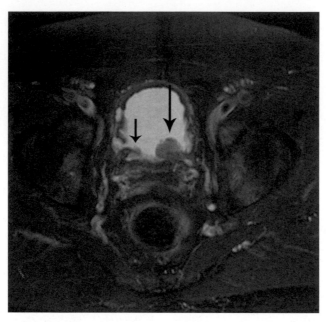

FIGURE 20-10   Malignancy simulates inflamed ureteroceles. Smoothly configured nodules (*arrows*) are perched at each ureteral orifice on fat-suppressed T2-weighted image. Both were high-grade transitional cell carcinoma at resection.

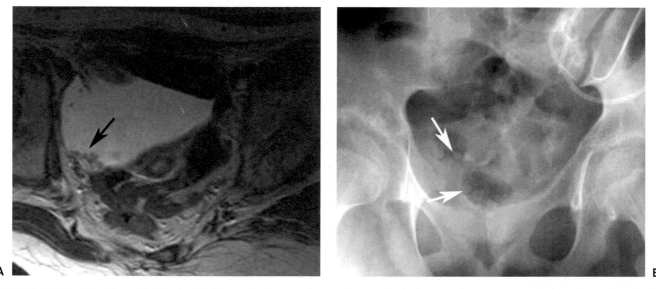

FIGURE 20-11   Bladder calculi. A: Bladder calculi (*arrow*) may be overlooked since they are typically signal voids. Bladder distension helps with conspicuity. **B:** Correlating radiograph shows the radiopaque calculi (*arrows*).

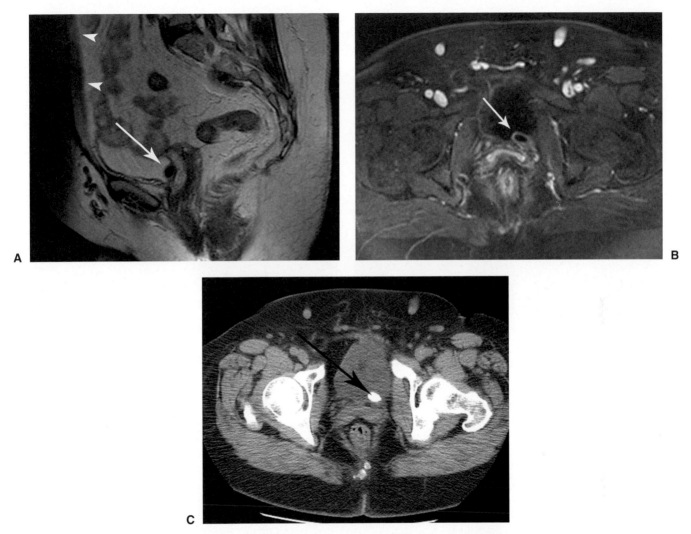

FIGURE 20-12 Stone in ureterocele. A: Sagittal T2-weighted image shows extremely hypointense material (*arrow*) in the vicinity of the ureteral orifice (*Anterior saturation band = arrowheads*). **B:** Axial T1-weighted contrast-enhanced image shows strong enhancement of the ureterocele wall, but signal void inside the ureterocele. **C:** The unconvinced urologist then ordered a CT, which confirmed the stone (*arrow*).

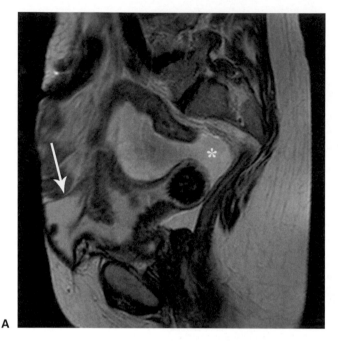

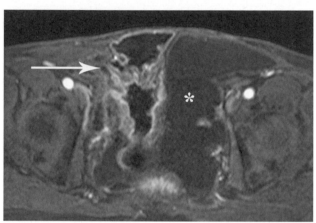

FIGURE 20-13 Neobladder constructed from cecum. The neobladder (*arrows*) simulates a necrotic mass after cystectomy on **(A)** sagittal T2-weighted image and **(B)** axial enhanced, fat-suppressed T1-weighted image. Notice the large amount of free fluid (*asterisk*) from an anastomotic leak.

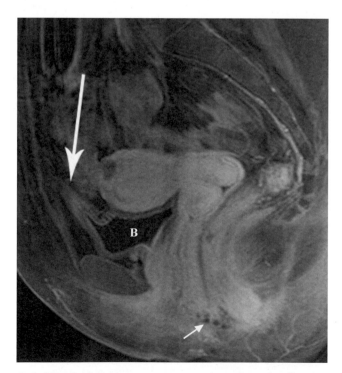

FIGURE 20-14 Small vesicourachal diverticulum in an asymptomatic patient. Small outpouching from the bladder (*B*) at its junction with the urachal remnant (*arrow*). Urachal remnant disease can sometimes be clinically quite significant. Notice suture artifact in the perineum (*short arrow*).

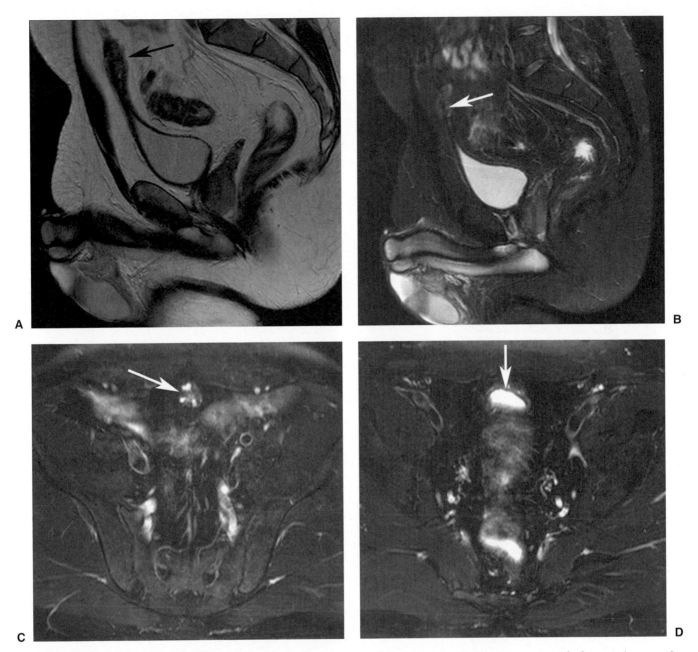

FIGURE 20-15 Urachus. **A** and **B:** Sagittal images show a urachal remnant or diverticulum (*arrows*), with the anterior-superior bladder wall tapering toward the umbilicus. **C:** Axial FSE T2-weighted image shows a small amount of fluid in the urachus (*arrow*), consistent partial patency. **D:** Image obtained more inferiorly shows the altered contour of the anteriorly positioned bladder (*arrow*).

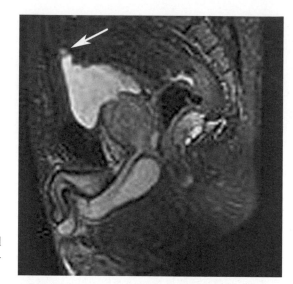

FIGURE 20-16 Urachal diverticulum. Sagittal FSE T2-weighted image shows a diverticulum (*arrow*) originating from the urachus.

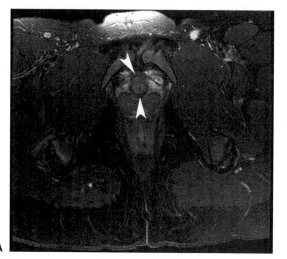

A

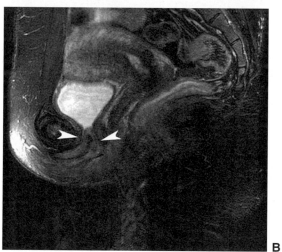

B

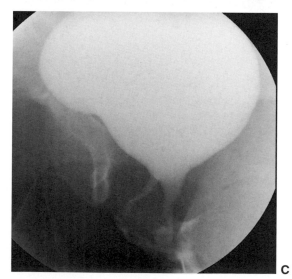

C

FIGURE 20-17 Urethral duplication. A: Axial and (**B**) sagittal FSE T2-weighted images show two separate urethrae (*arrowheads*). **C:** Voiding cystogram confirms this normal variant.

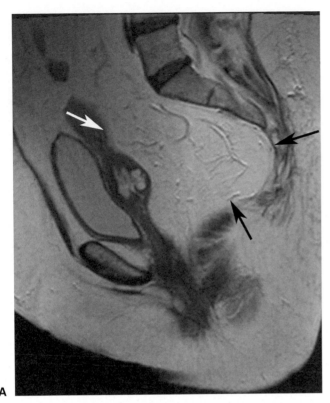

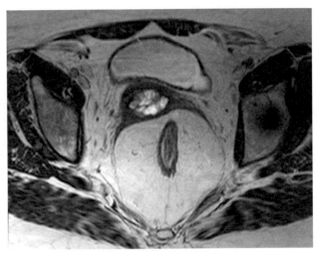

FIGURE 20-18 **Pelvic lipomatosis. A:** Sagittal and **(B)** axial T2-weighted images show extensive perirectal pelvic lipomatosis (*arrows*) with anterior displacement of the vagina, uterus, and bladder.

◼ Vascular and Artifacts

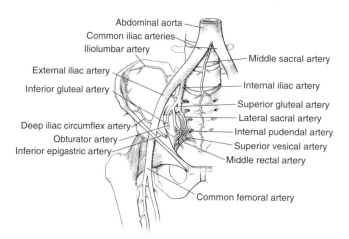

Abdominal aorta
Common iliac arteries
Iliolumbar artery
External iliac artery
Inferior gluteal artery
Deep iliac circumflex artery
Obturator artery
Inferior epigastric artery

Middle sacral artery
Internal iliac artery
Superior gluteal artery
Lateral sacral artery
Internal pudendal artery
Superior vesical artery
Middle rectal artery
Common femoral artery

FIGURE 20-19 Pelvic arterial anatomy. Illustration of the typical arterial anatomy within the pelvis.

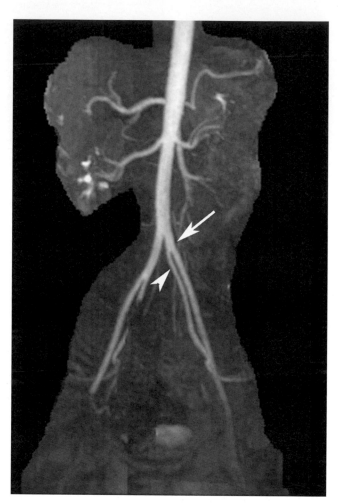

FIGURE 20-20 High origin of left internal iliac artery. Coronal MRA shows a high origin of the left internal iliac artery (*arrowhead*) from the common iliac artery (*arrow*).

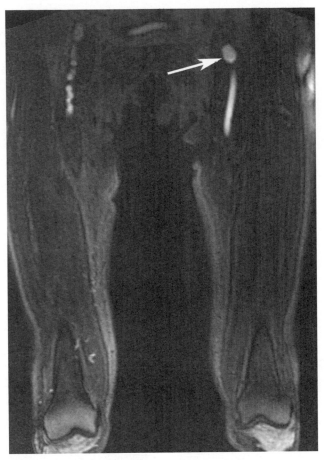

FIGURE 20-21 Dilated left profunda femora origin after endarterectomy. Coronal source image from MRA demonstrates the expected prominence of the left profunda femora origin (*arrow*) after an endarterectomy for atherosclerotic stenosis.

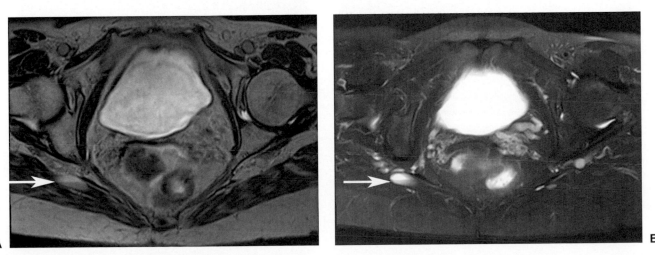

FIGURE 20-22 Prominent gluteal vein. Axial T2-weighted images **(A)** without and **(B)** with fat suppression show a fluid–fluid level (*arrows*) within a prominent right gluteal vein, which could be confused with a mass.

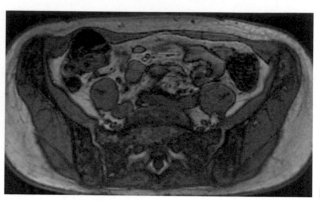
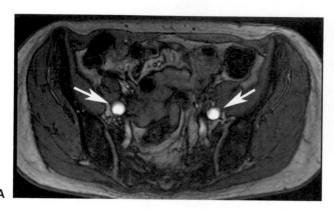

FIGURE 20-23   In-flow enhancement. A: The first image from axial pelvic imaging shows intense signal within the common iliac arteries (*arrows*). **B:** This did not persist on the remaining images and represented entry phenomenon artifact, in which bright signal in these vessels is observed due to blood flowing into the slice after multiple radiofrequency (RF) pulses have decreased the signal (due to incomplete longitudinal relaxation) in the stationary tissue. This is also called *entry slice phenomenon* and *flow-related enhancement.*

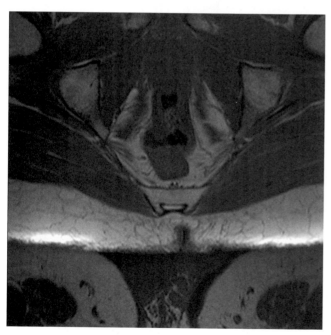

FIGURE 20-24   Signal wrap/aliasing. The anterior pelvis and perineum are misregistered posterior to the gluteal region, since signal outside of the field-of-view has wrapped back in due to poor patient positioning. This occurs when the frequency of the proton spins (outside the field-of-view) is not adequately sampled.

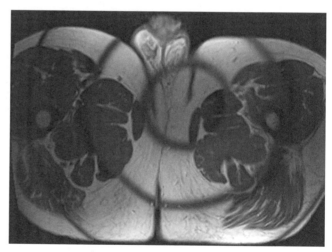

FIGURE 20-25   Field fall-off. Dark bands related to scanning tissue in regions of fall-off of the main magnetic field. This is more prevalent with short-bore systems, in which the magnetic field falls off very rapidly beyond the recommended scanning range in the Z direction.

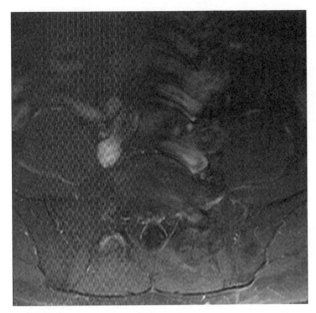

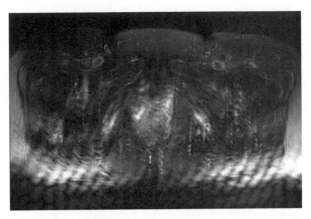

FIGURE 20-27 Ghosting. Ghosting has occurred at the bottom of this image but not at the top. This is likely caused by a system instability related to the signal received by the posterior radiofrequency (RF) coil which does not affect the signal from the anterior RF coil.

FIGURE 20-26 Radiofrequency (RF) interference, pulsation. Artifacts due to RF interference are observed on the left of this image, while ghosting artifacts due to pulsation are observed near the middle of this image.

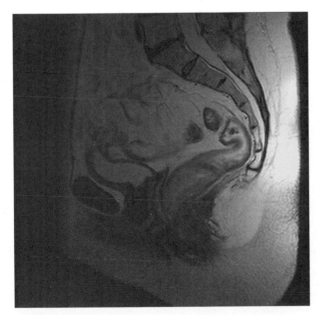

FIGURE 20-28 Anterior surface coils inadvertently turned off. Notice gradual signal loss from posterior to anterior.

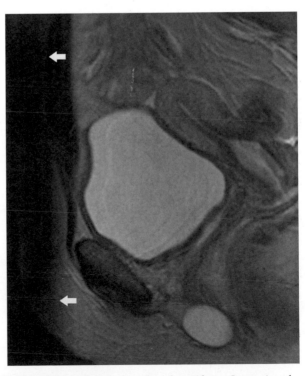

FIGURE 20-29 Saturation band artifact. Saturation band (*arrows*) over the anterior abdominal wall fat was placed to reduce ghosting. Saturation bands are also used above and below imaging plane to reduce flow-related artifact.

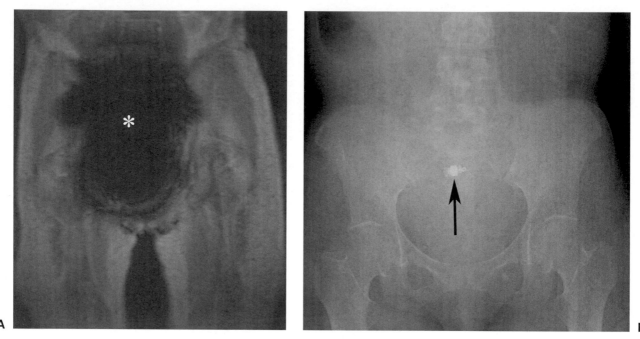

A **B**

FIGURE 20-30   Artifact from video capsule in the small bowel. A: Coronal scout image was markedly degraded by susceptibility artifact (*asterisk*) and examination was subsequently terminated. Spin dephasing and distortion is observed due to differences in magnetic susceptibility of the metal endoscopy capsule compared to that of tissue and air. **B:** Radiograph more clearly depicts the small metal video capsule (*arrow*) which had been lodged for months in the distal small bowel.

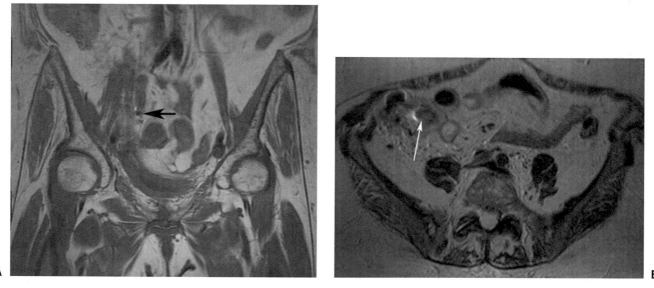

A **B**

FIGURE 20-31   Metallic clip artifact. A and **B:** Spin dephasing and distortion is observed due to differences in magnetic susceptibility of a metal clip (*arrows*) compared to that of tissue and air.

Suggested Readings

Amano Y, Gemma K, Kawamata H, et al. Fat-suppressed gadolinium-enhanced three-dimensional magnetic resonance angiography adequately depicts the status of iliac arteries following atherectomy and stent placement. *Cardiovasc Intervent Radiol*. 1998;21(4):345–347.

Bae KS, Jeon SH, Lee SJ, et al. Complete duplication of bladder and urethra in coronal plane with no other anomalies: Case report with review of the literature. *Urology*. 2005;65(2):388.

Bergman RA, Thompson SA, Afifi AK, et al., ed. *Compendium of human anatomic variation*. Baltimore: Urban & Schwarzenberg; 1988.

Boechat MI. MRI of the pediatric pelvis. *Magn Reson Imaging Clin N Am*. 1996;4(4):679–696.

Cappele O, Sibert L, Descargues J, et al. A study of the anatomic features of the duct of the urachus. *Surg Radiol Anat*. 2001;23(4):229–235.

Cardinot TM, Aragao AH, Babinski MA, et al. Rare variation in course and affluence of internal iliac vein due to its anatomical and surgical significance. *Surg Radiol Anat*. 2006;28:422–425.

Daniel BL, Shimakawa A, Blum MR, et al. Single-shot fluid attenuated inversion recovery (FLAIR) magnetic resonance imaging of the bladder. *J Magn Reson Imaging*. 2000;11(6):673–677.

Faure JP, Doucet C, Rigouard P, et al. Anatomical pitfalls in the technique for total extraperitoneal laparascopic repair of inguinal hernias. *Surg Radiol Anat*. 2006;28:486–493.

Kibbe MR, Ujiki M, Goodwin AL, et al. Iliac vein compression in an asymptomatic patient population. *J Vasc Surg*. 2004;29:937–943.

Lapointe SP, Wei DC, Hricak H, et al. Magnetic resonance imaging in the evaluation of congenital anomalies of the external genitalia. *Urology*. 2001;58(3):452–456.

Lesbats-Jacquot V, Amoretti N, Cucchi JM, et al. Subumbilical parietal cystic images. *Clin Imaging*. 2007;31(5):340–342.

Mallampati GK, Siegelman ES. MRI of the bladder. *Magn Reson Imaging Clin N Am*. 2004;12(3):545–555.

Michaely HJ, Attenberger UI, Kramer H, et al. Abdominal and pelvic MR angiography. *Magn Reson Imaging Clin N Am*. 2007;15(3):301–314.

Nael K, Ruehm SG, Michaely HJ, et al. Multistation whole-body high-spatial resolution MR angiography using a 32-channel MR system. *AJR Am J Roentgenol*. 2007;188:529–539.

Ozel LZ, Talu M, User Y, et al. Coexistence of a Meckel's diverticulum and a urachal remnant. *Clin Anat*. 2005;18:609–612.

Strouse PJ. Magnetic resonance angiography of the pediatric abdomen and pelvis. *Magn Reson Imaging Clin N Am*. 2002;10(2):345–361.

Chapter 21

Musculoskeletal

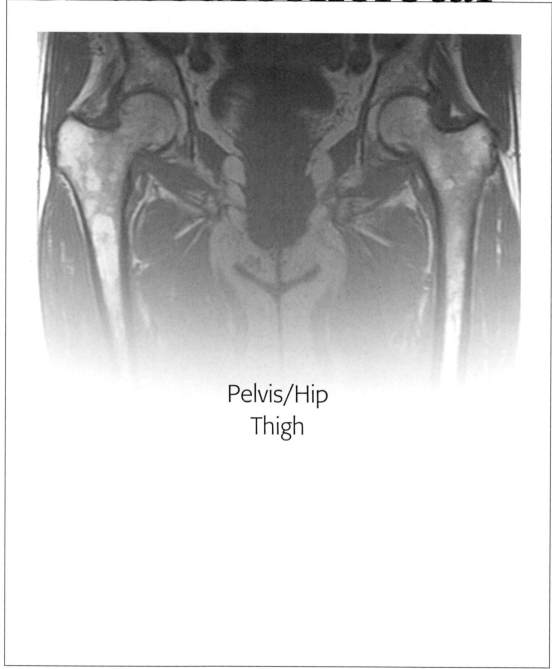

Pelvis/Hip
Thigh

Laura W. Bancroft and John E. Kirsch

■ Pelvis/Hip

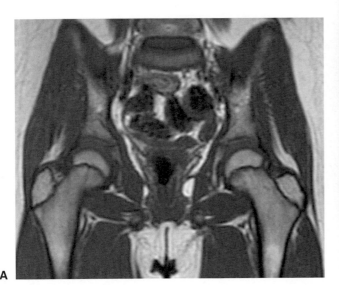
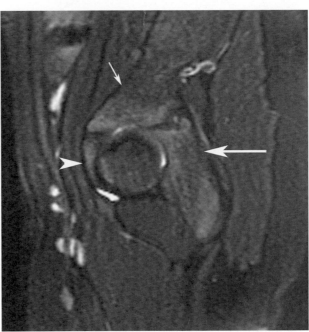

FIGURE 21-1 **Pediatric pelvis. A:** Coronal T1-weighted image shows the normal MR appearance of the pediatric pelvis. **B:** Sagittal FSE T2-weighted fat-suppressed image through the hip shows the pubis (*arrowhead*), ilium (*small arrow*) and ischium (*large arrow*) about the triradiate cartilage.

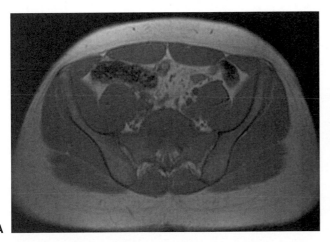
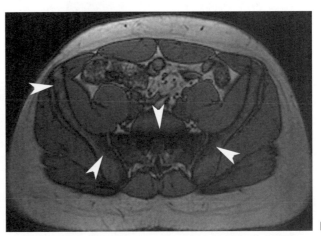

FIGURE 21-2 **Normal in- and out-of-phase imaging. A:** In- and **(B)** out-of-phase imaging demonstrates signal loss (*arrowheads*) in marrow that contains both fat and water content in the same voxel. Failure to drop in signal with out-of-phase imaging would be worrisome for a marrow replacing lesion.

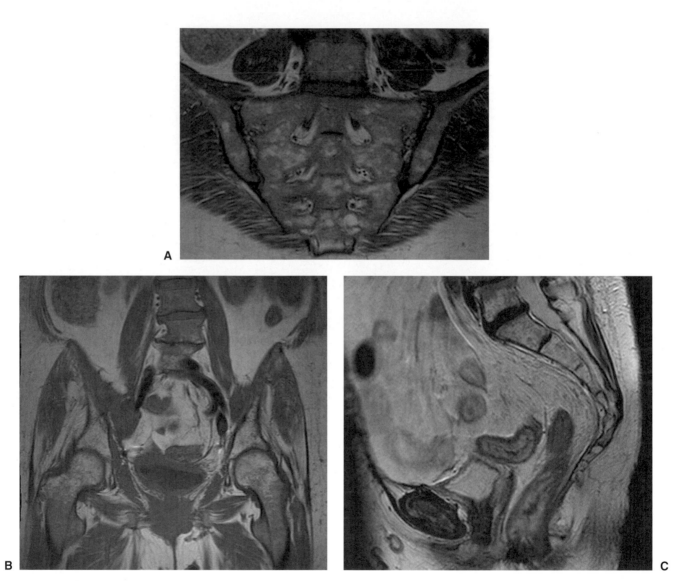

FIGURE 21-3 Heterogeneous marrow. **A–C:** There can be a variable mix of red and yellow marrow in the adult pelvis.

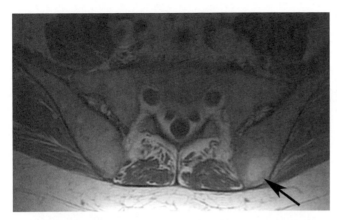

FIGURE 21-4   Focal fat in left ilium. Axial T1-weighted image shows focal fat (*arrow*) in the posterior left ilium, which is a normal finding.

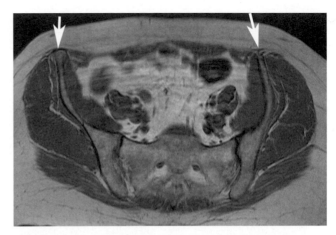

FIGURE 21-5   Asymmetric iliac bones. Mild asymmetry of the pelvis (*arrows*) can be seen without any underlying pathology.

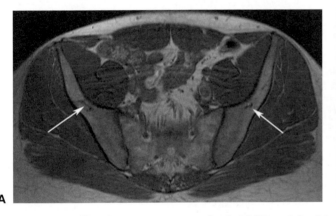

A

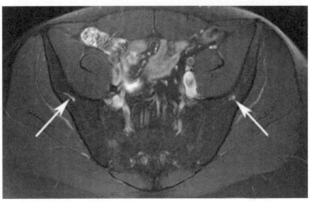

B

FIGURE 21-6   Iliac intraosseous vessels. Axial T1-weighted images **(A)** pre- and **(B)** postcontrast demonstrate symmetric iliac nutrient vessels (*arrows*), which can be quite prominent.

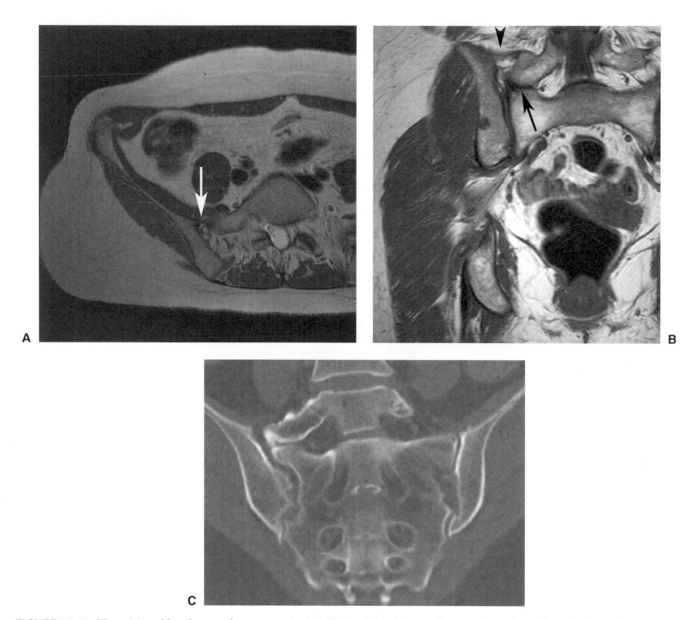

FIGURE 21-7 Transitional lumbosacral segment. A: Axial T1-weighted image shows unilateral pseudoarticulation (*arrow*) at site of transitional lumbosacral segment. Transitional vertebrae are present in approximately 20% of the population and often involve the lumbosacral junction. **B:** Coronal T1-weighted image shows the pseudoarticulation (*arrow*) as well as the iliolumbar ligament (*arrowhead*), signifying a sacralized lumbar segment. **C:** Coronal CT reconstruction correlation shows the elongated transverse process of the transitional segment articulating with the superior sacroiliac (SI) joint and the adjacent sacrum.

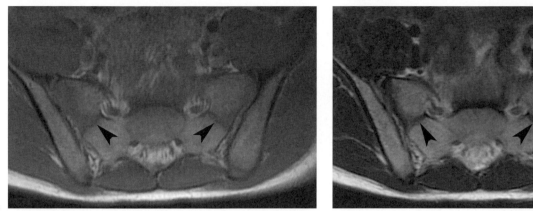
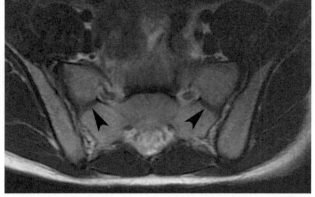

FIGURE 21-8 Pediatric sacrum. A and **B:** Axial imaging shows the normal articulations between the sacral segments (*arrowheads*) in a child. During childhood development, five central ossification centers become the vertebral bodies, six centers form the sacral ala, the costal ossifications centers form the lateral masses, and the neural ossification centers develop posteriorly.

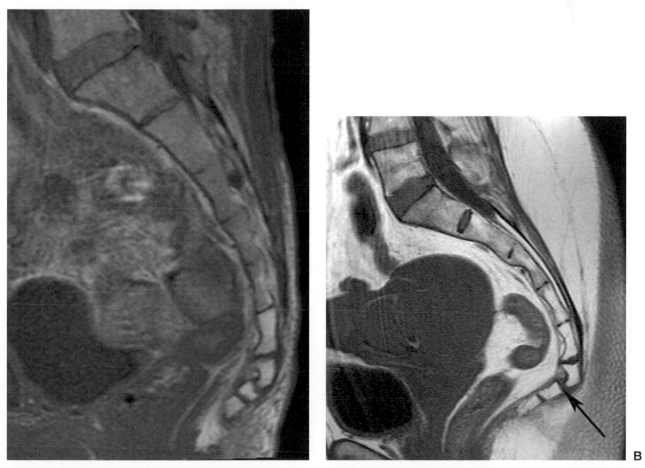

FIGURE 21-9 Variation in sacrococcygeal angulation and shape. In the sagittal plane, the sacrum and coccyx may be **(A)** relatively straight or **(B)** acutely angulated (*arrow*).

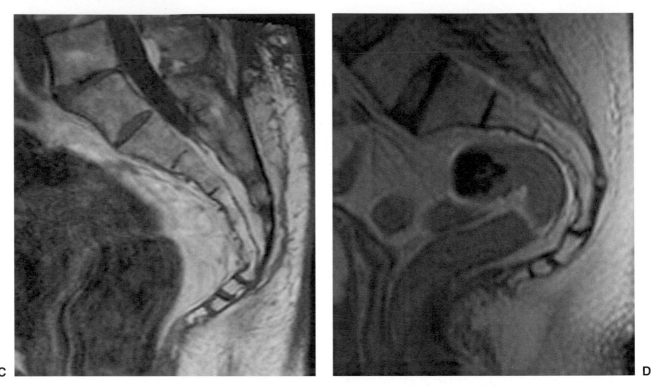

FIGURE 21-9 **Variation in sacrococcygeal angulation and shape.** (*continued*) **C** and **D**: The sacrum and coccyx may be **(B)** moderately or **(C)** markedly curved. The sacrum is typically broader and less curved in women, and narrower and more curved in men.

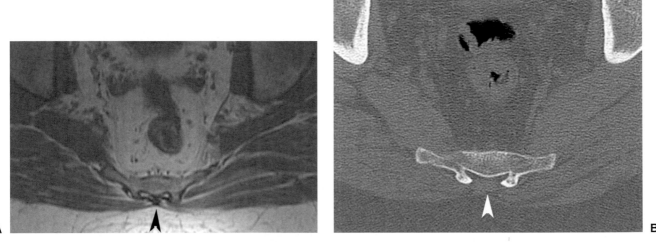

FIGURE 21-10 **Absence of sacral dorsal arches.** The sacral laminae may fail to meet in the dorsal midline (*arrowheads*), as demonstrated on **(A)** axial T1-weighed image and **(B)** correlating CT. Approximately 1% of the population will have the sacral canal completely open.

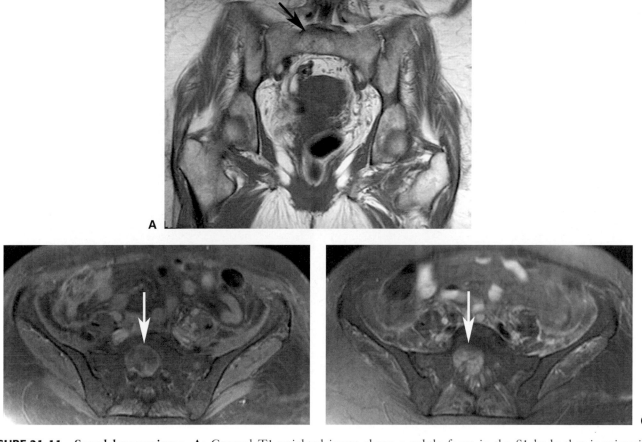

FIGURE 21-11 **Sacral hemangioma. A:** Coronal T1-weighted image shows a subtle focus in the S1 body that is primarily comprised of fat (*arrow*) with areas of coarsened trabeculae, consistent with an hemangioma. Axial **(B)** T2-weighted and **(C)** enhanced T1-weighted images show marked heterogeneity and enhancement of the hemangioma, which could be confusing without an unenhanced T1-weighted sequence.

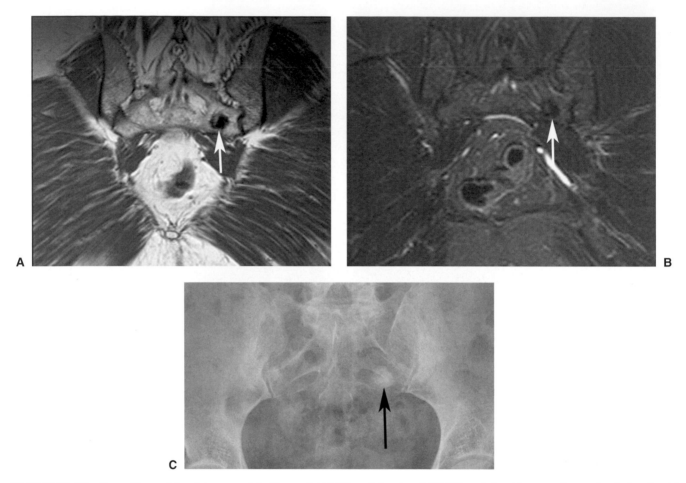

FIGURE 21-12 Sacral bone island (enostosis). Coronal **(A)** T1-weighted and **(B)** T2-weighted images show a focal signal void (*arrows*) with spiculated margins and some central fatty marrow, consistent with a bone island. No enhancement or increased fluid-sensitive signal was present. **C:** Correlating radiograph shows the classic appearance of a bone island (*arrow*).

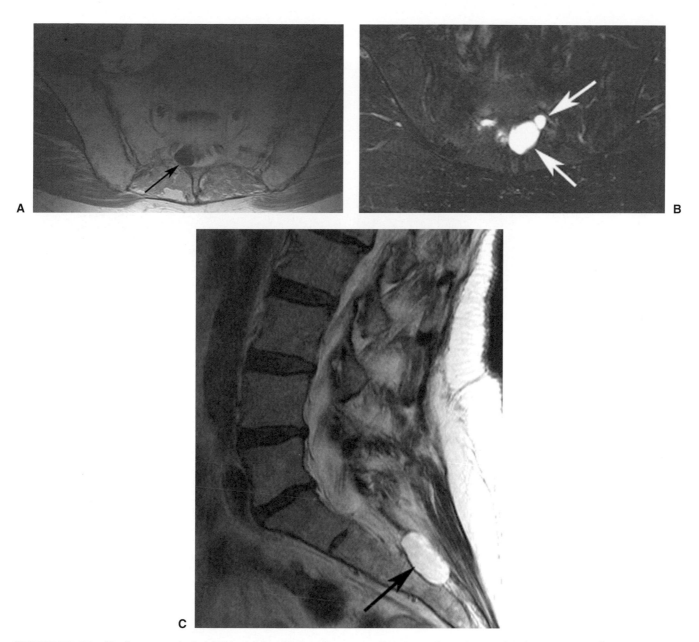

FIGURE 21-13 Tarlov cysts. A: Axial T1-weighted image shows a small perineural cyst (*arrow*). Tarlov cysts typically communicate freely with the subarachnoid space. **B:** Axial and (**C**) sagittal fluid sensitive images show larger sacral Tarlov cysts (*arrows*).

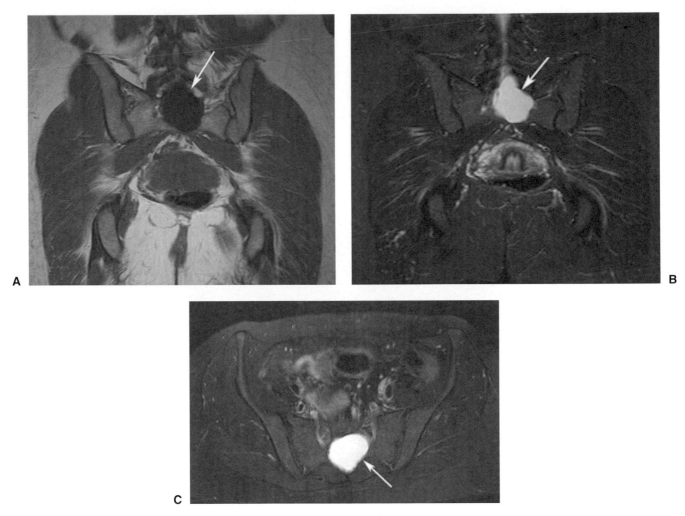

FIGURE 21-14 Occult sacral meningocele. A and **B:** Coronal and **(C)** axial FSE T2-weighted fat-suppressed images show an occult sacral meningocele (*arrows*). Pulsations of the cerebrospinal fluid or raised intraspinal pressure can erode or remodel the adjacent sacral canal or foramen. Although this patient was symptomatic, some patients can complain of pain and cyst aspiration may be performed.

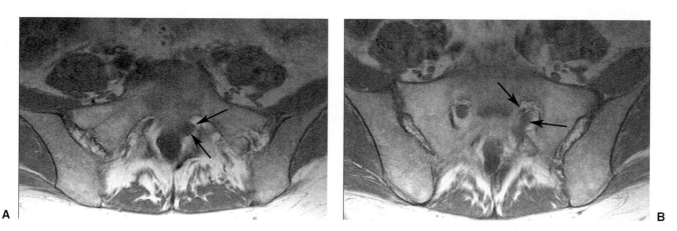

FIGURE 21-15 **Conjoined left S1-2 nerve roots. A** and **B:** Axial images through the sacrum show conjoined left S1 and S2 nerve roots (*arrows*).

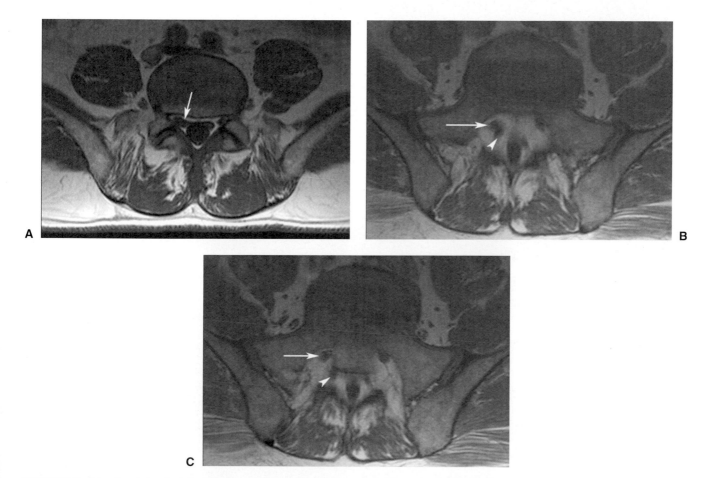

FIGURE 21-16 **Conjoined right S1-2 nerve roots. A:** Axial image shows a common origin of the right S1 and S2 nerve roots (*arrow*). **B** and **C:** More inferiorly, the S1 (*arrow*) and S2 (*arrowheads*) nerve roots become divided.

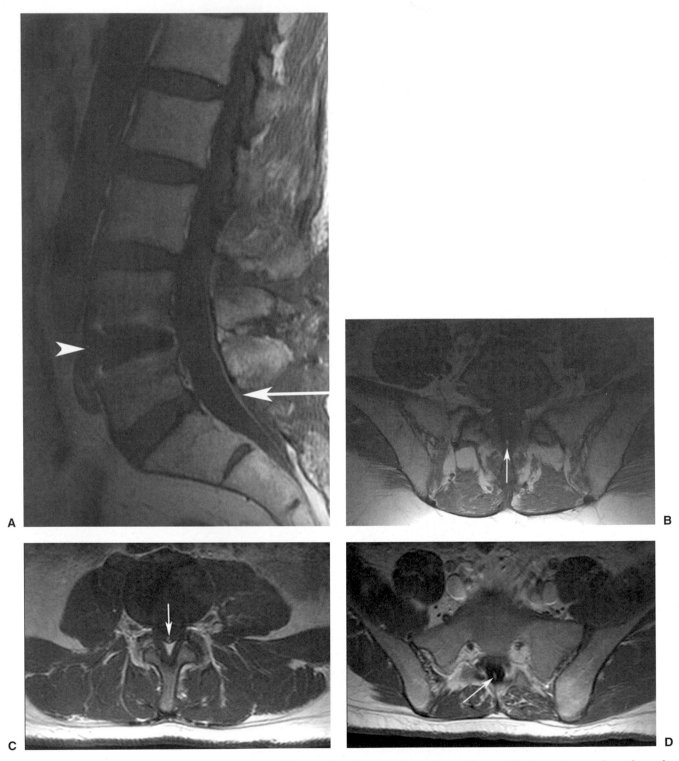

FIGURE 21-17 **Fatty filum. A:** Sagittal and **(B)** axial T1-weighted images show a linear focus of fat (*arrows*) extending along the posterior canal, which is a fatty filum. This finding can be seen in less than 1% of normal patients, and is occasionally associated with tethered cord and low-lying conus medullaris. Note the artifact from L4-5 intervertebral disc spacer (*arrowhead*). **C** and **D:** Axial T1-weighted images in different patients show fatty fila (*arrows*).

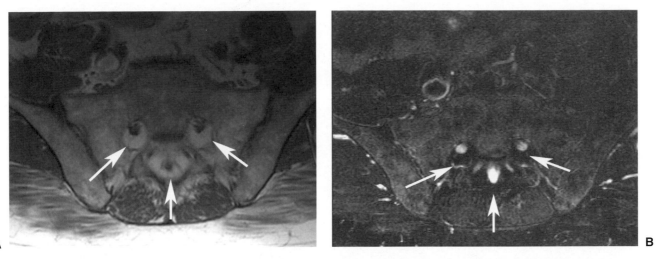

FIGURE 21-18 **Sacral epidural lipomatosis.** Axial **(A)** T1-weighted and **(B)** FSE T2-weighted fat-suppressed images demonstrate prominent epidural fat (*arrows*), of no clinical significance.

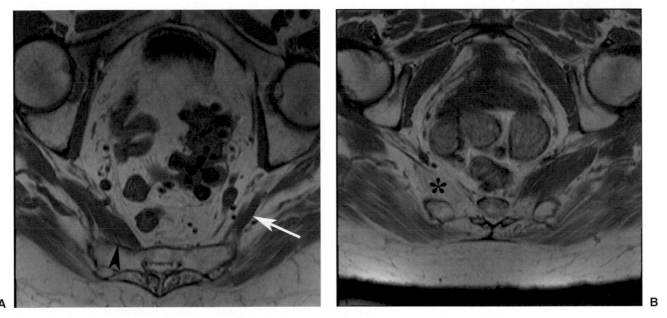

FIGURE 21-19 **Asymmetric piriformis muscle size and attachments.** **A:** The right piriformis (*arrowhead*) in this patient is larger than the left (*arrow*) and has a broader attachment onto the sacrum. Asymmetry of piriform thickness up to 8 mm has no reliable correlation to sciatic pain. **B:** Axial image in a different patient shows an almost ghostlike appearance of the atrophic right piriformis muscle (*asterisk*). Such degree of atrophy can be associated with nerve entrapment at the level of the sciatic notch.

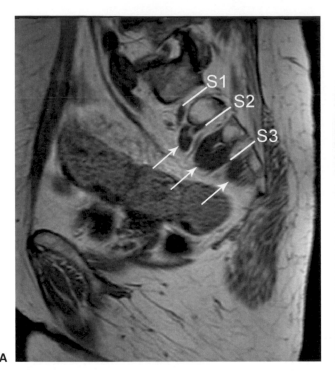

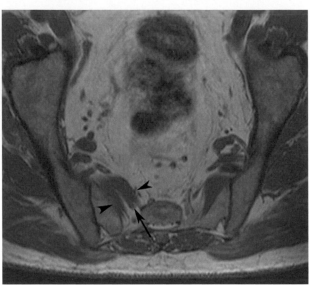

FIGURE 21-20 **Right S2 and S3 nerve roots extend through piriformis. A:** Sagittal image through the sacrum show the S2 and S3 nerve roots extending through the piriformis muscle. Approximately 75% of S2 nerve roots and 97% of S3 nerve roots will extend through the piriformis. **B:** Axial oblique image through the posterior pelvis delineates extension of the right S2 nerve root (*arrows*) through muscle fibers of the piriformis (*arrowheads*).

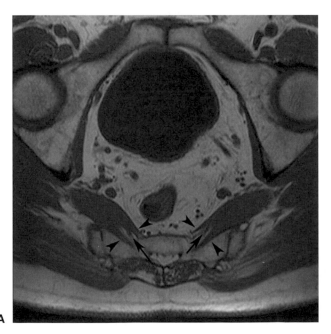

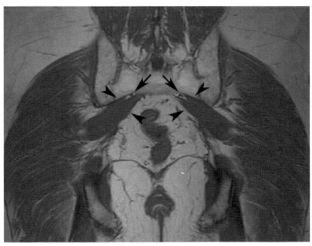

FIGURE 21-21 **Bilateral S2 nerve roots extend through piriformis. A:** Coronal and **(B)** axial oblique images through the posterior pelvis delineate extension of both S2 nerve roots (*arrows*) through fibers of the piriformis muscles (*arrowheads*).

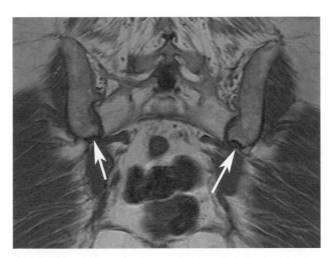

FIGURE 21-22 **Preauricular (paraglenoid) sulci.** Coronal T1-weighted image shows differing sizes of the normal preauricular sulci (*arrows*), which are the sites of ligamentous attachments and vascular conduits in females.

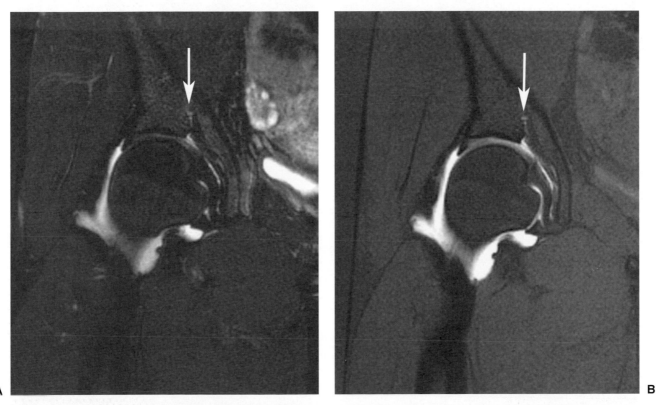

FIGURE 21-23 **Normal supraacetabular vascular channels.** Coronal **(A)** T2-weighted and **(B)** MR arthrographic images show a prominent supra-acetabular vascular channel (*arrow*).

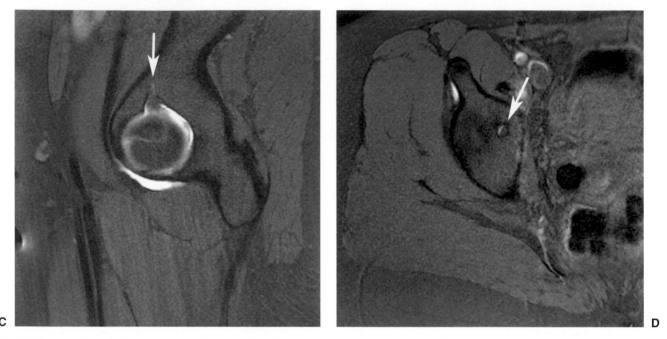

FIGURE 21-23 **Normal supraacetabular vascular channels.** (*continued*) This normal structure has a more **(C)** conical configuration (*arrow*) in the sagittal plane and **(D)** rounded appearance (*arrow*) in cross-section.

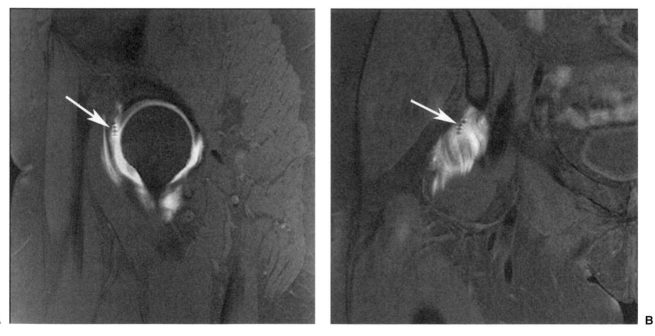

FIGURE 21-24 **Intra-articular bubbles from MR arthrogram. A:** Sagittal and **(B)** coronal images show several tiny foci of artifact (*arrows*) in the non-dependent joint space, consistent with inadvertently injected air during MR arthrogram.

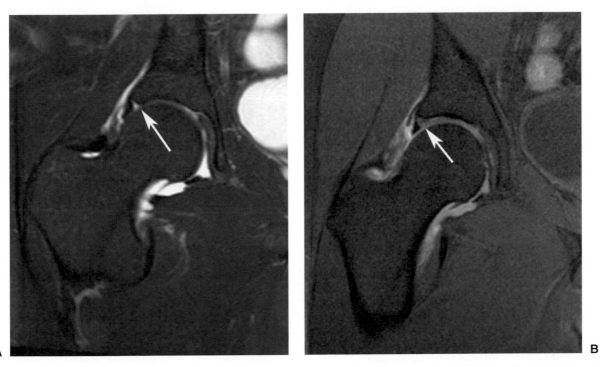

FIGURE 21-25 **Prominent sublabral cartilage simulating recess or partial labral detachment. A:** Coronal FSE T2-weighted fat-suppressed image shows high signal (*arrow*) extending between the superior labrum and acetabulum. **B:** However, coronal MR arthrographic image shows prominent intermediate signal cartilage (*arrow*) in this interval. No contrast extended either within or beneath the labrum.

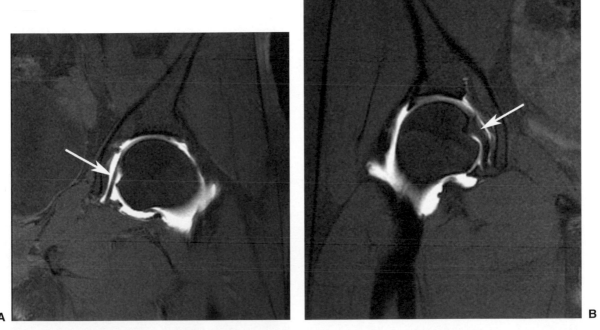

FIGURE 21-26 **Ligamentum teres. A** and **B:** The normal ligamentum teres (*arrows*) can vary somewhat in thickness. The ligamentum teres arises from the margins of the acetabular notch and the transverse acetabular ligament, is extracapsular, and may provide some stability to the hip joint in the presence of labral pathology.

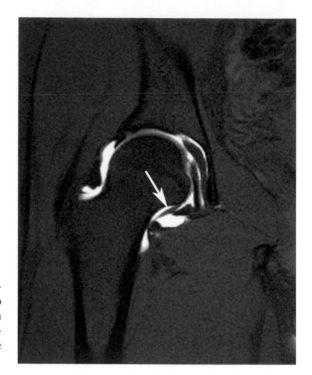

FIGURE 21-27 Pectinofoveal fold. The pectino-foveal fold is identified in the vast majority of hip MR arthrograms. About half of these folds will have a smooth contour, and the other half will have an irregular contour. The pectinofoveal fold inserts onto the capsule more often than onto the femur.

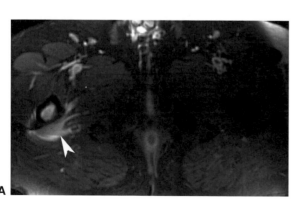

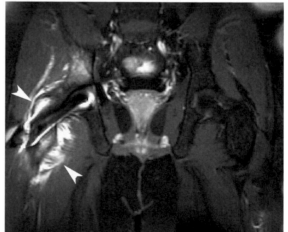

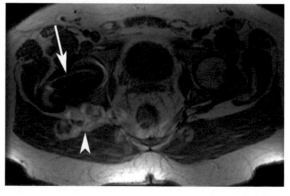

FIGURE 21-28 Field inhomogeneity due to metal. A: Axial and **(B)** coronal FSE T2-weighted images were obtained with chemical fat suppression, as opposed to obtaining a fast short tau inversion recovery (STIR) technique. However, signal outside of the field-of-view has wrapped (*arrowhead*) in the phase-encoding direction due to placement of the patient's hands anterior to the pelvis, rather than to the side. This occurs when the frequency of tissue proton spins (outside the field-of-view) is not adequately sampled (*Hip screw = arrow*).

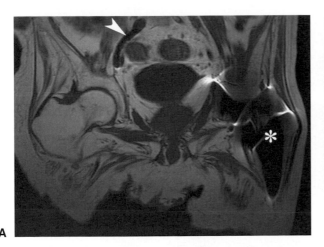
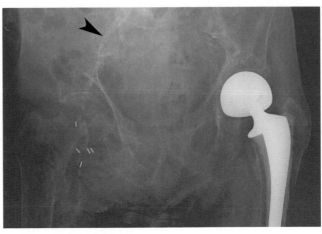

FIGURE 21-29 **Artifact from bipolar hip arthroplasty and iliac stent. A:** Coronal T1-weighted image shows substantial misregistration from metal susceptibility artifact due to left bipolar hip arthroplasty (*asterisk*), but little artifact from the right common iliac stent (*arrowhead*). Spin dephasing and distortion is observed due to differences in magnetic susceptibility of a metal implant compared to that of tissue. **B:** Correlating radiograph.

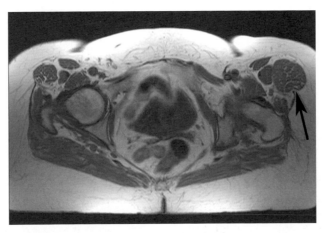

FIGURE 21-30 **Enlarged tensor fascia lata muscle.** Axial image shows hypertrophy of the left tensor fascia lata muscle (*arrow*), which should not be mistaken for a soft tissue mass. This should be differentiated from pseudohypertrophy, which occurs with denervation and shows a greater proportion of fat between the muscles.

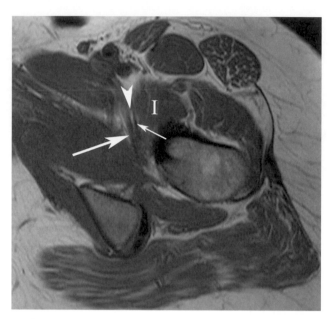

FIGURE 21-31 Distinct iliacus and psoas tendon attachments. Axial T1-weighted image shows two distinct paralleling structures, the psoas tendon (*large arrow*) and intramuscular portion of the iliacus tendon (*small arrow*). Fatty fascia from the iliopsoas tendon (*arrowhead*) accounts for the intervening increased signal. The psoas tendon attaches onto the lesser trochanter and the majority of the iliacus muscle (*I*) attaches onto the proximal femoral shaft without a tendon.

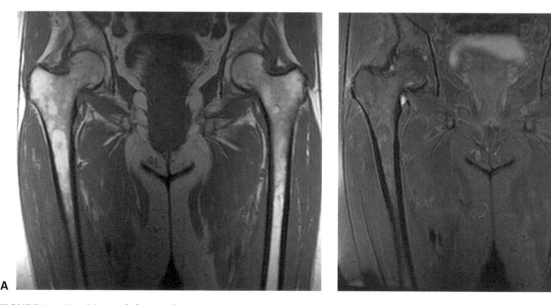

FIGURE 21-32 Normal femoral marrow. A: There can be variable ratios of red and yellow marrow within the femora. On T1-weighted images the red marrow is hypointense to fat, but hyperintense to skeletal muscle. **B:** Red marrow is hypointense to muscle on T2-weighted images.

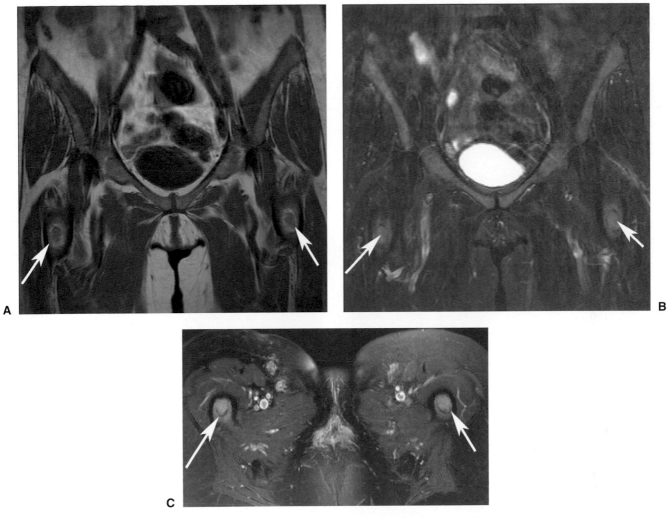

FIGURE 21-33 **Target sign in the proximal femora. A–C:** The presence of both red and yellow marrow can normally produce a "target sign" (*arrows*) in the subtrochanteric femora. This should not be confused with marrow replacing lesions.

▪ Thigh

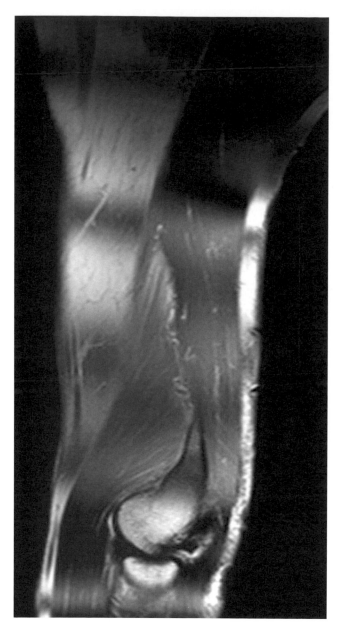

FIGURE 21-34 Poor shim. The banding in this image is due to an extremely poor shim of the magnetic field while applying a fat saturation technique. From top to bottom, a transition from fat saturation to water saturation to no saturation can be observed.

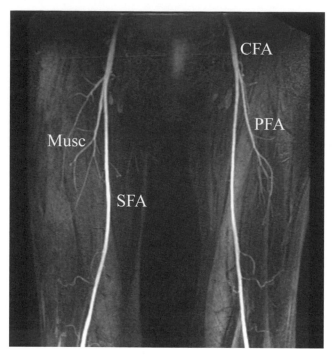

FIGURE 21-35 MRA of the thighs. Conventional anatomy of the arterial supply to the thigh (*Common femoral artery = CFA, Profunda femoris artery = PFA, Superficial femoral artery = SFA, Muscular branches = Musc*).

Table 21-1 Muscle variations in the pelvis/hip
Iliopsoas (third head = iliacus minor/iliocapsularis)
Psoas minor (absent, variable origin)
Tensor fascia lata (divided, accessory slips, fuse with gluteus maximus)
Gluteus maximus (accessory slips = ischiofemoral muscle, coccygeofemoral, fuse with tensor fascia lata)

(Compiled from Bergman RA, Thompson SA, Afifi AK, et al. *Compendium of human anatomic variation*. Baltimore: Urban and Schwartzenberg; 1988.)

Table 21-2 Muscles of the pelvis and their functions

Muscle	Origin	Insertion	Function	Innervation
Vastus medialis	Medial posterior femur	Medial tendon of rectus femoris	Extensor of knee	L3-4
Vastus intermedius	Anterior mid femur	Upper posterior patella	Extensor of knee	L3-4
Pectineus	Superior pubic ramus	Pectineal line femur	Thigh flexor	Femoral nerve (L2, L3)
Adductor longus	Anterior pubic bone	Medial linea aspera	Thigh adductor	Obturator nerve (L2-3)
Adductor brevis	Pubic bone and inferior ramus	Upper linea aspera	Thigh adductor	Obturator nerve (L2-3)
Adductor magnus	Ischium and inferior pubic ramus	Linea aspera Adductor tubercle	Thigh adductor	Obturator and tibial nerve (L3-5)
Gracilis	Inferior pubic ramus near symphysis	Upper anterior tibia	Thigh adductor	Obturator nerve (L3-4)
			Medical rotator thigh	
Obturator externus	Outer margins obturator foramen	Intertrochanteric fossa	Lateral rotator	Obturator nerve (L3-4)
Semitendinosus	Posteromedial ischial tuberosity	Upper anterior tibia	Thigh extensor	Tibial side of sciatic (L5-S1)
			Knee flexor	
Biceps femoris	Long head: posteromedial ischial tuberosity	Fibular head	Extend thigh	Long head: tibial side of sciatic nerve (L5-S1)
	Short head: lateral lip linea aspera	Fibular head	Flex knee	Short head: peroneal side of sciatic nerve (L5-S2)
Semimembranosus	Posterolateral ischial tuberosity	Posteromedial upper tibia	Thigh extensor	Tibial side of sciatic nerve (L5-S2)
			Accessory medial rotator and thigh adductor	

From Berquist TH. *MRI of the Musculoskeletal System.* 5th ed. Lippincott 2006.)

Suggested Readings

Pelvis/Hip

Abe I, Harada Y, Oinuma K, et al. Acetabular labrum: Abnormal findings at MRI in asymptomatic hips. *Radiology.* 2000;216:576–581.

Aihara T, Takahashi K, Ogasawara A, et al. Intervertebral disc degeneration associated with lumbosacral transitional vertebrae: A clinical and anatomical study. *J Bone Joint Surg Br.* 2005;87(5):687–691.

Anson BJ, ed. *Morris' human anatomy,* 12th ed. New York: The Blakiston Division, McGraw-Hill; 1966.

Atlihan D, Jones DC, Guanche CA. Arthroscopic treatment of a symptomatic hip plica. *Clin Orthop Relat Res.* 2003;411:174–177.

Bergman RA, Thompson SA, Afifi AK, et al., ed. *Compendium of human anatomic variation.* Baltimore: Urban & Schwarzenberg; 1988.

Böttcher J, Petrovitch A, Sörös P, et al. Conjoined lumbosacral nerve roots: Current aspects of diagnosis. *Eur Spine J.* 2004;13(2):147–151.

Carpineta L, Faingold R, Albuquerque PA, et al. Magnetic resonance imaging of pelvis and hips in infants, children, and adolescents: A pictorial review. *Curr Probl Diagn Radiol.* 2007;36(4):143–152.

Dinauer PA, Murphy KP, Carroll JF. Sublabral sulcus at the posteroinferior acetabulum: A potential pitfall in MR arthrography diagnosis of acetabular labral tears. *Am J Roentgenol.* 2004;183:1745–1753.

Gill JB. Fat suppression imaging in epidural lipomatosis: Case report. *J Surg Orthop Adv*. 2007;16(3):144–147.

Hughes RJ, Saiffusin A. Numbering of lumbosacral transitional vertebrae on MRI: Role of the iliolumbar ligaments. *AJR Am J Roentgenol*. 2006;187:W59–W66.

Hwang S, Panicek DM. Magnetic resonance imaging of bone marrow in oncology, Part 1. *Skeletal Radiol*. 2007;36(10):913–920.

Ilaslan H, Wenger DE, Shives TC, et al. Unilateral hypertrophy of tensor fascia lata: A soft tissue tumor simulator. *Skeletal Radiol*. 2003; 32(11):628–632.

Kershner DE, Binhammer RT. Lumbar intrathecal ligaments. *Clin Anat*. 2002;15:82–87.

Lee MJ, Kim S, Lee SA, et al. Overcoming artifacts from metallic orthopedic implants at high-field-strength MRI and multi-detector CT. *Radiographics*. 2007;27:791–803.

Lee EY, Margherita AJ, Gierada DS, et al. MRI of piriformis syndrome. *AJR Am J Roentgenol*. 2004;183(1):63–64.

Liney GP, Bernard CP, Manton DJ, et al. Age, gender, and skeletal variation in bone marrow composition: A preliminary study at 3.0 Tesla. *J Magn Reson Imaging*. 2007;26(3):787–793.

Loughenbury PR, Wadhwani S, Soames RW. The posterior longitudinal ligament and peridural (epidural) membrane. *Clin Anat*. 2006;19: 487–492.

Medina LS, Al-Orfali M, Zurakowski D, et al. Occult lumbosacral dysraphism in children and young adults: Diagnostic performance of fast screening and conventional MRI. *Radiology*. 1999;211:767–771.

Montazei JL, Divine M, Lepage E, et al. Normal spinal bone marrow in adults: Dynamic gadolinium-enhanced MRI. *Radiology*. 2003;229: 703–709.

Newell RLM. The spinal epidural space. *Clin Anat*. 1999;12:375–379.

O'Driscoll CM, Irwin A, Saifuddin A. Variations in morphology of the lumbosacral junction on sagittal MRI: Correlation with plain radiography. *Skeletal Radiol*. 1996;25(3):225–230.

Petersilge CA. Chronic adult hip pain: MR arthrography of the hip. *Radiographics*. 2000;20:S43–S52.

Polster JM, Elgabaly M, Lee H, et al. MRI and gross anatomy of the iliopsoas tendon complex. *Skeletal Radiol*. 2008;37(1):55–58.

Roberts N, Hogg D, Whitehouse GH, et al. Quantitative analysis of diurnal variation in volume and water content of lumbar intervertebral discs. *Clin Anat*. 1998;11:1–8.

Russell JM, Kransdorf MJ, Bancroft LW, et al. MRI of the sacral plexus and piriformis muscles. *Presented at 2007 Radiologic Society of North America*. North America, 2007.

Schemmer D, White PG, Friedman L. Radiology of the paraglenoid sulcus. *Skeletal Radiol*. 1995;24:205–209.

Whitlow CT, Mussat-Whitlow BJ, Mattern CWT, et al. Sacroplasty versus vertebroplasty: Comparable clinical outcomes for the treatment of fracture-related pain. *AJNR Am J Neuroradiol*. 2007;28:1266–1270.

Windisch G, Braun EM, Anderhuber F. Piriformis muscle: Clinical anatomy and consideration of the piriformis syndrome. *Surg Radiol Anat*. 2007;29:37045.

Zoga AC, Morrison WB. Technical considerations in MRI of the hip. *Magn Reson Imaging Clin N Am*. 2005;13(4):617–634.

Thigh

Kadir S. Arterial anatomy of the lower extremities. In: Kadir S, ed. *Atlas of normal and variant angiographic anatomy*. Philadelphia: WB Saunders; 1991:123–160.

Nael K, Ruehm SG, Michaely HJ, et al. Multistation whole-body high-spatial resolution MR angiography using a 32-channel MR system. *AJR Am J Roentgenol* 2007;188:529–539.

Rao BV, Chaudhuri JD, et al. Unusual termination of the great saphenous vein. *Clin Anat*. 2006;19:718–719.

Saadeh FA, Haikal FA, Abdel-Hamid FAM. Blood supply of the tensor fasciae latae muscle. *Clin Anat*. 1998;11:236–238.

Tanaka C, Ide MR, Junqueira A, et al. Anatomical contribution to the surgical construction of the sartorius muscle flap. *Surg Radiol Anat*. 2006;28:277–283.

Traxler H, Windisch A, Surd R, et al. Arterial supply of the gracilis muscle and its relevance for the dynamic graciloplasty. *Clin Anat*. 1999;12:159–163.

Tubbs RS, Salter G, Oakes WJ. Femoral head of the rectus femoris muscle. *Clin Anat*. 2004;17:276–278.

Tubbs RS, Salter EG, Oakes WJ, et al. Dissection of a rare accessory muscle of the leg: The tensor fasciae suralis muscle. *Clin Anat*. 2006; 19:571–572.

Willan PLT, Ransome JA, Mahon M. Variability in human quadriceps muscles: Quantitative study and review of clinical literature. *Clin Anat*. 2002;15:116–128.

Section VI

THE LOWER EXTREMITY

Chapter 22

Knee

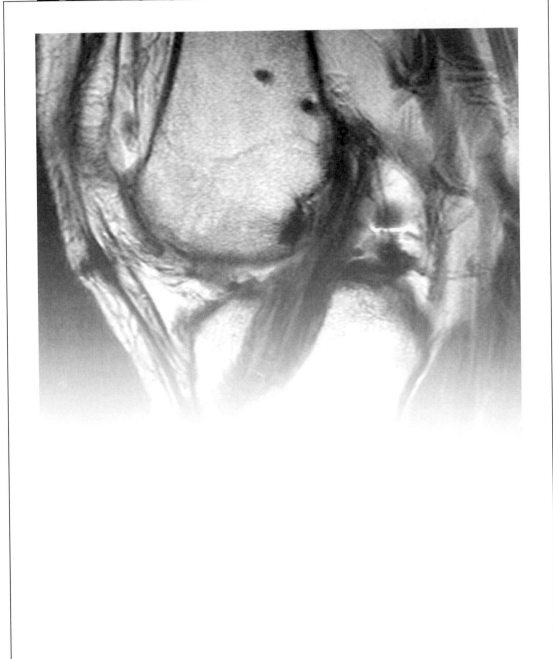

Laura W. Bancroft and Patrick T. Liu

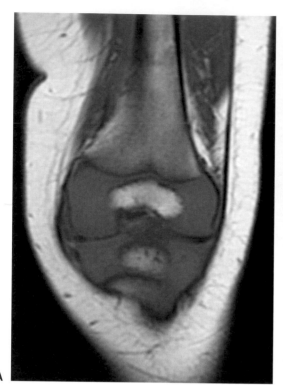

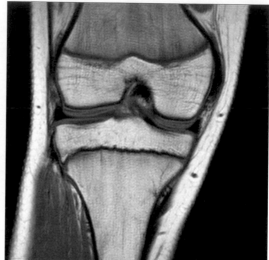

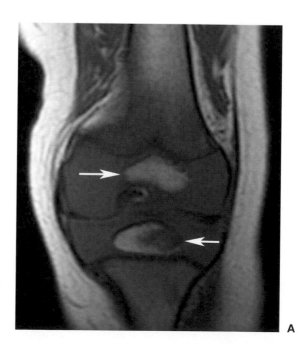

FIGURE 22-1 Normal pediatric physes and marrow development. Normal thicknesses of the physes in **(A)** 14-month old, **(B)** 11-year-old, and **(C)** 17-year-old children. Also notice the normal conversion of red to yellow marrow with age.

FIGURE 22-2 Normal pediatric ossification centers. Normal appearances of the ossification centers (*arrows*) in a 15-month-old child on **(A)** coronal T1-weighted image.

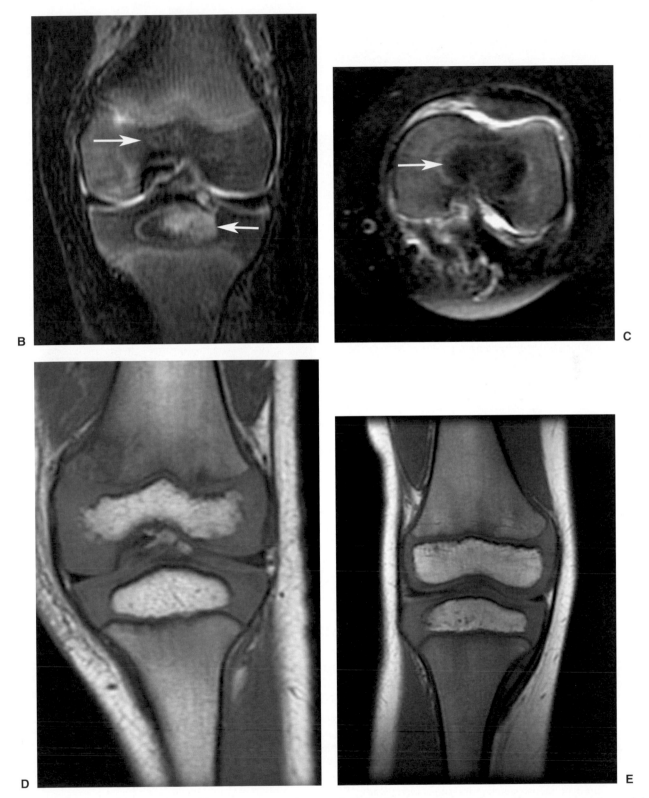

FIGURE 22-2   Normal pediatric ossification centers. (*continued*) Normal appearances of the ossification centers (*arrows*) in a 15-month-old child on **(B)** short tau inversion recovery (STIR) and **(C)** axial FSE T2-fat-suppressed images. **(D)** Normal growth of the centers in a 2.5-year-old child. **(E)** Normal growth of the centers in a 5-year-old child.

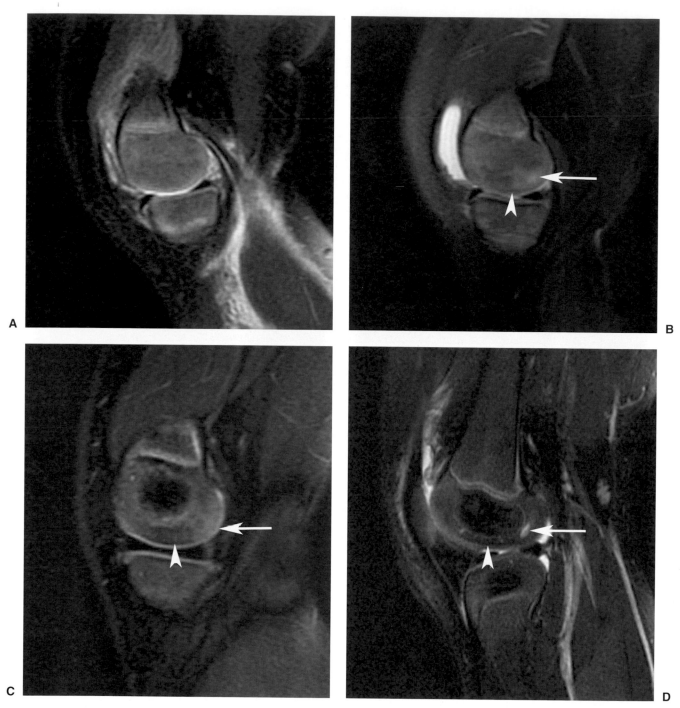

FIGURE 22-3 **Normal maturation of distal femoral epiphyseal cartilage.** There is a normal progression of the T2-weighted signal intensity of the distal femoral cartilage in children, which may be related to weight-bearing and normal maturation. **A:** The cartilage is relatively featureless in this normal 14-month-old. Normal developmental subchondral low signal (*arrowheads*) in the weight-bearing condyles and stippled hyperintense signal (*arrows*) in the posterior condyles have developed in these **(B)** 15-month-old and **(C)** 18-month-old children. **D:** More focal, hyperintense signal (*arrow*) is now present in this nearly 3-year-old child, along with persistent hypointense subchondral signal (*arrowhead*).

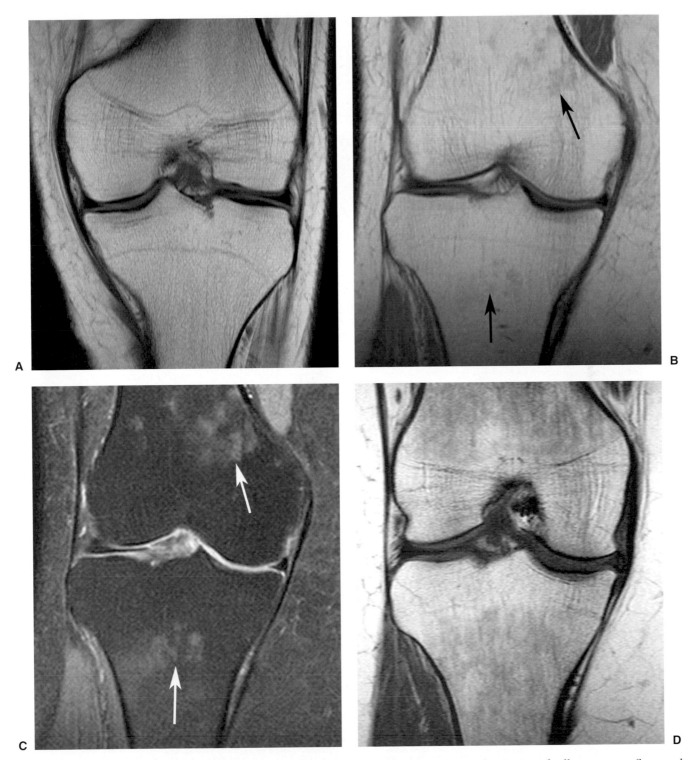

FIGURE 22-4 **Normal adult marrow. A:** MRI of the knee in adults typically shows a predominance of yellow marrow. Scattered rests of red marrow (*arrows*) can be seen in adults on **(B)** T1- and **(C)** double echo steady state (DESS) images. **D:** More red marrow reconversion occurs if there is increased oxygen demand (i.e., anemia, high performance athlete, smoker, obese, living at high altitude).

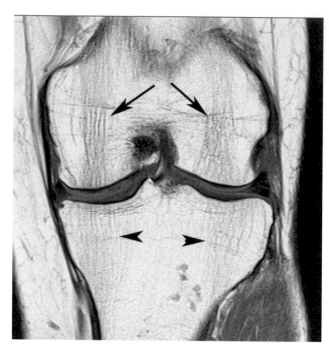

FIGURE 22-5 Prominent trabeculae in osteopenia. Coronal T1-weighted image shows prominent trabeculae in the femur (*arrows*) and to a lesser extent in the tibia (*arrowheads*) due to reactive changes in the presence of osteopenia. Incidental note is made of enchondroma in the proximal tibia.

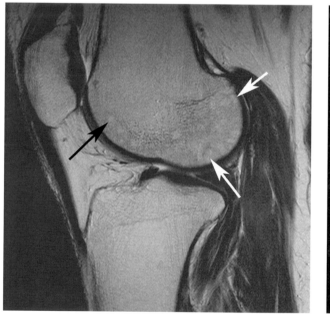
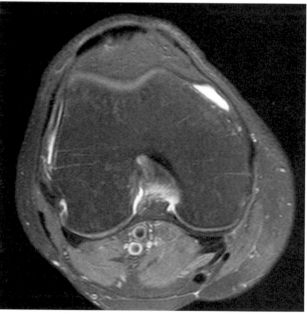

A   B

FIGURE 22-6 Marrow heterogeneity due to osteopenia. A: Sagittal FSE T2-weighted image demonstrates multiple tiny rounded foci of signal (*arrows*) that are slightly hyperintense to the remaining trabeculated marrow in this patient with osteopenia. **B:** Axial FSE proton density (PD) fat-suppressed (FS) image through the distal femoral subchondral bone shows diffuse areas of hyperintense signal, which are more conspicuous due to the fat suppression.

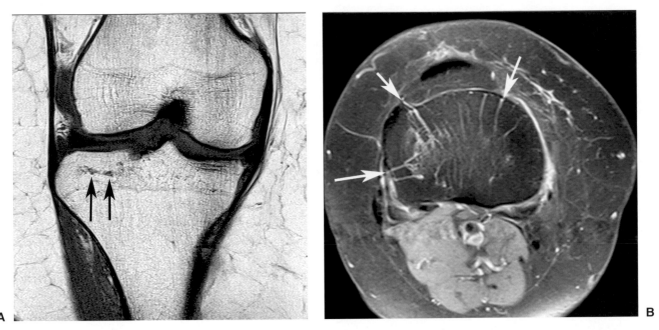

FIGURE 22-7 Prominent intraosseous vessels. A: Axial FSE proton density (PD) fat-suppressed (FS) image through the proximal tibia demonstrates prominent radiating intraosseous vessels (*arrows*), normal variant. **B:** Coronal T1-weighted image shows the vessels (*arrows*) in cross section.

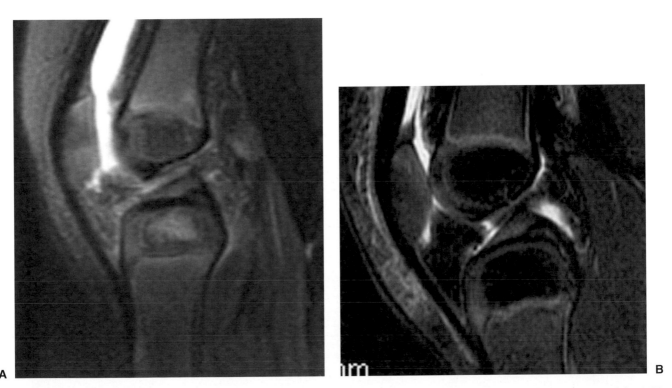

FIGURE 22-8 Normal pediatric anterior cruciate ligament (ACL). Sagittal images display the normal appearances of the ACL in **(A)** 15-month-old and **(B)** 2.5-year-old children. Note the joint effusion in images A and B.

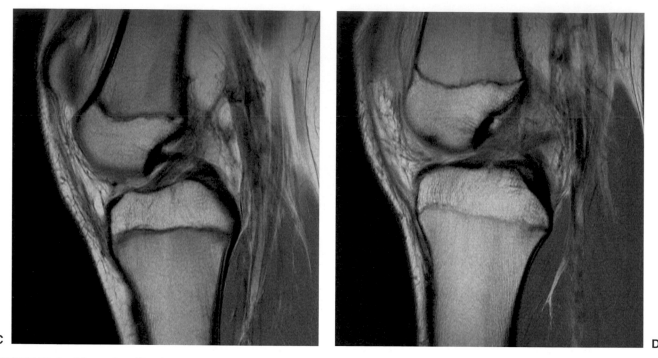

FIGURE 22-8   Normal pediatric anterior cruciate ligament (ACL). (*continued*) Sagittal images display the normal appearances of the ACL in **(C)** 14-year-old and **(D)** 16-year-old children.

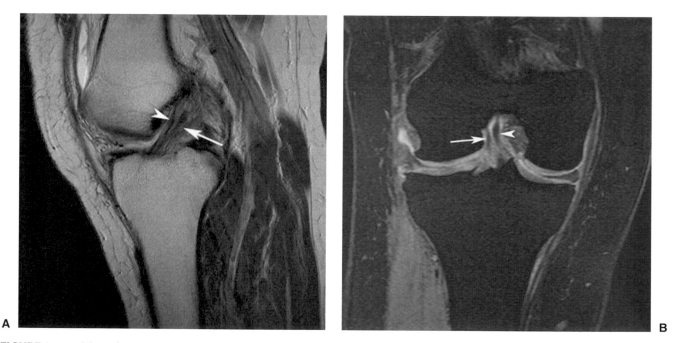

FIGURE 22-9   Two discrete bands of the normal anterior cruciate ligament (ACL). A and **B:** The normal posterolateral (*arrow*) and anteromedial (*arrowhead*) bundles of the ACL can be seen as two discrete bands, and should not be mistaken as a mid-substance tear.

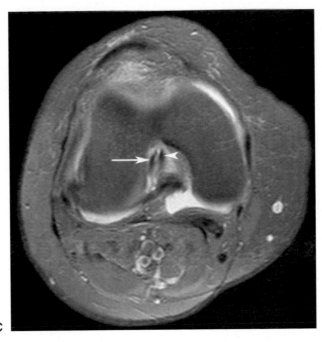

FIGURE 22-9 Two discrete bands of the normal anterior cruciate ligament (ACL). (*continued*) **C:** The normal posterolateral (*arrow*) and anteromedial (*arrowhead*) bundles of the ACL can been seen as two discrete bands, and should not be mistaken as a mid-substance tear.

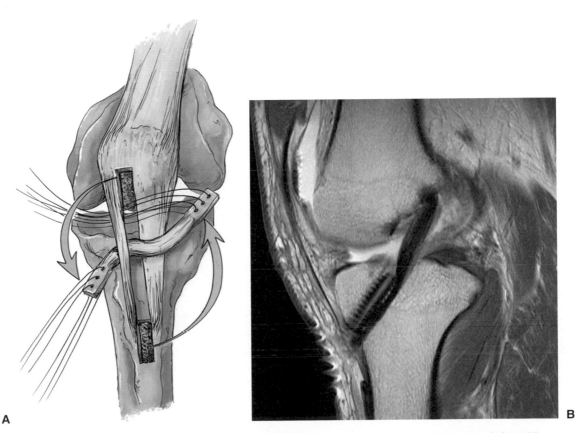

FIGURE 22-10 Anterior cruciate ligament (ACL) reconstructions. **A:** Illustration of patellar autograft for ACL reconstruction, with harvesting of the middle third of the patient's patellar tendon and adjacent bone plugs. Arrows indicate rotation of the harvested patellar graft into the surgical site. **B:** Sagittal image of intact single bundle bone-patellar tendon-bone anterior cruciate reconstruction.

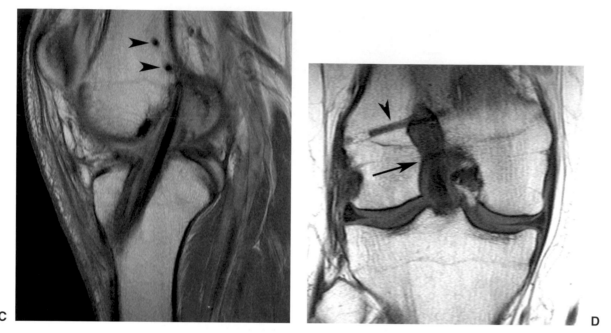

FIGURE 22-10 **Anterior cruciate ligament (ACL) reconstructions.** (*continued*) **C:** Sagittal image of intact single bundle bone-patellar tendon-bone anterior cruciate reconstruction shows uniform low signal throughout. Grafts may be of variable thickness, with intact thin graft in this patient (*Cross-pins = arrowheads*). **D:** A variety of screws, anchors, and cross-pins (*arrowhead*) can help secure the ACL graft (*arrow*).

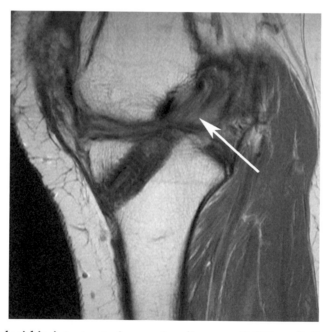

FIGURE 22-11 **Increased signal within intact anterior cruciate ligament (ACL) graft.** Focally or diffusely increased signal (*arrow*) within intact grafts may be present several months postoperatively due to "ligamentization" of the graft. ACL graft tear should not be suggested unless there is focal fluid signal within a defect or discontinuity of the graft.

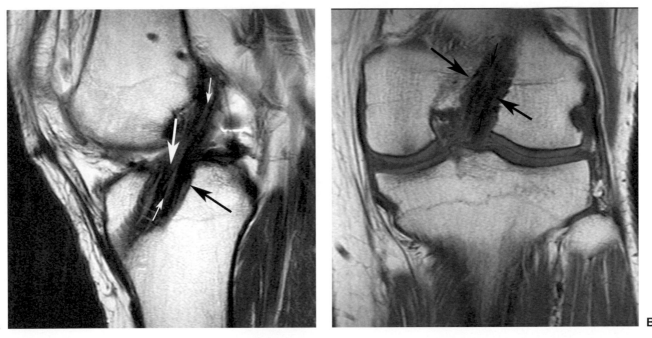

FIGURE 22-12 **Anterior cruciate ligament (ACL) reconstruction with hamstrings.** **A** and **B:** ACL graft from hamstring reconstruction shows multiple bundles (*large arrows*) of "folded over" ligaments. The normal interfaces between the bundles (*small arrows*) should not be misinterpreted as linear graft tears.

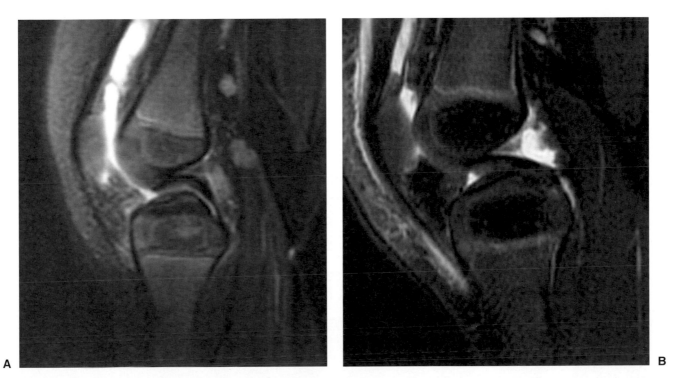

FIGURE 22-13 **Normal pediatric posterior cruciate ligament (PCL).** Sagittal images display the normal appearances of the PCL in **(A)** 15-month-old and **(B)** 2.5-year-old children. Note the joint effusion in images A and B.

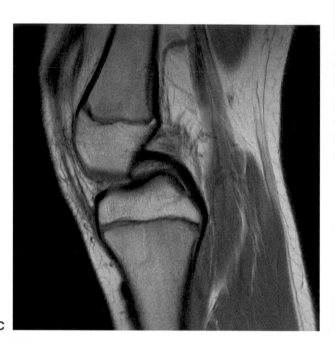

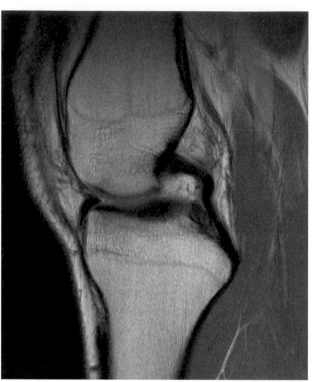

FIGURE 22-13   Normal pediatric posterior cruciate ligament (PCL). (*continued*) Sagittal images display the normal appearances of the PCL in **(C)** 11-year-old and **(D)** 17-year-old children. The buckled appearance of the PCL in **(D)** was due to slight hyperextension of the knee; the anterior cruciate ligament (ACL) was intact.

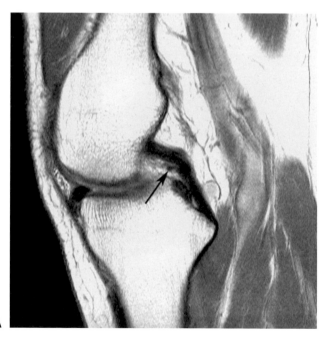

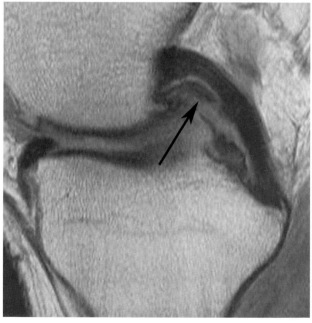

FIGURE 22-14   Ligaments of Humphrey and Wrisberg. Two sagittal proton density images through the intercondylar notch demonstrate the variably present meniscofemoral ligaments. **A:** Ligament of Humphrey (*arrow*) extends anterior to the posterior cruciate ligament (PCL). **B:** This ligament (*arrow*) could be potentially confused with a displaced bucket handle tear.

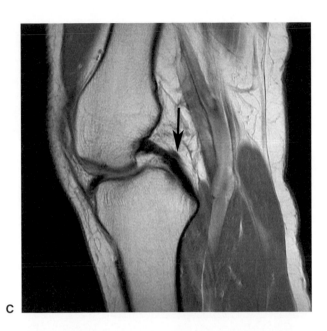

C

FIGURE 22-14 Ligaments of Humphrey and Wrisberg. (*continued*) **C:** Ligament of Wrisberg (*arrow*) extends posteriorly.

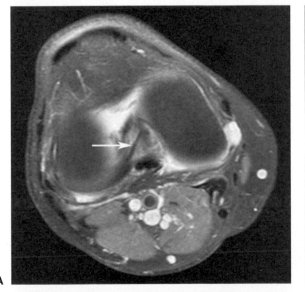

A

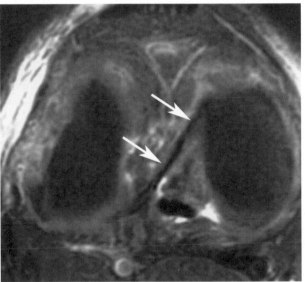

B

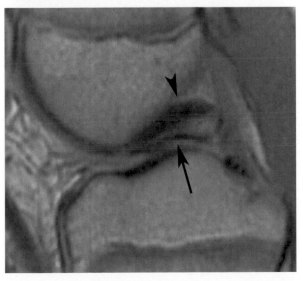

C

FIGURE 22-15 Oblique meniscomeniscal ligament. **A** and **B:** Axial proton density fat-suppressed images demonstrate the normal course of the oblique meniscomeniscal ligament (*arrows*). **C:** This normal structure (*arrow*) is seen alongside the posterior cruciate ligament (*arrowhead*) and should not be confused with a displaced linear meniscal fragment.

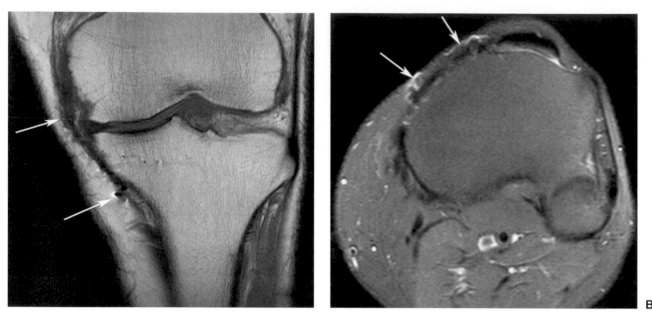

FIGURE 22-16 **Medial collateral ligament (MCL) repair artifact. A** and **B:** Artifact and mild thickening of the repaired MCL (*arrows*) are normal postoperative findings, and should not be confused with pathology.

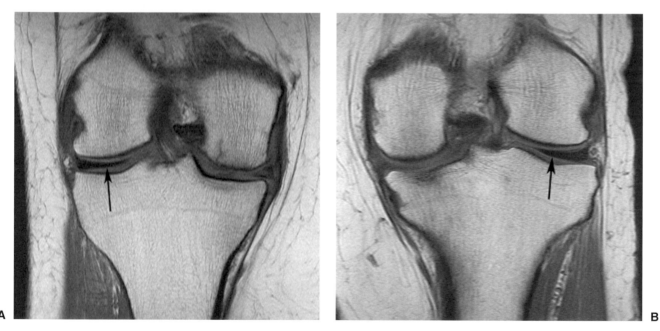

FIGURE 22-17 **Discoid meniscus. A** and **B:** Coronal T1-weighted images in two patients demonstrate lateral discoid menisci (*arrows*), with extension toward the intercondylar notch. Note made of medial meniscal tears.

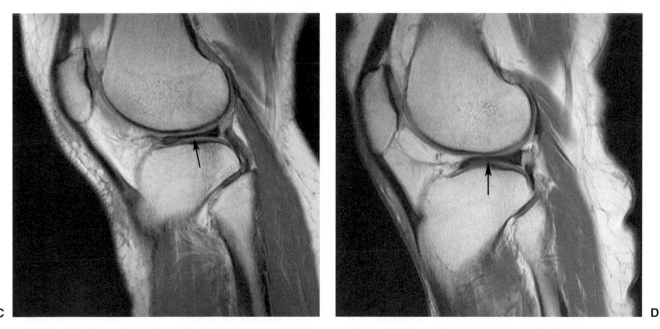

FIGURE 22-17 Discoid meniscus. (*continued*) **C** and **D:** Sagittal images show loss of the normal bow tie appearance of the meniscus (*arrow*). Visualization of the body of the meniscus on three or more consecutive sagittal images (obtained at 3-mm thickness) and/or a height difference greater than 2 mm between the lateral and meniscal horns are diagnostic for discoid meniscus.

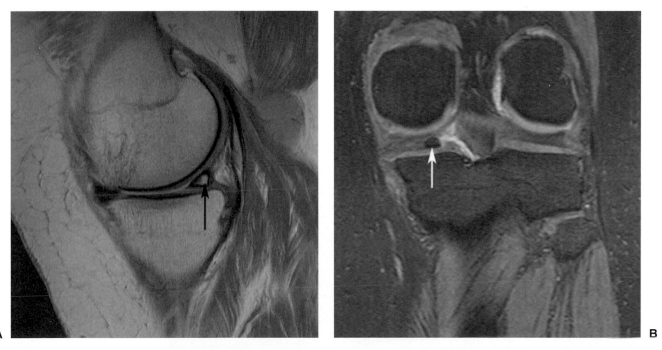

FIGURE 22-18 Meniscal ossicle. A: Sagittal proton density image shows a small hyperintense signal focus in the posterior horn of the medial meniscus (*arrow*), equivalent to marrow. **B:** Coronal double echo steady state (DESS) image shows it to be slightly hypointense (*arrow*) to marrow, due to gradient echo artifact from internal trabeculae.

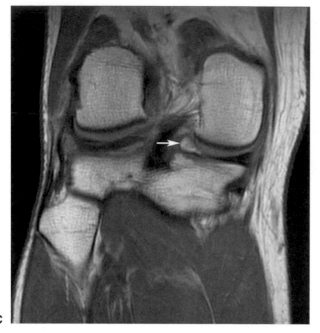

C

FIGURE 22-18   Meniscal ossicle. (*continued*) **C:** Coronal T1-weighted image in a different patient shows a larger, teardrop-shaped ossicle (*arrow*).

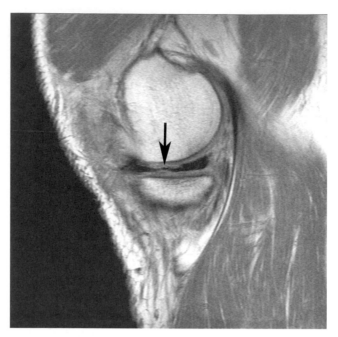

FIGURE 22-19   Meniscal flounce. Sagittal FSE proton density (PD) image demonstrates waviness (*arrow*) of the intact meniscus, termed *meniscal flounce*. This may be seen with MRI or at arthroscopy, dependent upon patient's knee position.

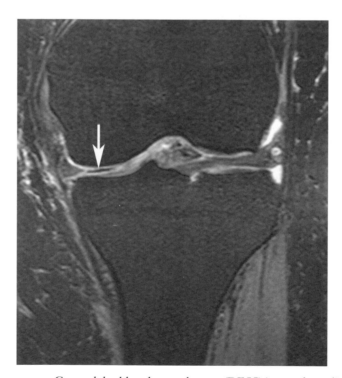

FIGURE 22-20   Vacuum phenomenon. Coronal double echo steady state (DESS) image shows linear artifact (*arrow*) from vacuum phenomenon that could be confused with a displaced meniscal fragment. Radiographs can confirm this finding.

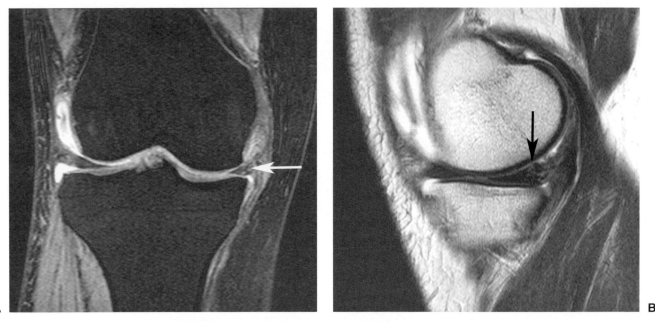

FIGURE 22-21   Repaired bucket handle tear. A: Coronal double echo steady state (DESS) and **(B)** sagittal FSE proton density images show persistent linear signal (*arrows*) that is less than that of fluid and artifact at site of repaired bucket handle tear.

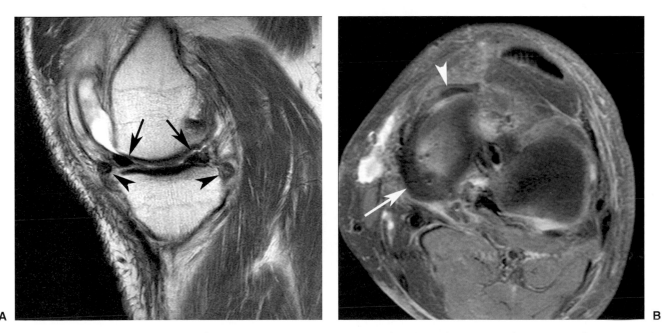

FIGURE 22-22   Meniscal transplant. Sagittal proton density (PD) **(A)** and axial PD fat-suppressed **(B)** images demonstrate the normal appearance of a medial meniscal transplant (*arrows*). Note the purposefully retained native meniscal remnants (*arrowheads*), onto which the transplant is partially attached.

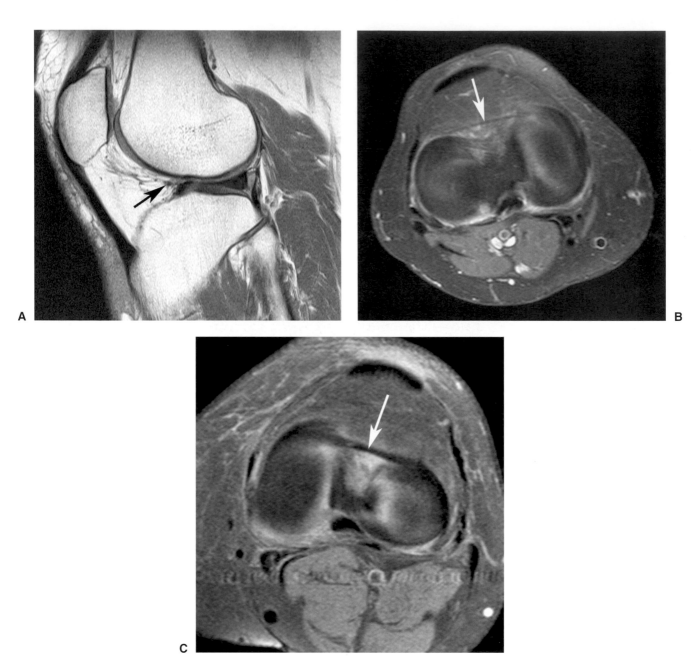

FIGURE 22-23 **Transverse geniculate ligament (anterior intermeniscal ligament).** Variable sizes of (**A** and **B**) thin and (**C**) thick transverse geniculate ligaments (*arrows*).

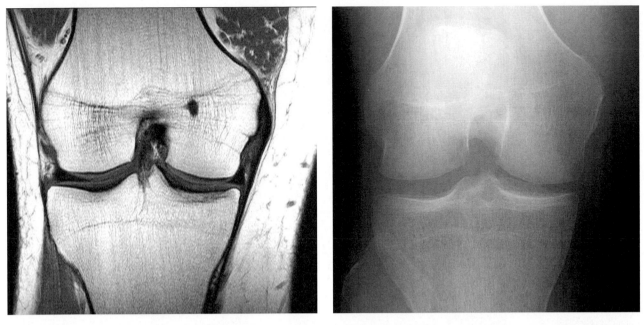

FIGURE 22-24 **Bone island. A:** Coronal T1-weighted image shows a typical bone island, which is a signal void that has spiculations that blend with the adjacent trabeculae, and is oriented along the longitudinal axis of the bone. **B:** Correlating radiograph.

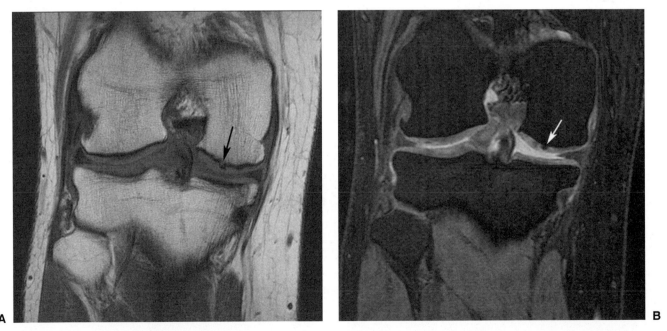

FIGURE 22-25 **Central (button) osteophyte.** Coronal T1-weighted **(A)** and double echo steady state (DESS) **(B)** images demonstrate a central "button osteophyte" (*arrows*) along the medial femoral condyle, variant location for an osteophyte. This should not be confused with other osteochondral pathology.

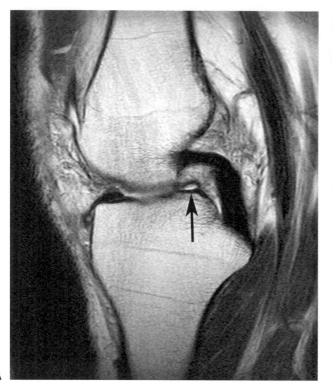

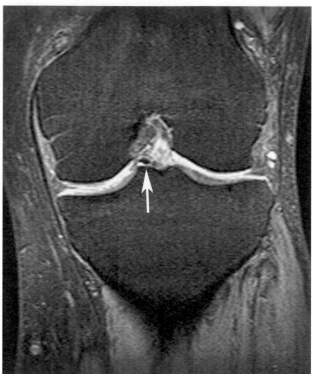

FIGURE 22-26 Accessory ossicle. A: Sagittal FSE proton density (PD) and **(B)** coronal double echo steady state (DESS) images demonstrate an accessory ossicle (*arrows*) at the fourth tubercle on the dorsal proximal tibia.

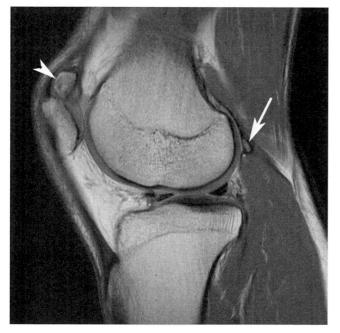

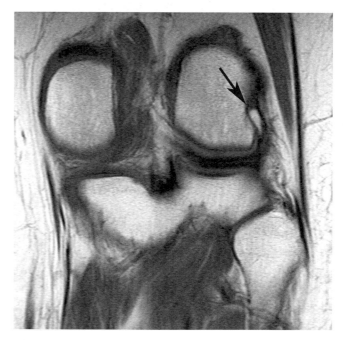

FIGURE 22-27 Fabella. The fabella (*arrow*) is the sesamoid of the lateral head of the gastrocnemius (*Bipartite patella = arrowhead*).

FIGURE 22-28 Cyamella. The cyamella (*arrow*) is the sesamoid of the popliteus tendon.

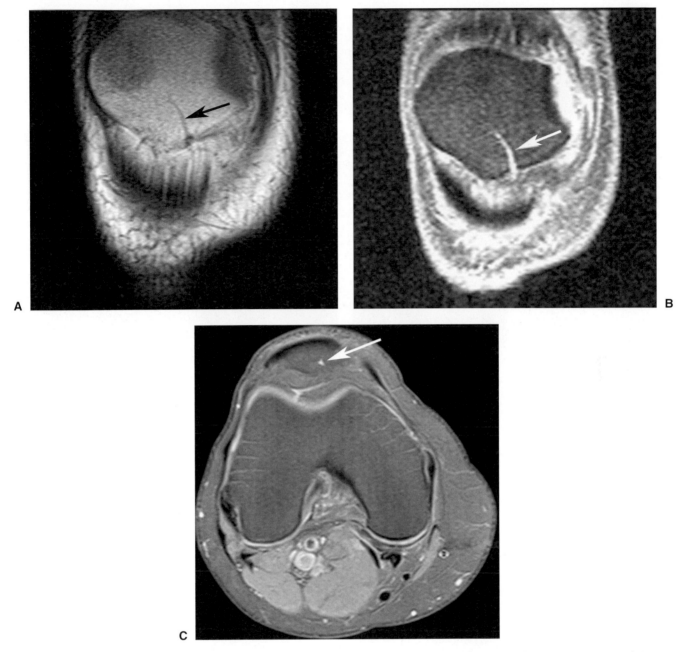

FIGURE 22-29 Patellar nutrient vessel. Coronal **(A)** T1- and **(B)** FSE T2-weighted images show a nutrient vessel (*arrows*) entering inferiorly, that should not be confused with a nondisplaced fracture on a single image. **C:** Axial FSE proton density fat-suppressed image shows the vessel (*arrow*) in cross section.

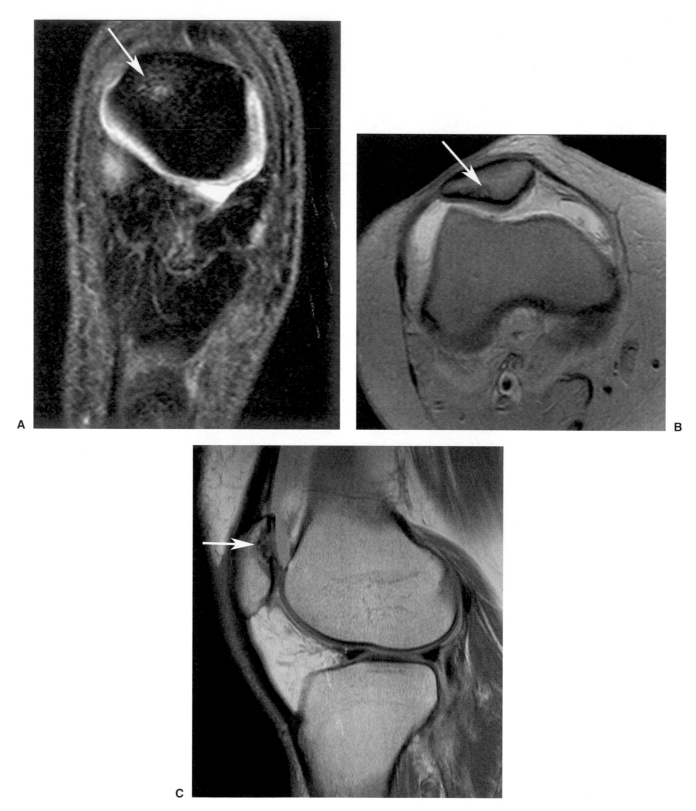

FIGURE 22-30 Dorsal defect of the patella. A–C: Small rounded defect (*arrow*) is present in the upper outer quadrant of the dorsal patella. This is the classic location for this benign, congenital variant.

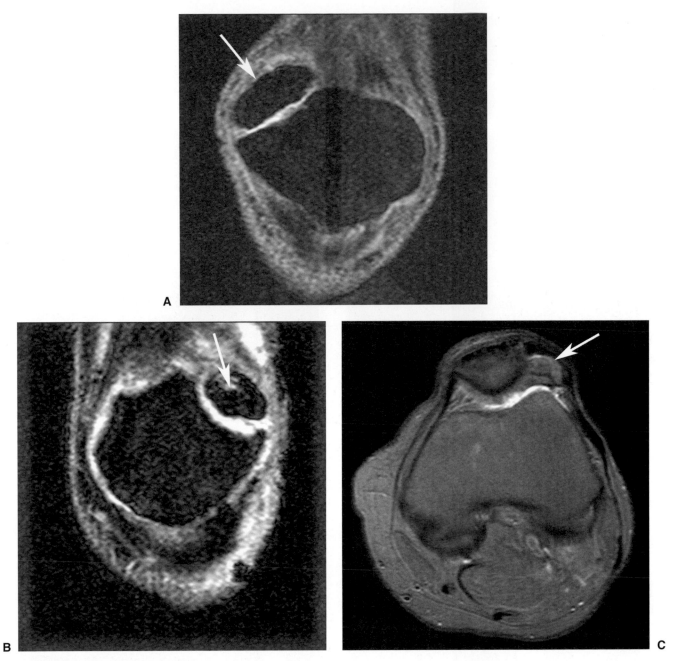

FIGURE 22-31 **Bipartite patella.** **A** and **B:** Coronal FSE T2-weighted fat-suppressed (FS) and **(C)** axial proton density (PD) images demonstrate a bipartite patella (*arrows*), in which the patella develops from two ossification centers, resulting in main and accessory bones. Bipartite patella is usually an incidental finding, and superolateral pole of the patella is the most common location of the accessory bone.

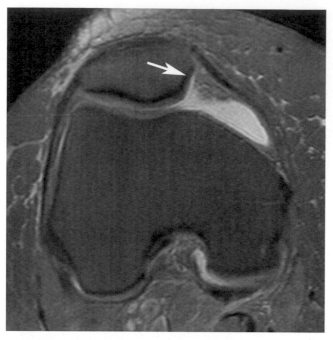

FIGURE 22-32   Odd (nonarticulating) facet of patella. Axial FSE proton density (PD) fat-suppressed (FS) image shows three patellar facets, one of which does not articulate (*arrow*).

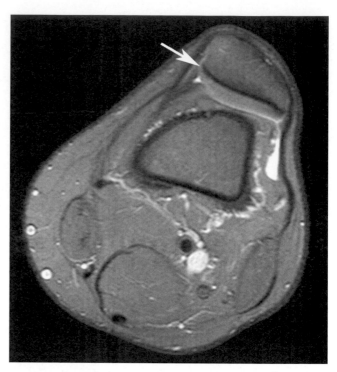

FIGURE 22-33   Flattened patellar configuration. Axial FSE proton density (PD) fat-suppressed (FS) image shows a flat posterior surface of the patella (*arrow*), a normal variant.

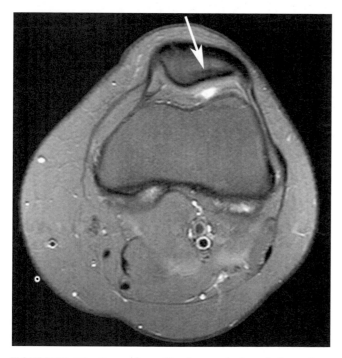

FIGURE 22-34   Lateral patellar facet subchondral condensation. A subchondral line of hypointense signal (*arrow*) can be seen with normal condensation of trabeculae.

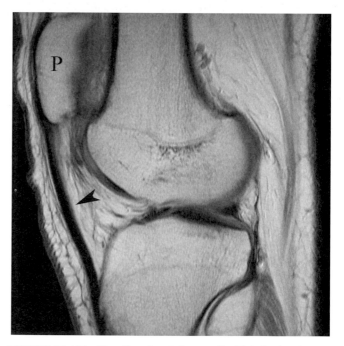

FIGURE 22-35   Patellar alta. The patella (*P*) is high riding in this patient with an intact patellar tendon (*arrowhead*). The MRI criterion for patellar alta is a patellar tendon to patella ratio of greater than 1.5. The MRI criterion for patellar baja is a patellar tendon to patella ratio of less than 0.74.

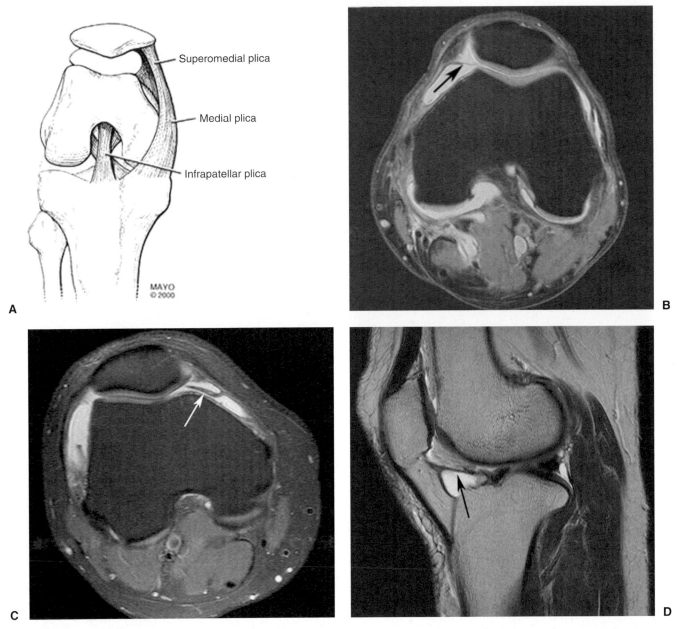

FIGURE 22-36 **Plica. A:** Illustration of the various plicae, which are normal remnants from embryologic development. **B:** Axial FSE proton density (PD) fat-suppressed (FS) image demonstrates a thin medial suprapatellar plica (*arrow*). **C:** Axial image delineates a thicker plica (*arrow*) in the same location. **D:** Sagittal FSE T2-weighted image shows the normal inferior patellar plica (*arrow*) outlined by joint fluid.

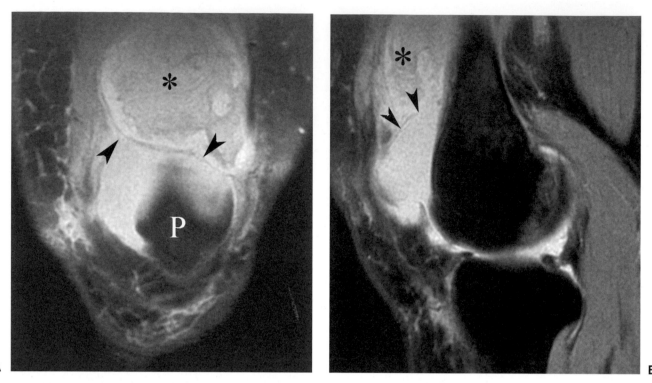

FIGURE 22-37 **Isolated suprapatellar bursa.** Coronal proton density (PD) fat-suppressed (FS) **(A)** and sagittal FSE T2-weighted FS images through the anterior knee demonstrate an isolated suprapatellar bursa (*asterisk*) caused by failure to resorb the suprapatellar plica (*arrowheads*) (*Patella = P*). Note the suprapatellar synovitis in this case.

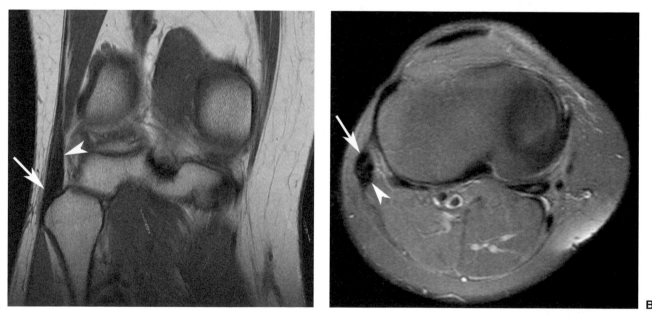

FIGURE 22-38 **Prominent conjoined tendon.** Coronal T1-weighted **(A)** and axial FSE proton density (PD) fat-suppressed (FS) **(B)** images demonstrate prominence of the conjoined tendon, comprised of the biceps tendon (*arrows*) and fibular collateral ligament (*arrowheads*).

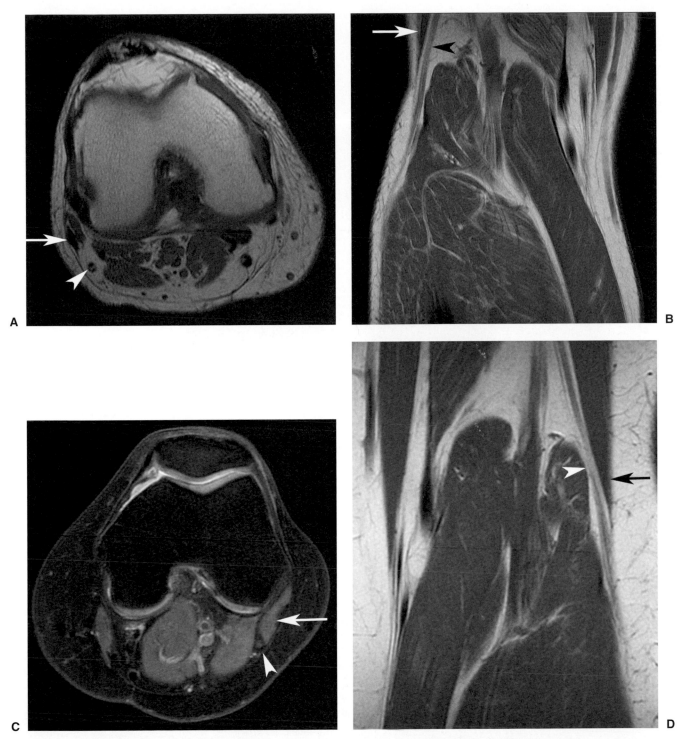

FIGURE 22-39 **Distal biceps configuration relative to the peroneal nerve. A** and **B:** The common peroneal nerve (*arrowhead*) may extend through a narrow, fatty tunnel (*Biceps = arrow*). **C** and **D:** Another variant at the level of the knee is a muscular tunnel, with distal and posterior extension of the short head of the biceps (*arrow*). This anatomic pattern may be associated with entrapment of the peroneal nerve (*arrowhead*).

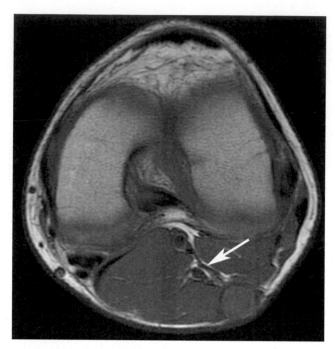

FIGURE 22-40 Accessory medial gastrocnemius muscle. Axial T1-weighted image shows a variant accessory slip of medial gastrocnemius muscle (*arrow*). This variant can be asymptomatic or associated with popliteal artery entrapment syndrome.

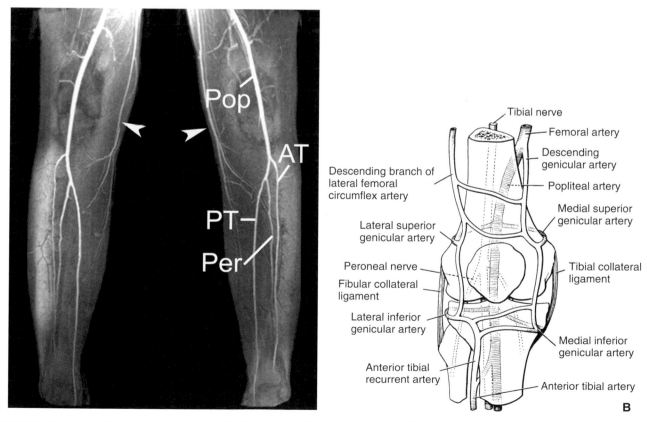

FIGURE 22-41 Arterial supply of the knee. A: Conventional arterial anatomy of the knee on MRA. Arrowheads signify venous contamination from filling of the greater saphenous vein and its branches (*Popliteal artery = Pop, Anterior tibial artery = AT, Posterior tibial artery = PT, Peroneal artery = Per*). **B:** Illustration of arterial supply of the knee.

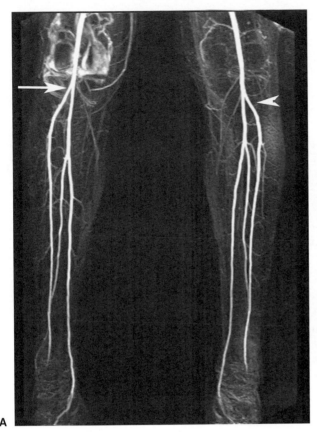

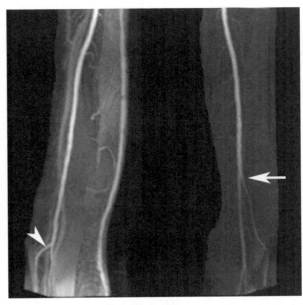

FIGURE 22-42 High anterior tibial artery origin above knee. A: MRA shows a slightly higher origin of the right anterior tibial artery (*arrow*) relative to the left side. **B:** MRA in a different patient shows a high left-sided anterior tibial artery origin (*arrow*) above the level of the knee (*Right anterior tibial artery = arrowhead*). Note made of hyperemia in right knee.

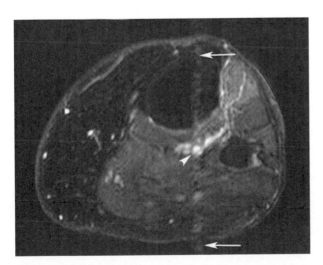

FIGURE 22-43 Pulsation artifact. Ghosting (*arrows*) from pulsation of blood flowing through the popliteal artery (*arrowhead*) is observed in the phase-encoding direction.

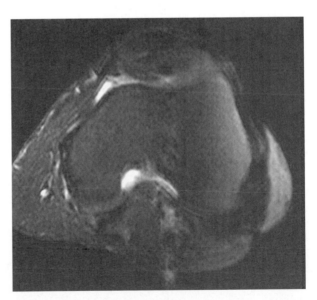

FIGURE 22-44 Pulsation artifact and poor fat saturation. Vertical ghosting due to pulsation from the popliteal artery is observed near the middle of this image. Poor fat saturation has occurred on the right side of the image with a transition (from left to right) of good fat saturation to water saturation to no saturation.

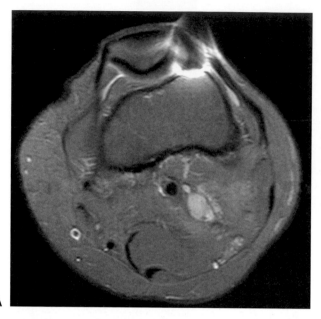

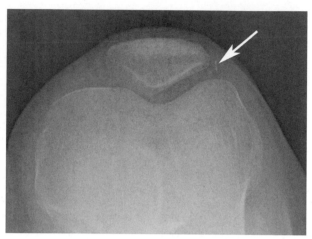

FIGURE 22-45 Susceptibility artifact. Susceptibility artifact in the lateral knee is more extensive on **(A)** proton density fat-suppressed image than expected from the tiny sliver of glass (*arrow*) demonstrated on **(B)** the radiograph. Susceptibility artifact is observed on MRI from glass with likely metallic content or coating. Differences in the magnetic susceptibility of the fragment and surrounding tissue produce changes in the local magnetic field causing distortion and spin dephasing.

Suggested Readings

Aigner F, Longato S, Gardetto A, et al. Anatomic survey of the common fibular nerve and its branching pattern with regard to the intermuscular septa of the leg. *Clin Anat*. 2004;17:503–512.

Bach FD, Carlier RY, Elis JB, et al. Anterior cruciate ligament reconstruction with bioabsorbable polyglycolic acid interference screws: MRI follow-up. *Radiology*. 2002;225:541–550.

Bejjani FJ, Jahss MH. Le Double's study of muscle variations of the human body. Part I: Muscle variations of the leg. *Foot Ankle*. 1985;6: 111–134.

Bergman RA, Thompson SA, Afifi AK, et al., ed. *Compendium of human anatomic variation*. Baltimore: Urban & Schwarzenberg; 1988.

Cogswell LK, Giele H. Anatomical study to investigate the feasibility of pedicled nerve, free vessel gastrocnemius muscle transfer for restoration of biceps function. *Clin Anat*. 2001;14:242–245.

Cross L, Hall J, Howdieshell TR, et al. Clinical anatomy of the popliteal blood vessels. *Clin Anat*. 2000;13:347–353.

Doda N, Peh WC, Chawla A. Symptomatic accessory soleus muscle: Diagnosis and follow-up on magnetic resonance imaging. *Br J Radiol*. 2006;79:129–132.

Duc SR, Wentz KU, Kach KP, et al. First report of an accessory popliteal muscle: Detection with MRI. *Skeletal Radiol*. 2004;33:429–431.

Garcia-Valtuille R, Abascal F, Cerezal L, et al. Anatomy and MRI appearances of synovial plicae of the knee. *RadioGraphics*. 2002;22:775–784.

Kadir S. Arterial anatomy of the lower extremities. In: Kadir S, ed. *Atlas of normal and variant angiographic anatomy*. Philadelphia: WB Saunders; 1991:123–160.

Kelly AM, Cronin P, Hussain HK, et al. Preoperative MR angiography in free fibula flap transfer for head and neck cancer: Clinical application and influence on surgical decision making. *AJR Am J Roentgenol*. 2007;188:268–274.

Kim YC, Chung IH, Yoo WK, et al. Anatomy and magnetic resonance imaging of the posterolateral structures of the knee. *Clin Anat*. 1997; 10:397–404.

Lee JH, Ehara S, Tamakawa Y, et al. Nutrient canal of the fibula. *Skeletal Radiol*. 2000;29:22–26.

Major NM, Helms CA. MRI of the knee: Findings in asymptomatic collegiate basketball players. *Am J Roentgenol*. 2002;179:641–644.

McCauley TR, Elfar A, Moore A, et al. MR arthrography of anterior cruciate ligament reconstruction grafts. *Am J Roentgenol*. 2003;181: 1217–1223.

Park JS, Ryu KN, Yoon KH. Meniscal flounce on knee MRI: Correlation with meniscal locations after positional changes. *Am J Roentgenol*. 2006;187:364–370.

Recondo JA, Salvador E, Villanúa JA, et al. Lateral stabilizing structures of the knee: Functional anatomy and injuries assessed with MRI. *RadioGraphics*. 2000;20:S91–S102.

Sakai H, Sasho T, Wada YI, et al. MRI of the popliteomeniscal fasciculi. *Am J Roentgenol*. 2006;186:460–466.

Shabshin N, Schweitzer ME, Morrison WB, et al. MRI criteria for patella alta and baja. *Skeletal Radiol*. 2004;33(8):445–450.

Singh K, Helms CA, Jacobs MT, et al. MRI appearance of Wrisberg variant of discoid lateral meniscus. *Am J Roentgenol*. 2006;187:384–387.

Varich LJ, Laor T, Jaramillo D. Normal maturation of the distal femoral epiphyseal cartilage: Age-related changes at MRI. *Radiology*. 2000;214: 705–709.

Vieira RLR, Rosenberg ZS, Kiprovski K. MRI of the distal biceps femoris muscle: Normal anatomy, variants, and association with common peroneal entrapment neuropathy. *Am J Roentgenol*. 2007;189: 549–555.

Zanetti M, Pfirrmann CWA, Schmid MR, et al. Clinical course of knees with asymptomatic meniscal abnormalities: Findings at 2-year follow-up after MRI-based diagnosis. *Radiology*. 2005;237:993–997.

Chapter 23

Calf

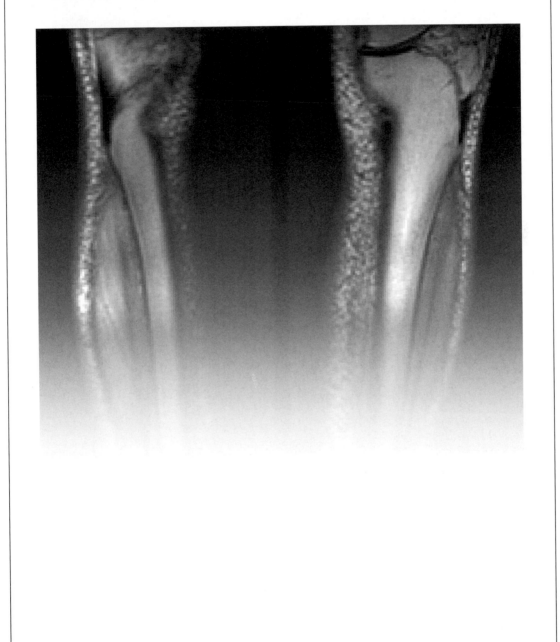

Laura W. Bancroft and Robert A. Pooley

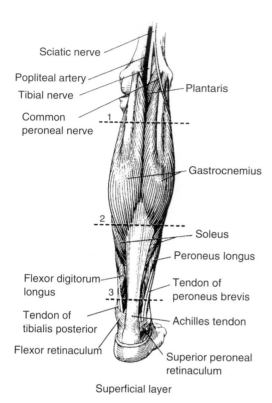

FIGURE 23-1   Illustration of superficial muscles of the calf. (From Berquist TH. *Radiology of the foot and ankle*, 2nd ed. Philadelphia: Lippincott Williams & Wilkins; 2000.)

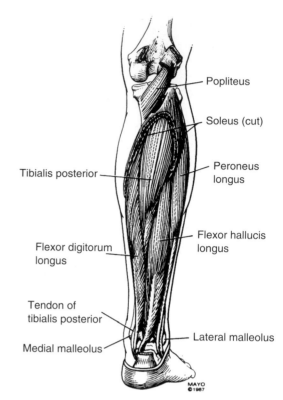

FIGURE 23-2   Illustration of deep muscles of the calf. (From Berquist TH. *Radiology of the foot and ankle*, 2nd ed. Philadelphia: Lippincott Williams & Wilkins; 2000.)

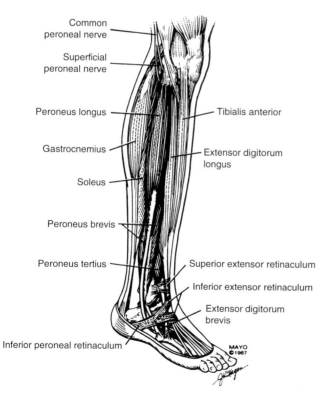

FIGURE 23-3   Illustration of lateral muscles of leg. (From Berquist TH. *Radiology of the foot and ankle*, 2nd ed. Philadelphia: Lippincott Williams & Wilkins; 2000.)

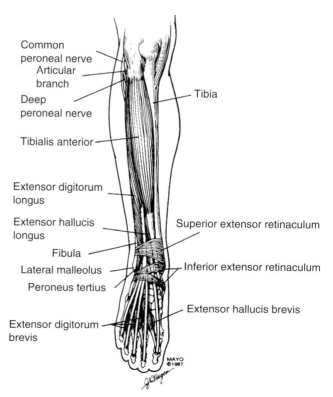

FIGURE 23-4   Illustration of anterior muscles of leg. (From Berquist TH. *Radiology of the foot and ankle*, 2nd ed. Philadelphia: Lippincott Williams & Wilkins; 2000.)

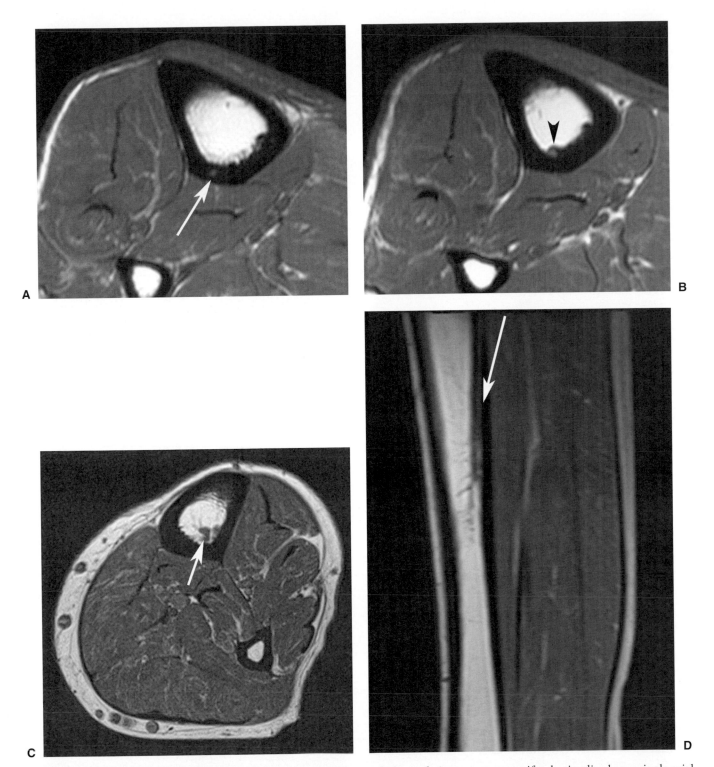

FIGURE 23-5 **Tibial nutrient foramen. A:** Nutrient foramina can have confusing appearances, if only visualized on a single axial image. T1-weighted axial image shows the intracortical portion of the vessel (*arrow*), which could possibly be confused with an osteoid osteoma or stress injury on a single image. Intramedullary extension of the normal vessel can be **(B)** rounded (*arrowhead*) or **(C)** irregular (*arrow*). **D:** Sagittal T1-weighted image in a different patient shows the typical orientation of nutrient vessels (*arrow*).

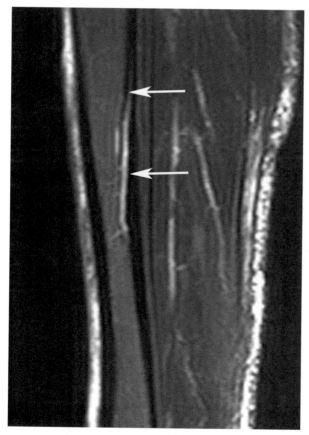

FIGURE 23-5 **Tibial nutrient foramen.** (*continued*) **E:** Sagittal FSE T2-weighted fat-suppressed image shows the typical orientation of nutrient vessels (*arrows*).

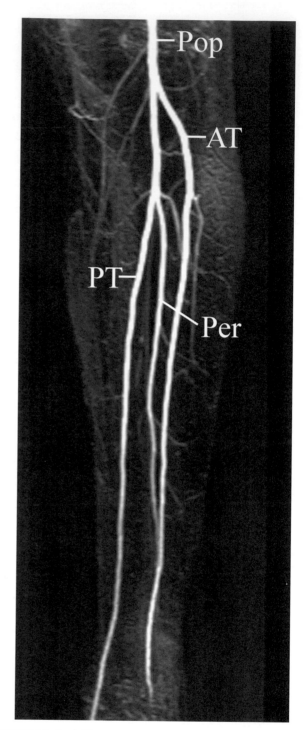

FIGURE 23-6 **MR angiography of the calf. A:** MR angiogram demonstrates the usual arterial supply to the calf (*Popliteal = Pop, Anterior tibial = AT, Posterior tibial = PT, Peroneal = Per*).

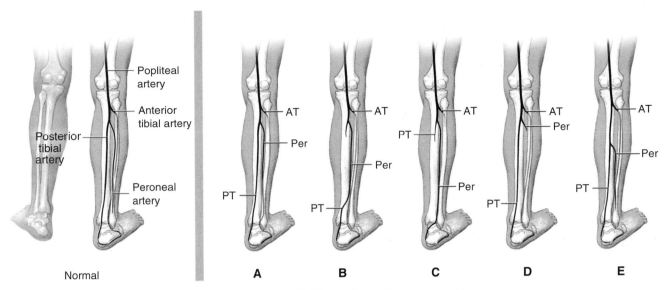

FIGURE 23-6 **MR angiography of the calf.** (*continued*) **B:** Illustrations of variant arterial anatomy.

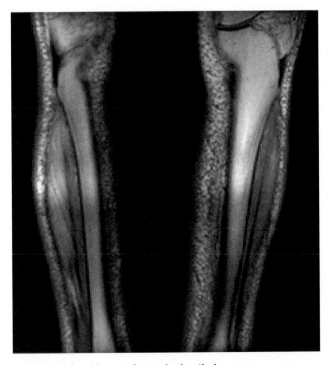

FIGURE 23-7 **Shading artifact.** Shading of the calves is due to bad coil elements.

Table 23-1 Muscles of the Leg, foot, and ankle

Location	Muscle	Origin	Insertion	Action	Innervation (segment)	Blood supply
Calf						
Superficial compartment	Gastrocnemius	Femoral condyles	Posterior calcaneus	Flexor of foot and knee	Tibial nerve (S1, S2)	Posterior tibial artery
	Soleus	Upper tibia and fibula	Gastrocnemius tendon	Plantar flexor of foot	Tibial nerve (S1, S2)	Posterior tibial artery
	Plantaris	Lateral femoral condyle and oblique popliteal ligament	Posteromedial calcaneus	Plantar flexes foot, flexes leg	Tibial nerve (L4-S1)	Posterior tibial artery
Deep compartment	Popliteus	Later femur and capsule of knee	Posterior tibia	Flexion and medial rotation of leg	Tibial nerve (L5, S1)	Posterior tibial artery
	Flexor hallucis longus	Posterior mid-fibula	Distal phalanx great toe	Flexor great toe and ankle	Tibial nerve (L5-S2)	Posterior tibial artery
	Flexor digitorum longus	Posterior tibia	Distal phalanges second to fifth toes	Flexes toes and foot and supinates ankle	Tibial nerve (L5, S1)	Posterior tibial artery
	Tibialis posterior	Posterior tibia, fibula, and interosseous membrane	Navicular, cuneiform, calcaneus, second to fourth metatarsals	Adduction of forefoot, hindfoot, inversion, plantar flexion	Tibial nerve (L5, S1)	Posterior tibial artery
Lateral compartment	Peroneus longus	Lateral fibula	First metatarsal and medial cuneiform	Evertor and weak plantar flexors	Superficial and deep peroneal nerve (L4-S1)	Peroneal artery
	Peroneus brevis	Lateral fibula	Base fifth metatarsal	Plantar flexion and eversion of foot	Superficial peroneal nerve (L4-S1)	Peroneal artery
Anterior compartment	Extensor digitorum longus	Upper tibia, fibula, and interosseous membrane	Lateral four toes	Dorsiflexes toes, everts foot	Deep peroneal nerve (L4-S1)	Anterior tibial artery
	Peroneus tertius	Distal fibula and interosseous membrane	Base fifth metatarsal	Dorsiflexes and everts foot	Deep peroneal nerve (L4-S1)	Anterior tibial artery
	Extensor hallucis longus	Distal fibula and interosseous membrane	Distal phalanx great toe	Extends great toe, weak invertor and dorsiflexion of foot	Deep peroneal nerve (L4-S1)	Anterior tibial artery
	Tibialis anterior	Lateral tibia and interosseous membrane	Medial cuneiform and first metatarsal	Strong dorsiflexion and invertor of foot	Deep peroneal nerve (L4-S1)	Anterior tibial artery

(From Berquist TH. *MRI of the musculoskeletal system*, 5th ed. Lippincott Williams & Wilkins; 2006.)

Suggested Readings

Bergman RA, Thompson SA, Afifi AK, et al., ed. *Compendium of human anatomic variation*. Baltimore: Urban & Schwarzenberg; 1988.

Kwon DS, Spevak MR, Fletcher K, et al. Physiologic subperiosteal new bone formation: Prevalence, distribution, and thickness in neonates and infants. *AJR Am J Roentgenol*. 2002;179:985–988.

Loh EY, Agur AM, McKee NH. Intramuscular innervation of the human soleus muscle: A 3D model. *Clin Anat*. 2003;16:278–382.

Mahakkanukrauh P, Chomsung R. Anatomical variations of the sural nerve. *Clin Anat*. 2002;15:263–266.

Mellado JM, Perez del Palomar L. Muscle hernias of the lower leg: MRI findings. *Skeletal Radiol*. 1999;28:465–469.

Nael K, Ruehm SG, Michaely HJ, et al. Multistation whole-body high-spatial resolution MR angiography using a 32-channel MR system. *AJR Am J Roentgenol*. 2007;188:529–539.

Potthast S, Bongartz GM, Huegli R, et al. Intraarterial contrast-enhanced MR aortography with and without parallel acquisition technique in patients with peripheral arterial occlusive disease. *AJR Am J Roentgenol*. 2007;188:823–829.

Rao KGM, Bhat MS. An additional muscle in the back of the leg. *Clin Anat*. 2006;19:724–725.

Uzel M, Gumusalan Y, Cetinus E, et al. Bilateral aplasia of the tibialis anterior and unilateral aplasia of the extensor hallucis longus muscles. *Skeletal Radiol*. 2007;36:83–86.

www.anatomyatlases.org.

Chapter 24

Ankle/Foot

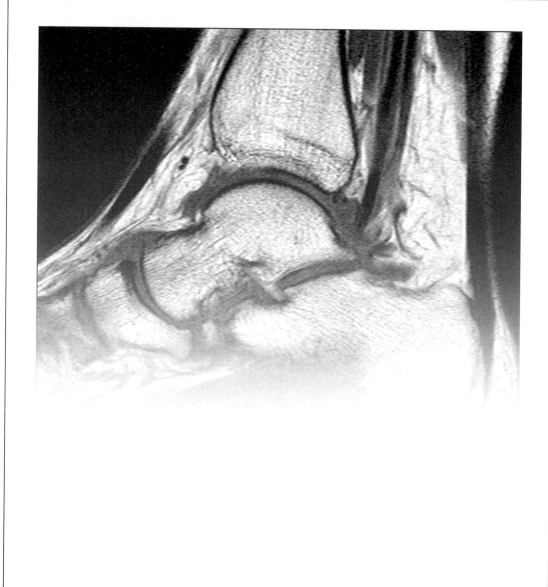

Laura W. Bancroft and William B. Morrison

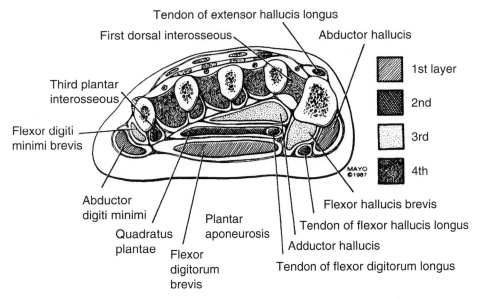

FIGURE 24-1 **Illustration of muscle layers in foot.** (From Berquist TH. *Radiology of the foot and ankle*, 2nd ed. Philadelphia: Lippincott Williams & Wilkins; 2000.)

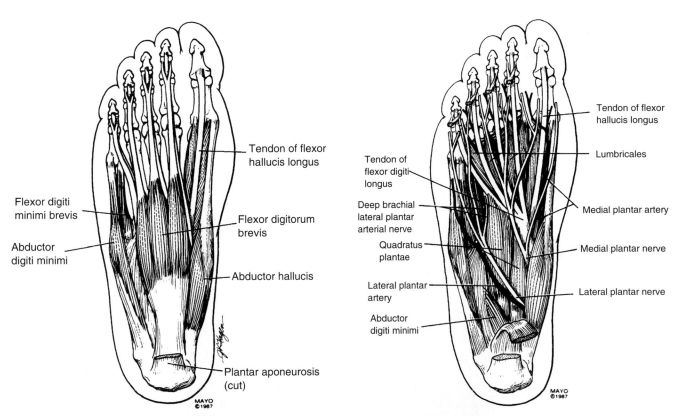

FIGURE 24-2 **Illustration of superficial muscle layers of foot.** (From Berquist TH. *Radiology of the foot and ankle*, 2nd ed. Philadelphia: Lippincott Williams & Wilkins; 2000.)

FIGURE 24-3 **Illustration of second muscle layer of foot.** (From Berquist TH. *Radiology of the foot and ankle*, 2nd ed. Philadelphia: Lippincott Williams & Wilkins; 2000.)

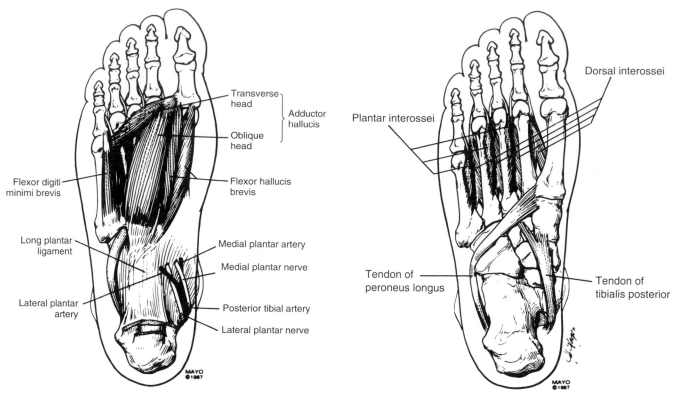

FIGURE 24-4 **Illustration of third muscle layer of foot.** (From Berquist TH. *Radiology of the foot and ankle*, 2nd ed. Philadelphia: Lippincott Williams & Wilkins; 2000.)

FIGURE 24-5 **Illustration of fourth muscle layer of foot.** (From Berquist TH. *Radiology of the foot and ankle*, 2nd ed. Philadelphia: Lippincott Williams & Wilkins; 2000.)

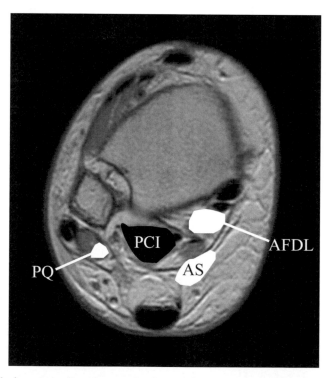

FIGURE 24-6 **Accessory muscle location.** Conglomerative image showing expected location of accessory muscles in the ankle (*Peroneus quartus* = PQ, *Peroneocalcaneus internus* = PCI, *Accessory flexor digitorum longus* = AFDL, *Accessory soleus* = AS).

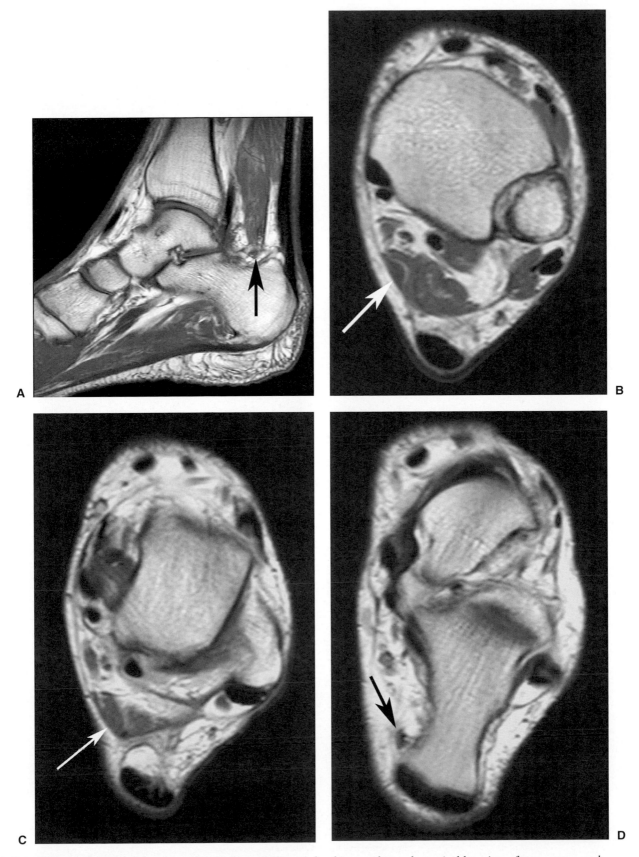

FIGURE 24-7 **Accessory soleus muscle. A:** Sagittal T1-weighted image shows the typical location of an accessory soleus muscle (*arrow*) in Kager's fat pad. **B–D:** Axial imaging of the accessory soleus (*arrows*) as it descends anteromedially to the Achilles tendon and attaches onto the posteromedial calcaneus.

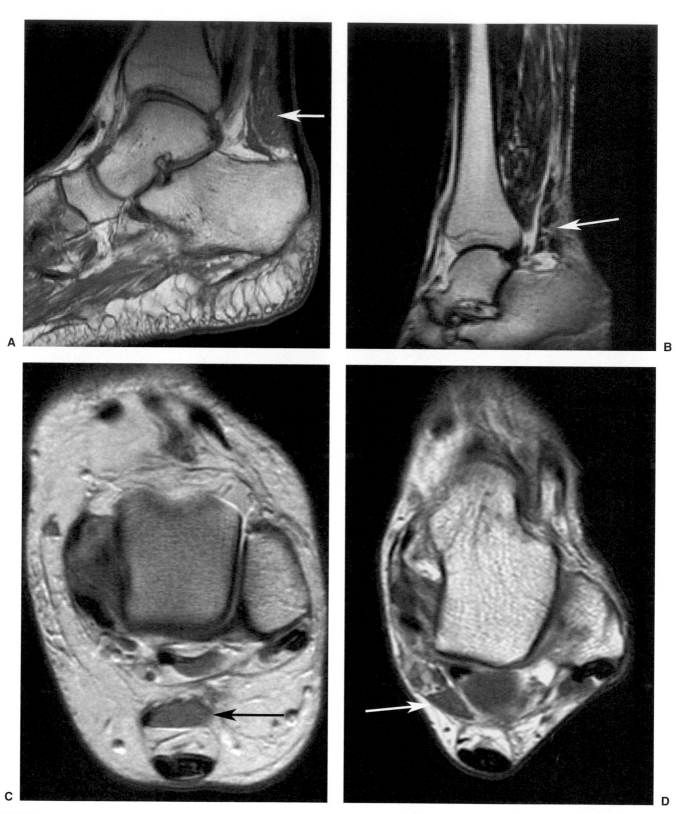

FIGURE 24-8 **Accessory soleus muscle.** Various appearances of accessory soleus muscles (*arrows*) in the **(A** and **B)** sagittal and **(C** and **D)** axial planes.

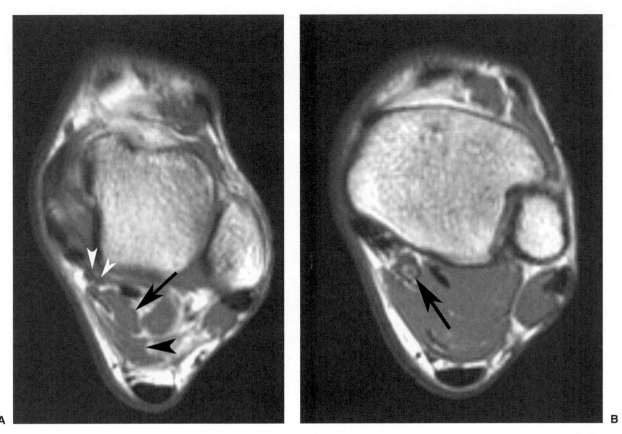

FIGURE 24-9 **Accessory soleus and accessory flexor digitorum longus muscles. A:** Axial T1-weighted image through the ankle demonstrates both accessory soleus (*black arrowhead*) and accessory flexor digitorum longus (*arrow*) muscles. The normally branching posterior tibial nerve (*white arrowheads*) should not be confused with an accessory muscle. **B:** Axial image obtained more superiorly demonstrates an enlarged posterior tibial nerve (*arrow*), consistent with neuropathy associated with the mass effect from the accessory muscles.

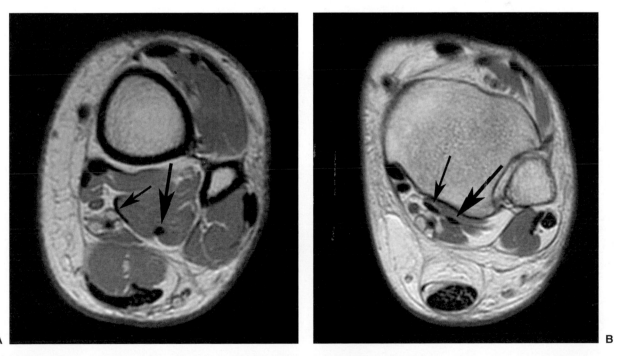

FIGURE 24-10 **Peroneocalcaneus internus. A** and **B:** Axial imaging shows an accessory muscle and tendon (*large arrow*) lateral to the flexor hallucis longus (*small arrow*), consistent with a peroneocalcaneus internus.

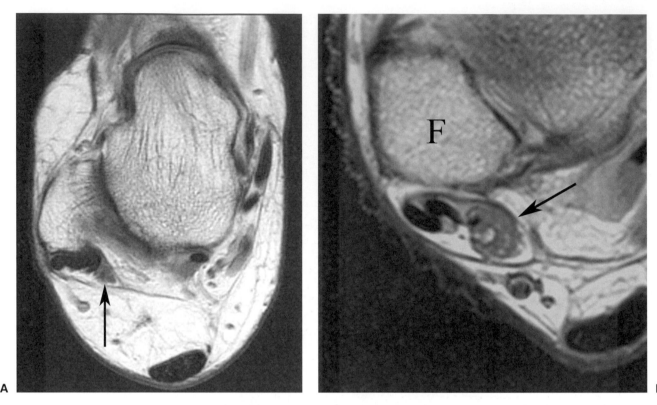

FIGURE 24-11   Peroneus quartus. A and **B:** The peroneus quartus (*arrows*) is an accessory muscle adjacent to the peroneus longus and brevis that has been shown to be present in approximately 10% to 15% of ankles. It has variable attachment onto the posterolateral calcaneus and peroneus brevis or longus tendons, and the cuboid (*F = fibula*).

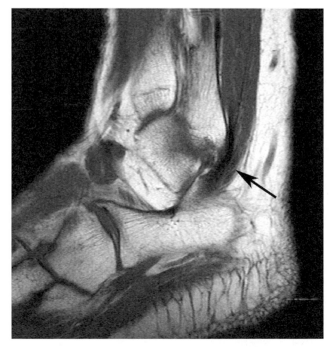

FIGURE 24-12   Low-lying peroneus brevis. The peroneus brevis muscle belly (*arrow*) can extend inferior to the tip of the lateral malleolus ("low-lying" peroneus brevis) and can result in mass effect upon the adjacent peroneal tendons.

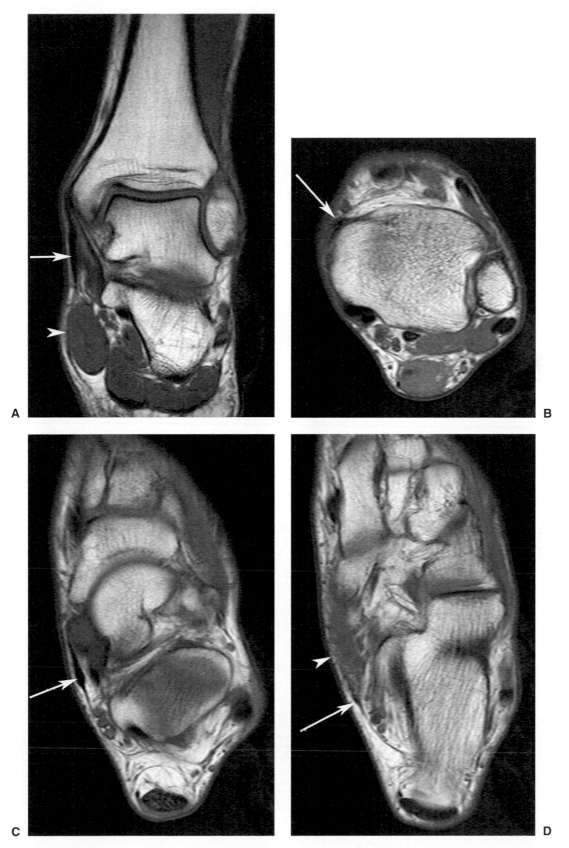

FIGURE 24-13 **Accessory abductor hallucis longus muscle. A:** Sagittal T1-weighted image shows an accessory muscle (*arrow*) extending between the tibia and the abductor hallucis longus muscle (*arrowhead*). **B–D:** Axial images show the superior to inferior extent of the accessory muscle (*arrows*) as it attaches onto the abductor hallucis longus muscles (*arrowhead*).

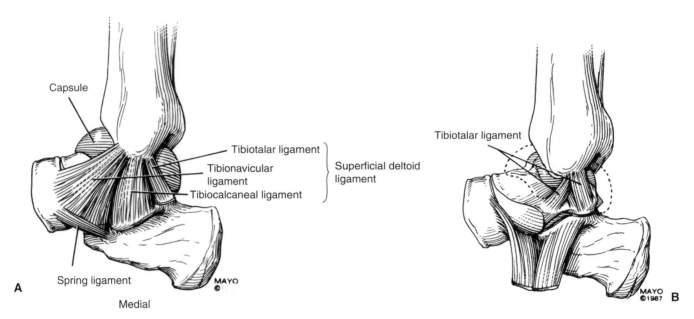

FIGURE 24-14 **Medial collateral ligaments.** Illustrations of the **(A)** superficial and **(B)** deep portions of the deltoid ligament. (From Berquist TH. *MRI of the musculoskeletal system*, 5th ed. Lippincott Williams & Wilkins; 2006.)

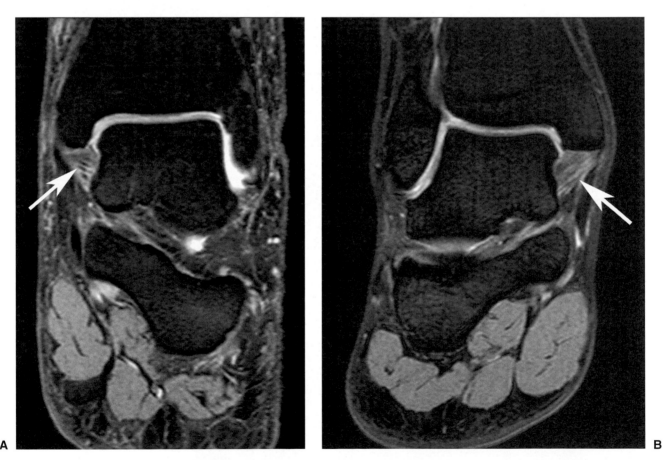

FIGURE 24-15 **Striated appearance of deltoid ligament. A** and **B:** The posterior tibiotalar (deep posterior) portions (*arrows*) of the deltoid ligament can have a striated appearance.

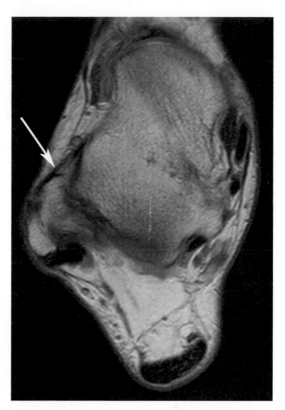

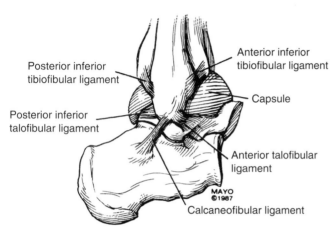

FIGURE 24-16 Lateral collateral ligaments. Illustration of the lateral collateral ligament complex of the ankle. (From Berquist TH. *Radiology of the foot and ankle*, 2nd ed. Philadelphia: Lippincott Williams & Wilkins; 2000.)

FIGURE 24-17 Anterior talofibular ligament. The normal anterior talofibular ligament (*arrow*) is composed of two or three bundles, which are variably appreciated on MRI.

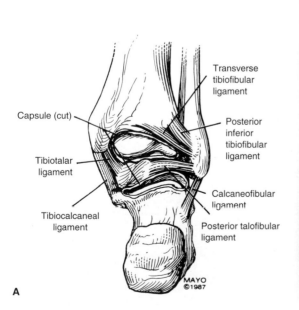

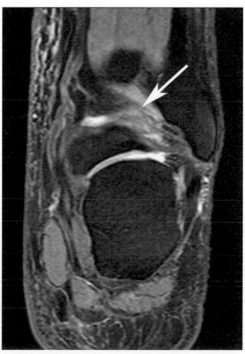

FIGURE 24-18 Posterior ankle ligaments. A: Illustration of ankle ligaments from posterior approach. (From Berquist TH. *Radiology of the foot and ankle*, 2nd ed. Philadelphia: Lippincott Williams & Wilkins; 2000.) **B:** The intermalleolar ligament (*arrow*) can be identified in approximately 80% of magnetic resonance studies. The medial attachment of this ligament is variable, and can be from the medial malleolus to the floor of the fibrous tunnel of the flexor hallucis longus.

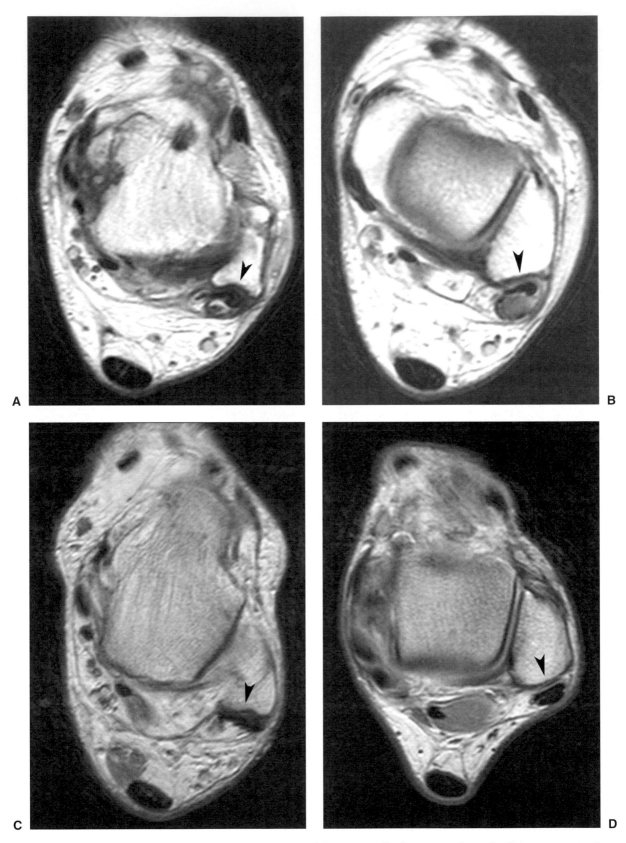

FIGURE 24-19   Fibular groove variants. Anatomic variants of the retromalleolar groove *(arrowhead)* in asymptomatic patients include **(A)** concave, **(B)** flat, **(C)** irregular and **(D)** convex.

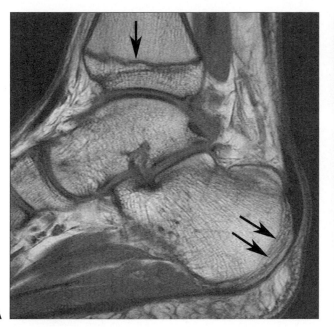

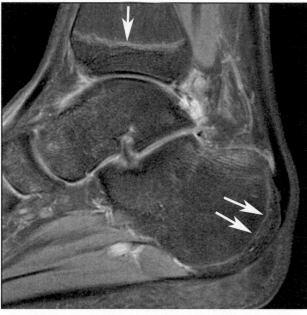

FIGURE 24-20 Pediatric ankle. Sagittal **(A)** T1-weighted and **(B)** FSE T2-weighted fat-suppressed images in a 14-year-old patient show the age-appropriate unfused distal tibial physis (*arrows*) and calcaneal apophysis (*double arrows*). The distal tibial physis typically fuses in a medial-to-lateral direction.

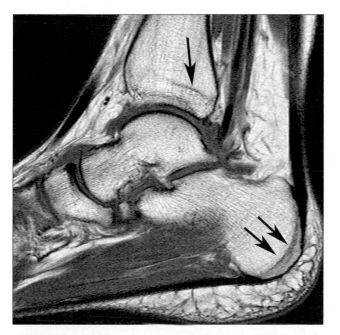

FIGURE 24-21 Physeal and apophyseal scars. Sagittal T1-weighted image shows a partially visible distal tibial physeal scar (*arrow*) and persistent calcaneal apophyseal scar (*double arrows*) in an adult patient.

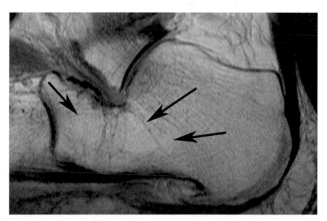

FIGURE 24-22 Decreased trabeculae in anterior calcaneus. Sagittal T1-weighted image shows relative paucity of trabeculae (*arrows*) in the anterior calcaneus, which should not be confused with a true lesion.

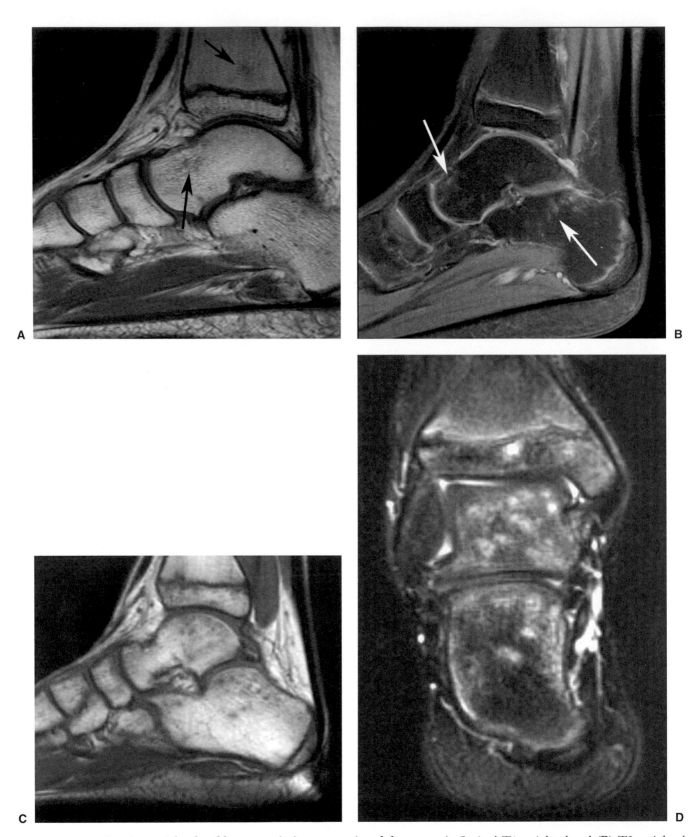

FIGURE 24-23 Persistent islands of hematopoietic marrow in adolescents. A: Sagittal T1-weighted and **(B)** T2-weighted images in an adolescent shows small signal foci (*arrows*) of prolonged T1 and T2 relaxation time. These signal foci in pediatric foot and ankle bone marrow typically disappear after 15 years of age, and likely represent residual hepatopoietic marrow. **C:** Sagittal T1 and **(D)** coronal short tau inversion recovery (STIR) images show much more dramatic signal heterogeneity.

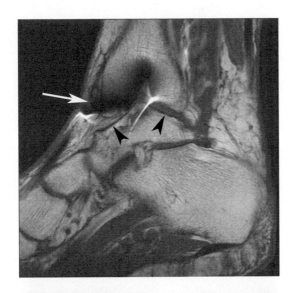

FIGURE 24-24 Metal artifact. Spin dephasing and distortion of the talar dome (*arrowheads*) is observed due to differences in magnetic susceptibility of a metal staple (*arrow*) compared to that of tissue.

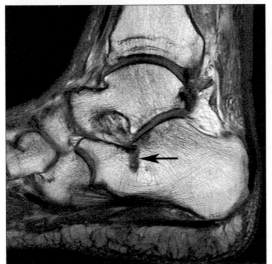

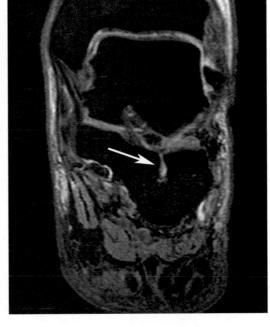

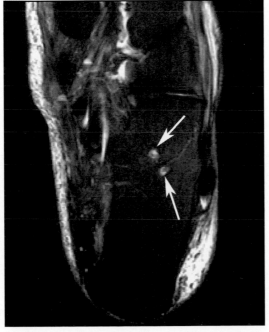

FIGURE 24-25 Prominent calcaneal vascular remnants. A–C: Calcaneal cyst-like foci (*arrows*) near sinus tarsi due to vascular remnants can be seen in 75% of patients younger than 30 years and approximately 90% of patients older than 50 years.

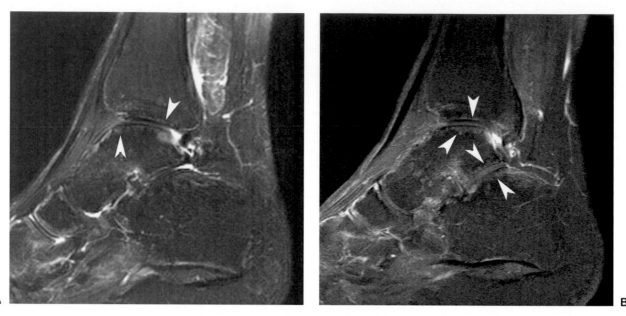

FIGURE 24-26 ▪ Osteopenia. Sagittal **(A)** FSE T2-weighted fat-suppressed and **(B)** enhanced T1-weighted fat-suppressed images show small subcortical foci (*arrowheads*) of increased signal and enhancement in this osteopenic patient. This is the equivalent of Hawkins' sign described on radiographs and should not be confused with erosions.

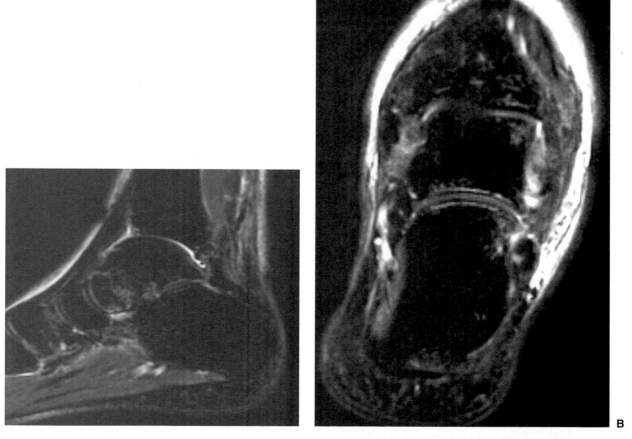

FIGURE 24-27 ▪ Immobilization edema. A: Sagittal and **(B)** coronal short tau inversion recovery (STIR) images show mottled subcortical marrow hyperintensities in this patient who has been immobilized after trauma. Also notice the dorsal ankle and foot subcutaneous edema.

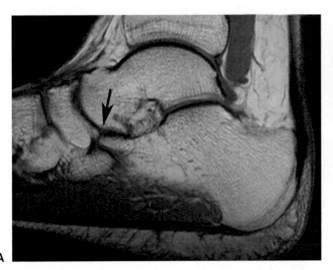
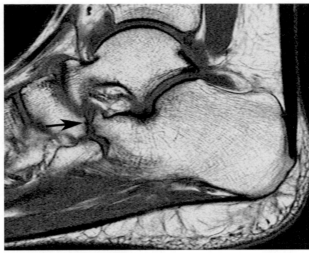

FIGURE 24-28 Calcaneonavicular coalition. A and **B:** Calcaneonavicular fibrous coalition (*arrows*) is the most common type of coalition of the foot. Although coalitions are present at birth, they do not become symptomatic until the teenage and young adult years.

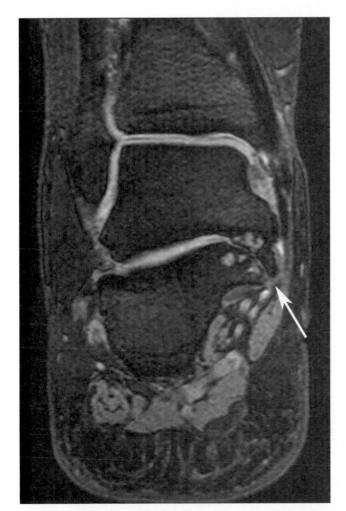

FIGURE 24-29 Subtalar coalition. This typical fibrous subtalar coalition (*arrow*) shows anomalous orientation of the joint and extensive degenerative change, and should not be confused with simple osteoarthrosis.

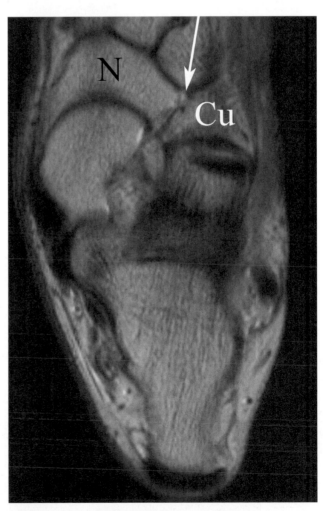

FIGURE 24-30 Cuboid-navicular coalition. Long axis T1-weighted image through the foot shows a fibrous coalition (*arrow*) between the cuboid (*Cu*) and the navicular (*N*).

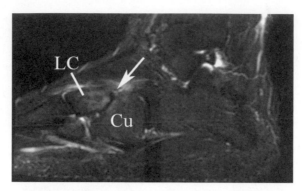

FIGURE 24-31 Cuboid-cuneiform coalition. Sagittal FSE T2-weighted image shows a fibrous coalition (*arrow*) between the cuboid (*Cu*) and lateral cuneiform (*LC*), with reactive signal changes in the adjacent bone.

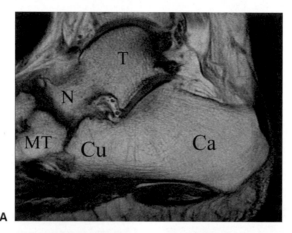

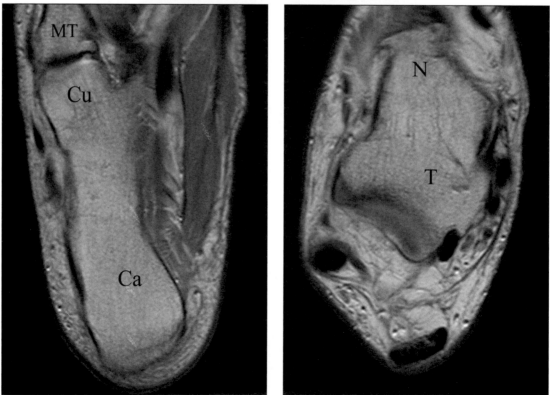

FIGURE 24-32 Multiple tarsal coalitions. A–C: One could easily overlook these rare calcaneocuboid and talonavicular coalitions on MRI (*Calcaneus = Ca, Cuboid = Cu, Talus = T, Navicular = N, Metatarsus = MT*).

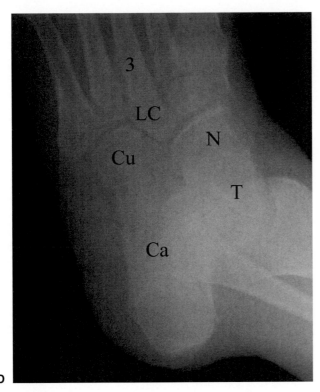

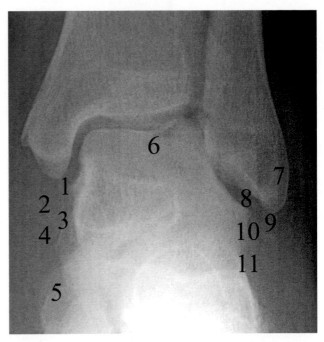

FIGURE 24-32 **Multiple tarsal coalitions.** (*continued*)
D: Note the additional fusion of the lateral cuneiform (*LC*) and third metatarsal (*3*), which was beyond the field of view for the MRI (*Calcaneus = Ca, Cuboid = Cu, Talus = T, Navicular = N*).

FIGURE 24-33 **Accessory ossicles about the ankle.** Location of various accessory ossicles about the ankle (1 = *intercalary bone between medial malleolus and talus, 2 = os subtibiale, 3 = talus accessorius, 4 = os sustentaculi, 5 = os tibiale externum, 6 = os trigonum, 7 = os retinaculi, 8 = intercalary bone between the alteral malleolus and talus, 9 = os secundarius, 10 = talus secundarius, 11 = os trochleare calcanei*).

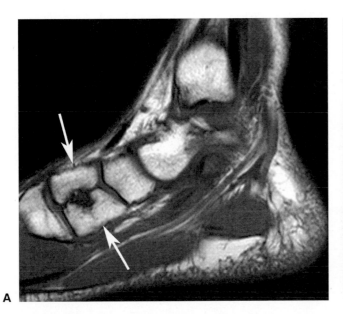

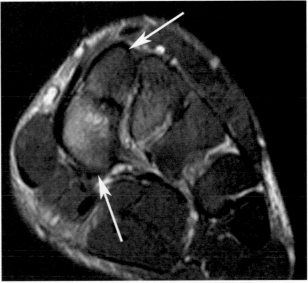

FIGURE 24-34 **Bipartite medial cuneiform. A:** Sagittal and (**B**) coronal images show a bipartite medial cuneiform (*arrows*), a normal variant.

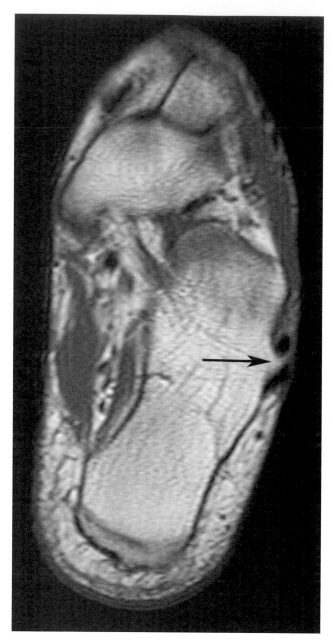

FIGURE 24-35 Peroneal tubercle. Axial image shows a prominent peroneal tubercle (*arrow*) separating the peroneus brevis and longus. Peroneal tubercles are present in approximately half of ankles and the vast majority measure 4.6 mm or smaller in asymptomatic patients.

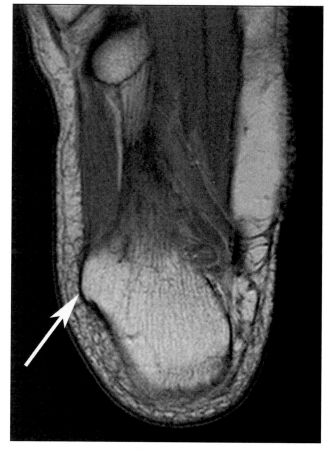

FIGURE 24-36 Retrotrochlear eminence of the calcaneus. Retrotrochlear eminences are universally present and average 3.4 mm in men and 2.5 mm in women. This represents an enlarged retrotrochlear eminence (*arrow*).

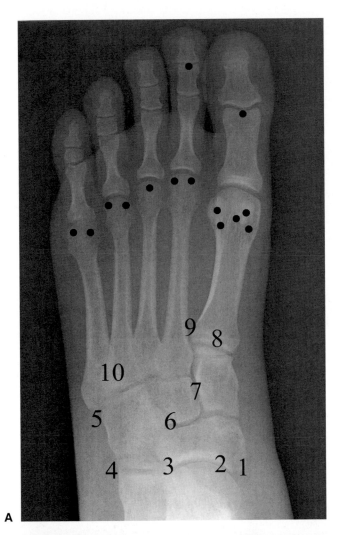

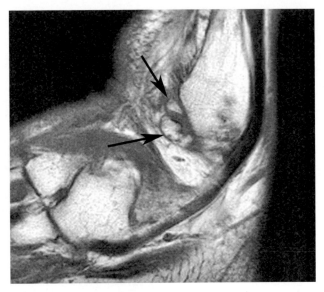

FIGURE 24-37 Accessory ossicles near lateral malleolus. Accessory ossicles (*arrows*) adjacent to the lateral malleolus are common.

FIGURE 24-38 Accessory ossicles and sesamoids. A and **B:** Illustrations of the numerous accessory ossicles and sesamoids in the foot (1 = *os naviculare* [*os tibiale externum*], 2 = *os supratalare*, 3 = *cuboides secondarium*, 4 = *os peroneum*, 5 = *os vesalianum*, 6 = *processus uncinatus*, 7 = *os intercuneiforme*, 8 = *pars peronea metatarsalia*, 9 and 10 = *os intermetatarseum*, 11 = *os trigonum*, 12 = *os talotibale*, 13 = *talus accessorius*, 14 = *os sustentaculum*, 15 = *calcaneus secondarius*, 16 = *os subcalcis*, 17 = *os supranaviculare*, ● = *sesamoids*).

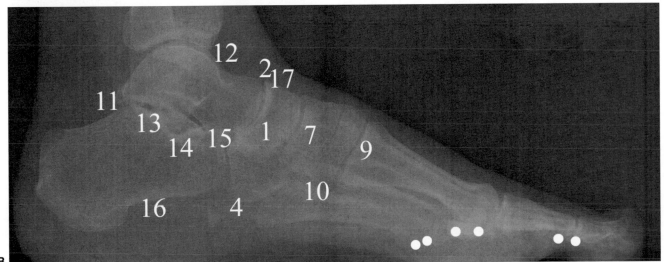

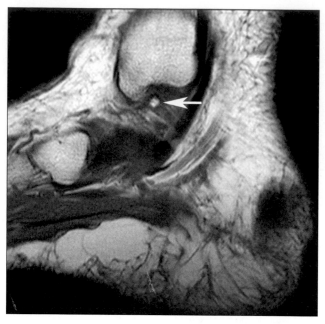

FIGURE 24-39 **Accessory ossicle near medial malleolus.** Accessory ossicles (*arrow*) adjacent to the medial malleolus are also common, and can sometimes be confused with remote avulsion fractures.

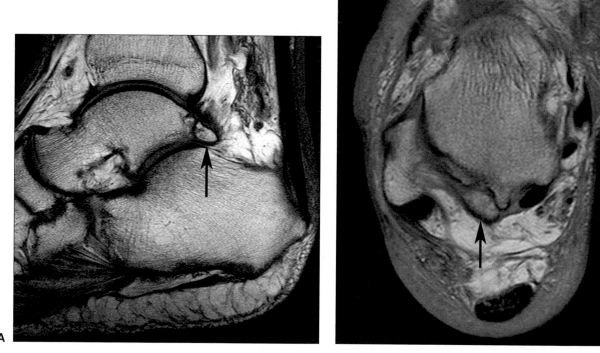

FIGURE 24-40 **Os trigonum. A** and **B:** Os trigonum (*arrows*) is the unfused Stieda process of the calcaneus. This can be of variable size, may be multiple, and may be asymptomatic or associated with impingement symptoms in the posterior ankle.

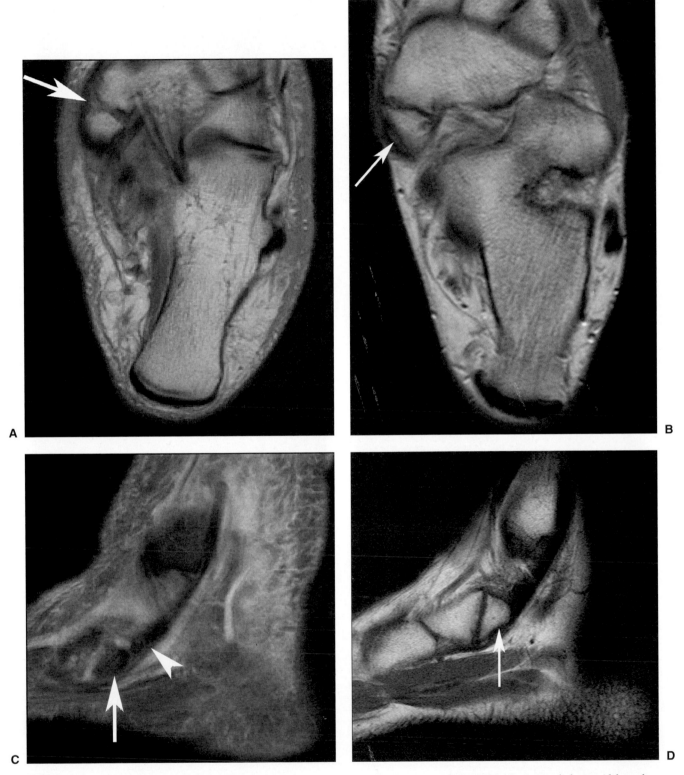

FIGURE 24-41   Accessory navicular. A–D: Accessory navicular bones (*arrows*) can be variable in size and shape. Although most cases of os naviculare are incidental, patients may become symptomatic if there is motion at the synchondrosis or tendon injury at the posterior tibial tendon attachment (*Posterior tibial tendon = arrowhead*).

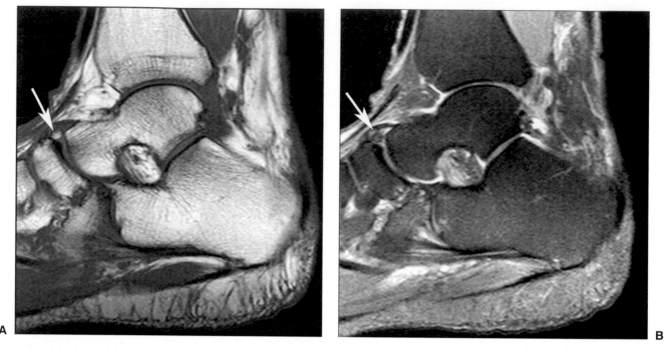

FIGURE 24-42 **Os supranaviculare.** Sagittal **(A)** T1- and **(B)** FSE T2-weighted images show an accessory ossicle (*arrows*) located dorsal to the talonavicular joint. This should not be confused with a loose body in the absence of degenerative change.

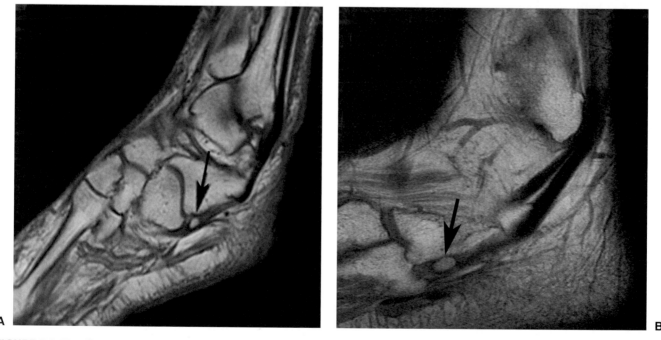

FIGURE 24-43 **Os peroneum.** **A** and **B:** Os peronei (*arrows*) are shown on sagittal T1-weighted images in two patients. At least one os peroneum is present in most of the population. In the absence of prior studies, multiple os peronei could be confused with fragmented ossicles and underlying peroneus longus injury.

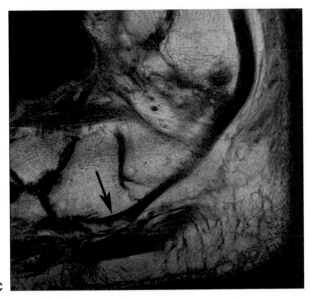

C

FIGURE 24-43   Os peroneum. (*continued*) **C:** Larger, crescentic shaped os peroneum (*arrow*) is shown in a different patient.

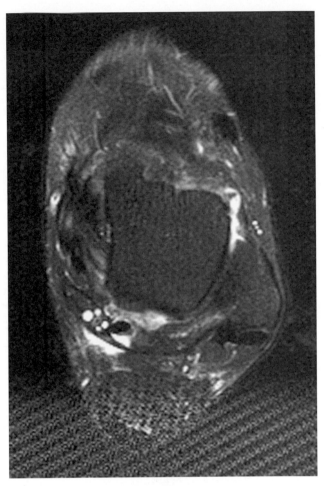

FIGURE 24-44   Radiofrequency (RF) interference. The artifact at the bottom of this image is the result of broadband RF interference.

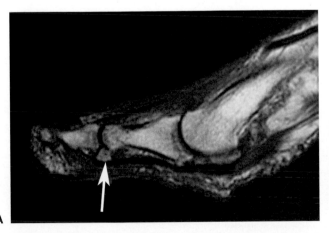

A

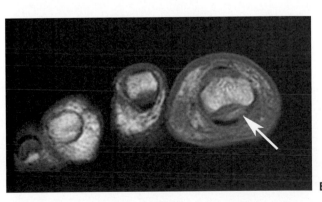

B

FIGURE 24-45   Sesamoid near first interphalangeal joint. Sesamoid bones are less common in more distal locations. However, sesamoids (*arrows*) within the flexor hallucis longus tendon are seen with some frequency.

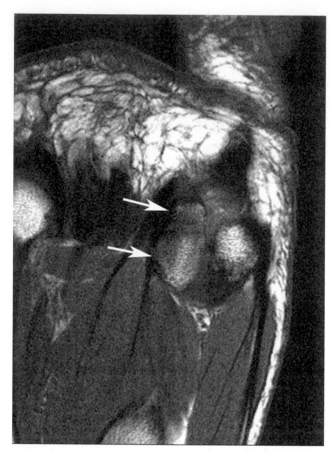

FIGURE 24-46 Bipartite sesamoid. Sesamoids subjacent to the first metatarsal head are frequently bipartite (*arrows*), especially the lateral one. These can be differentiated from fracture by lack of marrow edema-like signal, well-corticated margins, and lack of symptoms.

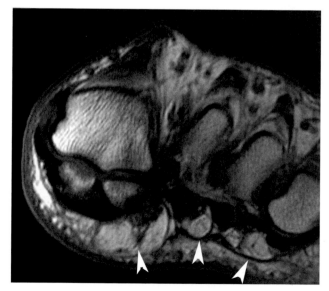

FIGURE 24-47 Plantar fat. Axial T1-weighted images show the variable lobules of fat (*arrowheads*) divided by septa in the plantar foot.

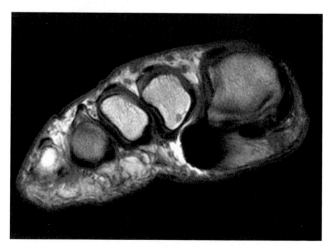

FIGURE 24-48 Artifact. Artifact from foreign body in the first webspace should not be confused with a Morton's neuroma.

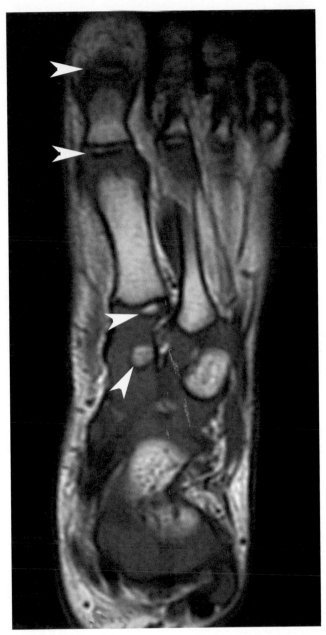

FIGURE 24-49 Pediatric foot. Long axis T1-weighted image in a child shows the mineralized ossification centers (*arrowheads*) and hypointense cartilage throughout the foot.

Table 24-1 Muscles of the foot

Location	Muscle	Origin	Insertion	Action	Innervation (Segment)	Blood Supply
Plantar						
Superficial first layer	Abductor hallucis	Medial calcaneus, plantar aponeurosis, and flexor retinaculum	Proximal phalanx great toe	Flexor and abductor MTP joint great toe	Medial plantar nerve (L5, S1)	Medial plantar artery
	Flexor digitorum brevis	Medial calcaneus plantar fascia	Middle phalanges second to fifth toes	Flexor of toes	Medial plantar nerve (L5, S1)	Medial plantar artery
	Abductor digiti minimi	Lateral process calcaneal tubercle	Lateral base proximal phalanx small toe	Abductor and flexor small toe	Lateral plantar nerve (S1, S2)	Lateral plantar artery
Second layer	Quadratus plantae	Medial and lateral calcaneal tuberosity	Flexor digitorum longus tendon	Flexes terminal phalanges two to five	Lateral plantar nerve (S1, S2)	Lateral plantar artery
	Lumbricals	Flexor digitorum longus tendon	MTP joints two to five	Flexes MTP joints	Medial and lateral plantar nerve (S1, S2)	Medial and lateral plantar arteries
Third layer	Flexor hallucis brevis	Cuboid, cuneiform	Great toe	Flexor great toe	Medial plantar nerve (L5, S1)	Medial and lateral artery
	Adductor hallucis	Second to fourth metatarsal bases and third to fifth capsules transverse leg	Great toe	Adductor great toe, maintains transverse arch	Lateral plantar nerve (L5, S1)	Lateral plantar artery
	Flexor digiti minimi brevis	Cuboid and fifth metatarsal base	Proximal phalanx fifth toe	Flexes fifth toe	Lateral plantar nerve (S1, S2)	Lateral plantar artery
Fourth layer	Interossei dorsal	Metatarsal bases	Bases of second to fourth proximal phalanges	Abduct toes	Lateral plantar nerve (S1, S2)	Lateral plantar artery
	Plantar	Metatarsal bases	Bases of third to fifth proximal phalanges	Abduct toes	Lateral plantar nerve (S1, S2)	Lateral plantar artery
Dorsal	Extensor digitorum brevis	Superior calcaneus, lateral talocalcaneal ligament, extensor retinaculum	Lateral first to fourth toes	Extends toes one to four	Deep peroneal nerve (L5, S1)	Dorsalis pedis artery

MTP, metatarsophalangeal.

(From Berquist TH. *MRI of the musculoskeletal system*, 5th ed. Lippincott Williams & Wilkins; 2006; Best A, Giza E, Linklater J, et al. Posterior impingement of the ankle caused by anomalous muscles: A report of four cases. *J Bone Joint Surg Am.* 2005;2075–2079; Brenner E. Insertion of the tendon of the tibialis anterior muscle in feet with and without hallux valgus. *Clin Anat.* 2002;15:217–223; Fernandes R, Aguiar R, Trudell D, et al. Tendons in the plantar aspect of the foot: MRI and anatomic correlation in cadavers. *Skeletal Radiol.* 2007;36:115–122; Kanatli U, Ozturk AM, Ercan NGT, et al. Absence of the medial sesamoid bone associated with metatarsophalangeal pain. *Clin Anat.* 2006;19:634–639.)

Table 24-2 Muscle variations in the foot

Quadratus plantae (flexor accessorius) (small, absent head or complete, accessory slip)

Lumbricals (absent, doubled, variant attachment, slips from flexor digitorum longus and flexor hallucis longus)

Flexor digitorum brevis (little toe absent or defective, end in fascia, accessorius quadratus plantae)

Abductor hallucis (anomalous slips)

Adductor of second toe (supernumerary muscle)

Abductor digiti minimi (accessory slip, supernumerary muscle = abductor ossis metatarsi digiti quinti and abductor accessorius digiti minimi)

Flexor hallucis brevis (anomalous slips)

Adductor hallucis caput obliquum (accessory slips)

Adductor hallucis caput transversum (transversus pedis) (absent)

Flexor digiti minimi brevis (pedis) (anomalous slips)

Opponens hallucis (supernumerary muscle)

(Compiled from Berman RA, Thompson SA, Afiti AK, et al. *Compendium of human anatomic variation*. Munchen, Baltimore: Urban and Schwartzenberg; 1988; Bejjani FJ, Jahnss MH. Le Double's study of muscle variations of the human body. Part II: Muscles variations of the foot. *Foot Ankle*. 1986;6:157–176.)

Suggested Readings

Ankle

Andreisek G, Plammatter T, Goepfert K, et al. Peripheral arteries in diabetic patients: Standard bolus-chase and time-resolved MR angiography. *Radiology*. 2006;242:610–620.

Barberini F, Bucciarelli-Ducci C, Zani A, et al. Unusual extended fibular origin of the human soleus muscle: Possible morpho-physiologic significance based on comparative anatomy. *Clin Anat*. 2003;16:383–388.

Bergman RA, Thompson SA, Afifi AK, et al., ed. *Compendium of human anatomic variation*. Baltimore: Urban & Schwarzenberg; 1988.

Bernaerts A, Vanhoenacker FM, Van de Perre S, et al. Accessory navicular bone: Not such a normal variant. *JBR-BTR*. 2004;87:25–252.

Best A, Giza E, Linklater J, et al. Posterior impingement of the ankle caused by anomalous muscles: A report of four cases. *J Bone Joint Surg Am*. 2005;87:2075–2079.

Bodily KD, Spinner RJ, Bishop AT. Restoration of motor function of the deep fibular (peroneal) nerve by direct nerve transfer of branches from the tibial nerve: An anatomical study. *Clin Anat*. 2004;17:201–205.

Bottger BA, Schweitzer ME, El-Noueam KI, et al. MRI of the normal and abnormal retrocalcaneal bursae. *AJR Am J Roentgenol*. 1998;170:1239–1241.

Brown RB, Rosenberg ZS, Schweitzer ME, et al. MRI of medial malleolar bursa. *AJR Am J Roentgenol*. 2005;184:979–983.

Buschmann WR, Cheung Y, Jahss MH. Magnetic resonance imaging of anomalous leg muscles: Accessory soleus, peroneus quartus and the flexor digitorum longus accessorius. *Foot Ankle*. 1991;12:109–116.

Chepuri NB, Jacoson JA, Fessell DP, et al. Sonographic appearance of the peroneus quartus muscle: Correlation with MRI appearance in seven patients. *Radiology*. 2001;218:415–419.

Doda N, Peh WC, Chawla A. Symptomatic accessory soleus muscle: Diagnosis and follow-up on magnetic resonance imaging. *Br J Radiol*. 2006;79:e129–e132.

Downey MS, Siegerman J. Accessory soleus muscle: A review of the literature and case report. *J Foot Ankle Surg*. 1996;35:537–543.

Eberle CF, Moran B, Gleason T. The accessory flexor digitorum longus as a cause of flexor hallucis syndrome. *Foot Ankle Int*. 2002;23:51–55.

Elias I, Zoga AC, Schweitzer ME, et al. A specific bone marrow edema around the foot and ankle following trauma and immobilization therapy: Pattern description and potential clinical relevance. *Foot Ankle Int*. 2007;28(4):463–471.

Elias I, Zoga AC, Raikin SM, et al. Incidence and morphologic characteristics of benign calcaneal cystic lesions on MRI. *Foot Ankle Int*. 2007;28(6):707–714.

Fleming JL, Dodd L, Helms CA. Prominent vascular remnants in the calcaneus simulating a lesion on MRI of the ankle: Findings in 67 patients with cadaveric correlation. *AJR Am J Roentgenol*. 2005;185:1449–1452.

Joshi SD, Joshi SS, Athavale SA. Morphology of peroneus tertius muscle. *Clin Anat*. 2006;19:611–614.

Kadir S. Arterial anatomy of the lower extremities. In: Kadir S, ed. *Atlas of normal and variant angiographic anatomy*. Philadelphia: WB Saunders; 1991:123–160.

Kouvalchouk JF, Lecocq J, Parier J, et al. The accessory soleus muscle: A report of 21 cases and a review of the literature. *Rev Chir Orthop Reparatrice Appar Mot*. 2005;91:232–238.

Soila K, Karjalainen PT, Aronen HJ, et al. High-resolution MRI of the asymptomatic Achilles tendon: New observations. *Am J Roentgenol AJR*. 1999;173(2):323–328.

Lohman M, Kivisaari A, Vehmas T, et al. MRI abnormalities of foot and ankle in asymptomatic, physically active individuals. *Skeletal Radiol*. 2001;30:61–66.

Lysack JT, Fenton PV. Variations in calcaneonavicular morphology demonstrated with radiography. *Radiology*. 2004;230.493–497.

Marshall H, Howarth C, Larkman DJ, et al. Contras-enhanced magic-angle MRI of the Achilles tendon. *AJR Am J Roentgenol*. 2002;179:187–192.

Mellado JM, Rosenberg ZS, Beltran J, et al. The peroneocalcaneus internus muscle: MRI features. *AJR Am J Roentgenol*. 1997;169:585–588.

Mellado J, Rosenberg ZS, Beltran J. Low incorporation of soleus tendon: A potential diagnostic pitfall on MRI. *Skeletal Radiol*. 1998;27:222–224.

Moroney P, Borton D. Multiple accessory peroneal muscles: A cause of chronic lateral ankle pain. *Foot Ankle Int*. 2004;25:322–324.

Muhle C, Frank LR, Rand T, et al. Collateral ligaments of the ankle: High-resolution MRI with a local gradient coil and anatomic correlation in cadavers. *RadioGraphics*. 1999;19:673–683.

Oh CS, Won HS, Hur MS, et al. Anatomic variations and MRI of the intermalleolar ligament. *AJR Am J Roentgenol*. 2006;186:943–947.

Oyedele O, Maseko C, Mkasi N, et al. High incidence of the os peroneum in a cadaver sample in Johannesburg, South Africa: Possible clinical implications? *Clin Anat*. 2006;19:605–610.

Raveendran SS, Kumaragama KGJL. Arterial supply of the soleus muscle: Anatomical study of fifty lower limbs. *Clin Anat*. 2003;16:248–252.

Roberts CC, Towers JD, Spangehl MJ, et al. Advanced MRI of the cruciate ligaments. *Magn Reson Imaging Clin N Am*. 2007;5(1):73–86.

Rosenberg ZS, Beltran J, Bencardino JT. MRI of the ankle and foot. *RadioGraphics*. 2000;20:S153–S179.

Ruhli FJ, Solomon LB, Henneberg M. High prevalence of tarsal coalitions and tarsal joint variants in a recent cadaver sample and its possible significance. *Clin Anat*. 2003;16:411–415.

Saupe N, Mengiardi B, Pfirrmann CWA, et al. Anatomic variants associated with peroneal tendon disorders; MRI findings in volunteers with asymptomatic ankles. *Radiology*. 2007;242:509–517.

Shabshin N, Schweitzer ME, Morrison WB, et al. High-signal T2 changes of the bone marrow of the foot and ankle in children: Red marrow or traumatic changes? *Pediatr Radiol*. 2006;36(7):670–676.

Sora M-C, Strobl B, Staykov D, et al. Evaluation of the ankle syndesmosis: A plastination slices study. *Clin Anat*. 2004;17:513–517.

Taser F, Shafiq Q, Ebraheim NA. Anatomy of lateral ankle ligaments and their relationship to bony landmarks. *Surg Radiol Anat*. 2006;28:391–397.

Wang XT, Rosenberg ZS, Mechlin MB, et al. Normal variants and disease of the peroneal tendons and superior peroneal retinaculum: MRI features. *RadioGraphics*. 2005;25:587–602.

Ward KA, Willcott J, Paxton S, et al. Reconstruction of the articular facets of the subtalar and talonavicular joints from volumetric magnetic resonance data. *Clin Anat*. 2001;14:272–277.

Yu JS, Resnick D. MRI of the accessory soleus muscle appearance in six patients and a review of the literature. *Skeletal Radiol*. 1994;23:525–528.

Foot

Akita K, Niiro N, Murakami G, et al. First dorsal interosseous muscle of the foot and its innervation. *Clin Anat*. 1999;12:12–15.

Bejjani FJ, Jahnss MH. Le Double's study of muscle variations of the human body. Part II: Muscles variations of the foot. *Foot Ankle*. 1986;6:157–176.

Boyd N, Brock H, Meier A, et al. Extensor hallucis capsularis: Frequency and identification on MRI. *Foot Ankle Int*. 2006;27:181–184.

Brenner E. Insertion of the tendon of the tibialis anterior muscle in feet with and without hallux valgus. *Clin Anat*. 2002;15:217–223.

Davies MB, Abdlslam K, Gibson RJ. Interphalangeal sesamoid bones of the great toe: An anatomic variant demanding careful scrutiny of radiographs. *Clin Anat*. 2003;16:520–521.

Fernandes R, Aguiar R, Trudell D, et al. Tendons in the plantar aspect of the foot: MRI and anatomic correlation in cadavers. *Skeletal Radiol*. 2007;36:115–122

Kanatli U, Ozturk AM, Ercan NGT, et al. Absence of the medial sesamoid bone associated with metatarsophalangeal pain. *Clin Anat*. 2006;19:634–639.

Kadir S. Arterial anatomy of the lower extremities. In: Kadir S, ed. *Atlas of normal and variant angiographic anatomy*. Philadelphia: WB Saunders; 1991:123–160.

Lohman M, Kivisaari A, Vehmas T, et al. MRI abnormalities of foot and ankle in asymptomatic, physically active individuals. *Skeletal Radiol*. 2001;30:61–66.

Macchi V, Tiengo C, Porzionato A, et al. Correlation between the course of the medial plantar artery and the morphology of the abductor hallucis muscle. *Clin Anat*. 2005;18:580–588.

Miller TT, Staron RB, Feldman F, et al. The symptomatic accessory tarsal navicular bone: Assessment with MRI. *Radiology*. 1995;195:849–853.

O'Sullivan E, Carare-NNadi R, Greenslade J, et al. Clinical significance of variations in the interconnections between flexor digitorum longus and flexor hallucis longus in the region of the Knot of Henry. *Clin Anat*. 2005;18:121–125.

Ozer MA, Govsa F, Bilge O. Anatomic study of the deep plantar arch. *Clin Anat*. 2005;18:434–442.

Pal CR, Tasker AD, Ostlere SJ, et al. Heterogeneous signal in bone marrow on MRI of children's feet: A normal finding? *Skeletal Radiol*. 1999;28:274–278.

■ Index

Index

Index